Cultural Pressures and Mental Health Challenges in Gen Z's Digital World

Viana Hassan
https://orcid.org/0000-0002-7372-5059
European Tourism and Events Training Academy, Malta

Amrik Singh
https://orcid.org/0000-0003-3598-8787
Lovely Professional University, India

IGI Global
Scientific Publishing
Publishing Tomorrow's Research Today

Vice President of Editorial Melissa Wagner
Director of Acquisitions Mikaela Felty
Director of Book Development Jocelynn Hessler
Production Manager Mike Brehm
Cover Design Jose Rosado

Published in the United States of America by
IGI Global Scientific Publishing
701 East Chocolate Avenue
Hershey, PA, 17033, USA
Tel: 717-533-8845 | Fax: 717-533-7115
Website: https://www.igi-global.com E-mail: cust@igi-global.com

Library of Congress Cataloging-in-Publication Data

LCCN: 2025027256 (CIP Data Pending)
ISBN13: 979-8-3373-4516-1
Isbn13Softcover: 979-8-333-4517-8
EISBN13: 979-8-3373-4518-5

British Cataloguing in Publication Data
A Cataloguing in Publication record for this book is available from the British Library.

Table of Contents

Detailed Table of Contents

Bangladesh's digital awakening has catalyzed social media influencers across platforms shaping the aspirations, self-perception, and mental well-being of Gen Z. The study aimed to understand the impact of influencer culture on aspirations and self-perception among them. Three main themes emerged: how impactful the influencers were, participants' coping mechanisms, and how cultural factors fared in this journey. The research suggests that Gen Z should adopt a supportive attitude and familial openness, periodic digital detoxes, and mindful consumption. Additionally, educators and policymakers should opt for media literacy, mental health awareness, and regulatory frameworks to guide ethical influencer practices. As the million-dollar industry is still deregulated, policymakers and the business community must collaborate to establish quality standards, codes of conduct, and provide training. By fostering open dialogue between generations, and embedding safeguards, Bangladesh can harness influencer culture as a positive force while protecting Gen Z's mental health and identity.

The influence of “social media figures on youngsters, adolescents, and children” is undeniable. Although its influence may yield favorable outcomes for “inspiration, education, and community development,” it is not without disadvantages. It is essential for young individuals to acquire critical thinking and “media literacy skills” to effectively navigate the virtual landscape. Influencers, akin to “celebrities,” have a moral “obligation and responsibility to disseminate truth, diversity, and ethical principles.” The culture of “social media influencers” can exert both helpful and

Z, essential for operations development in Bangladesh's competitive food service industry, by understanding their tastes and customizing menus, improving online visibility, and optimizing ease variables, including place and service speed. This knowledge enables restaurants to better customize their menus and marketing tactics to this critical customer base, which promotes customer retention and business growth.

The study will explore the scope of spa and wellness tourism as a new and potential trend which shape and promote the tourism and hospitality industry in India. Spa and wellness tourism can help to increase the economy of the country which enhances customer experience within the hospitality sector and provide a different opportunity for guest to rejuvenate with a new experience. The personalized guest interactions, optimization of revenue, difference of operation style, and overall experience of guest satisfaction through spa resorts. The latest trend in information technology and AI can be a supporting factor to improve wellness tourism. It gives an exceptional experience of new trends of culinary skills linked with medicinal properties or with health and wellness options. The spa sector facilitates increasing more job opportunities, by improving infrastructure to develop the new market and supporting local businesses to develop. To promotes sustainability by emphasizing environmental conservation and mingling with cultural and heritage of India in contributing to long-term economic and social wellbeing. Therefore, the study makes recommendations based on new tourist demands and new processes and protocols for the operation of wellness tourism sector. Hospitality Sector can make it customized to guests who are willing to spend more for a better experience and wellness of body and mind. Significantly Spa and wellness tourism can be significantly beneficial to local economies by attracting tourists.

In the age of digital epoch, where the phenomenon of digitalisation is revolutionising every facet, and social media platforms are occupying primary space, starting from interacting people, fitness regime, entertainment, watching and scrolling reels, news, educational engagement, and product acquisition, life revolves around social media only. The existence of individuals, especially Gen Z entirely depends upon social media for all requirements, whether it is interaction, exploration, consumption etc. These platforms are designed in such a way that they are engaging attention by sharing and commenting. At one end they are streamlining and facilitating our lives, but on the other having a negative effect on emotional wellbeing, self-perception, mental wellbeing of Genz because of too much usage and reliance on these social media platforms. This in result starts giving rise to the social and cultural comparison, which in turn increases anxiety, esteem issues and even lead to severe mental disorders, depression. This chapter critically examines how these social media platforms engender emotional and mental challenges, how these influencers are influencing Gen z and increasing peer comparison pressure that adversely affects self-esteem. It is time to rethink and to devise strategies in such a way that aims to create a safe digital landscape.

Awesh Khati, Lakshmibai National Institute of Physical Education, India
Sohom Saha, Lakshmibai National Institute of Physical Education, India
Namchan Norbu Bhutia, Jadavpur University, India
Rintu Saibya, University of Kalyani, India

This chapter explores the impact of digital culture on the athletic identity and mental well-being of Generation Z athletes. As digital natives, Gen Z engages with sport through social media and interactive platforms, redefining fandom, athlete branding, and performance expectations. Athletes now balance physical training with maintaining a curated online presence. While digital tools enhance visibility and engagement, they also introduce stressors such as comparison culture, screen overuse, disrupted recovery, and heightened performance anxiety. Constant connectivity and public scrutiny further intensify these challenges. The chapter emphasizes the need for digital literacy, mental health awareness, and institutional support to help athletes build resilience and set healthy boundaries. It offers a framework to understand and support Gen Z athletes as they navigate the complex demands of sport in a digitally saturated environment.

Indian adolescents are paying a silent and hefty price for being connected on social media. The chapter investigates how SMPs shape Indian teenagers' self-worth and body image, exposing the hushed crisis playing out on Indian screens. The adolescents are settling in a vicious circle of competition. It poses a question: What becomes of a generation growing up hooked on digital validation? The study is based on two theories: the Social Comparison Theory and Theory of Mimetic Desire. Teens want to be wanted because they see their peers being desired. These experiences within larger systems, soft power, platform capitalism, and digital colonialism, shape digital adolescent identities and desires. The results show a negative correlation between the usage frequency of SMPs and self-esteem. The study revealed a positive correlation between SMPs usage and body dissatisfaction. The females reported higher levels of body dissatisfaction and social comparison behaviours, indicating gendered differences. SMP users exhibited aspirational identification, reported higher digital beauty anxiety.

The rapid proliferation of digital platforms has significantly shaped Gen Z's social and psychological landscape, with digital identity and online validation emerging as critical factors influencing mental health. This study explores how the construction and curation of digital identities on social media, coupled with the pursuit of online validation through likes, comments, and followers, impact the mental well-being of Gen Z individuals. Drawing on psychological and sociological frameworks, the research examines the pressures of performative self-presentation, the effects of social comparison, and the role of algorithmic reinforcement in shaping self-esteem, anxiety, and depressive symptoms. Findings suggest that while digital platforms offer opportunities for self-expression and community building, the relentless pursuit of validation and exposure to idealized online personas can exacerbate feelings of inadequacy, social isolation, and mental distress. The study highlights the need for targeted interventions, including digital literacy programs and platform design changes.

In the age of influencer-led social media platforms in the digital age, the Gen Z cohort is at a crossroads where deep digital interaction intersects with psychic fatigue. This chapter explores the scroll fatigue phenomenon, which is a digital burnout derived from incessant consumption of carefully curated content, idealized life, and interesting brand pitches. Through the psychological and emotional implications of influencer marketing, the article highlights the impact of extended exposure on Gen Z's mental well-being, self-concept, and shopping habits. Drawing on the synthesis of media psychology, digital marketing, and youth cultural studies perspectives, the analysis illustrates the intricate dynamics between algorithm-controlled content dissemination, social comparison effects, and societal norms. This article also critically analyzes the ways in which influencer marketing insidiously shapes attitudes and creates decision fatigue. It provides insights into how Gen Z can promote more sustainable online behaviors and how brand strategists can embrace more ethical approaches.

This chapter examines the cultural pressures of Generation Z from the viewpoint called the perfect me trap, a two-dimensional pressure of performance (unending self-curation) and passivity (endless algorithm-driven consumption of content), which define Gen Z's digital culture. It draws from peer-reviewed research, ethnographic studies, and cultural commentary to explore how performance imperatives fuel perfectionism, identity fragmentation, and the commercialization of authenticity, while passive scrolling drives overstimulation, disengagement, and isolation. The analysis integrates frameworks, like social comparison, the pursuit of attention and validation, and the need for self-determination, to reveal the psychological drivers of the performance, and the pull of social platform designs, algorithmic authority, and emotional disengagement to explore the slide into passivity. With emerging strategies, the chapter concludes by foregrounding the need for intentional authenticity and embracing human imperfections as deliberate shifts that are possible.

This chapter explores the potential of interconnected regional tourism in South Asia, focusing on Sri Lanka, Maldives, Nepal, and India. The study aims to examine international tourists' perspectives on the feasibility and attractiveness of multi-country travel in the region, drawing comparisons with successful integrated tourism models in Europe. Using the Push–Pull Motivation Theory as a framework, the chapter employs a qualitative design based on 85 semi-structured interviews with international tourists visiting Sri Lanka between May and August 2024. The findings reveal key motivations, perceived benefits, and barriers influencing tourists' willingness to participate in interconnected travel. Insights on visa facilitation, transportation connectivity, and collaborative marketing strategies are also presented. The study concludes with recommendations for policymakers and tourism stakeholders on enhancing regional cooperation to drive sustainable growth and visitor flow across South Asia.

Preface

In an era defined by seamless connectivity and boundless digital expression, Generation Z stands at the epicenter of a profound cultural transformation. As true digital natives, Gen Z navigates a world where social media platforms, influencer economies, and algorithm-driven content shape not only their aspirations and identities but also their mental well-being. *Cultural Pressures and Mental Health Challenges in Gen Z's Digital World* delves into this intricate interplay, examining how curated online personas, relentless social comparisons, and performative lifestyles exacerbate psychological strains while intersecting with traditional cultural heritage, tourism dynamics, and athletic pursuits.

This volume brings together diverse scholarly voices from across South Asia, Europe, and beyond to illuminate the multifaceted challenges facing Gen Z. From the unregulated allure of influencer culture in Bangladesh to the scroll fatigue induced by marketing tactics, and from the body image crises among Indian adolescents to the mental conditioning needs of Gen Z athletes, these chapters reveal a shared narrative: the digital realm amplifies cultural pressures, often at the cost of authentic self-worth and emotional resilience. Yet, amid these challenges lie opportunities—for media literacy, ethical platform design, intergenerational dialogue, and sustainable tourism practices that honor cultural roots while fostering mental health.

Edited by Viana Hassan and Amrik Singh, this collection advocates for collaborative action. Policymakers, educators, influencers, and communities must unite to cultivate mindful digital habits, regulatory safeguards, and inclusive environments. By harnessing the positive potential of technology while mitigating its pitfalls, we can empower Gen Z to thrive in their digital world—not as passive consumers, but as resilient architects of their futures.

We extend our gratitude to all contributors for their insightful analyses and to readers for engaging with this vital discourse. May this book spark meaningful change in safeguarding Gen Z's mental health amid cultural and digital evolution.

Chapter Overview

Chapter 1 examines influencer culture's impact on aspirations and self-perception in Bangladesh, revealing coping mechanisms, cultural influences, and recommendations for media literacy, digital detoxes, and ethical regulations.

Chapter 2 assesses both positive (inspiration, education) and negative effects on young people, emphasizing critical thinking, media literacy, and influencers' ethical responsibilities to foster symbiotic audience relationships.

Chapter 3 investigates Bangladesh's cultural tourism challenges using secondary data and stakeholder perspectives, proposing collaborative approaches to enhance economic benefits while ensuring authenticity and community involvement.

Chapter 4 reviews literature through dramaturgical and social comparison theories, addressing identity fatigue and burnout in algorithm-driven platforms, with multi-stakeholder recommendations for sustainable digital environments.

Chapter 5 analyzes how social media platforms amplify self-perception through constant comparison, transforming personal introspection into a psychologically intense, frequency-driven phenomenon beyond traditional interactions.

Chapter 6 quantitative survey-based study in Bangladesh identifying preferences for diverse cuisines, online reviews, peer influence, and affordability, offering strategies for restaurants to enhance retention and growth.

Chapter 7 critical analysis of Alleppey's spa sector in Kerala, highlighting job creation, infrastructure development, sustainability, and AI-enhanced personalization for improved guest experiences and local economies.

Chapter 8 explores how likes, shares, and influencer-driven comparisons fuel anxiety, low self-esteem, and depression, advocating strategies for a safer digital landscape through ethical platform redesign.

Chapter 9 investigates digital culture's effects on athletic identity, including comparison stress and screen overuse, with frameworks for digital literacy, mental health support, and resilience-building boundaries.

Chapter 10 reveals negative correlations with self-esteem and positive links to body dissatisfaction via Social Comparison and Mimetic Desire theories, noting gendered differences and digital beauty anxiety.

Chapter 11 analyzes performative self-presentation and algorithmic reinforcement's role in anxiety and isolation, recommending digital literacy programs and platform changes for healthier self-expression.

Chapter 12 synthesizes media psychology to unpack burnout from curated content consumption, social comparison, and decision fatigue, providing insights for sustainable behaviors and ethical brand strategies.

Chapter 13 examines performance (self-curation) and passivity (scrolling) pressures using social comparison and self-determination frameworks, advocating intentional authenticity to counter perfectionism and isolation.

Chapter 14 details tailored mental skills like visualization and mindfulness, technology tools, and support systems to address stress, injury, and stigma, illustrated with evidence-based case studies.

Chapter 15 explores intersections of societal norms, academic aspirations, and constant comparison in digital spaces, proposing nuanced interventions targeting both cultural expectations and online vulnerabilities.

Chapter 16 qualitative study on Sri Lankan Gen Z using Push-Pull Theory, examining how heritage shapes social media identities and regional tourism potential through tourist interviews and policy recommendations.

This collection underscores a critical truth: Gen Z's digital world, while innovative and connective, often magnifies cultural pressures that erode mental well-being. Yet, through the collective wisdom of these chapters, a clear path emerges—empowering Gen Z with media literacy, ethical digital frameworks, and culturally sensitive support systems. By bridging generational divides and prioritizing authentic self-expression over performative perfection, societies can transform digital challenges into opportunities for resilience and growth. The future of Gen Z's mental health rests not in disconnection, but in mindful, collaborative navigation of their vibrant digital landscape.

Viana Hassan
European Tourism and Events Training Academy, Malta
American University of Malta, Malta
Amrik Singh
Lovely Professional University, India

Chapter 1
Exploring the Impact of Influencer Lifestyles on the Self-Esteem of Generation Z: A Qualitative Study in Bangladesh

Zarjina Tarana Khalil
https://orcid.org/0000-0001-6350-9443
North South University, Bangladesh

Samira Rahman
North South University, Bangladesh

ABSTRACT

Bangladesh's digital awakening has catalyzed social media influencers across platforms shaping the aspirations, self-perception, and mental well-being of Gen Z. The study aimed to understand the impact of influencer culture on aspirations and self-perception among them. Three main themes emerged: how impactful the influencers were, participants' coping mechanisms, and how cultural factors fared in this journey. The research suggests that Gen Z should adopt a supportive attitude and familial openness, periodic digital detoxes, and mindful consumption. Additionally, educators and policymakers should opt for media literacy, mental health awareness, and regulatory frameworks to guide ethical influencer practices. As the million-dollar industry is still deregulated, policymakers and the business community must collaborate to establish quality standards, codes of conduct, and

DOI: 10.4018/979-8-3373-4516-1.ch001

provide training. By fostering open dialogue between generations, and embedding safeguards, Bangladesh can harness influencer culture as a positive force while protecting Gen Z's mental health and identity.

INTRODUCTION

Over the past 30 years, the advent of the internet has radically transformed the way people communicate and interact with one another. The new digital communities like social media platforms, blogs and vlogs have enabled people to share knowledge and have been a catalyst for shifting the paradigm of how individuals consume content. As the media landscape became more fragmented, the concept of influencer marketing emerged. Social media influencers are individuals who are "followed" due to their knowledge, interest or expertise in certain topics. Their primary motive or purpose is to influence people to buy certain brands or products (like beauty or fashion), to engage in certain lifestyle choices (like fitness or nutrition), to seek life experiences (like travel or adventure sports) or to be part of a community (like gaming or racing). This is done by regular posting of content on social media platforms. However, since this depiction is behind a screen, oftentimes the content is curated to perfection, depicting unrealistic beauty standards and lifestyles. Given that the majority of the followers are young individuals, such "perfectly manicured" depictions create unrealistic expectations, thereby resulting in dissatisfaction and impacting their mental health.

Bangladesh, an emerging economy in South Asia, has seen a rapid rise in digitization over the decade. Data shows that the majority of the social media handles experienced rapid growth in terms of usage between 2024-2025. The increase in ad reach for each of the platforms are Facebook (+13.3%), Instagram (+15.4%), Tiktok (+24.5%), LinkedIn(23.8%) and Youtube (32.7%) (https://datareportal.com/reports/digital-2025-bangladesh). With an internet penetration rate of 44.5% in January 2025 and nearly a quarter of the population being Generation Z (between ages 13-28), it is only natural that the influencer culture seeped into the social media landscape of the country.

Teenagers typically spend 7 hours and 22 minutes in front of a device, with a large portion of their time spent watching short reels on websites like YouTube Shorts, Facebook reels, and TikTok (Peash, 2025). This tendency suggests that people are less interested in reading more in-depth material and prefer shorter, more aesthetically pleasing content. In this category, influencer content is highly valued. Fashion, beauty, technology, food, and lifestyle are some of the major industries where influencers are important trend-setters.

The Self-Esteem Paradox:

Influencer content often emphasizes visuals, idealist lifestyles, and viral trends over substantive content. Although many young people see this as a viable career, they do face setbacks from families, as the culture of Bangladesh is more collectivist, and societal values of strong academics and career progression in "stable jobs" are a priority. Additionally, as mentioned before, the "flowery" lives depicted on social media often cause anxiety and distress in young individuals, leading to loss of self-control, self-esteem, and identity (Peash, 2025). Social roles and expectations are interconnected with individual identity. Social Identity Theory (Tajfel & Turner, 1979) posits that individuals derive self-esteem from their affiliation with various groups. The confirmation of one's identity by others in the group leads to an upsurge in self-esteem. Gen Z users may align with influencer communities and derive self-worth based on perceived acceptance. Farivar and Wang (2022) discovered that identification with influencer groups can either elevate or undermine self-esteem, depending upon the relevance between follower identity and influencer messaging.

Although the prevalence of influencer impact in Bangladesh is acknowledged, there is limited academic research on the impact of influencer lifestyles on young followers, particularly with regard to mental well-being. However, this is a critical concern because mental health awareness and access to mental health resources are both limited in the Bangladesh context, intensifying concerns regarding the psychological impact of online engagement. Additionally, the lifestyle depicted by influencers focusing on freedom and independence is seen to be in contrast to the core traditional values of the mass majority. This cultural interplay has also not been addressed in existing literature.

Research Objectives:

The purpose of this chapter is to examine how Gen Z views these influencers, the kind of relationships they have, how they are impacted by influencers, how they cope with psychological pain, and how culture and family shape their preferences. The following research questions will be addressed:

Q1. How are influencer lives viewed and internalized by Gen Z followers?

Q2. How do they cope with anxiety or problems related to self-esteem?

Q3. How do cultural elements—like familial pressure in Bangladesh—affect their choices about how to interact online?

LITERATURE REVIEW

Unlike traditional celebrities, social media influencers are known for their activity and content creation on social media (https://influencermarketinghub.com/what-is-an-influencer/). The content is readily available, short, and trendy, resulting in greater views, but regular exposure to these highly edited and idealized images of peers and influencers on social media platforms often negatively impacts users' self-confidence. According to Tiggemann & Slater (2013), constant comparisons with idealized depictions result in feelings of low self-esteem and identity crisis.

Internalizing unrealistic beauty standards also leads to a lack of confidence and a constant fear of "I am not good enough" (Fardouly et al., 2015). Since Gen Z is the first generation to have grown up with social media, the impact on their mental health and identity crisis is more evident. Examining the intricate connections among social media use, self-esteem, and mental health has become even more crucial in the post-pandemic era, since, according to research, the rise in social media use during the pandemic exacerbated negative psychological and sociocultural factors (Gao, 2023).

The early use of the internet enabled cultural globalization by allowing communities from varied geographic regions to interact. This interaction resulted in local cultures merging with global elements, resulting in a hybridization of cultural identities (Castells, 2000). People started to engage in virtual spaces, resulting in the emergence of the "digital human" (Issa, 2025). With time, social media platforms evolved, resulting in the transition from anonymous online communities to individual user profiles, where the digital identities could be viewed by others (Issa, 2025).

According to Issa 2025, some of the key anthropological transformations in the social media era are,

1. Digital Self-Presentation: social media encourages self-representation, where individuals can create their profiles for social approval
2. Virtual Communities: Online communities became popular amongst people with shared interests, values, and identities. These platforms also enabled people to bond irrespective of their geographic location
3. Effect on Generational Identity: social media has a major role in defining Generation Z's identity by influencing their activism, global knowledge, and immediate communication.

Gen Z is the first group of people considered as fully digital-native due to their exposure to the digital world from their childhood. As they are exposed to social media from a very young age, they have been frequently exposed to emotionally and intellectually mature content—ranging from trauma narratives to complex social issues—long before they have the cognitive or emotional maturity to process it meaningfully. Developmental psychology stresses that emotional maturity depends on the gradual exposure to age-appropriate experiences, overseen by parental guidance, education, and cultural context. However, this digital native generation has extensive knowledge but this untimely exposure induces cognitive-emotional dissonance; adolescents may grasp facts yet lack the necessary cognitive and emotional maturity or life experience to interpret the information meaningfully. Metaphorically, this is akin to "dressing an infant in a 12-year-old's clothing"— inappropriate and potentially harmful. In the absence of adequate coping mechanisms from their environment —be they educational, familial, or cultural—this dissonance may lead to existential incomprehension, emotional instability, and increased vulnerability.

Researchers have been looking more closely at the psychological effects of social media on Gen Z, especially on self-esteem, which is how a person feels about their worth (Rosenberg, 1965). This literature review examines the influence of influencer culture on Gen Z's self-esteem by integrating psychological theories, qualitative research, and socio-cultural viewpoints.

The rise of the Comparison Culture - Social Comparison Theory (SCT) and Elaboration Likelihood Model (ELM)

People who are active on social media platforms participate for connection or validation from their networks. Certain individuals are also passive consumers, for whom viewing content is the core activity, without any direct participation. However, this continuous viewing of "perfect" visuals and lifestyles can influence users' self-perception and overall well-being. The social comparison leads to feelings of inferiority due to the unrealistic beauty standards and peer pressure. Additionally, negative comments and trolls also result in cyberbullying, all of which are detrimental to mental well-being. To make matters worse, the rampant use of filters, image editing tools, and artificially generated content on social media platforms may contribute to a distorted perception of reality among users, as they may compare their natural appearance to digitally enhanced images presented online (Gao, 2023).

Festinger (1954) posited that individuals evaluate their self-worth by comparing themselves with others. Influencers who display curated, idealized lifestyles promote upward comparisons for the followers that frequently undermine self-esteem and body satisfaction, particularly among adolescents (Vogel et al., 2015; Fardouly et al., 2015).

Petty and Cacioppo (1986) identified two ways of persuasion: central and peripheral. Influencer visuals serve as peripheral signals. When Gen Z is just scrolling through their feeds without consciously engaging with the content, they are more likely to accept beauty norms unconsciously, which reinforces their standards and results in negative self-evaluation. The Elaboration Likelihood Model shows how passive engagement makes these effects worse, which is especially relevant for Gen Z's browsing habits, whereas Social Comparison Theory explains the mental processes that lead to self-esteem problems caused by influencers.

Gen Z has had access to platforms like Instagram, Facebook and TikTok that often displays mature, often emotionally complex content and these exposures from early childhood are harmful leading to a cognitive-emotional mismatch. Bonfanti et al. (2025) conducted a comprehensive meta-analysis of 83 studies with over 55,000 participants, revealing a positive correlation between online social comparison and body image concerns. The results highlight the impact of comparing oneself to idealized images on social media, which can diminish self-esteem and foster anxiety-driven behaviors, especially in young people, even in the absence of direct bullying. Even indirect exposure to traumatic or mature content via media can produce vicarious trauma. Research shows that individuals who consume extensive coverage of disasters—through news and social media—may exhibit stress reactions similar to those who were directly involved (Holman et al., 2013).

Bangladesh-Specific Dynamics

According to the "Digital 2025: Bangladesh" report published by DataReportal - Global Digital Insights, there are 60 million active social media users, representing one-third of the population. This rise of social media has reduced the preference for traditional media. Although television, radio, and digital platforms have the power to influence public thought, the majority of the outlets now focus on entertainment and sensationalism, to be trendy and viral. However, in the recent past, it has also been seen that students utilized social media to call upon each other for community action. Therefore, this new shift is a proverbial double-edged sword, whereby there are possible positive outcomes but there are also significant negative impacts (Peash, 2025).

Since entering the digital economy is fairly simple with two basic requirements, a smartphone and internet connection, the youth are attracted to the prospects of gaining recognition as an influencer (Rahman, 2025). This is also shaping the concept of employment and social interaction, and the youth are veering towards it while moving away from higher education and traditional jobs. By embracing this as a profession, they are also enjoying financial independence at an early age (Rahman 2025).

The accumulation of social capital is another intangible benefit derived from social media popularity. The fame and recognition help in building a strong network that can be leveraged for future opportunities. The democratic environment of social media allows people to share their opinions and also showcase their talents

(Rahman 2025). For a lot of the youngsters, the core appeal of being an influencer is freedom. Content creation allows for more flexibility and control over one's brand and activities. Creators can also decide their topics, collaborations and how they want to present their content (Sultana, 2025).

Even though this career and transition may seem lucrative in many ways, there are also significant challenges. Firstly, there is a constant pressure of being consistent and authentic. Audiences look forward to content that strikes a chord with them, but due to the overall short attention span, they are always looking for something new. Additionally, although influencers have to focus on creating new content to be trendy and viral, taking it up as a profession requires long-term vision and focus (Sultana, 2025). Given the sector is still informal in the country, changes in platform policies or account suspensions create income instability if there is over-reliance on monetization (Rahman, 2025).

Although this field may give instant popularity, sustaining it is a constant challenge. Even if they have a very strong start, there needs to be a lot of hard work and focus to thrive on popularity. They need to keep innovating, understanding the market and keep working on the content (Billah, 2022). For those driven to this profession by the quick fame and fun lifestyle as depicted on social media, the lack of adequate knowledge about digital security or financial management serves as a major hindrance. They are more susceptible to online fraud or mismanaged earnings due to a lack of financial planning, thereby limiting the scope of a sustainable career (Rahman 2025).

With the rising popularity of influencers, the youth are looking at it as an aspirational career- mirroring global trends. They are lured by the prospects of fame, freedom and independence. However, this trend has long term implications- since influencers are often in the limelight, many traditional professions and social values become sidelined. Another alarming fact is that it reduces interest in essential careers like teaching and healthcare (Peash 2025).

Over the past few years, there has been a downward trend in reading habits among Bangladeshi youth, who now prefer quick digital content rather than in - depth reading. The trend toward passive entertainment consumption reduces opportunities to interact with complex ideas, ultimately undermining the culture of learning and thoughtful debate among the younger generation (Peash 2025). With regards to influencers, oftentimes their inability to gather knowledge restricts their chances of flourishing in their career (Billah 2022). There is also significant pressure - maintaining the online persona, dealing with online harassment, bullying and gender-based comments. Some of them also have to deal with family resistance towards such activities (Rahman 2025).

From the audience's perspective, this culture poses a significant threat to the mental well-being of the youth. Various studies have associated social media addiction with elevated stress levels, heightened anxiety, depressive symptoms, and reduced self-esteem. For example, Woods and Scott (2016) conducted an extensive survey-based study that demonstrated a significant correlation between extensive social media engagement during adolescence and heightened anxiety, depression, diminished self-esteem, and inferior sleep quality. Similarly, Marino et al. (2018) conducted a thorough synthesis of various empirical studies, revealing a consistent trend: problematic or addictive social media usage is significantly associated with psychological distress, particularly evidenced by low self-esteem, anxiety, and depressive symptoms, with a marked impact on youth demographics.

Blindly following trends leads to identity confusion and stress, compromising mental sanity. This shift fosters a culture that prioritizes superficial knowledge over deep understanding. The obsession with ephemeral fads and viral content has also led to the erosion of traditional values like academics, poetry, art and culture (Peash 2025).

Bangladesh faces significant deficiencies in mental health infrastructure as well as stigma and COVID-19 made matters worse. The country is struggling with an alarming rise in mental issues (18.7%) and a huge caveat in the treatment gap of 92.4% as of 2019. It is a largely ignored domain, where lack of awareness is prevalent and the bigger issue is, lack of action- 92% of patients do not seek professional help. There is limited understanding about this topic and driving down action is even more challenging due to cultural barriers and social taboos (BRAC Mental Health Strategy 2020-2030. (2021)). Even today, for the majority of families, going to a therapist indicates they are beyond repair and they perceive this as being embarrassing.

Mental Health Situation in Bangladesh

Mental health is an integral part of human health and well-being. Globally, mental health disorders account for a significant pressure on public health. Studies by the American Psychological Association (APA) and others reported that Gen Z is more anxious, stressed, and lonely than their previous generations. Research indicates that their augmented digital engagement correlates with heightened emotional vulnerability, fear of missing out (FOMO), and incessant validation-seeking (Sherlock & Wagstaff, 2018).

For low and middle-income countries, the pressure on public health for mental health disorders is even more intense as they are exacerbated by factors like low awareness, social stigma, lack of expertise, lack of willingness to accept, and a dearth of mental health professionals (Islam, 2015). The mental health of university students is a growing concern worldwide. The concern has gained deeper attention in Bangladesh following some mental health-related incidents (Mamun et al., 2019, Siddique et al., 2022).

The majority of the NGOs working in Bangladesh focus on chronic non-communicable diseases, but mental health has been neglected in the past. Therefore, there is both scarcity in data related to mental health as well as preparedness for treating mental health (Islam, 2015). In one of the studies on university students, it was noted that there is insufficient knowledge and high levels of stigma regarding mental issues. Although many students were aware of mental health in general, they did not have proper knowledge, and hence did not know how to deal with these issues. Moreover, anxiety, stress, and depression were common amongst this segment (Siddique et al., 2022). Mamun et al., 2019 also state that, spending more time on the internet has direct impact on depression, anxiety, insomnia, loneliness and lower self-esteem.

Although, recently, mental health awareness has been gaining momentum in the country, it is still an under-researched area with limited data (Mamun et al., 2019, Siddique et al., 2022). Additionally, with regards to the influencer industry, there has been a shift from traditional marketing practices, but the overall impact is hard to gauge as sufficient data is not available (Billah, 2022). Also, the majority of the works cited on Generation Z is on western country perspective. Research focusing on cultural interplay in the local context is rare and limited. This study is an exploration to look into these gaps.

METHODOLOGY

Research Design

This study employed a qualitative, interpretive methodology grounded in hermeneutic phenomenology (Heidegger, 1962) to explore Generation Z's lived experiences of influencer culture and its impact on mental health. Laverty (2003) and Van Manen (2016) assert that hermeneutic phenomenology aims to comprehend the subjective meanings of participants without imposing stringent analytical criteria. This study aims to explore complex emotional and social phenomena, including self-esteem, self-comparison, and psychological well-being, thereby considering this approach as particularly appropriate (Corbin & Strauss, 2008; Yilmaz, 2013).

Qualitative research was selected due to its ability to facilitate an in-depth analysis of participants' narratives, which provides a deeper understanding of their emotions, perceptions, and behaviors that are not possible to document through exclusively quantitative methods (Belk, 2017). Semi-structured interviews and focus group discussions (FGDs) were used to facilitate both individual reflection and interactive dialogue, ensuring richer, multi-layered data.

Participants and Sampling

The research comprised 20 comprehensive interviews and 3 focus group discussions (each consisting of 4–6 participants), yielding insights from a varied cohort of Generation Z individuals aged 20–25 living in Dhaka, Bangladesh. Participants included both university students and young professionals. Initially a purposive sampling method was used to ensure participants were active in Facebook, Instagram or TikTok users who follow at least three influencers. Subsequently, snowball sampling (Etikan et al., 2016) was subsequently used to expand the pool by referrals. This combination increased both relevance and diversity in the sample. Participation was voluntary, and informed consent was obtained prior to each interview or discussion. The following table shows the participant profile:

Table 1. Participant Profile

Participant	Age	Code	Occupation
1	23	P1	Student
2	23	P2	Student/Business
3	25	P3	Customer Service Manager/Student
4	24	P4	Student
5	24	P5	Student
6	22	P6	Student/Business
7	24	P7	Student
8	25	P8	Business
9	23	P9	Student/Food Blogger
10	24	P10	Fashion Influencer
11	23	P11	Student/Make up Artist/Ex influencer
12	24	P12	Student
13	23	P13	Student /Customer Service Executive
14	24	P14	Student
15	25	P15	Copyrighter at Marketing Agency
16	23	P16	Business owner and tutor
17	25	P17	Student
18	25	P18	Marketing executive
19	24	P19	Student
20	23	P20	Student

Data Collection:

Semi-structured interview guides and FGD protocols were designed based on the research objectives and prior literature on influencer culture, self-esteem, and mental health. Example guiding questions included:

1. How frequently do you engage with influencer content on Instagram/TikTok/Facebook?
2. In what ways has influencer content affected your mood or self-image?
3. Can you describe a time you compared yourself to an influencer?
4. Do you perceive this comparison as positive, negative, or both? Why?
5. What strategies do you use to cope with negative emotions after viewing influencer content?

All interviews and FGDs were conducted either face-to-face or via Zoom, depending on participant preference. Sessions lasted between 45–60 minutes. With permission, they were audio-recorded and transcribed verbatim for analysis.

Ethical Considerations:

Ethical approval was obtained before data collection commenced. All participants were briefed about the research objectives, methods, and their rights, including voluntary participation and the option to withdraw at any point. Confidentiality was maintained through pseudonymization of all identifying information.

Data Analysis

The analysis followed thematic analysis principles as outlined by Braun and Clarke (2006), with guidance from Saldaña (2021) on coding and theming. According to Saldaña (2021, p. 14), *"a theme is an outcome of coding, categorization, and analytic reflection, capturing and unifying the nature of the data's experiences or processes."*

The analytic steps were as follows:

1. Familiarization – reading transcripts multiple times to immerse in the data.
2. Initial Coding – assigning descriptive and interpretive codes to meaningful segments of text. Saldaña (2021, p. 13) notes that coding is *"a method of organizing and retrieving the most significant data segments for further analysis."*
3. Pattern Coding – grouping related codes into categories that summarize broader patterns (Saldaña, 2021).

4. Theme Development – reviewing and refining categories into overarching themes that represent recurring ideas and meanings. Saldaña (2021, p. 339) explains that *theming the data* involves identifying *"salient, essence-capturing, and recurring patterns across the dataset."*
5. Review and Interpretation – integrating themes with existing literature to develop an interpretive narrative that aligns with the research objectives.

An inductive approach was adopted so that themes emerged naturally from participants' own words rather than being imposed by pre-existing frameworks. Themes were supported with verbatim quotations to preserve authenticity and contextual meaning.

FINDINGS

Through thematic analysis, three main themes emerged, which summarized our three research questions: how the participants viewed the influencers and how impactful the influencers were, what their coping mechanisms were in dealing with social media, and how cultural factors fared in this journey. The table below shows the themes and the subthemes.

Table 2. The Themes and Subthemes

Theme	Description	Subthemes
1. **Influencer Impact on Aspirations & Self-Perception**	This theme explores how influencers shape Gen Z's self-perception, aspirations, and emotional well-being.	**1.1 Aspirational Role Models and Lifestyle Inspiration** **1.2 Perception of Influencer Authenticity** **1.3 Social Comparison and Internal Conflict** **1.4 Influencing as an Empowering or Viable Career Path** **1.5 Idealization vs. Realistic Self-Assessment** **1.6: Parasocial Relationships and Emotional Bonds**
2. **Coping Mechanisms & Emotional Resilience**	This subtheme examines the coping mechanisms utilized by Generation Z, detailing how they implement intentional strategies—such as digital detoxification, cognitive reframing, and affirmations—to maintain agency over their mental health.	**2.1 Digital Detox & Limiting Exposure** **2.2 Critical Reflection and Self-Awareness** **2.3 Affirmations and Mental Grounding**
3. **Identity & Social Expectations**	This theme examines how influencer culture relates to participants' developing sense of identity, particularly about family expectations, cultural norms, and peer perceptions. It highlights the dynamics between self-expression and external influences on individuals' online behavior.	**3.1 Support Networks: Friends & Family Grounding** **3.2 Personal Identity vs. Influencer Identity** **3.3 Cultural & Generational Gap in Understanding Influencer World**

Theme 1: Influencer Impact on Aspirations & Self-Perception

This theme explores how influencers shape Gen Z's self-perception, aspirations, and emotional well-being. As this was one of the main motives of the research, the researchers delved deeply into the participants' psyche and extracted a range of experiences—from inspiration and career motivation to envy, identity confusion, and parasocial bonds. Six sub-themes evolved from this theme and each of them are described below

1.1 Aspirational Role Models:

Since influencers are mostly popular with Gen Z, their presence and content are considered to be highly aspirational. Some of them have a mini celebrity status and are often requested for photos, videos, and selfies when they are in public places.

Participants shared that influencers who depict success, independence, and authenticity often leave an indelible mark on their minds. Several quotes highlighted how they were inspired by content about travel, fitness, academic performance, and entrepreneurship. Some key quotes include

"I follow a fitness influencer and he is from Russia. The reason I follow him is because he mostly encourages a lot of viewers to prioritize our goals, whether it comes to fitness, or whether it comes to doing my academic performance, whether it goes to any other priorities on my to-do list." **(P5)**

"I think it's booming and it's a great way of marketing. Seven to eight years ago, they used to make fun contents only. Now, we get to see a lot of things. Educational, traveling, business-related, marketing-related. Let's say, Ayman Sadiq, he teaches a lot of good things. And to be honest, I got influenced by him as well because he said some good things like How to make a strategy or how to do Excel properly, So, that's how I think that they are doing good." **(P13)**

Other participants also focused on positive vibes as there was already too much negativity in social media - so the vibes attracted them to the influencers

"The people I follow, they give me happy vibes and they inspire me. For example, her name is Sumayya. She is also a decent hijabi influencer. So, she motivates and tells a lot of inspirational things. And in an Islamic way too. And also Sunehra Tasnim is a very good, chill and happy personality person. So, she also inspires me." **(P11)**

For some of the participants, the lifestyles depicted almost represented a fantasy, particularly those related to travel, success and aesthetics.

"I envy Nadir on the go... His lifestyle, he travels a lot. I like to travel as well, but I do not have that time." **(P1)**

For others, the content was highly motivational, as they were inspired to adopt practices pertaining to discipline and risk-taking. One participant who is a customer service executive shared how an influencer influenced his thought process

"So, he specially talks about how to think about the problems people usually face and how to pitch to people the solution you are making. So, this helps me shape my thinking process and also helps me communicate better with people and empathize with people better to go to the deep root cause that people are actually facing" **(P3)**

One participant also mentioned that the influencers were setting the benchmark for success in this generation.

"I do feel like it would have been great if I were in that position. You know, everyone knowing me, everyone praising me for something." **(P13)**

1.2 Authenticity Perception:

The conversations provided rich insights into how the participants perceive influencer authenticity. Most participants emphasized that transparency in content enhanced the influencer's credibility. Some of the ways in which the influencers "felt real" were when they shared personal struggles, vulnerability, were open in talking about topics like family issues and mental health, as well as sharing behind-the-scenes videos/photos. These contents depicted genuineness.

"I follow an influencer whose content feels "very real" as it showcases everyday activities (cooking, home decor) and business growth without excessive glamour. It is genuine because it includes mundane tasks and long-term struggles (e.g., balancing studies and business). **(P8)**

Contents that were excessively polished frequently garnered feelings of skepticism among participants, with several noting that perceived "inauthentic" content adversely affected their self-esteem. Many users chose to unfollow influencers who lacked authenticity or showcased high levels of "perfection". Additionally, some participants reported internalizing feelings of being "not good enough", when comparing themselves to highly idealized online personas

One participant shared

"They are not really very realistic. And I myself was an influencer back in 2020-2022. And I was a model too for a fashion brand. So, I faced a lot of discrimination and I feel like that the influencers are more of, they show fake things or fake personalities in the gram or Facebook. That's why I also was mentally hampered a little bit. I was told that I look very aged and I need to lose weight and that scarred me" **(P11)**

Some participants also demonstrated maturity and literacy in understanding the reasons behind the curation, which is a good development as it means they are not blind to reality. For example, one participant shared

"Yes, curated content does bother me. As I've been following him (a fitness influencer) for quite a while, initially his videos were very raw and it looked legit, It's like no editing. Then with time and competition, they realized they needed to be more eye-catching. It seems like you need to put a bit of work into it, maybe some editing, skills and stuff like that. So he kind of got diverted to curation from his true skills." **(P4)**

Participants felt that providing authentic content is a core responsibility of the influencer, and there needs to be regulations in place to monitor this in the country.

"Obviously that reality check is very important. Like I mean you are a content creator and this is your responsibility to provide the authentic information. And also, the real fact whether it's good or bad you have to provide to your audience. That's your responsibility. But in terms of most of the content creators in Bangladesh they are actually not doing it. I have to give due respect actually to whom I follow, compared to other influencers I found him to be authentic." **(P15)**

1.3 Social Comparison:

Although many of the participants saw influencers as motivational, they also agreed that subconsciously, they often found themselves comparing their lives to the influencers. This comparison often triggered self-doubt and emotional struggles, which included feelings of low self-esteem, hurt or jealousy at others' achievements, and feeling inferior in college One participant also shared a very pertinent and relatable feeling of guilt and demotivation, due to excessive consumption like buying things from watching content online. When unable to process all the information, participants also questioned the authenticity of influencers' displays of success, reflecting internal conflict.

Participants who were influencers themselves shared feelings of being distressed with the pressure of being popular.

"I faced many discriminations among the influencers. I was working with other brands also. So, when there was a lot of influencers who were very popular. And I was just starting at that time. So, I was a little bit new in that industry. So, they preferred the other influencers more. And it was very visible in front of me. That's why I think that impacted me a lot. I did compare myself subconsciously with them and that also impacted my self-esteem." **(P11)**

Underperforming content often made them question their self-worth. To some of them, seeking validation seemed emotionally draining, and being constantly preoccupied with "likes" "followers" and "hashtags" led to mental exhaustion and burnout. This excessive chase for numbers and validation resulted in feelings of isolation as participants sometimes found themselves completely detached from real-life interactions, like

"Seeing their success made me question myself" **(P1).**

When asked, what message the participant would like to give the junior GenZ, the reply was

"I would firstly recommend to them that whatever they see on the internet is mostly not real. And they cannot never follow a particular person to relate themselves with them, nobody's story is the same." **(P5)**

1.4 Influencing as Career:

Influencing is increasingly being recognized as a legitimate and motivating profession. Participants highlighted its financial prospects and entrepreneurial nature and identified travel influencing as a feasible career option. It is worth noting that the participants acknowledged the creativity, perseverance, and diligence required in this field, and they are hoping to communicate the same to their parents. They believe that going forward, exploring journalism and fitness as careers was an option they would consider, illustrating its empowering impact.

"Business needs creators to spread the message of what they are. If there is a shift in branding, if there is a shift in the production or how they are building the product. So, they need creators because it's not just the era of celebrities anymore." **(P18)**

Based on the quotes, the following are the key findings:

- **Career Paradigm Shift:** Influencers are shaping the industry
  - *"I think they have done great for our industry from setting the bar of remuneration, and how brands are going to look at us. Not as models but as creators. So, we can charge fixed amount of money from them and they have decided the bar." **(P10)***
- **Skill Development:** Participants reported acquiring practical skills as a result of their engagement in this space.
  - ***P8*** shared, *"I started learning editing because of them."*
- **Entrepreneurial Mindset:** There is an increasing perception of influencing as a credible business endeavor.
  - As ***P17*** observed, *"They run teams, studios."*

This shift in the career thought process is understandable because when participants see "someone like them" overcome challenges, they find it more relatable and therefore it boosts their confidence. Also, transparency regarding the journey (e.g. claims like "my first video got only 10 views") further amplifies the credibility. They also understand and acknowledge that it is not easy being an influencer and it requires significant time and effort.

"I think I love what they do. But I think it is not that easy for everyone to do that. I think it's kind of a talent. Like, promoting a brand, it's not that easy. It takes a lot of time. It takes creativity. And I think the influencers that I follow are very good at it. And other than that, I think it takes a lot of investment as well. Like, it takes up your time. It takes some costs, like, you know, a good mic, a good camera. And let's say I'm a food reviewer. It takes investment to buy the food. And I know that these are quite expensive." **(P13)**

For some participants, the influencers have also instilled confidence and they aim to reach higher levels in their careers based on the guidance of the influencers.

"Yes, he helps me to be inspired to be someone better and shoot for the CXO roles or like chief executive officer roles like I should be someone like him. People would know my name." **(P3)**

1.5 Idealization vs. Reality:

Gen Z's progression from idealization to self-acceptance is characterized by an initial recognition that influencer content is often carefully curated and intentionally performed. This awareness of cyber-perfection reduces their propensity for self-blame and encourages a more pragmatic perspective. Subsequently, individuals begin to value authenticity and reject universal standards and redefine achievements through the lens of personal growth rather than social media highlights. This transformative process signifies a move from passive content consumption to active, empowered self-definition, whereby embracing one's genuine and unfiltered experiences becomes more acceptable against digital idealizations.

Participants who were influencers themselves also shared that with time they have grown to understand the process better and therefore are better at dealing with the uncertainties of the industry as depicted by the following insight

*"Social media algorithms are very unpredictable. I can create something larger than life and magnificent. But somehow, there are days when the algorithm doesn't just work for you. It's not your content. It's just something, it's not reaching out to people. It's technology and you cannot have 100% control over it. But content creation is something you don't stop. The next one doesn't work. But right after that, another one will work. So, you have to keep trying posting and engaging with your audience." **(P10)***

1.6 Parasocial Relationships and Emotional Bonds

This subtheme explores the emotional connections Gen Z develops with influencers, where participants often view content creators as friends, mentors, or the proverbial "boro bhai" (elder brother in the Bangladesh context). Several participants admitted to having a very strong one-sided connection to the influencers, despite not having any actual relationship. This highlights the pertinent phenomenon, how digital interactions can influence Gen Z's social connections, sometimes blurring the boundaries between online and offline relationships. Some of the highlights based on the interviews are:

- **One-Sided Intimacy:** Participants described deep, friend-like attachments
  - (P17: *"Cried for influencers like family"*).
- **Emotional Dependency:** Influencers' lives affected moods
  - (P13: *"I miss them when they're gone"*).
- **Illusion of Reciprocity:** *Despite knowing the relationship was asymmetrical, participants felt seen and understood*
  - *(P10: "When they replied to my comment, I felt they cared").*

Theme 2: Coping Mechanisms & Emotional Resilience

This subtheme explores the mechanisms used by Generation Z to deal with social media stressors. The mechanisms reflect intentional strategies—such as digital detoxification, critical thinking- to get to the base of the matter, and positive affirmations—to achieve calmness and sanity. This structured approach shifts responses from reactive avoidance to proactive resilience in managing social media pressures, thereby supporting long-term self-regulation.

2.1 Digital Detox & Limiting Exposure

Participants agreed that being online 24/7 is exciting and useful but can also take a toll on mental and emotional health. In order to protect their mental well-being and prevent the constant preoccupation with social media, many participants actively limited their engagement with social media. Some of them muted accounts or deactivated Instagram from time to time to ease their minds, while others took breaks by deleting apps altogether. They stressed the benefits of "deplugging" from triggering content, as the reduced exposure helped them stabilize their mindspace. Given the plethora of content available at the fingertips, it is very easy to get into a loop of doomscrolling - continuous scrolling of triggering content, which resulted in wasted hours, emotional burden, and guilt of not controlling screen time- so the detox worked well, and they strongly advocated these temporary breaks. One participant also felt the influencers need to take a break from the internet as well.

"Constant scrolling does tire me out if it's too many but as I have told you I don't spend too much time on social media, so it doesn't bother me a lot. Still sometimes, especially influencers from western culture, there's so many influencers coming in my feed, that they're doing so many activities, so many tests, but sometimes I feel like they should also take a break from the internet." **(P5)**

"I uninstall apps when I feel overwhelmed. Even if it's just for a week, it helps." **(P1)**

With regards to certain influencers, they chose to unfollow them, if anything was unsetting, as shared by a participant.

"I used to watch an influencer many years ago, I don't like him anymore. His personal life is very chaotic and he lost his credibility due to some dubious publicly controversial actions so I find him inconsistent with the values he used to promote." **(P17)**

2.2 Critical Reflection and Self-Awareness

This subtheme highlights a critical development necessary for the Gen Z- the ability to identify the emotional impact of social media and to critically analyze the content they encounter. Rather than engaging passively with influencer representations and absorbing whatever is demonstrated, these individuals engage in reflective practices that prompt them to question depictions, consider issues of authenticity (linked to Subtheme 1.2), and assess their own situation. This heightened self-awareness helps them to avoid potential feelings of inadequacy or distress and fosters a positive and thoughtful engagement with social media platforms.

Self-awareness stems from the realization that "highlight reels" are not reality, and also exposing oneself to negative triggers is a form of self-harm. Participants also mentioned that they started to critically analyze the content rather than just plain comparison, and in the process, they acknowledged the fact that not everything they viewed was necessarily real or right for them.

"First, I would take these external factors like fitness, nutrition, then my education, academic performance, then maintaining my religion. Then I'm going to match the way I was raised with the influencers and keep myself as morally positive and right." **(P5)**

Key Quotes:

- *"I actively remind myself they're showing 10% of their life."* **(P11)**
- *"I train my brain to reject their version of success" **(P7).***

These reflections in this subtheme demonstrate a journey, starting with development of personal resilience by taking a deliberate stand against the emotional manipulation in influencer content. There is also a shift from being reactive to being proactive through critical thinking. This is a powerful coping mechanism — depicting growth through emotional maturity and digital literacy.

"I take notes, I make a checklist, I also paste sticky notes in front of my table so that I know about important deadlines and something important that I need to do, communicate. So, previously the checklist used to come from other people that they expect these things to be done. But now the checklist I myself make. Yes, I have more control over my life, more control over the priorities and I question a lot of things." **(P3)**

2.3 Affirmations and Mental Grounding

This subtheme elaborates on how participants utilize both internal and external tools to control their emotions and, in the process, build resilience in response to idealized or triggering online content. Instead of complete withdrawal, they implement strategies to 'deal with' what is shown to them. Some of the common strategies described include gratitude journaling (which helps them appreciate what they have), self-talk (which acts as a pep-talk, assuring them that things are ok), mantras (which help them remain focused and steadfast), and mindfulness (which helps them to remain balanced). All these activities eventually help them to maintain self-worth rooted in real-life experiences. These protective routines help manage emotional challenges such as comparison, idealization, and digital overload.

Key Quotes:

- *"Gratitude journaling really shifts my mindset. Even when I'm anxious, I list 3 good things."* ***(P14)***
- *"Sometimes I look at my own wins, not just followers or views. That helps me stay grounded."* ***(P16)***
- *"I keep a board of things I've achieved, not likes, real things. That's what helps when I feel off."* ***(P5)***
- *"I listened to a motivational speaker and it really helped me deal with my issues of anxiety and overthinking- particularly when he explained that what is meant to happen will happen, we just have to try our best and leave it up to Almighty, that really helped me reach attain a calmness."* ***(P13)***

Positive affirmations like sticky notes to praise oneself, breathing exercises and relaxing music helped the participants to achieve inner peace. Additionally, some of them also sought therapy whilst others found talking to friends and peers therapeutic.

"During the lockdown I was very mentally distressed. I even took counselling sessions from the university counselling center, they helped me a lot but I needed some purpose, I needed some goal in my life and just getting regular salaries or having a nice job did not feel enough. The counsellor suggested that I was being very limited in my circle, I am living in my own bubble and I am not letting new ideas come into me. So, I have to be more open, I have to go into more circles, know more people and make my environment diverse so that I always have something in my plate that helped me look beyond the immediate horizon." **(P3)**

These strategies reflect a proactive effort to maintain emotional health and affirm self-worth beyond social comparison. Rather than disengage entirely from digital life, participants are creating psychological filters—mental habits that buffer the self from external pressures. Such practices also indicate a growing understanding of mental health literacy and a willingness to actively manage self-esteem through positive internal dialogue.

Theme 3: Identity & Social Expectations

This theme explores how participants imbibe influencer culture and develop their sense of identity. Given Gen Z is the first generation growing up with social media, the challenge to strike a balance between their online and offline persona is particularly applicable to them. This challenge becomes even more acute in a collectivist culture like Bangladesh where high levels of family expectations, cultural norms, and peer perceptions are prevalent. The theme highlights the dynamics between self-expression and external influences on individuals' online behavior. Several participants reported that aligning their online presence with their personal values, as well as navigating differing generational perspectives in an increasingly digital society adds a lot to their mental stress. The subthemes that evolved are as follows:

3.1 Support Networks: Friends & Family Grounding

One of the main emphases of the participants has been on the vital role of supportive relationships in their lives. These relationships include close friends and family, who often serve as a safe zone for them and provide emotional grounding. Conversations and venting with this group help them reaffirm their self-worth based on real-world interactions. Participants mentioned that there were times, when the only support they were looking for was having someone to "listen" to them. It is also worth mentioning that, often, few things are difficult to share with family members, so having a close circle of friends is almost like a lifeline. Being part of a network helps them fulfill their belongingness needs, gives them periodic reality checks, and helps them remain grounded, thereby reducing the self-esteem threats of upward social comparisons (Theme 1.4). In summary, a strong support network performs the following functions

- Support networks act as emotional anchors and provide reality checks.
  - *"You're comparing your chapter 2 to someone's chapter 20." **(P7's cousin)***
  - *"My friends remind me that I'm more than what my profile shows." **(P9)***
- A strong support network also helps in validation and acts as a cushion from harsh reality
  - *"My friends don't judge me when I say I feel insecure." **(P10)***
  - *"Sometimes I just talk to my mom and I feel better than after hours online." **(P19)***
- A strong support network also helps in showing alternative indicators of success
  - *"Success doesn't need to be flashy." **(P14's father)***

- *"My parents don't care about followers. They care if I'm eating well and sleeping okay." (P11)*

3.2 Personal Identity vs. Influencer Identity

Participants mentioned that they often experienced burnout at times, when trying to keep up with their online personalities. They often felt that there was a split personality in who they were and who they show on their respective handles. Maintaining an image that wasn't actually theirs often resulted in feelings of loss of identity.

- Some participants experienced identity erosion, whereby they felt they were losing their authentic self.
  - *"I felt like I was copying others. It wasn't me anymore."* **(P12)**
- Excessive fixation with influencer-based content resulted in feelings of self-doubt, thereby harboring feelings of being "not good enough".
  - *"Sometimes I wonder if I post because I want to, or because I feel I have to." (P20)*
- Other participants mentioned that they made a conscious effort to stop losing themselves and start rebuilding autonomy.
  - *"You need to stop shaping your life for the camera instead of the other way around." (P17)*
  - *"It took effort to unlearn influencer-speak." (P19)*

3.3 Cultural & Generational Gap in Understanding Influencer World

As a country, Bangladesh has a collectivitist culture, where familial honor, desires and ties are held very strongly. Therefore, parental (and sometimes even for extended family) wishes and consent are considered when making major life decisions like career and family. Therefore, traditional careers like medicine, engineering and civil services are most coveted and preferred, although in recent years, entrepreneurship and few unconventional career paths are gaining momentum (e.g. make-up artists, chefs, bakery etc.).

Therefore, members of Generation Z who pursue influencer-related careers often experience differing perspectives from older generations. Participants reported that some parents referred to content creation as *"useless job"* or *"screen addiction,"* indicating that they are not willing to recognize digital work as a form of employment". There are "differential perspectives of Gen Z and older generations, particularly regarding digital engagement, mental health awareness, and emerging career paths like content creation. Several participants mentioned the uneasiness they experience due to the limited understanding or support from family members, typically due to the proverbial "generational gap".

- Dismissal of Digital Careers: Older generations devalue online work.
    - *"It's hard to talk about content creation as a career when no one around you even sees it as work." **(P18)***
    - *"Because in our country, in our society, they don't get the difference between a content creator and a model." **(P10)***
- Lack of Understanding of Online Platforms .
    - *"My parents don't understand the pressure that comes with online visibility." **(P13)***
    - *"They think social media is just a waste of time. But for us, it's a way to express and connect." **(P6)***
    -
- Social Isolation: Participants hide interests to avoid conflict.
    - *"I have to hide my passions." **(P12)***
    - *"I had to lie about my page because my family wouldn't get it." **(P16)***

Additionally, even in terms of content, there are cultural differences and participants did acknowledge that family values and understanding is crucial in shaping how they react on internalizing content. One participant shared

"If I talk about cultural perspectives in Russia, they're really open minded, like, they are really open with their relationships, with others. We try to maintain a certain boundary among us, but they don't do that because they openly approach everyone. And even if it's the opposite gender, that is sometimes his video shows that they're a bit too open about how they expressed themselves in their cultural setting, whereas in our culture, it's not an appropriate thing. So that's why I kind of do think those are the few drawbacks of following him." **(P4)**

DISCUSSION

The reflections from the participants highlight the fact that, in the Bangladeshi context, social comparison is further amplified by our collectivist culture. Theme 1 shows that the seeping of influencer culture is a proverbial double-edged sword, whereby influencers are seen as aspirational figures, but also contribute to undermining self-esteem. For example, a participant mentioned that they loved an influencer's nighttime routine (Subtheme 1.1), and felt frustrated as they couldn't replicate it, not just for the elaborate rituals but also for lack of time (Subtheme 1.4). However, the authenticity of the influencer (Subtheme 1.2) also acted as a mitigating factor when the influencer admitted that they also struggle with maintaining their routines.

The relationship between authenticity (Subtheme 1.2) and parasocial relationships (Subtheme 1.6) reveals another critical dynamic: influencers who are perceived as authentic or real harbor a healthy one-sided attachment. Those who depict more curated lifestyles add to distress and frustration. However, with time (and given our interviewees represented the older sect of GenZ), participants moved from imitation (Subtheme 1.1) to critical differentiation (Subtheme 1.5), which highlights a developmental arc in media literacy. Authenticity is also linked to participants' career plans, whereby participants mentioned that influencers who are transparent about their journey are almost like mentors since they show how to build something from scratch.

With regards to career aspirations, most participants agreed that this is evolving into a lucrative career option but it still needs time to become a formal sector for employment. Since the older generation is still not fully understanding of the prospects, many participants agreed that they see influencing as a more side hustle as opposed to a full time employment, and they are willing to complete their education so there is always a back up.

- *"I would suggest being an influencer can be a part-time thing. But you have to have the first option."* ***(P2)***
- *"Even if content creation works out, I want to finish my degree first."* ***(P18)***

The findings of theme 2 depict a hierarchy in coping mechanisms. It starts with Tier 1- Avoidance, which comprises quick fixes like app deletion and unplugging from social media. It then moves to Tier 2- Cognitive, which depicts a reframing of their minds by critical reflection through journaling and Tier 3- Embodied - regular activities like positive validation. Hence, it can be seen that participants progress from being reactive (deactivating apps) to being proactive (writing positive notes about themselves). The cognitive reframing through critical reflection is an important skill that acts as a buffer against depression and anxiety. The following key quote pairings from two participants demonstrate the change.

Table 3.

	1.3 Social Comparison and internal conflict	**2.2 Critical reflection and self awareness**
P6	*"When I look at them, I feel they are so far ahead of me"*	*"When I looked at my achievements, I started to understand that success isn't linear or universal."*
P14	*"Often, social media is a daily reminder of what I don't have."*	*"Gratitude journaling shifts my mindset. I list 3 good things."*

Theme 3 revealed how GenZ juggled between identity, cultural expectations and self-worth in a time where influencers are an integral part of their daily lives. The reflections implied that identity formation is actually layered, not just from what users consume but also by the expectations and judgments of those around them. It highlighted the importance of social support, the dissonance in identity of online and offline persona and the generational divides in valuing online world or career. The theme showcases identity as a battleground as influencers are seen to threaten the self-concept (Subtheme 3.2), but offline networks (Subtheme 3.1) and critical reflections (Subtheme 2.2) helps to restore balance. While influencers model new paths of self-expression, young people are still navigating deeply rooted cultural frameworks and a desire for genuine belonging—both online and off.

Although both subtheme 1.3 Social comparison and internal conflict and Subtheme 3.2 Personal identity vs influencer identity involves comparison, they are in different layers. Subtheme 1.3 focuses more on immediate emotional consequences of comparing oneself to users - some examples include

- **Envy**: "*Seeing their bodies/lifestyle makes me feel like I am lacking something*" ***(P18)***
- **Guilt**: "*I feel like I am lazy seeing their productivity*'' ***(P15)***
- **Anxiety**: "*You suddenly feel anxious for no good reason*'' ***(P12)***

However, from the conversations, it could be inferred that these reactions were more episodic or short term, usually happening during scrolling. On the other hand, subtheme 3.2 focuses on longer term impact on personality through loss of identity. Some examples include

- **Loss of self**: "*I dressed/talked like them until I didn't recognize myself*' ***(P10)***
- **Value substitution**: "*I reshaped my dreams based on their content*" **(P12)**
- **Existential doubt**: "*Am I boring because I am not loud like them*" **(P3)**

Therefore, unmanaged social comparisons do have the power to make long term impacts on identity. However, the coping mechanisms of Theme 2 along with the support networks in Subtheme 3.1 are crucial for minimizing this damage.

The support networks in Subtheme 3.1 mitigate the identity erosion in Subtheme 3.2 and have a reanchoring effect on the participants. Family and friends provided a real picture to the participants and following key quotes help to illustrate this phenomenon.

"*My cousin said you are comparing your chapter 2 to their chapter 20.*" **(P7)** 3.1 counters "*I was reshaping dreams based on what they show.*" **(P12)** 3.2

Subtheme 3.3 also highlighted an important dimension of cultural and generational gap in understanding the influencer world. Although Subtheme 1.4 showcased influencing as a viable career, in subtheme 3.3 it can be seen that the older generation has a dismissive attitude towards digital careers. Parents are often dismissive and have rigid career expectations. This creates a tension between digital native aspirations and traditional expectations leading to secrecy and frustration. However, some participants also mentioned that their parents were adaptable and willing to listen and learn more about influencing.

"My mom now asks, 'what did you learn from that content creator'? instead of judging, which makes me more comfortable in discussing with her" ***(P14).***

"They are like 50s… now they are understanding the perspective of the influencers too." **(P2)**

This is an important development as parents who listen (rather than dismiss) can become allies in media literacy, and the learning process will benefit both generations. Although support groups are crucial, the reality is that not all support groups are the same. Participants also shared instances when sharing with friends did not yield the desired responses so they had to resort to motivational speakers.

"I did talk to both friends and family about my overthinking issue. My family suggested to do my side. But whenever I tried talking to my friends, they started overthinking as well. That's why I did not further have any discussions about it with them- but online motivational speakers helped." **(P13)**

Participants also mentioned that there should be policies regarding age limits and content quality, and parents should be monitoring the social media behaviour of the younger Gen Zs.

"I think there should be an age barrier. There should be a quality as well. I would suggest, if I could suggest their parents, I would have said to monitor them. Because sometimes for social media, I did not prepare myself for mid-terms, diseases and other things and it literally has impacted me a lot. And I am literally suffering for it. So, I would say, to understand what is needed, to understand that there is a limit to everything. I should not over exceed." **(P13)**

CONCLUSION & RECOMMENDATIONS

The influencer culture is here to stay and it is a reality that needs to be understood by Gen Z and their parents. Our discussions with the participants reveal that many of the influencers are highly aspirational, and members of Gen Z look up to them and form a parasocial bond with them. However, authenticity is a key factor that determines the level of aspiration or bonding that participants feel. Authentic influencers are also perceived as mentors, and their success stories are seen as benchmarks that also shape the participants' career aspirations. However, looking at curated lifestyles often results in social comparison, which leads to feelings of frustration, distress, and low self-esteem. Oftentimes, blindly following the influencers also results in an identity crisis and the loss of self.

Participants shared several ways of coping with these distressful feelings. Some temporary solutions include digital detox - by deleting apps, unfollowing influencers, or deactivating their own social media handles. But over time, they also reshaped their critical thinking through practices like journaling, self-reflection, and positive validations.

Most participants emphasized the importance of having a strong support group - friends and family to constantly give reality checks, reassurance, and grounding. However, one concern was that, for some participants, making the parents understand the significance of social media was a challenge as they do not understand the dynamics of the digital world.

Given that this is an evolving concept that will become more and more ubiquitous in the coming days, several actions can be taken to make the experience smooth for all. There should be media literacy programs to help the audience understand the difference between authentic and curated content. There should also be discussions about healthy comparison and self-worth in digital spaces. Influencers should be encouraged to balance aspirational and authentic storytelling. To nurture a healthy parasocial bond, they may share more real content like "day in my life" or "get ready with me" which will give the audience a glimpse of their real life. In other words, rather than just focusing on outcomes, they can also run through a process (e.g. weight loss journey or spending time with their own family).

The influencer industry in Bangladesh is worth above USD 100 Million (Khan, 2024). However, it is still highly informal and deregulated, with no proper regulations regarding policy, payment, and protection. To leverage the growth of this sector, the business community and policymakers must collaborate to fund education and training programs to address evolving aspects of digital marketing. As influencer marketing grows, ensuring authenticity and transparency will become more critical (Khan, 2024).

Platforms can also contribute to the well-being of their audience by taking a few responsible actions, such as incorporating "break reminders" when they notice someone is watching content incessantly. Additionally, they may also embed reality check prompts like "Remember this is a highlight reel" when users linger on aspirational content.

Parents need to be more empathetic in understanding the influencer culture and Gen Z. Rather than being rigid and dismissive towards digital careers or personalities, having an open conversation and willingness to learn about this development is likely to be helpful. This will encourage the younger generation to openly discuss their thoughts and ideas, as well as their struggles and insecurities. Co-consuming content and sharing feedback will also help both sides share their perspectives, thereby creating a better understanding. Parents do not need to understand the influencer culture perfectly- they need to affirm their child's inherent worth, while gently questioning curated ideas.

Viewers (Gen Z) should be mindful when consuming content and understand the reality. They should be cognizant of their values and goals and follow influencers who align with their values. They also need to be proactive in media literacy and not fall for everything that they see on social media. To have a more solid mental grounding, they should opt for periodic digital detox sessions and self-reflection. Additionally, whenever they feel overwhelmed or pressured due to social media, they should seek out their support group, including friends, family, or professional help. Given the collectivist culture of Bangladesh, family will play a key role- hence, trying to have open communication is healthy.

On a macro-level, regulatory frameworks should be established to prevent deceptive marketing practices, and businesses must invest in cybersecurity measures to protect sensitive customer data. Efforts should also be made to formalize the influencer industry with proper guidelines and a code of conduct that will specify influencer responsibilities and legal bindings. This would include parental guidance, mandating infleuncer qualifications (as recently done in China), remuneration, remuneration, control of content, age restrictions and platform regulations. By investing in digital literacy, infrastructure, ethical guidelines, and cybersecurity, Bangladesh can navigate the digital realm with confidence, leveraging the power of influencers as digital entrepreneurs and creating new career opportunities for Gen Z.

Limitations and Future Research

This study focused on "Zillenials", the older echelon of Generation Z. This means that they already have a longer duration of exposure to social media and have worked on coping with the issues they faced. Given, mental health issues were more pervasive on university students, this study focused on this particular segment. Also, all the participants of the study were based in Dhaka, the capital city, which is most digitally advanced. Future studies could focus on younger GenZs and also incorporate communication with schools regarding what can be done to make this transition easier for the next generation. Also, despite the prevalent urban-rural and digital divide in the country, some social media platforms like TikTok are becoming increasingly popular outside Dhaka. This is an important factor that needs attention as they are more likely to be outside formal regulations and understanding the impact on the youth is a challenge but is of utmost importance.

REFERENCES

Belk, R. W. (2017). Qualitative research in advertising. *Journal of Advertising, 46*(1), 36–47. DOI: 10.1080/00913367.2016.1201025

Billah, M. (2022, December 7). The rise of the "influencer" market in Bangladesh. *The Business Standard*. https://www.tbsnews.net/long-read/rise-influencer-market-bangladesh-546854

Bonfanti, R. C., Melchiori, F., Teti, A., Albano, G., Raffard, S., Rodgers, R., & Lo Coco, G. (2025). The association between social comparison in social media, body image concerns and eating disorder symptoms: A systematic review and meta-analysis. *Body Image, 52*, 101841. DOI: 10.1016/j.bodyim.2024.101841 PMID: 39721448

BRAC Mental Health Strategy 2020-2030. (2021). In https://www.brac.net/program/mental-health/. BRAC Mental Health Strategy Working Group. Retrieved June 7, 2025, from https://www.brac.net/program/wp-content/uploads/2021/09/BRAC-mental_-health_strategy-2020-2030.pdf

Braun, V., & Clarke, V. (2006). Using thematic analysis in psychology. *Qualitative Research in Psychology, 3*(2), 77–101. DOI: 10.1191/1478088706qp063oa

Castells, M. (2000). Globalisation, identity and the state. *Social Dynamics, 26*(1), 5–17. DOI: 10.1080/02533950008458682

Corbin, J., & Strauss, A. (2008). *Basics of Qualitative Research* (3rd ed.). Techniques and Procedures for Developing Grounded Theory., DOI: 10.4135/9781452230153

Etikan, I. (2016). Comparison of convenience sampling and purposive sampling. *American Journal of Theoretical and Applied Statistics, 5*(1), 1. DOI: 10.11648/j.ajtas.20160501.11

Fardouly, J., Diedrichs, P. C., Vartanian, L. R., & Halliwell, E. (2015). Social comparisons on social media: The impact of Facebook on young women's body image concerns and mood. *Body Image, 13*, 38–45. DOI: 10.1016/j.bodyim.2014.12.002 PMID: 25615425

Farivar, S., & Wang, F. (2022). Effective influencer marketing: A social identity perspective. *Journal of Retailing and Consumer Services, 67*, 103026. DOI: 10.1016/j.jretconser.2022.103026

Festinger, L. (1954). A theory of social comparison processes. *Human Relations, 7*(2), 117–140. DOI: 10.1177/001872675400700202

Gao, M. (2023). Social media's influence on eating disorders. *Modern Economics & Management Forum*, *4*(4), 107. DOI: 10.32629/memf.v4i4.1489

Holman, E. A., Garfin, D. R., & Silver, R. C. (2013). Media's role in broadcasting acute stress following the Boston Marathon bombings. *Proceedings of the National Academy of Sciences of the United States of America*, *111*(1), 93–98. DOI: 10.1073/pnas.1316265110 PMID: 24324161

Islam, A. (2015). Mental Health and the health system in Bangladesh: Situation analysis of a neglected domain. *American Journal of Psychiatry and Neuroscience*, *3*(4), 57. DOI: 10.11648/j.ajpn.20150304.11

Issa, A. (2025). Digital Anthropology: Navigating Human Experience in the Age of Artificial Intelligence and Social Media. *Digital Humanities, Social Sciences and Cultural Preservation*. https://doi.org/DOI: 10.2139/ssrn.5258483

Khan, S. R. (2024, January 1). Traversing the power of digital and influencer marketing in apparel industry. *Textile News, Apparel News, RMG News, Fashion Trends*. https://www.textiletoday.com.bd/traversing-the-power-of-digital-and-influencer-marketing-in-apparel-industry

Laverty, S. M. (2003). Hermeneutic Phenomenology and Phenomenology: A comparison of historical and methodological considerations. *International Journal of Qualitative Methods*, *2*(3), 21–35. DOI: 10.1177/160940690300200303

Mamun, M. A., Hossain, M. S., & Griffiths, M. D. (2019). Mental health problems and associated predictors among Bangladeshi students. *International Journal of Mental Health and Addiction*, *20*(2), 657–671. DOI: 10.1007/s11469-019-00144-8

Marino, C., Gini, G., Vieno, A., & Spada, M. M. (2018). The associations between problematic Facebook use, psychological distress and well-being among adolescents and young adults: A systematic review and meta-analysis. *Journal of Affective Disorders*, *226*, 274–281. DOI: 10.1016/j.jad.2017.10.007 PMID: 29024900

Peash, M. N. H. (2025, May 26). Influencer culture among our youth on the rise -. *The Daily Observer*. https://www.observerbd.com/news/527197#:~:text=Influencer%20culture%20has%20contributed%20to,fleeting%20fads%20and%20viral%20content%20

Petty, R. E., & Cacioppo, J. T. (1986). Communication and persuasion. In *Springer eBooks*. https://doi.org/ DOI: 10.1007/978-1-4612-4964-1

Rahman, M. (2025, May 23). Social media influencers & the new youth economy. *The Financial Express*. https://thefinancialexpress.com.bd/views/views/social-media-influencers-the-new-youth-economy

Rosenberg, M. (1965). Society and the adolescent Self-Image. In *Princeton University Press eBooks*. https://doi.org/ DOI: 10.1515/9781400876136

Saldana, J. (2021). *The Coding Manual for Qualitative Researchers*. Sage Publications Limited.

Sherlock, M., & Wagstaff, D. L. (2018). Exploring the relationship between frequency of Instagram use, exposure to idealized images, and psychological well-being in women. *Psychology of Popular Media Culture*, *8*(4), 482–490. DOI: 10.1037/ppm0000182

Siddique, M. B., Ovi, M. R., Ahammed, T., Chowdhury, M. B., & Uddin, M. J. (2022). Mental health knowledge and awareness among university students in Bangladesh. *Heliyon*, *8*(10), e11084. DOI: 10.1016/j.heliyon.2022.e11084 PMID: 36303905

Sultana, N. (2025, January 14). Understanding the rise of influencers. *Dhaka Tribune*. https://www.dhakatribune.com/opinion/op-ed/370760/under-the-rise-of-influencers

Tajfel, H., & Turner, J. C. (1979). An integrative theory of intergroup conflict. In Austin, W. G., & Worchel, S. (Eds.), *The social psychology of intergroup relations* (pp. 33–37). Brooks/Cole.

Tiggemann, M., & Slater, A. (2013). NetGirls: The Internet, Facebook, and body image concern in adolescent girls. *International Journal of Eating Disorders*, *46*(6), 630–633. DOI: 10.1002/eat.22141 PMID: 23712456

Van Manen, M. (2016). *Researching lived experience: Human Science for an Action Sensitive Pedagogy*. Routledge.

Vogel, E. A., Rose, J. P., Okdie, B. M., Eckles, K., & Franz, B. (2015). Who compares and despairs? The effect of social comparison orientation on social media use and its outcomes. *Personality and Individual Differences*, *86*, 249–256. DOI: 10.1016/j.paid.2015.06.026

Woods, H. C., & Scott, H. (2016). #Sleepyteens: Social media use in adolescence is associated with poor sleep quality, anxiety, depression and low self-esteem. *Journal of Adolescence*, *51*(1), 41–49. DOI: 10.1016/j.adolescence.2016.05.008 PMID: 27294324

Yilmaz, K. (2013). Comparison of Quantitative and Qualitative Research Traditions: Epistemological, theoretical, and methodological differences. *European Journal of Education*, *48*(2), 311–325. DOI: 10.1111/ejed.12014

Chapter 2
A Comprehensive Analysis of the Relevance of Social Media Influencer Culture and Its Consequences on Youth

Varun Kesavan
https://orcid.org/0000-0002-2373-2613
VIT Business School, VIT University, Vellore, India

Aruna Polisetty
https://orcid.org/0000-0002-9391-6442
VIT Business School, VIT University, Vellore, India

Viana Imad Hassan
https://orcid.org/0000-0002-7372-5059
European Tourism and Events Training Academy, Malta

ABSTRACT

The influence of "social media figures on youngsters, adolescents, and children" is undeniable. Although its influence may yield favorable outcomes for "inspiration, education, and community development," it is not without disadvantages. It is essential for young individuals to acquire critical thinking and "media literacy skills" to effectively navigate the virtual landscape. Influencers, akin to "celebrities," have a moral "obligation and responsibility to disseminate truth, diversity, and ethical principles." The culture of "social media influencers" can exert both

DOI: 10.4018/979-8-3373-4516-1.ch002

helpful and detrimental impacts on contemporary "youth"; however, the adverse effects can be mitigated by fostering a symbiotic relationship between "influencers and their audience."

1. INTRODUCTION

The term "influencer" has grown prevalent in the digital realm, particularly in social media marketing. Tasks formerly performed by celebrities are now assumed by ordinary individuals with substantial followings on social media platforms. We refer to these individuals as influencers, and they have established a novel sector of marketing: influencer marketing (Influencer Marketing Hub, 2025).

An influencer is someone capable of impacting the purchasing choices of others due to their authority, expertise, status, or rapport with their audience. Influencers typically engage on social media platforms such as Facebook, YouTube, X, TikTok, and Instagram.

Each influencer is generally recognised for a particular specialisation, such as fashion, travel, gaming, beauty, food, fitness, or other areas of interest. They generate content pertinent to their niche, attracting an audience specifically interested in that subject matter (Influencer Marketing Hub, 2025).

According to Justin Welsh, a successful entrepreneur,

"An influencer is an individual who has the power to affect the purchasing decisions of others because of their authority, knowledge, position, or relationship with their audience" (Influencer Marketing Hub, 2025).

Social media has emerged as a key and unavoidable aspect of adolescent existence, with influencers occupying a central role. Influencers in fashion, beauty, and fitness significantly affect teenagers' perceptions, attire, and self-esteem. Influencers are widely recognised as both inspirational and potentially harmful, even hazardous. Comprehending the mechanisms of influencers and establishing limits is essential for both adolescents and parents in successfully navigating the digital landscape (Stern, 2025).

"Social media has transformed communication, information sharing, and self-perception, as well as our understanding of the surrounding world." Prominent entities in the digital realm include "social media influencers—individuals" with substantial followings who can influence "opinions, trends, and behaviours." For contemporary youth, these influencers serve as "role models, trendsetters, and sources of inspiration," transcending their "status as mere online personalities" (Bhorkar, 2024).

In the contemporary technological landscape, "youth's daily lives are centred around their engagement with social media." Social-media-influencers have become a prominent subject of discourse within the "social media landscape." These "celebrities, bloggers, and social media influencers" have amassed millions of followers and have considerable influence across several sectors, including "fashion, beauty, fitness, and lifestyle" (Murtaza, 2023). The impact of "social media influencers on youth" is a disputed matter. This discussion will analyse the merits and demerits of this trend among young people and assess its societal influence. This article explores the significant impact of "social media influencers" on "youth culture and identity," emphasising the merits and demerits of this trend among "young individuals" and analysing its broader societal implications. It is supported with factual examples that illustrate their influence on the youth.

2. BACKGROUND OF THE STUDY.

Social media has emerged as a significant influence on communication patterns, cultural norms, and the formation of self-identity, especially among youth in the digital age. The rise of social media influencers (SMIs) has transformed the ways in which individuals, particularly adolescents and young adults, interact with media, view themselves, and engage with their surroundings (Bhorkar, 2024). In contrast to traditional celebrities, influencers achieve recognition by demonstrating relatability, authenticity, and engaging actively with their audiences on platforms like Instagram, TikTok, YouTube, and X (formerly Twitter) (Murtaza, 2023). Influencers have emerged as significant opinion leaders, influencing consumer behaviour, fashion trends, lifestyle choices, and political and social discussions (Zhang et al., 2022).

The emergence of influencer culture is linked to the growing accessibility of digital technologies and the participatory characteristics of social media platforms that promote user-generated content (Shah et al., 2022). For many youths, influencers serve not only as sources of entertainment but also as role models and aspirational figures who represent success, beauty, and personal expression (Bhorkar, 2024). Murtaza (2023) asserts that the daily routines of young individuals are significantly linked to digital media consumption, with influencers playing a pivotal role in shaping perceptions of identity, lifestyle, and community belonging.

Social media influencers have a multifaceted impact. Although they can promote inspiration, education, social awareness, and community development, their curated and often idealised representations of life may also lead to unrealistic standards, body dissatisfaction, anxiety, and diminished self-esteem among youth (Jung et al., 2022; Bhorkar, 2024). Research indicates that continual exposure to idealised online images results in social comparison and self-objectification, adversely affecting mental health (Holland & Tiggemann, 2016). The "Instagram vs. Reality" trend arose to challenge idealised representations online and emphasise the necessity for authenticity in social media environments (Bhorkar, 2024).

Despite these challenges, influencers can also serve as agents of social change. They have mobilised massive audiences for causes such as climate activism, mental health awareness, and gender equality (Bhorkar, 2024; Ampornklinkaew, 2025). Greta Thunberg exemplifies effective activism, as her social media efforts have catalysed a worldwide youth movement focused on environmental sustainability and policy reform. Influencers possess the capacity to generate significant societal impact that extends beyond mere commercial endorsements (Ampornklinkaew, 2025).

The relationship between social media influencer culture and youth development requires thorough academic investigation. Previous studies have explored influencer marketing and audience engagement; however, there is a lack of critical analysis regarding its psychosocial effects and ethical considerations for youth identity development and behaviour (De Veirman et al., 2019). This study aims to analyse the relevancy of social media influencer culture and its effects on youth, considering both positive and negative outcomes. This work underscores the significance of media literacy and critical thinking as essential tools for youth to responsibly negotiate the complex digital landscape (Bhorkar, 2024).

3. RESEARCH GAP

In the last ten years, social media influencers (SMIs) have had a significant effect on youth culture, lifestyle goals, and consumer behaviour. The current literature predominantly focuses on influencer marketing, online branding, and audience engagement (Casaló et al., 2018; Kim & Kim, 2022). Nonetheless, a considerable deficiency persists in the comprehensive understanding of how the ubiquitous influencer culture impacts youth identity development, psychological health, and value systems, both positively and negatively (Bhorkar, 2024; Murtaza, 2023).

Prior research has predominantly concentrated on the commercial and promotional dimensions of influencer engagement, including brand partnerships, purchase intentions, and consumer trust (De Veirman et al., 2019; (Lou & Yuan, 2018). This marketing-focused viewpoint neglects the wider sociological and psychological effects of influencer culture on youth audiences. As a result, there is a scarcity of research examining the impact of influencers on self-perception, moral development, social accountability, and digital literacy in adolescents and teenagers (Jung et al., 2022).

Moreover, current research tends to be platform-specific, concentrating on individual platforms such as Instagram or TikTok, and failing to provide cross-platform comparison analyses that reflect the interconnected digital environment experienced by youth (Suganya & Bawa, 2024). The growing convergence of social media platforms, where influencers engage across several channels, restricts our understanding of the multifaceted influence of influencer culture on teenage behaviour and cognition.

Moreover, although numerous studies have highlighted the beneficial functions of influencers as educators, motivators, and agents of change in areas such as mental health advocacy and environmental activism (Lee & Chung, 2025; Bhorkar, 2024), there is a lack of thorough investigation into how these positive outcomes coexist or conflict with negative effects, including body image concerns, unrealistic life expectations, social comparison, and anxiety (Holland & Tiggemann, 2016). The dual nature of influence—its capacity for both empowerment and detriment—remains inadequately examined within a cohesive theoretical framework.

A further inadequately addressed aspect is the ethical and moral accountability of influencers as public personalities. While certain scholars have addressed the authenticity and transparency of influencer-audience dynamics (Casaló et al., 2018), limited research has focused on the ethical aspects of influence—specifically, how influencers view their social responsibility and how young audiences interpret the moral implications within influencer content (Murtaza, 2023; De Veirman et al., 2019).

Finally, although there is increasing acknowledgement of the necessity for media literacy and critical thinking among young social media users (Bhorkar, 2024), empirical studies linking media literacy instruction to the reduction of influencer-related harms are limited. This underscores a significant deficiency in comprehending how educational institutions, families, and digital platforms can jointly empower adolescents to critically assess influencer content and responsibly navigate the digital environment.

In summary, contemporary academia often dissects influencer culture, categorising it either as a business phenomenon or as a distinct psychological concern. There is an absence of thorough, multidisciplinary research that synthesises the sociological, psychological, and ethical aspects of influencer culture and its intricate effects on youth development. This study seeks to systematically and impartially assess the impact of social media influencer culture on teenage behaviour, identity, and social responsibility, thereby enhancing the comprehension of digital influence in contemporary society.

4. AIM OF THE STUDY

This study aims to analyse the relevance and various consequences of social media influencer culture for contemporary youth, focussing on psychological, sociocultural, and behavioural dimensions. This study examines the influence of social media influencers (SMIs) on the attitudes, identities, consumption patterns, and moral reasoning of young individuals in a rapidly changing digital environment (Bhorkar, 2024; Murtaza, 2023).

The study seeks to investigate the dual role of influencers, focusing on their function as sources of inspiration, education, and social engagement, alongside their contribution to pressures concerning body image, materialism, and self-esteem in adolescents and young adults (Perloff, 2021; Holland & Tiggemann, 2016). This analysis aims to offer a comprehensive understanding of the positive and negative impacts of influencer culture on youth development and well-being.

This research investigates the ethical and moral responsibilities of influencers as digital opinion leaders, focusing on their roles in promoting truth, inclusivity, diversity, and social accountability (Bhorkar, 2024). This study integrates perspectives from media studies, psychology, and sociology to demonstrate that influencers can be viewed not only as trendsetters or marketers but also as agents of social change capable of promoting community development and civic awareness (Lee & Chung, 2025).

The study emphasises the significance of media literacy and critical thinking among youth as essential tools for responsibly navigating the complexities of influencer-driven content. This study aims to identify strategies that educators, parents, and policymakers can employ to enhance digital resilience among youth, enabling them to differentiate between authentic influence and performative or commercially driven behaviour (Bhorkar, 2024; De Veirman et al., 2019).

This study seeks to enhance the existing academic discourse on youth digital culture by exploring the influence of social media influencers on personal development, societal values, and collective consciousness in the 21st century. This study aims to analyse the relevance and various consequences of social media influencer culture for contemporary youth, focussing on psychological, sociocultural, and behavioural dimensions. This study examines the influence of social media influencers (SMIs) on the attitudes, identities, consumption patterns, and moral reasoning of young individuals in a rapidly changing digital environment (Bhorkar, 2024; Murtaza, 2023).

The study seeks to investigate the dual role of influencers, focusing on their function as sources of inspiration, education, and social engagement, alongside their contribution to pressures concerning body image, materialism, and self-esteem in adolescents and young adults (Holland & Tiggemann, 2016). This analysis aims to offer a comprehensive understanding of the positive and negative impacts of influencer culture on youth development and well-being.

This research investigates the ethical and moral responsibilities of influencers as digital opinion leaders, focusing on their roles in promoting truth, inclusivity, diversity, and social accountability (Bhorkar, 2024). This study integrates perspectives from media studies, psychology, and sociology to demonstrate that influencers can be viewed not only as trendsetters or marketers but also as agents of social change capable of promoting community development and civic awareness (Lee & Chung, 2025).

The study emphasises the significance of media literacy and critical thinking among youth as essential tools for responsibly navigating the complexities of influencer-driven content. This study aims to identify strategies that educators, parents, and policymakers can employ to enhance digital resilience among youth, enabling them to differentiate between authentic influence and performative or commercially driven behaviour (Bhorkar, 2024; De Veirman et al., 2019).

This study seeks to enhance the existing academic discourse on youth digital culture by clarifying the influence of social media influencers on personal development, societal values, and collective consciousness in the 21st century.

5. LITERATURE REVIEW

The emergence and influence of social media influencers

Social media influencers (SMIs) have emerged as significant cultural figures by utilising platforms like Instagram, TikTok, YouTube, and X to engage extensive youth audiences and influence tastes, norms, and purchasing behaviours (Engel et al., 2023). Evidence indicates that adolescents often trust influencers and incorporate their recommendations into everyday choices, making SMIs powerful intermediaries between brands and youth consumers (RTC Networks, 2025).

Influencer marketing and consumer behaviour.

A significant body of literature investigates the relationships between influencers and brands, focusing on the impact of sponsored content on purchase intentions, perceived credibility, and parasocial relationships. Influencer marketing integrates entertainment and advertising, enhancing persuasive effectiveness among younger audiences, who may exhibit diminished capacity to identify commercial intent (Lin et al., 2025). Research demonstrates that the effectiveness of persuasion is contingent upon perceived authenticity and source credibility; individuals are more inclined to respond to influencer recommendations when they regard the influencer as authentic (Hartmann et al., 2025).

Identity development and adolescent culture

Adolescence represents a critical phase of identity formation, during which the lifestyles showcased by influencers provide templates for appearance, behaviour, and values that numerous adolescents seek to replicate. Research indicates that influencers serve as role models and social referents, influencing self-presentation norms, style choices, and aspirational identities among adolescents and young adults (Lajnef, 2023).

Mental health, body image, and psychosocial outcomes are interrelated factors that significantly influence individual well-being and social functioning.

Empirical research increasingly associates exposure to influencer content with adverse psychosocial effects among certain youth, such as body dissatisfaction, social comparison, anxiety, and depressive symptoms. Recent meta-analyses and reviews underscore the connection between social media exposure, particularly content focused on appearance, and negative body image outcomes. These effects are significant in adolescent girls, although they are also observable across different genders (Engel et al., 2023). Furthermore, platform algorithms have the capacity to amplify hazardous trends, such as diet fads, and foster echo chambers that exacerbate harm.

Influencers serve as catalysts for civic engagement and social transformation.

Influencers have the capacity to engage audiences in support of prosocial initiatives. Numerous studies and reviews indicate that "green leaders," or activist influencers, can enhance awareness, influence public discourse, and catalyse collective action, as exemplified by the climate mobilisation efforts surrounding Greta Thunberg. The social impact of these figures is contingent upon perceived authenticity, message framing, and the level of follower engagement (Mede & Schroeder, 2024).

Media literacy, ethical considerations, and accountability for influencers

Recent policy and practice reports emphasise that both creators and audiences exhibit deficiencies in fact-checking and ethical training. UNESCO and various organisations advocate for enhanced verification training for content creators, while psychological and educational research supports media-literacy interventions aimed at fostering critical thinking and digital resilience in youth. Empirical interventions designed to teach critical consumption skills demonstrate potential in decreasing vulnerability to misinformation and enhancing adolescents' media habits (Milmo, 2024).

6. METHODOLOGY

The present study has only employed a qualitative research design. This study uniquely examines several features and techniques employed by social media influencers to persuade youth culture towards specific brands or products, as indicated by the existing literature on the subject.

7. THE UPSURGE OF SOCIAL MEDIA INFLUENCERS

"Social media influencers" have arisen from platforms such as "Instagram, TikTok, YouTube, and Twitter." They encompass "beauty experts, fashion influencers, gamers, fitness aficionados, and lifestyle bloggers." In contrast to conventional "celebrities, influencers frequently cultivate their audience through genuineness and relatability." They convey their "experiences, perspectives, and knowledge, fostering a sense of closeness and trust with their audience." "Charli D'Amelio, a teenage dancer who achieved prominence on TikTok, currently has over 150 million followers. Her engaging content and dance routines have made her a household name among Gen Z, influencing dance trends, fashion preferences, and even consumer behaviour" (Bhorkar, 2024).

8. INFLUENCERS IN THE WORLD OF SOCIAL MEDIA

"Social media influencers" are those "who have garnered a substantial following on platforms" such as "Instagram, YouTube, TikTok, and Twitter." Regardless of whether their enthusiasm lies in "fashion, video games, travel," or another domain, they frequently generate and distribute relevant information. Influencers use "social media platforms, including posts, videos, and stories, to engage and sway their followers." The dual impact of "social media influencers on youth" is clearly evident (Murtaza, 2023).

9. SEMINAL DRIFTS AND CONSUMER BEHAVIOR

"Social media influencers" prominently influence trendsetting. "Influencers determine trends" in "fashion, beauty, fitness, and travel." "Brands" recognize this influence and frequently partner with influencers to endorse their products, a tactic referred to as influencer marketing.

Examine the instance of "Kylie Jenner, whose cosmetics firm, Kylie Cosmetics, achieved remarkable success in part due to her extensive social media influence. Her cosmetic tutorials, product releases, and endorsements on Instagram and YouTube have influenced millions of young people to imitate her style and purchase her products." This example illustrates how influencers can shape customer behaviour and provide profitable commercial opportunities (Bhorkar, 2024).

10. INFLUENCERS AND YOUTH INDIVIDUALITY

In addition to trends, "social media influencers" significantly influence the formation of "youth identity." "Adolescence is a developmental stage" during which individuals investigate their interests, values, and self-identity. Influencers, via their curated content, offer paradigms of identity and "lifestyle that youth" frequently emulate or aspire to. "Emma Chamberlain, a prominent YouTuber, is recognised for her honest and unvarnished vlogging style. Her honesty resonates with numerous youthful viewers who perceive her as a sincere and relatable individual. Emma's impact transcends design and lifestyle; she advocates for self-acceptance and "mental health awareness," motivating her followers to embrace their uniqueness and well-being" (Bhorkar, 2024).

11. THE DOUBLE-EDGED SWORD OF INSPIRATION

The impact of "social media influencers" can be beneficial, although it also presents potential drawbacks. The meticulously produced and frequently idealised representations of life in "social media can establish unattainable benchmarks for beauty, prosperity, and pleasure." Such ideals may result in problems such as "body image issues, anxiety, and diminished self-esteem in adolescents. An exemplary instance is the emergence of "Instagram vs. Reality" posts, wherein influencers underscore the disparity between their curated "online image and their actual look. These posts seek to counteract the demand for perfection while highlighting the pervasive impact of social media on self-image" (Bhorkar, 2024).

12. INFLUENCERS AS AGENTS OF SOCIAL CHANGE

Influencers are not merely "trendsetters and commercial promoters;" they may also serve as significant "agents of societal change." Numerous influencers use their platforms to champion "social justice, environmental sustainability, mental health," and other significant causes. Their capacity to engage and mobilise extensive audiences makes them significant partners in fostering awareness and promoting collective action. "Greta Thunberg, a youthful climate campaigner, epitomises this impact. Her social media presence has mobilised a worldwide youth movement to advocate for action on climate change. Her posts, talks, and advocacy have motivated millions of young individuals to engage in the cause, illustrating the capacity of influencers to bring about significant change" (Bhorkar, 2024).

13. CIRCUMNAVIGATING THE INFLUENCER LANDSCAPE

Young individuals must employ "critical thinking and media literacy to navigate the influencer world." Although influencers can offer significant insights, amusement, and inspiration, it is crucial to acknowledge the artificiality of their work and the monetary motivations that may be behind it (Bhorkar, 2024). "Educators and parents" may significantly influence adolescents to critically interact with "social media and make educated decisions."

14. THE IMPACT OF SOCIAL-MEDIA INFLUENCERS

14.1 POSITIVE IMPACTS

- **INSPIRATION AND MOTIVATION:** "Social media influencers" can serve as a significant source of "inspiration and motivation for youth." Influencers motivate their audiences to emulate them by sharing their "experiences and accomplishments" (Murtaza, 2023). The impact of "social media influencers on youth" is paramount.
- **EDUCATIONAL CONTENT:** Numerous prominent individuals disseminate "awareness and understanding regarding significant issues such as mental health, body positivity, and environmental concerns" through the content they share on "social media." This content has the capacity to broaden young people's perspectives and stimulate discussions on urgent societal issues (Murtaza, 2023). The impact of "social media influencers on youth" should not be underestimated.

- **EXPERTISE IN A PARTICULAR FIELD:** Numerous individuals with substantial "social media" followings are specialists in specific domains. Through the provision of "reviews, recommendations, and guidance," they assist young individuals in making informed decisions regarding "purchases and pastime pursuits" (Murtaza, 2023). "Social media influencers exert a considerable influence on contemporary teenage culture."
- **COMMUNITY BUILDING:** An influencer cultivates a sense of community among their followers through the communities established around their content. These groups facilitate interactions among "young individuals, enabling discussions on shared interests and providing support" (Murtaza, 2023).
- **EQUIPPING WITH RESOURCES:** In addition to "knowledge, influencers provide a range of valuable resources to their followers." By presenting their "audience with tools, products, and services that offer superior quality and competitive rates" (Ansari, 2023). This approach facilitates the "enhancement of experiences" as improved options become increasingly accessible to individuals.
- **INCLUSIVITY:** Numerous influencers advocate for "inclusiveness and diversity." They use their platforms to emphasise topics pertaining to "equality, foster discourse, and enhance knowledge regarding social and cultural matters" (Ansari, 2023).
- **PROMOTING CREATIVITY:** "Creativity" thrives in the aftermath of "influencer culture" (Ansari, 2023). "Social media influencers frequently advocate for artistic expression, motivating their followers to investigate their creativity and pursue their passions."
- **ENHANCED WELL-BEING:** Individuals who engage with "social media figures" and share similar interests or activities report an increased sense of "self-congruity and enhanced overall well-being" (Ansari, 2023). This collective enthusiasm cultivates a "sense of community and facilitates individual development."

14.2 NEGATIVE IMPACTS

- **UNREALISTIC STANDARDS OF BEAUTY:** Critics of "social media influencers" assert that they establish an unrealistic benchmark of attractiveness for their fans. The constant exposure of "young individuals to altered and filtered images may adversely affect their self-esteem" (Murtaza, 2023).
- **MATERIALISTIC VALUES:** Influencers frequently endorse "products and promote a consumerist culture due to their focus on material possessions (Murtaza, 2023). Adolescents may cultivate an unhealthy fixation on

aesthetics and material possessions as a result of exposure to widespread advertising."

- **CULTURE OF INFLUENCERS:** Adolescents may disproportionately prioritise online notoriety and validation, jeopardising authentic relationships and personal growth. The mental well-being and interpersonal connections of individuals excessively engaged in their digital personas are endangered (Murtaza, 2023).
- **LACK OF AUTHENTICITY:** Influencers, pressured to maintain a meticulously curated "online persona, may portray a disingenuous self, lacking sincerity." Such behaviour may distort "young people's perception of reality, hindering their ability to cultivate good connections and embrace self-acceptance" (Murtaza, 2023).
- **DECEPTIVE PORTRAYALS:** The ostensibly flawless lives that "influencers portray can be deceptive." This facade may cause certain spectators to feel dejected regarding their lives, since they perceive themselves as inadequate in contrast (Ansari, 2023). Nonetheless, the influencers may not possess the "ideal" life they portray.
- **MENTAL HEALTH IMPACT:** Continuous exposure to influencers and their ostensibly perfect lives might engender detrimental "self-comparisons" (Ansari, 2023). These situations can lead to "mental health problems, including anxiety and despair, as individuals perceive themselves as insufficient compared to controlled online identities."
- **PARASOCIAL RELATIONSHIPS:** Followers frequently cultivate "parasocial relationships (PSR) with influencers," experiencing a profound "connection despite the unidirectional nature of these interactions. These unidirectional relationships can result in detrimental emotional dependence and disillusionment when the influencer does not fulfil the audience's expectations" (Ansari, 2023).

15 THE PHASES TO ALLEVIATE THE OUTCOME OF SOCIAL MEDIA INFLUENCERS ON YOUTH

- **MEDIA KNOWLEDGE EDUCATION:** "Schools that incorporate media literacy" into their "curricula empower pupils to assess information for credibility and recognise instances of distortion" (Murtaza, 2023). The "training should encompass influencer marketing and the potential impacts of social media on mental health."
- **DIVERSE DEPICTION:** Encouraging "influencers to advocate for diversity and inclusiveness in their content may facilitate the challenge of cultur-

al traditions and assumptions" (Murtaza, 2023). "Influencers" can promote "tolerance and appreciation for diversity by showcasing individuals from diverse backgrounds."

- **ACCOUNTABLE INFLUENCER-BRAND COLLABORATIONS:** It is imperative for "influencers to disclose their agreements with firms transparently" (Murtaza, 2023). They can cultivate their "fans' trust" by being candid regarding sponsored content and providing impartial evaluations.
- **SELF-AWARENESS AND DIGITAL DETOX:** The adverse "consequences of excessive exposure to influencer content can be alleviated by self-awareness and digital detox," wherein young individuals are urged to disengage from "social media and concentrate on self-care, hobbies, and face-to-face interactions" (Murtaza, 2023).

15.1 RESEARCH FACTS ON INFLUENCER ADVERTISING

- 91% of "customers exhibit greater trust in influencers compared to conventional advertisements" (Deepika M, 2025).
- Seventy per cent of "adolescents engage with a minimum of one influencer" (Deepika M, 2025).
- "Brands are allocating billions in influencer marketing to engage youthful demographics" (Deepika M, 2025).

15.2 THE SHADY SIDE OF INFLUENCER CULTURE

Influencers frequently experience significant "strain, contending with mental health challenges stemming from the necessity of sustaining an impeccable online persona." Recent instances of "influencers grappling with melancholy, anxiety, or suicidal ideation underscore the adverse aspects of internet notoriety." This fosters an environment in which "young followers may juxtapose themselves with these influencers and experience insecurity regarding their lives" (Deepika M, 2025). For instance, certain influencers experience "exhaustion, anxiety, or even despair while striving to uphold an impeccable image." The impact on youth is substantial. "Adolescent followers engage in self-comparison and experience insecurity" regarding their lives (Deepika M, 2025).

15.3 THE REPERCUSSION EFFECTS OF SOCIAL MEDIA INFLUENCERS ON YOUTH'S BEHAVIOR

"Social media influencers" significantly influence "young individuals' thoughts, behaviours, and decision-making processes." Their influence is unequivocal, ranging from "brand promotion to lifestyle choice alteration."

- **YOUTH INFLUENCERS**

A multitude of influencers are "youthful, rendering them more relatable to their audience."

For instance, "Prajakta Koli, recognised online as MostlySane, began her career as a YouTuber" and rapidly became one of India's most cherished "digital creators." Her relatable "comedic sketches and vlogs have amassed millions of followers" (Deepika M, 2025).

- **SOCIAL MEDIA INFLUENCE**

Influencers dictate trends on "Instagram, YouTube, and Twitter via viral challenges, filters, and fashion styles." "Social media networks amplify their reach through the promotion of highly engaging content, resulting in increased likes and shares." For instance, "Bhuvan Bam, the originator of the YouTube channel BB Ki Vines, generates hilarious footage that has garnered a substantial audience" (Deepika M, 2025). His influence "extends beyond the entertainment sphere. He participates in charity endeavours and promotes awareness of social concerns, influencing the opinions of his younger audience."

- **INFLUENCER POWER**

Influencers have the capacity to alter "fashion trends, dietary habits, lifestyles, and political perspectives." For instance, "Virat Kohli, the former captain of the Indian cricket team, boasts over 270 million social media followers (Deepika M, 2025). His endorsements and lifestyle choices, encompassing exercise regimens and apparel goods, significantly influence his followers' inclinations."

- **YOUTH CULTURE**

Influencers shape the "development of youth culture by presenting novel trends, lifestyles, and social conventions." For instance, "Jaya Kishori utilises social media platforms to disseminate spiritual guidance and teachings, amalgamating traditional spirituality with modern trends, thus impacting youth culture" (Deepika M, 2025).

- **INFLUENCER MARKETING**

"Brands partner with influencers to truly promote products, by utilising their credibility and audience reach" (Deepika M, 2025). For instance, "Malini Agarwal has garnered numerous awards, including being #1 on Impact's 50 Most Influential Women in Media, Marketing, and Advertising in 2017 and being acknowledged as a prominent business leader on Fortune India's 40 Under 40 List."

- **YOUTH BEHAVIOR**

The information consumed influences actions, goals, and lifestyle decisions.

For instance, "Ajey Nagar first uploaded videos on YouTube at the age of 10, initially concentrating on football tutorials and then on gaming content (Deepika M, 2025). He attained significant success through his comedic roasting videos and accumulated over 43 million subscribers."

- **SOCIAL MEDIA TRENDS**

Influencers generate and disseminate trends that swiftly capture the interest of the youth.

"Kusha Kapila, a digital creator, presented comedic personas that critique society conventions (Deepika M, 2025). Her content-initiated trends in comedy narrative, resulting in the extensive emulation of analogous structures by other authors and audiences."

- **YOUTH ENGAGEMENT**

Young individuals dedicate several hours each day to viewing influencer videos, perusing posts, and participating in debates. For instance, "CarryMinati (Ajey Nagar), a prominent YouTuber recognised for his roast videos and live broadcasts, captivates millions of young viewers with engaging material that incites conversations and arguments within the community" (Deepika M, 2025).

15.4 INFLUENCERS VS. CELEBRITIES

Influencers have emerged as "digital celebrities; however, they significantly differ from those in television, film, and other entertainment sectors." Due to influencers expanding their following and establishing "ties and trust, their followers are more inclined to make purchases based on an influencer's recommendations rather than those of a prominent celebrity." The "Trust in Influencer Marketing report revealed that 61% of participants place greater trust in sponsored posts from influencers compared to traditional celebrity endorsements, underscoring a shift in trust dynamics towards influencers." Although a renowned "actor or musician may exert influence, their impact is significantly less compared to that of prominent influencers who have independently achieved celebrity status." "Conventional celebrities no longer exclusively invite influencers to events. They have emerged as the biggest names at significant athletic events and as interviewers during award presentations" (Izea, 2024). Brands are recognising the significant impact that influencers possess and their potential effectiveness.

15.5 THE OUTCOME OF INFLUENCERS ON THE SOCIETY

The culture of influencers has significantly influenced multiple facets of society:

- **TRENDS**

Influencers frequently establish or "popularise trends in fashion, beauty, fitness, cuisine," and other domains. Their adherents seek "guidance on contemporary styles, products, or activities, resulting in viral trends that can disseminate worldwide" (Izea, 2024).

- **LIFESTYLES**

Influencers frequently disclose their daily "routines, dietary habits, exercise regimens, and personal experiences," thereby impacting their "followers' lifestyles." A "health and fitness influencer may motivate followers to embrace healthier dietary practices or initiate a new exercise regimen" (Izea, 2024).

- **CONSUMER HABITS**

Influencers significantly influence "customers' behaviour." They frequently endorse "products or businesses among their followers, impacting their purchasing choices." This paper elucidates why "influencer marketing has emerged as a potent instrument for enterprises" (Izea, 2024). Research indicates that "customers frequently place equal or greater faith in recommendations from influencers compared to those from friends or family."

- **SOCIETY**

Influencer culture has significantly "influenced society's standards and expectations." It has fostered "the "selfie" culture and the focus on personal branding" (Izea, 2024). The phenomenon has generated discussions on "authenticity since several influencers have faced criticism for endorsing unrealistic standards or lifestyles."

- **MENTAL HEALTH**

The influencer culture has adversely "affected mental health, correlating with phenomena such as fear of missing out (FOMO), social media addiction, and diminished self-esteem," all of which are associated with the incessant exposure to idealised lives frequently depicted by influencers. "Mental health advocates have emerged on social media to create support communities for individuals dealing with similar issues." Influencers can cultivate "supportive online groups that foster understanding and alleviate feelings of isolation" (Izea, 2024). These networks can be particularly "advantageous for individuals confronting mental health challenges who may lack access to similar assistance in their offline environments."

- **ECONOMY**

The emergence of influencers has generated novel "economic prospects. Influencers can generate revenue from their platforms via brand collaborations, sponsored content, and goods, which enhances the gig economy" (Izea, 2024). Although "influencer culture has many advantages, it is crucial to remain cognisant of its possible drawbacks, including the promotion of unattainable standards, consumerism, and the risk of disinformation."

15.6 LEGAL CONSIDERATIONS FOR SOCIAL MEDIA INFLUENCERS INFLUENCE ON YOUTH

- **PROTECTING MINORS**

Numerous social media networks have age limitations; yet, young users frequently devise methods to bypass these regulations. "Influencers must be cognisant of the content they produce and ensure compliance with legislation pertaining to children, including avoiding explicit material and adhering to child labour laws" (Lawfluencers, 2024).

- **FALSE ADVERTISING AND ENDORSEMENTS**

"Adolescents and teenagers are very impressionable and frequently rely on the endorsements of their preferred influencers." Influencers must use caution while "promoting products or services to avoid engaging in deceptive advertising" (Lawfluencers, 2024). Exaggerating a "product's efficacy, misrepresenting its advantages, or promoting things without adequate scrutiny may all amount to deceptive advertising, resulting in legal consequences."

- **DATA PRIVACY AND SECURITY**

"Social media influencers significantly influence the digital landscape, especially among the youth demographic." Nonetheless, their impact has "legal obligations, especially regarding data privacy and security" (Lawfluencers, 2024). By complying with rules such as "the Digital Personal Data Protection Act 2023 in India, the GDPR in the European Union, and the CCPA in the United States," influencers can "safeguard the privacy rights of their audience while preserving trust and credibility."

15.7 THE WAYS IN WHICH PARENTS CAN CARE CHILDREN FROM DROPPING FROM THE INFLUENCER CULTURE

The notion of "marketing strategy and advertising is inherently challenging for adults to comprehend." "Influencer culture involves influencers creating an illusion of intimacy, making followers feel connected to their lives, despite merely doing their professional duties and promoting businesses through their posts" (Obe et al., 2024).

- **SAY NO TO INFLUENCER GOODS**

The "younger children" are, the less they can and should comprehend this concept. "Parents and other trustworthy people are responsible for safeguarding children" (Obe et al., 2024). In this scenario, it may entail repeatedly declining "the purchase of their preferred influencer's goods."

- **TALK ABOUT INFLUENCER COMMERCIALS**

As "children mature, particularly from Year 5 onwards," "parents may begin to discuss the concepts of influence and advertising with them. It is essential to acknowledge that of-ups frequently succumb to such phenomena as well" (Obe et al., 2024). Examine posts from "influencers and children and categorise them repeatedly. Although we may irritate them, some aspect will resonate."

- **STAY ON TOP OF WHO THEY FOLLOW**

Understanding "the individuals and influencers that children follow is crucial for parents to engage effectively in relevant discussions." This task is ongoing and necessitates considerable patience Obe et al. (2024).

15.8 ADVICES TO UNDERSTANDING INFLUENCER CULTURE

- **REALIZE THAT INFLUENCERS GET PAID**

An influencer frequently "receives compensation for endorsing content, either monetarily or through complimentary products. Influencers must label any promotional posts with the hashtag '#ad' to help followers differentiate between advertising and personal content" (Obe et al., 2024).

- **CRITICALLY THINK ABOUT CONTENT**

Irrespective of their "follower level or verification status, it remains essential to thoroughly evaluate the messaging or content an influencer endorses" (Obe et al., 2024).: Influencers have distinct "perspectives and beliefs that may not correspond with your values."

- **RECOGNISE PHOTOS ARE EDITED**

Users encounter a multitude of "heavily manipulated or filtered photographs on social media." Instruct your "child to consider this when viewing influencer or any online content" (Obe et al., 2024). Significant "effort may be required to render a single photograph 'perfect', and the original image may appear markedly different."

- **USE PLATFORM TOOLS LIKE MUTE**

It is inherent in human nature to engage in "self-comparison with others." "Children and adolescents are indistinguishable in this regard." If individuals discover that "social media adversely impacts their mental health or diminishes their self-esteem," then a hiatus may prove beneficial. Advise your "child to unfollow or mute any profiles that negatively impact their welfare and consistently communicate their feelings to someone" (Obe et al., 2024).

- **EMBRACE THE POSITIVES**

Numerous influencers utilise their platforms for "positive purposes, serving as an excellent means to discover novel ideas and lifestyles or gain insights into diverse cultures." Motivate "your child to select and disseminate accounts that evoke positive emotions and promote uplifting messages online" Obe et al. (2024).

16 WHAT IS AN INFLUENCER ON SOCIAL MEDIA?

An "influencer is a social media figure" who persuades their "audience to acquire the items or services they endorse." Their "social media profiles will feature a balanced combination of personal branding, content development, and promotion" (Worb, 2025).

16.1 THE DIFFERENCE BETWEEN INFLUENCERS AND CONTENT CREATORS

Although the phrases "influencer" and "content creator" are sometimes used synonymously, a distinction exists between them. A "content creator is an individual who produces digital material, while an influencer generates content to cultivate an audience and get brand collaborations" (Worb, 2025).

16.2 CATEGORIES OF SOCIAL MEDIA INFLUENCERS BY FOLLOWER COUNT

Influencers are typically classified into "four distinct levels according to their social media follower count" (Worb, 2025).

- **NANO SOCIAL MEDIA INFLUENCERS**

A "nano influencer is someone with 1,000 to 5,000 followers," such as the Toronto food influencer @MesseEats (Worb, 2025). "Nano influencers are optimal for small to medium-sized enterprises with constrained marketing resources."

- **MICRO SOCIAL MEDIA INFLUENCERS**

A "micro-influencer is an individual with 5,000 to 25,000 followers," such as @teelythefoodie. "Any brand or enterprise can gain advantages from collaborating with micro-influencers, particularly when aiming to access new, engaged audiences" (Worb, 2025).

- **MID SOCIAL-MEDIA-INFLUENCERS**

A "mid-tier influencer is an individual possessing between 25,000 and 100,000 followers, such as Kay Brown, known as @kayyorkcity, who is featured on our podcast," Beyond Influence. "Mid-tier influencers serve as optimal marketing partners for companies and businesses aiming to engage extensive audiences, as they possess the capacity to yield considerable exposure and conversions for their items or services" (Worb, 2025).

- **MACRO SOCIAL MEDIA INFLUENCERS**

A "macro influencer is defined as an individual possessing between 100,000 and 500,000 or more followers, exemplified by fitness and food creator @deannawoo." The objective of collaborating with "macro influencers is generally associated with enhancing brand awareness and driving sales. Macro-influencers are most effective for campaigns that have substantial budgets. In contrast to collaborations with nano- or micro-influencers, engagement will typically involve only one or two macro-influencers rather than multiple individuals" (Worb, 2025).

- **MEGA INFLUENCERS**

A "mega influencer is someone possessing 500,000 or more followers, typically including celebrities, athletes, or prominent creators. Consider celebrities such as @kimkardashian or @charlidamelio." "Mega influencers are optimal for firms and businesses aiming to enhance their "brand awareness on a large scale." Collaborating with prominent influencers on social media enables the amplification of reach and visibility swiftly, positioning brands before millions of individuals. What are the disadvantages? incurs a substantial cost. Consequently, mega influencers are typically allocated to firms with substantial expenditures for extensive campaigns" (Worb, 2025).

16.3 FORMS OF SOCIAL MEDIA INFLUENCERS BY INDUSTRY AND NICHE

- **FOOD INFLUENCERS**

"The phone takes precedence" is particularly applicable to culinary influencers.

These "influencers disseminate various content, including their optimal game-day meals, seasonal faves, and grocery budgeting strategies. Numerous innovative methods exist for engaging with them. Consider Folgers Coffee's recent collaboration with Meredith Hayden (also known as @wishbonekitchen)" (Worb, 2025). Given that "Meredith's content predominantly features morning recipes, Folgers represents a seamless and brand-aligned integration within her feed."

- **HEALTH AND WELLNESS INFLUENCERS**

The "health and wellness business" are thriving, particularly on "social media." Indeed, "47.6% of individuals use social media as their primary source of health information" (Worb, 2025). "Health and wellness influences encompass various subjects, including diet, fitness, exercise, sleep, stress management, mental health, and social relationships."

- **FASHION INFLUENCERS**

"Fashion influencer marketing involves the production of content centred on fashion-related themes." "Fashion influencers present daily style inspirations, disseminate current fashion trends, and showcase authentic hauls" (Worb, 2025). "Fashion influencers encompass a diverse array of fashion-related subjects; yet, it is evident that their followers seek inspiration, relatability, and advice from them."

- **LIFESTYLE INFLUENCERS**

"Lifestyle influencers" constitute a significant portion of the internet influencers you encounter. Due to their "lack of confinement to one niche, their content generally chronicles their daily activities, ranging from weekend excursions to their morning skincare regimen. (Worb, 2025). Chrissy Rutherford exemplifies a quintessential lifestyle influencer. She discusses fashion, expatriate life, mental health, travel, and her daily experiences. Lifestyle influencers are adaptable, making them a fantastic choice for most brand relationships."

- **MEMES AND POP CULTURE COVERAGE INFLUENCERS**

"Meme and pop culture influencers, albeit not novel, have surged in prominence recently." There are "compelling reasons to incorporate pop culture into your social strategy. These influencers concentrate on humour and entertainment from the perspective of television, film, and celebrity culture. Influencers such as "Alexandra Nikolajev (@lexniko)" and "Amanda Hirsch (@notskinnybutnotfat) frequently collaborate with lifestyle and performing firms." (Worb, 2025). Due to their appeal to a younger population, these "influencers are ideal for marketers aiming to engage a Gen-Z and Millennial audience."

- **TRAVEL INFLUENCERS**

"Travel influencers are transforming societal travel practices. Travel influencers produce premium material pertaining to various aspects of travel." (Worb, 2025). Some "travellers' influencers emphasise their preferred trips and destinations, while others focus on sharing travel tactics, bargains, and items."

- **FAMILY INFLUENCERS**

"Family influencers are individuals who concentrate on family life, parenting, and familial interactions. Mommy influencers constitute a subcategory within a substantial influencer niche." (Worb, 2025). Numerous "family influencers diversify their content across multiple platforms, including vlogging on YouTube and posting on Instagram and TikTok." They disseminate a "diverse array of content encompassing educational resources, parenting narratives, and their preferred brands or toys."

- **GAMING INFLUENCERS**

"Gaming influencers are individuals that specialise in video game content and frequently share it on platforms such as Twitch, YouTube, and TikTok." Followers, can generally anticipate "live streaming, game reviews, insights on forthcoming releases, and additional content.

Indeed, "89.5% of video game sales occur in the digital realm, making video game influencers highly profitable. Partnering with gaming influencers can result in innovative marketing that resonates with consumers." (Worb, 2025). Later and Chobani collaborated with "creators on Twitch to endorse a special game, resulting in a total of 7 million impressions."

- **ANIMAL INFLUENCERS**

"Animal influencers range from owners blogging on behalf of their dogs to influencers detailing the intricacies of their furry companions' lives." "Animal influencers disseminate content encompassing daily vlogs, product evaluations, training advice, grooming techniques, and pet nutrition." (Worb, 2025). The realm of "pet influencing and its burgeoning opportunities for creators, including Lindsay Van Bramer and her dog Beth, known as PardonThyFrench, were subsequently investigated."

- **BEAUTY INFLUENCERS**

The "beauty sector is poised for significant expansion, with projections indicating it will reach $716.3 billion by 2025." "Beauty influencers produce and disseminate material pertaining to makeup, skincare, haircare, and other beauty-related subjects. These influencers are regarded as authorities in the field and frequently possess the trust and confidence of their audience" (Worb, 2025). "Onboarding beauty influencers is the most effective method for a firm to authentically present its products. Audiences appreciate observing the functionality and application of products in practical scenarios."

17 THE TOP FOREMOST SOCIAL MEDIA INFLUENCERS

Since its inception over ten years ago, "Instagram has evolved into an essential social media platform and a fundamental component of any digital marketing plan. It is a social networking site where individuals have either attained instant celebrity status or established themselves as businesses due to their expanding follower base." As time passes, these "individuals and enterprises gain a unique status and become known as 'social media influencers'." The phrase has acquired new significance since "TikTok has emerged as one of the globe's most prominent social media platforms, owing to its extensive reach, diverse features, and high shareability" (Simon, 2025a, DMI).

17.1 ABOUT SOCIAL MEDIA INFLUENCER

A "social media influencer is someone who has gained authority in a certain sector, possesses a substantial audience, and can motivate others to act based on their endorsements. Indeed, influencer marketing is rapidly transforming into a crucial instrument in a company's repertoire when executed well" (Simon, 2025a, DMI). Influencers have "the resources and credibility to continuously draw visitors and can inspire others to broaden their social influence. They can range from a blogger to a superstar to an online business, leveraging a niche to achieve extensive credibility." "Instagram's content, presented as photographs or short-form videos, facilitates peer-to-peer sharing, enabling marketers to utilise storytelling through Stories to enhance their audience reach. Since its start, the quantity of brand-sponsored influencer posts on Instagram has increased significantly" (Simon, 2025a, DMI). Despite "TikTok's rising prominence, Instagram remains the most effective platform for social influencer marketing, as affirmed by 87% of top businesses, according to eMarketer."

17.2 EXAMPLES OF LEADING SOCIAL MEDIA INFLUENCERS

- **GARY VAYNERCHUK**

Baby "Boomers, Millennials, and Gen Z individuals alike hold 'Gary Vee', a 48-year-old entrepreneur, author, and motivational speaker, in high regard. Gary Vee, boasting a highly engaged Instagram following of 10.1 million and growing, is recognised for his distinctive approach to pragmatic counsel on business expansion, personal achievement, financial literacy, and maximising life's potential." (Simon, 2025a, DMI). "Gary Vee exemplifies authenticity by consistently producing a blend of rapid videos and impactful memes that offer actionable insights."

- **ZACH KING**

"Zach King, an illusionist and filmmaker, gained prominence through his vlogs and films. He possesses more than 29.3 million followers due to his uplifting narratives and 'magic vines' which elicit smiles. "He shares arbitrary videos, humorous content, and various entertaining sights." The Instagram star's more spectacular magic videos, including a recent illusion with Ed Sheeran, continue to astonish viewers and attract numerous new followers." (Simon, 2025a, DMI).

- **ADDISON RAE**

For anybody contemplating a career as an "internet personality with aspirations for a television contract, Addison Rae is the exemplar to emulate. Her lip sync videos generated significant attention upon their initial release on TikTok, and this success—coupled with her 35.9 million Instagram followers for beauty-related content—facilitated the acquisition of a Netflix show and the launch of a debut single." Since her "rise to prominence in 2021, Addison Rae has engaged in many brief endeavours, like serving as a UFC presenter and featuring in the 2023 slasher film, 'Thanksgiving'. Addison's association with Kourtney Kardashian, a prominent Instagram influencer, facilitated her rise in fame among an interested audience, and she continues to uphold a significant following on Instagram." (Simon, 2025a, DMI).

- **HUDA KATTAN/HUDA BEAUTY**

The "Oklahoma-born cosmetics specialist is among the most influential beauty authorities globally, possessing extensive social media exposure. She commenced her career as a blogger and has since turned her Instagram account, @hudabeauty, amassing 54.1 million followers with her makeup lessons." The determinants of

"Huda's success include showcasing effective cosmetics applications, developing trends, disseminating reviews, and producing instructional content. Following the establishment of her makeup line and its subsequent growth, Huda encountered difficulties over her brand's direction. As an empowered influencer, she is assuming charge of Huda Beauty as CEO, implementing a transformation that reflects her personal values." (Simon, 2025a, DMI). Her "Instagram profile features videos demonstrating cosmetic application, commercial endorsements, sporadic fashion counsel, and additional content."

- **KHABY LAME**

A "former Italian factory worker is rapidly ascending the Instagram influencer rankings. Following his job losses due to the coronavirus outbreak, Khaby Lame initially used TikTok to share creative videos. He established his presence on Instagram, amassing 79.7 million followers and continuing to grow. "What is the key to his success on Instagram?" He creates videos showcasing his reactions to life hacks, enhanced by his comedic facial expressions and snark." His most renowned "video demonstrates a convoluted method of peeling a banana with a knife, which he subsequently contrasts with the straightforward act of peeling the banana by hand. Following his ascent to prominence, baseless rumours about the influencer's demise circulated online in 2023 via fabricated videos and deceptive articles. However, the positive news is that Khaby is alive and in excellent health. Strangely, these peculiar rumours have only increased his Instagram following." (Simon, 2025a, DMI).

- **TAYLOR SWIFT**

As one of the "globe's most renowned pop artists, Taylor Swift need's minimal introduction. In addition to her record-breaking albums, extensive collection of Grammy trophies, and overall musical brilliance, not everyone is aware that Taylor possesses considerable commercial acumen." "Taylor's Instagram following of 283 million exemplifies her marketing acumen and substantial social media impact. The star's recent presence at the Super Bowl to support her boyfriend, Travis Kelce, incited a significant social media frenzy, while her distinctive visual aesthetic maintains the engagement of her Instagram followers." (Simon, 2025a, DMI).

- **KYLIE JENNER**

"Kylie Jenner has emerged as a formidable influencer, amassing 400 million followers. As a multifaceted woman, she showcases her modelling, socialite status, and makeup empire through her Instagram posts. She generates substantial income from sponsored posts and previously held the record for the most-liked Instagram post until it was surpassed by an egg. An impressive accomplishment within this distinguished group of social media influencers!" "Hopper HQ's Instagram Rich List indicates that Jenner earns approximately 1.8 million dollars for every sponsored Instagram post, positioning her among the highest-paid Instagram influencers." (Simon, 2025a, DMI).

- **SELENA GOMEZ**

For years, she was the most "followed individual on Instagram until celebrities like 'The Rock' and Cristiano Ronaldo surpassed her; Gomez is an exceptional celebrity influencer. The award-winning singer and actress, boasting over 449 million followers, frequently uses her social media platforms to advocate for charity initiatives, including her campaign against human trafficking, women's rights, and the protection of children from abuse. In addition to evident business endorsements, she frequently shares several personal photographs and videos to engage with her enormous fan following. In 2017, the celebrity underwent a kidney transplant due to a lupus diagnosis in 2015, an experience that Selena courageously chronicled, in part, on her Instagram feed." Following her "health challenges, Selena has recovered with the success of her cosmetics firm, Rare Beauty, which she is contemplating selling for an impressive $2 billion." (Simon, 2025a, DMI).

- **CRISTIANO RONALDO**

The "Juventus football icon and five-time Ballon d'Or recipient possesses the most substantial social media presence globally. Ronaldo is first on the list of highest-paid Instagram influencers, earning $3.23 million per sponsored post. His 625 million followers get access to these sponsored postings, which include his paid collaborations with brands such as Nike and others. He additionally publishes diverse items related to games and training, on-field action photographs, and family images. Wherever Ronaldo ventures, the world is certain to accompany him." (Simon, 2025a, DMI).

18 DISCUSSION

The findings of this study reinforce the complex and multifaceted role of social media influencer culture in shaping the attitudes, values, and behaviours of modern youth. The data demonstrate that influencers act as trendsetters, educators, and social agents, while potentially contributing to psychological distress and consumer conformity. The findings align with current research indicating that influencer culture enhances social connectivity and identity expression while simultaneously promoting unrealistic ideals and materialistic tendencies among young users. (Lajnef, 2023)

Authenticity and relatability are fundamental to influencer-follower relationships. The research indicates that perceived authenticity can be strategically managed, frequently integrating sincerity with commercial aims. The study emphasises the significant impact of influencers on the formation of youth's identities. Adolescence represents a developmental stage characterised by exploration and social comparison, with influencers acting as reference points for identity and lifestyle decisions (Agarwal, 2024).

This study confirms that, while influencers can promote positive emotions like motivation and belonging, excessive or idealised exposure may have adverse psychological consequences. "Instagram vs. Reality" campaigns have gained popularity to address these pressures; however, unrealistic beauty standards remain pervasive, significantly impacting young audiences, especially female users.

The dopamine-driven reward system of social media boosts influencer engagement, promoting emotional dependency and compulsive consumption (Casaló et al., 2018). Influencer culture functions as a dual mechanism, fostering emotional connections and simultaneously reinforcing cycles of digital validation. The research supports the notion that social media influencers have a substantial impact on consumer behaviour among young individuals.

The commercial dimension of influencer culture frequently obscures the distinction between genuine endorsement and compensated promotion. Many youth participants reported challenges in differentiating genuine endorsements from marketing, despite regulatory guidelines mandating the disclosure of sponsored content (Lajnef, 2023). This underscores the necessity for improved media literacy education to foster critical awareness of persuasive techniques in influencer marketing environments (Agarwal, 2024).

The research highlights the importance of media literacy education in countering the adverse effects of influencer culture. Media literacy serves as a protective measure against emotional manipulation, misinformation, and unrealistic self-comparison, thereby ensuring that the advantages of influencer culture—such as inspiration, education, and community—surpass its possible detriments.

19. CONCLUSION

The impact of "social media influencers" on teenage culture and identity is indisputable. They influence trends, "consumer behaviour, individual values, and self-perceptions." This impact can yield both beneficial and detrimental outcomes, serving as a distinguishing characteristic of modern adolescent culture. By comprehending and critically analysing this phenomenon, young individuals can leverage the advantages of “social media” while mitigating its possible drawbacks. In the contemporary digital era, influencers are not merely shaping youth culture; they are, in numerous respects, defining it.

Although influencers can inspire and empower, they may also disseminate detrimental values and adversely impact “mental health.” As followers, it is imperative to engage with these digital interactions critically, recognising the beneficial effects while remaining cognisant of the detrimental ones. Ultimately, our proficiency in manoeuvring through this influencer-centric era depends on our ability to recognise, adapt, and prioritise our own well-being.

The influence of media personalities on young people is a complicated and varied phenomenon. Although influencers can motivate and instruct youth, they can present dangers associated with unreasonable expectations, materialism, and false information. As “social media” evolves, it is essential for “parents, schools, and policymakers” to cultivate critical thinking abilities in adolescents, allowing them to navigate the influencer environment responsibly. By fostering “media literacy” and facilitating open dialogues regarding the content consumed by youth, society may use the beneficial elements of influencer culture while alleviating its adverse impacts. A balanced approach that highlights both the merits and demerits of influencer “culture” will enable young individuals to make educated decisions in their digital lives.

REFERENCES

Agarwal, N. A. (2024). The effect of social media in identity formation in adolescence. *World Journal of Advanced Research and Reviews*, *23*(3), 775–779. DOI: 10.30574/wjarr.2024.23.3.2685

Ahuja, M. (2025, May 1). *Top 60 Social Media Influencers: Who's Leading the Chart*. SocialPilot. Retrieved May 27, 2025, from https://www.socialpilot.co/blog/top-social-media-influencers

Ampornklinkaew, C. (2025). The role of social media influencers in influencing consumers' imitation intentions. *Digital Business*, *100143*(2), 100143. Advance online publication. DOI: 10.1016/j.digbus.2025.100143

Ansari, Z. (2023, September 18). The social media influencers impact on youth. *Locobuzz Solutions Private Limited*. Retrieved May 19, 2025, from https://locobuzz.com/blogs/social-media-influencers-impact-on-youth/

Bhorkar, R. (2024, November 14). *The influence of social media influencers on youth culture and identity*. Retrieved May 18, 2025, from https://www.linkedin.com/pulse/influence-social-media-influencers-youth-culture-identity-bhorkar-xybzc/

Casaló, L. V., Flavián, C., & Ibáñez-Sánchez, S. (2018). Influencers on Instagram: Antecedents and consequences of opinion leadership. *Journal of Business Research*, *117*, 510–519. DOI: 10.1016/j.jbusres.2018.07.005

De Veirman, M., Hudders, L., & Nelson, M. R. (2019). What is influencer marketing and how does it target children? A review and direction for future research. *Frontiers in Psychology*, *10*, 2685. Advance online publication. DOI: 10.3389/fpsyg.2019.02685 PMID: 31849783

Deepika, M. (2025, March 15). *The impact of social media influencers on youth behavior and culture in India.* The One Liner. Retrieved May 19, 2025, from https://theoneliner.in/the-impact-of-social-media-influencers-on-youth/

Designed and Developed by Will Earp, South West Grid for Learning Trust Ltd. (n.d.). *Impact of Influencer Culture – How to help young people create a more positive online space.* Retrieved May 19, 2025, from https://swgfl.org.uk/topics/digital-wellbeing/impact-of-influencer-culture-how-to-help-young-people-create-a-more-positive-online-space/

Engel, E., Gell, S., Heiss, R., & Karsay, K. (2023). Social media influencers and adolescents' health: A scoping review of the research field. *Social Science & Medicine*, *340*, 116387. DOI: 10.1016/j.socscimed.2023.116387 PMID: 38039770

Hartmann, P., Apaolaza, V., Paredes, M. R., & D'Souza, C. (2025). How Greenfluencers boost climate action: Why inspirational green leadership matters. *International Journal of Consumer Studies*, *49*(3), e70050. Advance online publication. DOI: 10.1111/ijcs.70050

Hayes, H. (2024, February 8). *The impact of influencers on young adults and teens*. Heather Hayes & Associates. Retrieved May 19, 2025, from https://heatherhayes.com/the-impact-of-influencers-on-young-adults-and-teens/

Holland, G., & Tiggemann, M. (2016). A systematic review of the impact of the use of social networking sites on body image and disordered eating outcomes. *Body Image*, *17*, 100–110. DOI: 10.1016/j.bodyim.2016.02.008 PMID: 26995158

Influencer Marketing Hub. (2025, October 1). *What is an Influencer? – Social Media Influencers Defined [Updated 2024]*. Retrieved October 3, 2025, from https://influencermarketinghub.com/what-is-an-influencer/

Influencity. (2024, August 9). Marketing with Kid Influencers: Benefits and Best Practices. *Influencity*. Retrieved May 19, 2025, from https://influencity.com/blog/en/marketing-with-kid-influencers-benefits-and-best-practices

Izea. (2024, December 13). *Impact and Influence: The Effects of Influencer Culture on Society - IZEA Worldwide, Inc*. IZEA Worldwide, Inc. Retrieved May 19, 2025, from https://izea.com/resources/impact-and-influence-of-influencer-culture-on-society/

Jung, J., Barron, D., Lee, Y., & Swami, V. (2022). Social media usage and body image: Examining the mediating roles of internalization of appearance ideals and social comparisons in young women. *Computers in Human Behavior*, *135*, 107357. DOI: 10.1016/j.chb.2022.107357

Khan, M. M. (2023, July 25). *The Power Of Social Media Influencers On Today's Youth*. Mentoria. Retrieved May 19, 2025, from https://mentoriablog.azurewebsites.net/the-power-of-social-media-influencers-on-todays-youth/

Kim, J., & Kim, M. (2022). Rise of Social Media Influencers as a New Marketing Channel: Focusing on the Roles of Psychological Well-Being and Perceived Social Responsibility among Consumers. *International Journal of Environmental Research and Public Health*, *19*(4), 2362. DOI: 10.3390/ijerph19042362 PMID: 35206553

Lajnef, K. (2023). The effect of social media influencers' on teenagers Behavior: An empirical study using cognitive map technique. *Current Psychology (New Brunswick, N.J.)*, *42*(22), 19364–19377. DOI: 10.1007/s12144-023-04273-1 PMID: 36742063

Lawfluencers. (2024, September 9). Social media influencers impact on youth - positive and negative. *Lawfluencers | Lawyers for Digital & Collaborative Economy*. Retrieved May 19, 2025, from https://lawfluencers.com/social-media-influencers-impact-on-youth/

Lee, A., & Chung, T. D. (2025). With great power comes great responsibility: The antecedents and outcomes of social media influencers' perceived social responsibility authenticity. *Journal of Business Research, 192*, 115300. DOI: 10.1016/j.jbusres.2025.115300

Lin, L., Chang, F., Huang, T., Yu, T., Chen, T., Chiu, C., Chen, P., Miao, N., Chuang, H., Chen, C., & Chen, H. (2025). Body dissatisfaction and unhealthy weight-control behaviors of adolescents: The roles of exposure to influencer marketing and use of dating apps. *Medicine, 104*(27), e43152. DOI: 10.1097/MD.0000000000043152 PMID: 40629583

Lou, C., & Yuan, S. (2018). Influencer Marketing: How message value and credibility affect consumer trust of branded content on social media. *Journal of Interactive Advertising, 19*(1), 58–73. DOI: 10.1080/15252019.2018.1533501

Mede, N. G., & Schroeder, R. (2024). The "Greta Effect" on Social Media: A systematic review of research on Thunberg's impact on digital climate change communication. *Environmental Communication, 18*(6), 801–818. DOI: 10.1080/17524032.2024.2314028

Media influence on pre-teens and teenagers: social media, movies, YouTube and apps. (2024, December 20). Raising Children Network. Retrieved May 19, 2025, from https://raisingchildren.net.au/pre-teens/entertainment-technology/media/media-influence-on-teens

Milmo, D. (2024, November 26). Online influencers need 'urgent' fact-checking training, warns Unesco. *The Guardian*. https://www.theguardian.com/media/2024/nov/26/online-influencers-need-urgent-fact-checking-training-warns-unesco?utm_source=chatgpt.com

Murtaza, G. (2023, May 24). *Understanding the role of social media influencers on youth*. Retrieved May 18, 2025, from https://www.linkedin.com/pulse/understanding-role-social-media-influencers-youth-ghulam-murtaza

Obe, S. M., Von Weiler, J., & Gardner, W. (2024, December 12). *What are the impacts of influencer culture on young people?* Internet Matters. Retrieved May 19, 2025, from https://www.internetmatters.org/hub/question/how-influencer-culture-affects-young-people-online/

Shah, D., Webster, E., & Kour, G. (2022). Consuming for content? Understanding social media-centric consumption. *Journal of Business Research, 155*, 113408. DOI: 10.1016/j.jbusres.2022.113408

Simon @ DMI. (2025a, February 5). 9 of the Biggest Social Media Influencers on Instagram. *Digital Marketing Institute*. https://digitalmarketinginstitute.com/blog/9-of-the-biggest-social-media-influencers-on-instagram

Simon @ DMI. (2025b, May 8). 20 surprising influencer marketing Statistics. *Digital Marketing Institute*. https://digitalmarketinginstitute.com/blog/20-influencer-marketing-statistics-that-will-surprise-you

Social media influencers' impact on youth today. (2025, May 29). RTC Networks. https://www.myrtcnetworks.com/news-releases/social-media-influencers-impact-on-youth-today/?utm_source=chatgpt.com

Stern, R. PhD. (2025, March 9). How social media is shaping teen identity. *Psychology Today*. https://www.psychologytoday.com/us/blog/power-in-relationships/202503/likes-and-lies-the-effects-of-influencers-on-teens

Suganya, R., & Bawa, S. A. (2024). Exploring the influence of social media influencers' credibility on consumer behavior: An empirical study. *ComFin Research, 12*(1), 82–92. DOI: 10.34293/commerce.v12i1.6815

The influencer impact - children and screens. (2024, August 16). Children and Screens. Retrieved May 19, 2025, from https://www.childrenandscreens.org/learn-explore/research/the-influencer-impact-a-parents-guide-to-influencers/

Walsh, S. (2025, January 31). *The top 30 social media influencers worldwide*. Search Engine Journal. Retrieved May 27, 2025, from https://www.searchenginejournal.com/top-social-media-influencers/475776/

Wood, A. (2024). Essay on the Impact of Media Influencers on Youth. *EssayGenius AI Essay Writer*. https://essaygenius.ai/essay/essay-on-the-impact-of-media-influencers-on-youth

Worb, J. (2025, March 13). *15 types of social media influencers you need to know in 2025*. Retrieved May 26, 2025, from https://later.com/blog/types-of-social-media-influencers/

yusralodi3@gmail.com & yusralodi3@gmail.com. (2024, February 29). *Influencer culture and its impact*. Youth Ki Awaaz. https://www.youthkiawaaz.com/2024/02/influencer-culture-and-its-impact/

Zhang, G., Chong, L., Kotovsky, K., & Cagan, J. (2022). Trust in an AI versus a Human teammate: The effects of teammate identity and performance on Human-AI cooperation. *Computers in Human Behavior*, *139*, 107536. DOI: 10.1016/j.chb.2022.107536

Chapter 3
Balancing Cultural Heritage and Tourism Development in Bangladesh

Mohammad Badruddoza Talukder
https://orcid.org/0009-0008-1662-9221
International University of Business Agriculture and Technology, Bangladesh

Firoj Kabir
https://orcid.org/0009-0001-3014-3163
Daffodil International University, Bangladesh

ABSTRACT

This chapter aims to develop how Bangladeshi cultural heritage tourism development balances the demands of community involvement and preservation. Bangladesh, a country rich in historical landmarks and cultural variety, struggles to preserve the authenticity of its legacy. The findings, which are based on secondary data from the body of existing literature and perspectives from stakeholders like local communities, government representatives, and tourism experts, show that while cultural tourism presents opportunities for cultural exchange and substantial economic benefits, there are also significant risks associated with problems like poor heritage management, inadequate infrastructure, and limited community involvement. The chapter suggests using strategic instruments to improve visitor experiences without sacrificing cultural integrity. It concludes that responsible cultural heritage tourism that protects Bangladesh's uniqueness and advances sustainable socioeconomic development requires a cooperative strategy involving legislators, local people, and tourist operators.

DOI: 10.4018/979-8-3373-4516-1.ch003

INTRODUCTION

Cultural heritage tourism is concerned with visiting historical and archaeological tourism for enjoyable experiences (Kabir & Rahman, 2020). In this context, heritage defines a visiting place or an area and ensures an extraordinary experience emerging from present accouterments associated with a site. Cultural heritage tourism emerged as a valuable economic and marketing tool when planning for competitive prospects in the tourism business sector. The enhancement of the tourism industry through heritage also provides the visitor with enjoyment and involvement and thus enhances the worth of the place (Bappy & Avi, 2021). But history discloses that Bangladesh has been the backbone of civilization, the nerve center of social dissemination, right from the dawn of the history of humanity. This South Asian country, which has significant heritage tourism attractions, has the potential to become an essential global heritage tourism destination despite few studies exploring the matter rigorously and directing towards a tactical blueprint for this segment's development (Amam, 2024).

However, a few issues can negatively affect Bangladesh's successful cultural heritage tourism development initiatives (Akthar & Hassan, 2021). That is why it is necessary to determine the existing conditions and challenges of heritage tourism in the country to set up a suitable promotion or development strategy to attract domestic and foreign tourists. Towards the above-said need, the scope of this chapter is to market effectively and brand heritage tourism in Bangladesh. Tourism management has been put through the trials of continuous growth plus concentration diversification over the decades in one of the quickest-growing economic sectors around the globe (Nasiche, 2024). Modern tourism tendencies relate to further development and the increase in the number of the latest and alternative directions. These demands have increased, making tourism a factor that leads to socio-economic growth (Tapera et al., 2024).

Therefore, cultural tourism is one of the oldest types and remains fundamental in most parts of the world. Due to available definitions of culture, the amount of cultural goods and services and the frequency of practicing culture has increased. Tourism, which involves visiting historical and archaeological attractions, is one of the everyday activities that most tourists engage in (Talukder, 2025). Heritage sites can be visited in almost every country. For that reason, the significance of heritage tourism is increasing daily (Sardar et al., 2021). Heritage tourism may, therefore, be defined as tourism governed by the sole purpose of acquiring knowledge or entertainment at historical and archaeological attractions. Bangladesh is a small South Asian country with diverse cultural, historical, and archaeological sites, the world's most important heritage sites. Accordingly, this country can develop an enormous potential to be one of the world's leading heritage tourism destinations.

Proper organization of marketing programs is inevitable in encouraging tourists to visit the heritage sites. Most developed and developing nations have applied and adopted marketing concepts and techniques to appeal to heritage tourists in their respective countries. The said concept of Marketing for heritage tourism has not got adequate attention in Bangladesh. As a result, the number of heritage tourists here is far lower than that of neighboring countries like Sri Lanka, Maldives, India, and Bhutan. This chapter investigates the current opportunities and challenges of heritage tourism marketing in Bangladesh.

LITERATURE REVIEW

Tourism is generally a communal, cultural, and economic phenomenon involving individuals' movement to different locations or countries outside their usual premises for personal or professional requirements. Tourism does not only reflect traveling to a specific target area but also embraces all activities undertaken during the stay. It also includes the option of day visits and excursions (Talukder et al., 2024). The concept of tourism is a relaxation action that includes the discretional utilization of time and cash, and entertainment is regularly the principal reason for participation in this industry. As per the Malaysian Tourism Promotion Board (2004), the concept of tourism can be divided into several categories, such as traveling on holidays, VFR (visiting friends and relatives), traveling for business, traveling for medical purposes, conferences, shopping, official travel, traveling for academic purposes, sports and so on. In fact, due to the rapid expansion of the globalization concept, tourism has contributed to the global economic outline. It has become a basic source of foreign revenues for many regions. Several studies also describe the association between tourism and economic growth in South Asian regions. Cultural tourism is a country or region's largest commercial and entertainment sector. The pool of traditional and cultural activities creates much interest for domestic and foreign tourists, especially cultural tourists. separated several attributes into three dimensions related to cultural destinations. Three dimensions that they use are destination environment (price level in the area, weather, accessibility, wilderness, remoteness, personal safety, transportation, culture), atmosphere (quality of service, lack of language barrier, relaxing, exotic atmosphere, and reputation), and tourism resource (natural attraction, activities offered in area and hospitality) (Kalenjuk Pivarski et al., 2023). Culture and heritage, as a crucial part of the demand for knowledge of the place visited, create the experience of the tourist's visit that permits us to possess the power to form the choice to return, recommend, and promote the destination as a prominent part of his historical heritage experience. Cultural and heritage-based tourism has long existed, but recent geographical, social, and cultural changes within the main source countries have opened many niche markets in destination countries, including culture-oriented holidays (Kabir & Rahman, 2020). Cultural tourism has been on a rapid and consecutive rise for many years, and most so now, the European Commission has designated 2018 as a year of cultural heritage. Many developing and developed countries have realized that cultural tourism is worth pursuing because it is a high-spending tourism involving highly educated individuals (Noaime, 2023). Cultural Tourism in Bangladesh includes experiencing regional urban or local cultural & traditional activities such as different types of cultural festivals, food, clothes, religious values, heritage, traditional drama, music and dance, cultural sports, museums, etc. It also encircles the lifestyle, monuments, heritage sites, and participation in arts-related activities in Bangladesh (Avi & Sardar, 2021). this chapter tried to formulate all the related contents & presented some new ideas by drawing a proposed model with a full explanation of cultural tourism in Bangladesh. The chapter indicates significant information in the International Tourism and Hospitality Journal about cultural tourism in Bangladesh; cultural tourists are more likely to use travel information sources to stay in Bangladesh, recall the communities they visited, engage in travel activities, and spend money. Consequently, it demonstrates how much tourists are interested in Bangladeshi culture tourism. The development areas and the value in terms of tourist destinations, as well as cultural and social interaction with the host communities of Bangladesh, are important (Kiarie, 2024). Bangladesh is historically rich with authentic cultural amusement activities, and its culture is thoroughly reflected in its lifestyle, art and architecture, language and literature, music, dance, painting, and clothing. Bangladesh's three primary religions (Hinduism, Buddhism, and Islam) have influenced its culture and history. The people of Bangladesh's way of life structure the culture of Bangladesh. ITHJ features a diverse culture that has evolved with influences from diverse social groups. The culture of Bangladesh refers to the way of life of the people of Bangladesh, which has evolved over the centuries and encompasses the cultural diversity of several social groups of the region. The Bengal Renaissance of the 19th and early 20th centuries noted that Bengali writers, authors, scientists, researchers, thinkers, music composers, painters, and filmmakers played a serious role in developing Bengali culture. It's illuminated in various forms, including music, dance, and drama; art, architecture, and craft; folklore; languages and literature; philosophy and religion; festivals and celebrations; moreover, as in a significantly distinct cuisine and culinary tradition. Therefore, Bangladesh can offer desirable tourism products, services, and experiences with infinite demands for finite government and non-government resources (Rössler, 2023). As a part of tourism, cultural tourism is making good demand & playing a great role in developing the economic sector in Bangladesh. The journey of people to specific cultural destinations that offer our Bangladeshi cultural attractions, including folklore, historic sites, artistic and cultural events, and shows, aims to disseminate and acquire new knowledge and experiences that meet the traveler's intellectual needs and individual growth. As a form of tourism, it immerses tourists in local cultural-related activities such as rituals and festivities. It leads the destination in providing opportunities for authentic cultural exchange between locals and visitors. The tourism industry includes all the socio-economic activities directly or indirectly involved in providing services to tourists (Kausar et al., 2024). Tourism can be classified into several distinct categories. They include holiday travel, visiting friends and relatives (VFR), business travel, health treatment, shopping, conferences, incentive travel, official mission, education, sport, and other travel. Tourism marketing is an integrated effort to satisfy tourists by providing the best possible services. It is a device to transform potential tourists into actual tourists. It is the safest way to generate demand and expand the market. As an important element of Marketing Mix, promotion is vital in tourism marketing, as with any product and service. Tourists want to know about the attractions and facilities of a particular destination. They also want to know about the information related to their visit to make the tour safe, secure, and enjoyable. When tourists plan a trip, they look for available information, services and facilities, tour operators, things to see and do, safety and security, accommodation and transportation, and other necessary information about the location from different sources. The Internet is the most used media for information in this modern age.

Heritage Tourism Products in Bangladesh

Both historical and architectural treasures may be found in abundance in Bangladesh. Many heritage places in this country have the potential to draw tourists from both inside the country and from other countries. However, due to the absence of intense advertising campaigns, these heritage destinations have become less appealing compared to other locations worldwide. Many medieval heritage sites in Bangladesh were created throughout the pre-Muslim and Muslim centuries. Badruddoza et al. (2024) explain the relationship between language migration and heritage tourism.

An overview of cultural heritage attractions of Bangladesh:

Archaeological Tourism Products

Lalbag Fort

The Aurangabad Fort, often called Lalbagh Fort, is Bangladesh's best example of Mughal architecture. It is located southwest of the city of Dhaka and faces Buriganga. The tomb of Bibi Pari, the purported daughter of Nawab Shaista Khan, a modest three-domed mosque, the governor's hammam, and the audience hall are all located there. This fort was more of a palace fort than a regular fort, as its primary function was to provide a protective perimeter for the interior's opulent buildings. Lalbagh Fort, located in Dhaka, Bangladesh, is an ancient Mughal fort sometimes called Fort Aurangabad (Bhuiyan & Bhuiyan, 2023). Under the Mughal Prince Muhammad Azam, construction started in 1678 but was abandoned when he was called back to Delhi. Essential features are the Diwan-i-Aam (Audience Hall) and the Tomb of Pari Bibi, a three-domed mosque. Following Pari Bibi's passing, the fort's construction was put on hold, which resulted in its abandonment. Lalbagh Fort is a well-liked tourist destination and an essential representation of Mughal history and architecture in Bangladesh today.

Ahsan Manzil

This majestic tower, named after his son Nawab Ahsanullah Bahadur, was first constructed in 1872 by Nawab Abdul Ghani as a palace on the site of an ancient French factory. It is located on the bank of the Buriganga River. Ahsan Manzil is a historically significant landmark that is now a museum. The official house of the Nawabs of Dhaka was Ahsan Manzil, a historic palace situated on the banks of the Buriganga River in Dhaka, Bangladesh. Its enormous dome and pink facade are striking examples of Indo-Saracenic architecture built in the 19th century. During the British Raj, social and political life revolved around the palace. After years of neglect, it was repaired and turned into a museum with Nawab-era artifacts and displays. According to Talukder et al. (2024), Ahsan Manzil is a well-known monument representing Dhaka's rich history.

Sonargaon

Sonargaon is Bengal's first known capital, around 26 miles from Dhaka. Up until the 13th century, it served as the Deva Dynasty's seat. Sonargaon served as the Sultanate of Bengal's secondary capital from that time till the arrival of the Mughals. The tomb of Sultan Ghiasuddin (1399–1409 A.D.), the shrines of Panjpirs and Shah Abdul Alla, and a stunning mosque in Goaldi village are a few of the historic sites that are still standing (Sonargaon, 2014). The ancient Bengal region's capital was Sonargaon, a historic town near Dhaka in Bangladesh. Sonargaon, well-known for its rich cultural legacy, was a bustling trade and business hub in the Middle Ages, especially when the Mughal and Sultanate empires ruled it. Numerous important locations may be found in the region, such as the Tomb of Sultan Ghiyasuddin Azam Shah, the Folk Art and Crafts Museum, and the historic Panam City. For people who want to learn more about Bangladesh's history and traditional arts, Sonargaon is a well-liked destination these days.

Wari Bateshwar

Northeastern Bangladesh's Wari-Bateshwar is home to an old fort built in 450 BC. This site dates back 2,500,00 years and is an important archaeological find. It refutes previous theories of Bangladesh's early urban civilization. Researchers claim that the finding of artifacts and, more significantly, Wari-Bateshawar's geographic position point to its connections with Southeast Asia and Rome. Situated in Bangladesh's Narsingdi region, Wari-Bateshwar is an ancient archaeological site thought to have been inhabited between 450 BCE and 300 CE during the early historic era. The location is noteworthy because it has traces of an old, fortified city that was a component of Bengal's early urbanization. Pottery, terracotta figures, and silver punch-marked coins have all been found during excavations, demonstrating the importance of Wari-Bateshwar as a center of regional commerce and cultural interchange. The location provides insightful information about Bengal's prehistoric past and civilization (Talukder, 2021).

Mainamati

"Mainamati," formerly known as "Samatata," refers to a region nearly level with the sea. This location is the vast hub of the Buddhist culture from the 7th to the 12th centuries, Salban Vihara. Over fifty ancient sites dotting the hills have been discovered during excavation at this UNESCO site; these sites mostly feature various sorts of Buddhist remnants from the eighth to the twelfth century A.D. Numerous Buddhist monasteries, temples, and stupas have been revealed during excavations at multiple locations. A vast assortment of artifacts that beautifully describe the magnificent cultural achievements of the time have also been unearthed. Mainamati, a significant archaeological site in Bangladesh close to Comilla, is well-known for its Buddhist past. It was a prominent Buddhist scholarship and culture hub from the 7th to the 12th century. More than fifty historic Buddhist villages can be found at the site, including the Salban Vihara, a sizable monastery complex, and the Mainamati Museum, a collection of relics with bronze sculptures, coins, and terracotta plaques on display. Mainamati is a crucial location for learning about the history and architecture of the ancient Buddhists.

Paharpur

Paharpur Vihara is a globally renowned historical site. Based on a collection of inscriptions on clay seals, it has been determined to be the purported Somapura Vihara of the illustrious Pala ruler Dharmapala. It is the only Vihara that is this big south of the Himalayas. With 177 monk cells around the courtyard, this massive quadrangular monastery is dominated by a tall pyramidal temple in the middle

(Sharmin, 2021). The typical collections of artifacts discovered from the region are kept at a site museum.

The unearthed items have also been conserved at Rajshahi's Varendra Research Museum. The historic Somapura Mahavihara, one of South Asia's biggest and most important Buddhist monastic complexes, is near Paharpur in northern Bangladesh. This UNESCO World Heritage Site was constructed in the eighth century under the Pala dynasty. It has a sizeable cruciform temple with elaborate clay ornamentation and a large courtyard encircled by many monk cells. Paharpur drew intellectuals and pilgrims from all over Asia since it was a significant hub of scholarship and spiritual activity. It still serves as a reminder of ancient Bengal's magnificent architecture and rich Buddhist legacy (Roy, 2021).

Mahasthangarh

Located on the western bank of the Karatoa River, Mahasthangarh is the earliest archaeological site in Bangladesh. The stunning site is a formidable landmark in the neighborhood, with its ancient remains arranged in a semicircle with a radius of around 8 kilometers. Several solitary mounds surround the walled city. This archaeological site dates to the third century B.C. and is still highly sacred to the Hindus. A trip to the Mahasthangarh site museum will reveal a variety of antiques. The Gokul Medh in the Mahasthangarh area and the Shah Sultan Bulkhi Mahisawar shrine are also famous. One of Bangladesh's earliest archaeological monuments, Mahasthangarh, is situated in Bogura and dates at least to the third century BCE (Talukder & Kaiser, 2024). In the past, it served as the capital of the Pundra Kingdom and was a major city under the Mauryan, Gupta, and Pala dynasties, among others. The site has old buildings, artifacts, and inscriptions that provide clues about the prehistoric history and culture of the area, along with the ruins of a walled city. A must-visit location for learning about Bangladesh's prehistoric past and early urban civilization is Mahasthangarh.

Kantaji's temple

Maharaja Pran Nath of Dinajpur constructed this temple close to the town 1752. Every square inch of the temple's exterior is exquisitely decorated with clay plaques that depict a staggering variety of modern social settings and favorite activities, as well as flora, fauna, geometric elements, and themes from mythology. The local museum and the Maharaja's Palace house artifacts from bygone eras are worthwhile excursions.

Shait Gombudge Mosque, Bagerhat

Ulugh Khan Jahan, a saint, established a Muslim colony close to the shore in the mid-fifteenth century. Today, this area is known as the Bagerhat district. Khan Jahan constructed many mosques, roads, tanks, and other public structures across his city. Among these is the Shait Gombudge mosque, the "60-domed Mosque," the most impressive brick mosque in Bangladesh. (Mosque Shait Gombudge. In Dinajpur, Bangladesh, there is a magnificent Hindu temple called Kantaji's Temple, sometimes called Kantanagar Temple. Maharaja Pran Nath constructed the temple in the 18th century, and it is well known for its exquisite terracotta decoration that covers the whole building. The temple is a marvel of late medieval Bengali architecture devoted to Krishna, also known as Kantaji in the local dialect. Its elaborate clay panels feature everyday life, floral patterns, and images from Hindu mythology. One of Bangladesh's best examples of temple building is Kantaji's Temple, which is praised for its aesthetic appeal.

Seven dome Mosque

The seventh dome mosque was made by Shaista Khan, a Subadhar and army general of the Mughal Empire in the Bengal region from 1664 to 1688. The mosque has a unique architectural value.

Binat Bibi Mosque

The square, one-domed Binat Bibi Mosque was constructed over 600 years ago. The mosque's architecture and construction are primarily influenced by Pre-Mughal elements (Yeamin Masum et al., 2024).

Star Mosque

The Armanitola neighborhood in Dhaka's historic district is home to Star Mosque, also called Tara Masjid. The mosque has blue star decorations and intricate embellishments (Sgroi, 2021). This mosque was initially a straightforward rectangular mosque and was constructed in the late 18th century by Mirza Golam Pir in the Mughal style (Lhendup, 2024).

Shrine of Hazrat Shah Paran

Famous Sufi saint "Shah Paran" (R) founded a khanqah near Khadim Nagar, approximately 7 km from Sylhet town, where he initiated Sufi spiritual activities and rituals (Sharma & Singh, 2024). His grave was next to his khanqah. Hordes of devotees have frequented his tomb for ages; this tradition is still in place today.

Konya Shah's mausoleum lies next to the Shah Paran major tomb complex, which worshippers also frequent.

Shrine of Hazrat Shah Jalal

In the center of Sylhet town, near Dargah Mahalla, lies the shrine dedicated to the famous Muslim saint Hazrat Shah Jalal (R.A.). Early in the fourteenth century, this saint introduced the Islamic faith to the area. Hazrat Shah Amanat's Dargah is East of Laldighi, Chittagong, and Hazrat Shah Sufi Amanat Shah's Dargah Sharif is east of the central prison. Additional items for religious tourism include the grave of Bibi Moriom Mughal Eid gah (Dhanmondi Eid gah), Choto Sona Mosque Hussaini dalan, Sultan Bayezid Bostami's mausoleum, and other examples of religious tourist items.

Central Shahid Minar

Symbol of Bengali nationalism, this monument was built to commemorate the martyrs of the historic language movement on 21st February 1952.

Martyred Intellectual Memorial

The Martyred Intellectuals Memorial honors the intellectuals who lost their lives during the Bangladesh Liberation War. The memorial may be found in Dhaka near Rayerbazar, Mohammadpur Thana (Wu, 2021).

National Poet's Grave

This is where revolutionary poet Kazi Nazrul Islam was buried after passing away on 29th August 1976. The Dhaka University Central Mosque is next to the cemetery (Beltramo et al., 2024).

Bahadurshah Park

This 1857 memorial site, which was once Victoria Park and is situated in the old city across from Jagannath University, was constructed to honor the heroes of the first liberation fight against British rule that took place in the years 1857–1859 (Nekmahmud & Hassan, 2021).

Curzon Hall

Following the initial division of Bengal in 1905, Curzon Hall was constructed in Dhaka, showcasing a harmonious amalgamation of Mughal and European aesthetics (Lin et al., 2024).

Baldha Garden

The garden is situated in Wari, Dhaka, founded in 1904 by the late Narendra Narayan Roy. This garden features a wide variety of both native and exotic species.

World War II Cemetery

Over 700 Second World War troops from Japan and the Commonwealth nations are interred in this well-kept cemetery in Chittagong.

Shilaidaha Kuthibari, Kushtia

The exquisite home honors the legacy of Nobel laureate poet Rabindranath Tagore (1861–1941), who resided here regularly to oversee the management of his Zamindari and contributed to the advancement of Bengali literature via his writings during that period. It is situated around 20 km away from

Kushtia town.

Other Historical Tourism Products There are other notable historical tourism products in Bangladesh, such as Suhrawardy Uddayan Old High Court Building Natore - Dighapatiya Rajbari (Palace), etc.

Tourism and hospitality contribution to tourism preservation in Bangladesh

Cultural heritage tourism in Bangladesh plays a crucial role in balancing tourism promotion with preserving cultural and historical sites for community development. The following factors are identified from the literature:

Conservation Efforts: The assistance of governmental and non-governmental organizations has allowed for the restoration and preservation of several heritage monuments, including Lalbagh Fort, Ahsan Manzil, and Somapura Mahavihara. These initiatives ensure that the sites' authenticity and integrity are preserved even as more people visit them.

Sustainable Tourism Practices: There are programs to encourage eco-friendly travel with the most minor adverse effects on historical monuments. For instance, restricted visitor numbers, appropriate waste disposal, and environmentally friendly infrastructure all aid in preventing injury and deterioration in these locations.

Cultural Awareness and Education: Educational initiatives that enlighten visitors and residents about a location's historical and artistic value are frequently a part of heritage tourism. This understanding fosters a sense of accountability and respect for preserving these historic sites.

Community Involvement: Incorporating local communities with tourism ensures they reap economic benefits from the flood of tourists while contributing to preservation initiatives. This might involve putting people to work as tour guides, supporting regional handicrafts, and supporting neighborhood-based conservation initiatives.

Government Policies and Regulations: The Bangladeshi government has established laws and rules to safeguard historical monuments. Important include prohibitions on buildings near important locations and fines for vandalism and other unlawful activity. By taking these steps, we can ensure that tourism development doesn't come at the price of cultural preservation.

Returns Reinvestment: The money received from tourism is frequently used to support ongoing conservation initiatives, which support the upkeep and restoration of historic sites. As a result, a cycle is established in which tourism directly aids historical preservation (Bhuiyan & Bhuiyan, 2023).

Bangladesh's cultural heritage tourism and hospitality play a crucial role in promoting tourism while preserving cultural and historical sites. Here's how this balance is achieved:

Sustainable Tourism Practices: There are programs to encourage eco-friendly travel with the most negligible adverse effects on historical monuments. For instance, restricted visitor numbers, appropriate garbage disposal, and environmentally friendly infrastructure all aid in preventing harm and deterioration to these locations (Firoj & Mohammad, 2024).

Cultural Awareness and Education: Heritage tourism often includes educational programs that inform tourists and locals about sites' historical and cultural significance. This awareness fosters a sense of responsibility and respect for preserving these heritage locations.

Community Involvement: Incorporating local communities with tourism ensures they reap economic benefits from the flood of tourists while contributing to preservation initiatives. Local crafts, community-led conservation initiatives, and guide training are examples of how to do this (Kumar et al., 2023).

Government Policies and Regulations: The government of Bangladesh has implemented policies and regulations to protect heritage sites, including restrictions on construction around these areas and penalties for vandalism or illegal activities(Mohammad & Fahmida, 2023). These measures help ensure that tourism growth does not come at the expense of cultural preservation.

Revenue Reinvestment: The money received from tourism is frequently used to support ongoing conservation initiatives, which support the upkeep and restoration of historical sites. As a result, a cycle is established in which tourism directly aids cultural preservation.

Problems of Heritage Tourism in Bangladesh

Guided Tours and Regulations: Using professionally led tours can help control tourist behavior and lower the possibility of heritage site damage (M. T. Islam, 2023). Regulations are put into place and enforced to manage access to vulnerable locations and guarantee that visitors adhere to preservation measures.

Cultural Festivals and Events: Organizing cultural festivals and events that showcase customary arts, crafts, and performances may boost travel while encouraging the preservation of cultural heritage. These activities promote responsible tourism by increasing knowledge of and respect for cultural assets (Karim, 2022).

Digital Documentation and Virtual Tours: Leveraging technology to create digital documentation and virtual tours of heritage sites allows people to experience and learn about these sites without physically visiting them. This approach reduces the physical strain on the sites and provides broader access to global audiences.

Partnerships with International Organizations: Collaborating with international heritage organizations, such as UNESCO and ICOMOS, helps Bangladesh benefit from global expertise and funding for conservation projects. These partnerships also bring international attention to the importance of preserving heritage.

Visitor Management Systems: Using sophisticated visitor management systems, such as timed entrance, reservation systems, and tickets, heritage buildings may save wear and tear by managing visitor flow and preventing overcrowding (N. Islam, 2023).

Community-Based Tourism Initiatives: Promoting community-based tourism endeavors, where local people design and oversee tourist experiences, cultivate a feeling of accountability and ownership for safeguarding their cultural legacy.

Educational Institutions and Research: Research and conservation studies conducted in collaboration with academic institutions advance our knowledge of historic places and help create practical preservation plans (Sarker, 2024).

Maintenance and Upkeep Programs: Regular maintenance and upkeep programs are crucial for preserving heritage sites. This includes repairs, cleaning, and monitoring to ensure that sites remain in good condition and are safe and enjoyable for visitors.

Promotion of Local Crafts and Traditions: Further combining preservation with tourism supports and promotes regional crafts and customs as part of the tourist experience, which helps maintain traditional skills and financially benefits craftsmen (Sarker, 2024).

Feedback Mechanisms: The provision of visitor feedback methods facilitates the gathering of viewpoints and recommends the enhancement of tourist operations and conservation initiatives. Plans may be guided by this input, which can also improve visitor experiences (Omi et al., 2024).

Figure 1. Interconnection of heritage products, tourism impacts, and sustainable development for balanced, inclusive cultural growth.

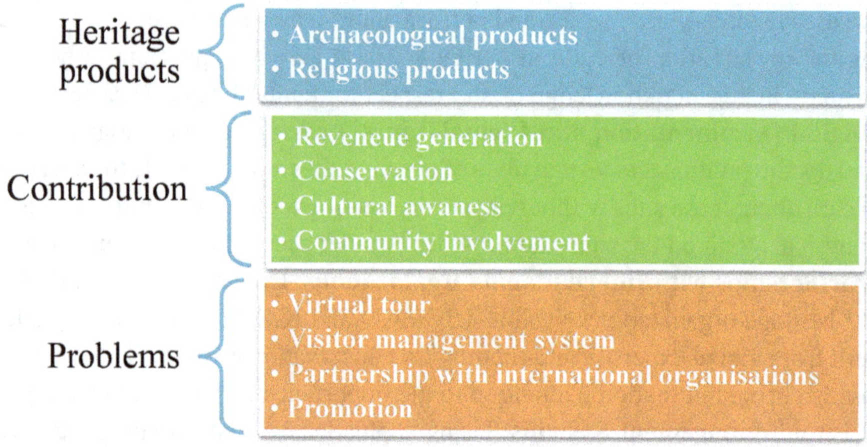

Source: Authors own

The figure presents three core dimensions: heritage products, which include Bangladesh's cultural, historical, and religious benefits, and the impacts of tourism. The figure highlights the importance of maintaining stability between utilizing heritage resources and addressing development challenges to ensure sustainable and inclusive growth. It advocates for a strategic and collaborative approach that leverages the potential of cultural heritage tourism while safeguarding cultural integrity and maximizing socio-economic benefits for local communities.

Recommendations

Here are some recommendations to address the problems facing cultural heritage tourism in Bangladesh:

1. **Implement Visitor Management Systems**: To regulate visitor numbers and reduce congestion at heritage sites, develop and implement visitor management methods, such as tickets, guided tours, and timed entrance.

2. **Enhance Infrastructure**: To promote tourist and preservation efforts, invest in upgrading the infrastructure surrounding heritage sites, such as better access roads, visitor centers, signs, and transit alternatives.
3. **Secure Conservation Funding**: To guarantee historic places' long-term protection and increase financing for conservation and restoration initiatives through public-private partnerships, foreign aid, and government support.
4. **Strengthening Regulations and Enforcement**: Strict rules should be established and upheld to stop graffiti, vandalism, and other types of damage. Establish sanctions for infractions to safeguard historical places.
5. **Promote Awareness and Education**: Start educating visitors and residents about preserving cultural heritage and practicing appropriate behavior when visiting historical places through awareness campaigns and educational initiatives.
6. **Develop Sustainable Tourism Practices**: Promote eco-friendly initiatives, trash management, and conservation-friendly tourism activities as examples of sustainable tourism practices that lessen their environmental influence.
7. **Support Community Involvement**: Involve local communities in developing and administrating tourism to guarantee that they gain financially from the industry while actively contributing to preserving their cultural legacy.
8. **Improve Site Management**: Improve site management procedures through employee training, detailed maintenance schedules, and the application of sensible visitor control techniques.
9. **Protect Against Environmental and Natural Threats**: Create plans for flood defense and disaster response to protect heritage assets from environmental hazards and natural catastrophes. Create flood defense and disaster response plans to protect heritage assets from environmental hazards and natural catastrophes.
10. **Promote Cultural Authenticity**: Avoid commercializing heritage, which might cause cultural deterioration, and strike a balance between the growth of tourism and the maintenance of genuine cultural practices and traditions.
11. **Foster International Collaboration**: Collaborate with global heritage organizations and specialists to access worldwide resources, expertise, and optimal conservation and tourism administration approaches.
12. **Create Economic Incentives**: Encourage the incorporation of regional crafts and customs into the tourism experience by offering financial incentives and assistance to local companies and artists that help preserve the area's cultural legacy.

Conclusion and future research

Striking a balance between heritage tourism and preserving cultural and historical assets in Bangladesh is a complex task that calls for an all-encompassing strategy. It is necessary to maintain the authenticity of heritage places and address problems such as excessive tourism, poor infrastructure, and inadequate financing for conservation. The adverse effects of tourism may be mitigated in Bangladesh by implementing efficient visitor management systems, improving infrastructure, acquiring money for conservation, and promoting environmentally responsible travel patterns. To further promote preservation efforts, strengthening rules, encouraging community engagement, and forming partnerships with international organizations are all examples of steps that may be taken. This will ultimately guarantee that Bangladesh's rich past continues to be a source of pride and educational value for future generations while also contributing to the growth of the nation's economy. This will be accomplished via a commitment to responsible tourism and cultural preservation. Several intriguing paths might be explored in the future study of heritage tourism and conservation in Bangladesh. Impact assessment studies might be used to examine the long-term consequences of tourism on heritage sites. These studies could provide insights into visitor behavior and site conditions, facilitating the development of more effective management techniques. Investigating sustainable tourism practices and technology may give answers to reducing the adverse effects on the environment and the physical environment while simultaneously improving tourists' experiences.

REFERENCES

Akthar, N., & Hassan, A. (2021). Demand Analysis of Tourism and Hospitality Products and Services in Bangladesh. In Hassan, A. (Ed.), *Tourism Products and Services in Bangladesh* (pp. 159–179). Springer Singapore., DOI: 10.1007/978-981-33-4279-8_8

Amam, M. (2024). Influence of Cultural Heritage Preservation on Tourism Development in Egypt. *American Journal of Arts. Social and Humanity Studies*, *4*(1), 22–32. DOI: 10.47672/ajashs.2063

Avi, Md. A. R., & Sardar, S. (2021). Application of Innovative Technologies in Bangladesh's Tourism and Hospitality Industry: Challenges and Suggestions. In A. Hassan (Ed.), *Technology Application in Bangladesh's Tourism and Hospitality Industry* (pp. 369–379). Springer Singapore. DOI: 10.1007/978-981-16-2434-6_22

Badruddoza Talukder, M., Kumar, S., Misra, L. I., & Firoj Kabir, . (2024). Determining the role of eco-tourism service quality, tourist satisfaction, and destination loyalty: A case study of Kuakata beach. *Acta Scientiarum Polonorum. Administratio Locorum*, *23*(1), 133–151. DOI: 10.31648/aspal.9275

Bappy, T. A., & Avi, Md. A. R. (2021). Technological Innovation Application in the Tourism and Hospitality Industry of Bangladesh. In A. Hassan (Ed.), *Technology Application in the Tourism and Hospitality Industry of Bangladesh* (pp. 63–77). Springer Singapore. DOI: 10.1007/978-981-16-2434-6_4

Beltramo, R., Duglio, S., & Mascadri, G. (2024). Mountain Tourism: Environmental Management for Fostering Tourism Destinations: From Context Analysis to Tourism Products. In Lagioia, G., Paiano, A., Amicarelli, V., Gallucci, T., & Ingrao, C. (Eds.), *Innovation, Quality and Sustainability for a Resilient Circular Economy* (pp. 509–515). Springer International Publishing., DOI: 10.1007/978-3-031-28292-8_62

Bhuiyan, M. R. U., & Bhuiyan, M. B. (2023). Crises and Conflicts on the Way to Sustainable Tourism Development: A Study of Cox's Bazar, Bangladesh. *Journal of Environmental Management and Tourism*, *14*(2), 320. DOI: 10.14505/jemt.v14.2(66).03

Das, I. R., Talukder, M. B., & Kumar, S. (2024). Implication of Artificial Intelligence in Hospitality Marketing. In Kumar, S., Talukder, M. B., & Pego, A. (Eds.), *Advances in Hospitality, Tourism, and the Services Industry* (pp. 291–310). IGI Global., DOI: 10.4018/979-8-3693-1978-9.ch014

Dogan, S., Mistry, T. G., & Nanu, L. (2024). Revolutionizing getaways: Automation and artificial intelligence's transformative journey in tourism and hospitality. *Worldwide Hospitality and Tourism Themes*, *16*(2), 248–251. Advance online publication. DOI: 10.1108/WHATT-03-2024-0075

Firoj, K., & Mohammad, B. T. (2024). Measuring sustainability in the broadcasting media industry in Bangladesh. *I-Manager's. Journal of Management*, *18*(3), 51. DOI: 10.26634/jmgt.18.3.20234

Islam, M. T. (2023). Disaster Management in Bangladesh: Historical Perspective. In M. T. Islam, *Disaster, Governance and Development* (pp. 33–59). Springer Nature Singapore. DOI: 10.1007/978-981-99-1631-3_3

Kabir, K., & Rahman, M. S.-U. -. (2020). General Tourism and Hospitality Education and Research in Bangladesh. In M. S.-U.- Rahman & A. Hassan (Eds.), *Tourism Policy and Planning in Bangladesh* (pp. 179–192). Springer Singapore. DOI: 10.1007/978-981-15-7014-8_11

Kalenjuk Pivarski, B., Grubor, B., Banjac, M., Đerčan, B., Tešanović, D., Šmugović, S., Radivojević, G., Ivanović, V., Vujasinović, V., & Stošić, T. (2023). The Sustainability of Gastronomic Heritage and Its Significance for Regional Tourism Development. *Heritage*, *6*(4), 3402–3417. DOI: 10.3390/heritage6040180

Kausar, D. R., Damanik, J., & Tanudirjo, D. (2024). Borobudur as priority tourism destination: How political economy affects world cultural heritage site management and heritage preservation. *IOP Conference Series. Earth and Environmental Science*, *1366*(1), 012057. DOI: 10.1088/1755-1315/1366/1/012057

Kiarie, E. (2024). Cultural Heritage Preservation in the Face of Globalization. *International Journal of Humanities and Social Science*, *3*(3), 1–14. DOI: 10.47941/ijhss.2081

Kumar, S., Talukder, M. B., Kabir, F., & Kaiser, F. (2023). Challenges and Sustainability of Green Finance in the Tourism Industry: Evidence From Bangladesh. In Taneja, S., Kumar, P., Grima, S., Ozen, E., & Sood, K. (Eds.), (pp. 97–111). Advances in Finance, Accounting, and Economics. IGI Global., DOI: 10.4018/979-8-3693-1388-6.ch006

Lhendup, K. (2024). *PhD Thesis Final Draftword-2 3*. DOI: 10.13140/RG.2.2.20121.63849

Lin, X., Shen, Z., Teng, X., & Mao, Q. (2024). Cultural Routes as Cultural Tourism Products for Heritage Conservation and Regional Development: A Systematic Review. *Heritage*, *7*(5), 2399–2425. DOI: 10.3390/heritage7050114

Mohammad, B. T., & Fahmida, K. (2023). Economic impact of river tourism: Evidence of Bangladesh. *I-Manager's. Journal of Management*, *18*(2), 47. DOI: 10.26634/jmgt.18.2.20235

Nasiche, N. (2024). The Role of Wellness Tourism in the Growth of the Hospitality Industry. *Journal of Modern Hospitality*, *3*(1), 53–64. DOI: 10.47941/jmh.1954

Nekmahmud, Md., & Hassan, A. (2021). Tourism Products and Services in Bangladesh: In Search of Policy and Development Frameworks. In Hassan, A. (Ed.), *Tourism Products and Services in Bangladesh* (pp. 3–24). Springer Singapore., DOI: 10.1007/978-981-33-4279-8_1

Noaime, E. (2023). *Historic Syrian Cities in the Post-War Period: Balancing Cultural Preservation and Tourism Investment*. DOI: 10.20944/preprints202303.0457.v1

Rössler, M. (2023). Balancing Tourism and Heritage Conservation: A World Heritage Context. In Cameron, C. (Ed.), *Evolving Heritage Conservation Practice in the 21st Century* (Vol. 5, pp. 207–218). Springer Nature Singapore., DOI: 10.1007/978-981-99-2123-2_13

Roy, M. (2021). Tourism Industry in Bangladesh: An Assessment of Advanced SWOT Model and TOWS Matrix. In Hassan, A. (Ed.), *Tourism in Bangladesh: Investment and Development Perspectives* (pp. 279–310). Springer Nature Singapore., DOI: 10.1007/978-981-16-1858-1_18

Sardar, S., Hossain, D. M. E., Kamruzzaman, D. M., & Ray, R. (2021). ICT APPLICATIONS IN TOURISM AND HOSPITALITY INDUSTRY OF BANGLADESH: A RESEARCH REVIEW. *IJRDO -. Journal of Business and Management*, *7*(6), 64–74. DOI: 10.53555/bm.v7i6.4404

Sgroi, F. (2021). Food products, gastronomy and religious tourism: The resilience of food landscapes. *International Journal of Gastronomy and Food Science*, *26*, 100435. DOI: 10.1016/j.ijgfs.2021.100435

Sharma, M., & Singh, A. (2024). Enhancing Competitive Advantages Through Virtual Reality Technology in the Hotels of India. In Kumar, S., Talukder, M. B., & Pego, A. (Eds.), *Advances in Hospitality, Tourism, and the Services Industry* (pp. 243–256). IGI Global., DOI: 10.4018/979-8-3693-1978-9.ch011

Sharmin, Z. (2021). Marketing Strategies and Suggestions for Tourism Products and Services in Bangladesh. In Hassan, A. (Ed.), *Tourism Products and Services in Bangladesh* (pp. 433–444). Springer Singapore., DOI: 10.1007/978-981-33-4279-8_19

Talukder, M. B. (2021). An assessment of the roles of the social network in the development of the Tourism Industry in Bangladesh. *International Journal of Business, Law, and Education*, *2*(3), 85–93. DOI: 10.56442/ijble.v2i3.21

Talukder, M. B. (2025). Climate change adaptation strategies for a tourism destination: A study of Kuakata beach. *Acta Scientiarum Polonorum. Administratio Locorum*, *24*(1), 165–179. DOI: 10.31648/aspal.10073

Talukder, M. B., Kabir, F., & Mia, Md. N., & Khan, M. R. (2024). Application of Smart Technologies in the Development and Promotion of Religious Tourism Destination: In R. A. Castanho & M. Franco (Eds.), *Advances in Hospitality, Tourism, and the Services Industry* (pp. 71–88). IGI Global. DOI: 10.4018/979-8-3693-3158-3.ch003

Talukder, M. B., & Kaiser, F. (2024). The Future of Adventure Tourism in Bangladesh. In Jermsittiparsert, K., & Suanpang, P. (Eds.), *Advances in Hospitality, Tourism, and the Services Industry* (pp. 325–347). IGI Global., DOI: 10.4018/979-8-3693-5903-7.ch016

Talukder, M. B., Kumar, S., Kaiser, F., & Mia, Md. N. (2024). Pilgrimage Creative Tourism: A Gateway to Sustainable Development Goals in Bangladesh. In M. Hamdan, M. Anshari, N. Ahmad, & E. Ali (Eds.), *Advances in Public Policy and Administration* (pp. 285–300). IGI Global. DOI: 10.4018/979-8-3693-1742-6.ch016

Tapera, J., Hamunakwadi, P., Mashapure, R., & Mukurazita, E. (2024). African Tourism and Hospitality Experience. In B. Nyagadza, F. Chigora, & A. Hassan, *Agritourism in Africa* (1st ed., pp. 119–144). Routledge. DOI: 10.4324/9781032696188-7

. Wu, Y. (2021). Design of Tourism Cultural and Creative Products Based on Regional Historical and Cultural Elements. *E3S Web of Conferences, 251*, 03004. DOI: 10.1051/e3sconf/202125103004

Chapter 4
Curated vs. Real Identity, Pressure, and Psychological Well-Being in Online Spaces

Arzoo Rai
https://orcid.org/0009-0000-8103-5819
Lovely Professional University, India

Amrik Singh
https://orcid.org/0000-0003-3598-8787
Lovely Professional University, India

ABSTRACT

In the era of algorithm-driven platforms, Generation Z faces increasing tension between authentic self-expression and curated self-presentation. This integrative literature review draws on psychology, sociology, and media studies to examine how digital identities are constructed, negotiated, and regulated. Using Goffman's dramaturgical theory, Festinger's social comparison theory, and Higgins' self-discrepancy theory, it situates identity performance along a curated–authentic continuum. The study explores platform design, constant comparison, and performative authenticity in an attention-driven economy, highlighting how context collapse and algorithmic incentives contribute to identity fatigue, self-worth erosion, and emotional burnout. It concludes with multi-stakeholder recommendations for educators, platform designers, policymakers, and users to foster ethical, inclusive, and psychologically sustainable digital environments.

DOI: 10.4018/979-8-3373-4516-1.ch004

INTRODUCTION

The widespread development of digital technologies and widespread sensation of social media have radically changed the way people formulate and understand themselves and the way they represent themselves. Online platforms are now used not just as interactional spaces, but also as performative platforms on which people act idealized versions of themselves in reaction to social norms, technological, and algorithmic incentives (Marwick & boyd, 2011; Zhao et al., 2008). This has led to what is known as a curated self; a bestowed digital personality that takes place through the selective creation of a digital identity, whose intent or objective is to gain validation or admiration. On the contrary, authentic identity would focus on congruence between oneself with the external action in an attempt to achieve authenticity in various circumstances. The social network sites by the definition of boyd and Ellison (2007) provide a frameworked arena of identity presentation as well as network keeping. White as it may be, digital environments are designed in a manner that in the process makes finding authenticity difficult. Controls, software-based feedback loops, social metrics, and audience convergence can tend to value curated content more than spontaneous expression (Kaplan & Haenlein, 2010). Users have therefore continued to find themselves in a panic of always being real and authentic and being viewed in idealised ways. To the first generation who were born with the digital age, identity construction is strongly coupled with the process of self-presentation in the online realm, and thus, they are inherently sensitive to the psychological aspects of identity error (Valkenburg et al., 2006; Nadkarni & Hofmann, 2012). Recent research underlines that digital well-being is not just a screen time issue but is also connected to the overall wellness issues, like the pressures within the healthcare tourism and the wellness industries (Hassan et al., 2025; Sharma & Singh, 2025). The given paper investigates the way in which users, and especially Gen Z, along with digital spaces, are negotiating the tension between the curated and authentic identities created by the technological structures and the demands of social settings. It is a synthesis of interdisciplinary literature in the fields of psychology, sociology, and media studies, and draws upon the Dramaturgical Theory of Goffman (1959), the Social Comparison Theory of Festinger (1954) and the Self-Discrepancy Theory of Higgins (1987). Focusing on creating a continuum between the perspectives of the emerging fields of AI, immersive platforms, and tourism studies, the paper frames the concept of the curated-authentic identity as the problem of a cultural and psychological challenge, which is also a problem of technology and organisation (Srivastava et al., 2025; Al Aqad et al., 2025). The theoretical aim would be to create a conceptual model that could underscore the curated- authentic identity continuum and its implications on mental health, autonomy on its end (user), and platform ethics, and to synthesize current as well as developing literature through which a holistic perspective can be achieved.

THEORETICAL FRAMEWORK

Figure 1. Conceptual framework

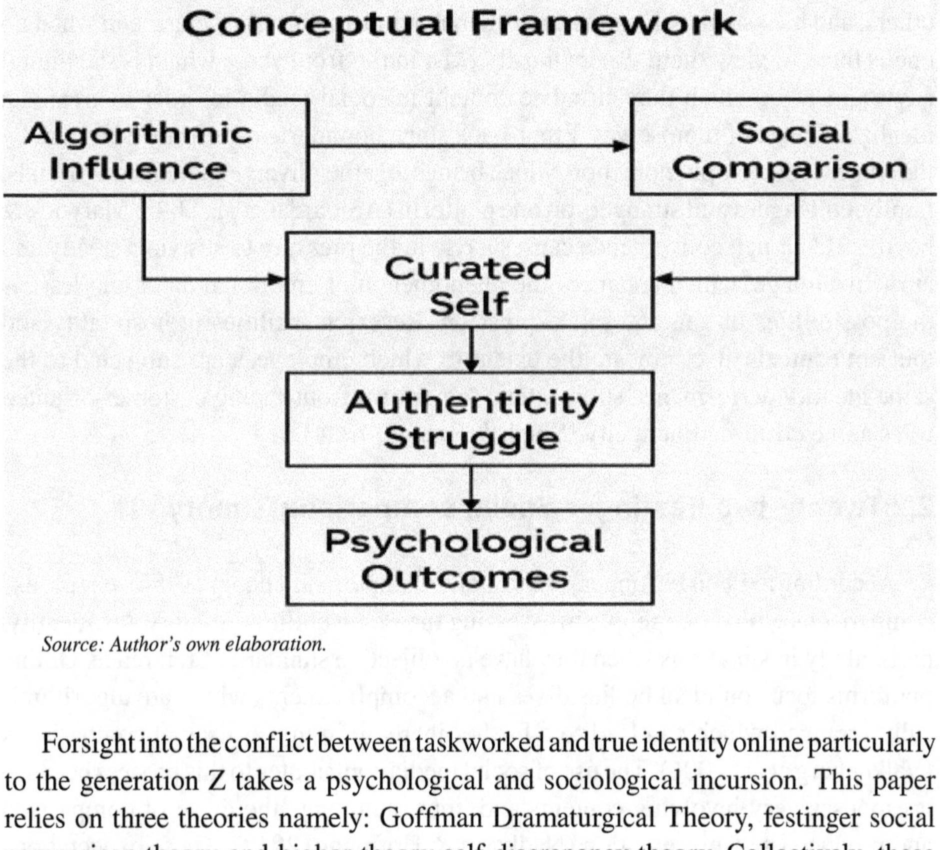

Source: Author's own elaboration.

Forsight into the conflict between taskworked and true identity online particularly to the generation Z takes a psychological and sociological incursion. This paper relies on three theories namely: Goffman Dramaturgical Theory, festinger social comparison theory and higher theory self-discrepancy theory. Collectively, these frameworks offer a multidimensional perspective to analyse psychological, social, and technological forces that determine identity performance in the virtual world (Ansari & Singh, 2023). The new work is also focused on considering the extension of these traditional theories with new contexts of identity experimentation and performance through immersive technologies such as AI, AR, and the Metaverse (Bhalla et al., 2023; Srivastava et al., 2025).

2.1 Dramaturgical theory, Goffman.

In Dramaturgical Theory (1959), Erving Goffman it is possible to think of social interaction in the Theatrical performance concept in resonance with Dramaturgical Theory, where one is always onstage presenting themselves in various ways, depending on audience and the situation. He makes a distinction between front stage behavior which refers to those behaviors that people use in public that aim to shape others, and backstage behavior which are behaviors that persons engage in when no one is there to view them. Users mostly exist in the front stage which is the digital environment in which they circulate content in social media in order to create an idealized image of themselves. Front-back stage boundaries are further obscure by the context collapse phenomenon, which brings together diverse audiences of friends, family, colleagues and strangers on one platform (Ambardar et al., 2023; Marwick & boyd, 2011). Such convergence causes a rise in the pressure to sustain a steady and attractive image, which enhances the phenomenon of emotional labor and lessens the possibilities of genuine self expression. Research facilities in hospitality and tourism contexts also indicate the extent to which employees are subjected to the same identity performance strains, tend to perform front-facing customer-oriented roles at the cost of authenticity (Singh & Supina, 2024).

2.2 Twenty-two Festinger Social comparison Theory.

According to Leon Festinger, in his Social Comparison Theory (1954), people use comparisons with other people in assessing their own abilities, dignity and identity, particularly in situations when they have no objective standard of reference. Online platforms focus on ideal bodies, lives and accomplishments which are algorithmically arranged which can lead to a further increase in upward social comparisons (Valkenburg et al., 2006). The use of social media contributes to this process because it espouses very involving contents and, thus, augments the cycle of comparison and produced self-presentation (Nadkarni & Hofmann, 2012). These expectations may also lead to lower self-esteem, dissatisfaction, and more performance anxiety in Gen Z, who has not yet formed his or her identity identity. Recent literature also shows that identity fatigue and emotional strain are exacerbated by the effects of social comparisons that are heightened through algorithm-driven immersion in digital platforms and the Metaverse, (Al-Romeedy et al., 2025; Srivastava et al., 2025).

2.3 Higgins Self-Discrepancy Theory.

The Self-Discrepancy Theory of E. Tory Higgins (1987) demonstrates the psychological uneasiness that comes along with discrepancies among various versions of the self: the actual self (the way one perceives oneself), the ideal self (the way one wants to be), the ought self (the way one feels he should be). Online, filtering, selectivity of stories and showing the preferred qualities, curated self-presentation can be a tactic to fill the divide between the real and ideal selves (Bargh et al., 2002). Although it can help reduce some discomfort, the chronological presence of a lack of alignment may result in an identity dissonance, an emotional exhaustion, and even impostor syndrome. As studies in hospitality and organizational psychology reveal, the same discrepancies occur in workplaces (Singh & Kumar, 2024; Singh, 2025). Employees tend to face the problem of not being able to reconcile those real and externally shared values, which may have a direct negative effect on mental health.

2.4 Synthesis of Theories

Combining all three models, one can have a multidimensional perspective on the curated-authentic identity continuum of Gen Z:Goffman describes revealment of digital interaction as being performative. Festinger lays emphasis on the societal influences outside that elicit comparison and self-presentation that has been curated.Higgins talks of the inner psychological tensions brought about by rubrics of identity.These theories highlight the fact that Gen Z does not manage their digital identity only as a stylistic decision; it is a profound psychological and sociological process, which is conditioned by platform design, the level of audience visibility, and culture. Modern literature applies this understanding to the virtual layer of immersivity and organizational strategies as well as tourism practice, and it validates that ICT mediation around the curated-authentic struggle is mediated by technological artifacts and institutional demands (Singh & Hassan, 2024; Supina & Singh, 2025). In consequence, any study of online identity should consider the interaction between external intersocial processes and personal self-management processes particularly where the latter are strongly associated with an individual who is yet to develop a sense of self.

Table 1. Key Theories, Focus Areas, and Digital Implications for Gen Z.

Theory	Focus Area	Digital Implication (Especially for Gen Z)
Goffman's Dramaturgical	Performance & audience interaction	Online personas shaped for front-stage visibility; identity fatigue in public spheres
Festinger's Social Comparison	Self-evaluation through comparison	Algorithmic content fuels upward comparison and social anxiety
Higgins' Self-Discrepancy	Internal identity conflict	Misalignment between actual and ideal self causes fatigue and confusion

Source: Author's own elaboration.

3. LITERATURE REVIEW

It has completely changed the concept of identity building, especially in the case of Generation Z (Gen Z), the first generation born into a totally hyper-connected, entirely algorithmically mediated world. Social, psychological, media studies, and communication theorist concur existing literature shows that online self-presentation is informed by psychological motives, platform features and cultural scripts that tend to drag users between resolved and natural portrayals of self. This review summarizes major theoretical frames, empirical results and new arguments on this continuum of curated-authentic identity. Recent research believes, too, in the way those dynamics are compromised by the technology innovations behind immersive spaces like the Metaverse, and by prevailing social forces observed in hospitality and tourism environments (Srivastava et al., 2025; Supina & Singh, 2024).

3.1 The Curated Self in Digital Contexts

The Dramaturgical Theory by Goffman (1959) is still one of the limiting assumptions, within which we can consider potential self-presentations as an act, a theatrical performance, wherein they control impressions to ensure that they conform to the expectations of others. This metaphor is enhanced in digital space, in social media platforms, the stage forms a constant, indexable and measurable space where performers create a lasting virtual stage of permanent retention. The front stage social-presenting posts, stories and profiles are socially favorable and back stage private messages, drafts, or "finsta" provide partial altruistic forgettances of the unedited self. Context collapse (boyd, 2010; Marwick & boyd, 2011) serves as the intensifier of the pressure to curate, blending friends, family, peers, employees into one homogeneous audience. This breakdown causes users to need to attack at the lowest common denominator, and reduce the risk of self expression in order to minimize risk of reputational harm. On this point of argument by indicating that the content promoted by, and popularized by, the algorithms running on a platform, encourage the self-presentation that is both socially and algorithmically programmed to be promoted. To Gen Z, the crafted personality is not a question of taste but an economic move in a visibility economy where a personal brand, career connections, or even the capacity to secure a job is which depends on the social media presence footprint (Hogan, 2010). Simultaneously, more recent researchers find that curated performances can also be applied to a workplace and service setting, and their employees have to practice digital self-presentation as well as be occupied with a customer facing position (Ambardar et al., 2023; Singh & Kumar, 2024).

3.2 Social Comparison and Identity Insecurity

Along with the emergence of curation, there has been the commodification of authenticity in digital culture. As being real is applauded, researchers caution of the fact that it tends to be performance authenticity carefully fighting not to appear as such but hoping to convey relatability (Warfield, 2014). The digital authenticity can sometimes lean more on sincerity, as well as strategic self-disclosure where it is still difficult to distinguish genuine performance, and calculated performance. There are different ways in which platform cultures have an impact on conventions of authenticity. Instagram promotes a sense of aesthetic authenticity whereby the everydayness of such aestheticism, casual messy hair, honesty postage posts are in actuality the result of a series of tries, and editing. In contrast, the algorithm in Tik Tok gives an incentive to spontaneity and humour, a more improvisational type of authenticity. Turkle (2011) warns though that it could be simulations that have been designed to look real but not to show more about the self. To the Gen Z generation, authenticity is dubious: demonstrating vulnerability can create a connection, but being too personal will be seen as judgmental or exploitative. This tension is what seems like authenticity is not a personal choice but experimental and negotiated in terms of the society and as a practice in which the platforms mediate its practice. Reported contemporary studies in the field of hospitality and organizational psychology indicate that the staff is also struggling with self-contradictions as they reconcile between demands of authentic engagement and conformity to performance as presented within professional expectations (Singh, 2025; Singh & Supina, 2024).

3.3 Social Comparison, Self-Discrepancy, and Psychological Strain

The Social Comparison Theory, by Festinger (1954), illustrates the psychological process through which, people compare themselves with other people. Online, comparisons of the upward type and downward comparisons with those who look better, less successful, or more socially tied, are usually prompted by the exposure to curated and ideal content (Vogel et al., 2014). The studies have also associated these upward comparisons with low self esteem (Valkenburg et al., 2006), dissatisfaction with their bodies (Yamamiya et al., 2005), and anxiety. The Self-Discrepancy Theory of Higgins (1987) is an addition to this: he pays attention to the emotional outcomes of the differences between the actual, the ideal, and the ought self. Deliberate exposure to curated content generates these gaps with ongoing exposure along with feelings of guilt, shame, or inadequacy (Bargh et al., 2002). According to Nadkarni and Hofmann (2012), social media enhances this effect since the conjunction of two psychological needs belongingness and self-presentation into a strengthening loop of validation-seeking and self-comparison is created in social media. To make the issue more complicated, a paradox of privacy (Debatin et al., 2009) demonstrates that users know the dangers but still tend to post personal content to gain social compensation. This contradiction is the cause of identity strain because the urge to be connected and the necessity to be safe are contrary. As recent AI research and Metaverse studies have suggested, algorithmically immersive environments only increase upward comparisons where the curated-authentic identity gap is at times even stronger (Al-Romeedy et al., 2025; Srivastava et al., 2025).

3.4 Platforms as Identity Architects

Social media sites are not neutral to the extent that they are the proactive creators of the norm of identities. Data colonialism as the production of personal and behavioral data as a resource. Both priorities algorithmic systems give to the material that generates the interest and users tend to prioritize emotion-inducing or emotional content more. According to Lupton (2016), self-tracking and quantification transforms into identity work integrating measurement into self-worth and digital measures. This is critiqued of visibility economy, in which a need to remain relevant demands one to produce platform-specific identity performances on an ongoing basis. This architecture imposes its rules covertly: the visible is rewarded and the invisible may socialise or not. In the case of Gen Z, where peer validation is playing a larger and larger role via these platforms, the algorithm becomes a spectator and a sawbwa. More current studies have also highlighted that AI, blockchain, and VR capacities are no longer regarded as peripheral requests in platform design, but the capabilities also influence what kinds of identities are able to be displayed, rewarded or suppressed (Francis et al., 2024; Singh & Hassan, 2024).

3.5 Navigating the Curated–Authentic Continuum

Violating structural pressures, users more so Gen Z adopt opportunistic measures to stabilize curated and authentic self-representations; boyd (2014) writes of how young people increasingly form private Instagram accounts known as finstas to share posts with specific audiences, or join underwriting interest online groups based on shared values, rather than mass appeal (Duffy & Hund, 2015). The other approach is selective vulnerability which helps in displaying some of the flaws under the guise of showing the authenticity at the same time avoids too much disclosure (Baym & boyd, 2012). Although such strategies might counter identity strain, they can also lead to identity fragmentation, and it becomes hard to have coherence among various online-based selves. According to recent studies that focus on cross-sectoral analysis, similar strategies apply in tourism and hospitality where individual and organizations weigh off curated branding and the necessity to present authenticity to clients (Singh & Bathla, 2023; Supina & Singh, 2025). The issue of curated-authentic continuum is thus not binary, but a negotiated area that varies due to the psychological needs, expectations of the audience, and the draws of the platform to engage in a particular activity. Under this fact, systemic intervention by design, policy and education is fundamental in creating environments that lead to the promotion of expressive freedom and psychological health. There is an increase in the calls that demand such systemic approaches, and scholars believe in the significance of integration between digital literacy, wellness procedures, and organizational ethics (Hassan et al., 2025; Sharma & Singh, 2025).

3.6 Generation Z, Tourism, and Curated Digital Identity

Gen Z can be characterised as one of the most transparent and diverse generations that combine personal identity with traveling and visibility online. They appreciate regardless, low-cost, individual, and culture- focus travel experiences; which are frequently purchased through AI-based or social-mediated services (Future Partners, 2025). Contrary to Millennial-motivated FOMO, Gen Z is shifting towards the authentic spontaneity and wants to experience a flexible and meaningful travel that fits their own values. The recent discoveries confirm the fact that Gen Z has highly identity-focused travel behavior: Marques et al. (2025) demonstrate that the age, gender and urban/rural living are key issues that provide women with the motivation to seek personal development and social connection whereas men attach great importance to the theme of nature and adventure. These motivations are not only stimulated by social media, and Gen Z travelers tend to become the drivers of such motivations (Suciu et al., 2024). In addition, being digital natives, they prefer to experience the authentic and sustainable and already understand immersive and Metaverse-capable types of travel (MDPI, 2024; MDPI, 2025).

4. RESEARCH GAPS

Although there is a good theoretical background given in the literature, some gaps still exist:

- Inadequate cross-cultural research: The majority of studies are western based and do not entirely reflect on Gen Z experience in non-west regions.
- Lack of longitudinal data: Not a lot of studies are longitudinal studies on the long-term psychological impact of identity curation in Gen Z.

- Platform-limited behaviors: These users should be analyzed more in comparison (i.e. LinkedIn vs. Tik Tok) and more among young users.
- Intersectionality/Gen Z: There is limited research on how gender, age, class, and ethnicity influence the identity practices individuals perform (specifically Gen Zers) when creating a curated identity.
- Combining with new technologies: Studies have not investigated, to the fullest, how AI, Metaverse spaces, and blockchain technologies step up the tension of curated-authentic identity (Al Aqad et al., 2025; Singh & Hassan, 2024).

5. METHODOLOGY

The research paper has adopted a qualitative integrative literature review research methodology to consolidate cross cutting views of interdisciplinary understanding of curated and authentic identity in cyberspace (Singh & Ansari, 2024). This approach facilitates the combination of theoretical formulations, conceptual theories, and empirical studies in the areas of psychology, sociology, communication and media studies. It aims to create an overall conceptual format on negotiating a digital identity through the extant research and theoretical bases (Hassan et al., 2025). The strategies of this type of integration are becoming more and more common in studies of hospitality, tourism, and digital wellness, where identity performance overlays with workplace psychology and self-presentation to customers.

5.1 Research Design

The paper takes the form of the qualitative integrative literature review method to bring together theoretical frameworks, conceptual understandings, and empirical studies about psychology, sociology, communication and media studies. In contrast to systematic reviews, is more quantitative, unlike systematic reviews, the method of the integrative review allows taking into consideration studies of various types, supports critical interaction with theoretical and empirical research (Whittemore & Knafl, 2005). This will be necessary because of the multidimensional nature of the phenomena which is often difficult to investigate, like the curated- authentic identity continuum. Following the latest methodological controversies, one can also communicate the way AI-generated environment and social interactions provided by the Metaverse transform the conventional concept of qualitative research (Al Aqad et al., 2025).

5.2 Data Sources and Selection Criteria

Using a set of search forms structured search of peer-reviewed articles in Scopus-indexed journals, academic book publishers (e.g., Oxford University Press, Yale University Press, Routledge, MIT Press), or databases such as Google Scholar, JSTOR, SpringerLink, ScienceDirect, and SAGE Journals, the literature was identified. Sources that were searched were in publication dates ranging between 2002 and 2024, including the fundamental theories as well as the modern research. Inclusion criteria were as under:Articles that deal with online self-representation, the digital self, authenticity, social comparison or influence by algorithms.Research that incorporated or used theoretical models like Dramaturgical Theory by Goffman (1959) social comparison theory developed by Festinger (1954), and self-discrepancy theory by Higgins (1987).Empirical research on the topic of social media networks (e.g., Instagram, Tik Tok, Facebook, LinkedIn) in terms of identity construction among the Gen Z.Non-peer-reviewed material, studies that were unrelated to identity performance, and unwork that was not theoretically supported were excluded (Rai & Singh, 2026). Recent research on professional branding through curated online identities in the workplace as well as its emerging scholarship was also taken into consideration wherever applicable (Singh & Kumar, 2024)

5.3 Analytical Framework

Thematic analysis was performed on the literature through an iterative coding process which identified recurring coding concepts, patterns and relationships. Three major theoretical approaches helped to execute the analysis: According to Goffman, Dramaturgical Theory (1959) to mean performative self-presentation as well as impression management at the online space.The importance of comparison in the development of curated identity behavior was investigated using the Social Comparison Theory by Festinger social comparison theory (1954).The Self-Discrepancy Theory of Higgins (1987) to test the psychological effects of identity misalignment. These frameworks were overlapped with the new notions, including context collapse (boyd, 2010), performative authenticity (Warfield, 2014), and algorithmic influence, and formed a coherent conceptual 3D map. To further the analysis, papers in hospitality, tourism and innovative digital terms were analyzed, these areas also point to the fusion of customer-facing curated identity and worker-centered well-being (Ambardar et al., 2023; Singh & Sihmar, 2025).

5.4 Limitations

As contrary to what is assumed by the empirical research, the method of the integrative review provides certain conceptual richness, but the lack of statistical generalizability. Cultural differences in the performance of digital identity have been underexplored because of the focus of Western-centric research. As well, the platform-specific behaviors can have a large variance that need more comparative and longitudinal studies. Additionally, it is evident that under stones recent studies regarding AI, wellness tourism, and interactions in the Metaverse (Sharma & Singh, 2025; Srivastava et al., 2025) propose that identity pressures are already increasing, but the evidence is new and lacking analysis.

5.5 Ethical Considerations

Since the study only utilizes secondary data by means of publicly accessible, peer reviewed scholarly references; there were no ethical clearance or human subject approval needs. Nevertheless, all sources are cited accordingly and the interpretations are based on scholarly rigor to shun prejudices and misappropriation.

6. DISCUSSION

The combination of the integrative literature review helps understand the intricate nature of digital self-presentation in which both cultured and authentic dimension of online personas tend to co-exist in conflict. In the case of Gen Z, who inhabit the focal point between reason and digital immersion, these tensions are not mere behavioral adherents, but profoundly psychological ones. Addressing both technological limitations, social pressures, and identity formation, the group particularly those, who belong to Gen Z, must address the challenges of expressing themselves using digital means even more after online technology is adopting a more and more significant role in mediating personal expression. This segment critically analyzes the results within the perspective of the chosen theories and provides an idea on the implication of curated identity performance on-line.

6.1 Identity as a Performed Necessity

The dramaturgical perspective designed by Goffman (1959) frames social interaction in everyday situations as a type of performance, with people practicing impression management so that their outer image is perpendicular to the expectations of the audience. In the digital realm, such performativity is enhanced under the influence of an algorithmic incentive system where high visibility, compelling, and aesthetically valuable pieces of information are valued. Leading social networks such as Instagram or Tik Tok articulate success in likes and shares as well as followers, which has something to do with a loop of feedback where the content that meets product trends in a social source is prioritized. Subsequently, users do shape their identities not just to express themselves but to satisfy the implicit requirements of the algorithm, and the explicit requirements or expectations of their audience. A similar treatment of performativity is now undertaken in the context of tourism and hospitality where service workers assume the role of different personas in an effort to fit the brand of an organisation (Singh, 2025; Supina & Singh, 2024). This is further complicated by the so-called phenomenon of context collapse where a varied audience (e.g., friends, family, colleagues, strangers, etc.) gathers on one platform (boyd, 2010; Marwick & boyd, 2011). Users are often being forced to select one, patio cleansing identity mainstream that attracts a wide market more than complex choices. Since Gen Z is still in the early years of identity formation, requiring an acceptable way of self-presentation in a very public place where to be judged is quite probable, presenting self-identity can be not only self-involuntary but also necessitates to conform to the demands of interpersonal communication.

6.2 Authenticity as a Commodity

Although authenticity is frequently promoted in the digital culture, the very concept became a source of commercializing it and utilizing it as the strategy to gain greater involvement. Performative authenticity involves the attempts by Warfield (2014) to produce trust and intimacy in the process of developing a relationship with an audience by staging such aspects of the self as vulnerability, relatability, or imperfection carefully. To provide an example, influencers post behind-the-scenes, or messy realities, which seem spontaneous, yet actually are edited with the idea of soliding parasocial relationships and keeping their audience membership. This is especially noticeable in influencer marketing, where fake claims of authentic either intention can be the camouflage of a commercial intent. Turkle (2011) warns that this kind of simulated authenticity poses a threat to displace authentic person to person interaction with simulation as an emotional performance that is an art-manufactured emotion release targeted at the mass market. Platform culture has its own concept of what is considered to be authentic. The culture of Tik Tok favors unpolished, unscripted and comedic content whereas the Instagram culture is more oriented to image perfection and idealism. This proves that authenticity is never an attractively wide-cut but it is platform resultant mode of performance that shapes itself to the expectations of audiences and algorithms. The new research has indicated that even in the context of tourism and wellness relating to healthcare practitioners, the concept of authentic experience is designed to conform to the consumption needs of the consumer, which indicates the process of larger cultural commoditating authenticity (Hassan et al., 2025; Pandey et al., 2025).

6.3 Psychological Costs of Identity Curation

Mental health is costly since people are under constant pressure to post paint something that makes them desirable to others on-line. The Social Comparison Theory by Festinger (1954) brings out how individuals will compare themselves whenever they need to do so against others without actually having any objective standards. These comparisons are of an upward nature in social media where most people feel exposed to idealized versions of lifestyles, achievements, and appearance. Studies indicate that this upward comparison is backed by low self esteem, dissatisfaction with the body and enhanced anxiety (Valkenburg et al., 2006; Yamamiya et al., 2005). Nadkarni and Hofmann (2012) also observe that social media sites generate two major psychological drives belongingness and self-presentation in a symbiotic cycle where social members will constantly change their identity to ensure social acceptance. The Self-Discrepancy Theory by Higgins (1987) provides the information on the emotional cost of these pressures. Mismatches between the actual self (perception one has of him/herself), the ideal self (perception one believes he/she should be) and the ought self (perception one believes he/she ought to be) tend to lead to inadequacy, impostor syndrome, and emotional burnout (Bargh et al., 2002). Moreover, privacy lowers and threat of unintended self disclosure (Debatin et al., 2009), which introduces an extra level of psychological tension as the user balances the urge to connect and fear of the loss of reputation (Al-Romeedy et al., 2025; Srivastava et al., 2025). Recent Metaverse research confirms that such incompatibilities are further amplified by the immersive digital space where the gap between the edited avatars and the real world is increased as a result of the physical space.

6.4 Platforms as Architects of Identity Norms

Digital spaces are not neutral intermediaries; they are social realities in action and determine which and who types of identities are visible, desirable and rewarded. Couldry and Mejias (2019) posit that platforms follow the principles of data colonialism as they build value by leveraging participation by users and organize online relationships in ways that enhance interactions. Curation by algorithm favors some aesthetic, behavioral, and cultural industry standards, which shapes the way users form vision of success and genuineness. As an example, a positive or negative reaction with a high emotional response has a greater tendency of being promoted thus supporting a performance based culture. Self-tracking technologies, e.g. fitness apps or productivity trackers are seen by Lupton (2016) as being part of innuendo of ever-present self-observation, in which personal value is pegged on behavioral indicators that are measurable. This structure promotes a feedback mechanism in, visibility turns into a means of payment, it regularly surpasses personal alignment or even emotional comfort. Such an environment does not just represent identity but also in co-construction with the logic of algorithm constructing the platform itself (Islam & Singh, 2025; Singh & Kumar, 2025). New studies indicate this has been carried into service and tourism sectors, where forms and applications determine the manner in which employees and organizations can present themselves to the clients.

6.5 Navigating the Curated–Authentic Continuum

Regardless of such structural and digital pressures, users particularly among Gen Z are not passive consumers. A variety use tactical self-presentation strategies to handle the curated-authentic continuum; boyd (2014) records how youth users maintain several accounts ("finstas" when friends access, and "rinstas" when others see) to segment their audience. Others engage in niche online communities in which a sense of authenticity is framed by normative standards as opposed to conventional measures of mainstream popularity. Deliberate disclosure of a selective vulnerability with intention to withhold other forms of vulnerability can also be one way of recovering some power in self-presentation. This may however become the site of identity fragmentation where one cannot integrate his various online identities with the offline counterparts. According to Baym and boyd (2012), even though such strategies can cushion the emotional well-being, they also play into maintaining the cycle of performance as they require ongoing audience management. Finally, the dilemma is the balance between the social capital acquired as a result of strategic self-presentation and emotional maintenance in a media ecosystem that is designed to advantage practice rather than authenticity systemically (Singh & Sihmar, 2025; Sharma & Singh, 2025). This stress highlights the significance of interventions at the educational, policy, and platform levels in order to design healthier digital identity practices. Raising awareness across sectors (e.g. of tourism, higher education, and workplace psychology) and implementing wellness strategies and company support (combined with cross sectoral awareness-e.g. of workplace psychology) to mitigate identity strain is being more and more made by scholars.

6.6 AI, Identity, and Mental Health

There are significant psychological effects of AI personalization. Individual self-esteem has been found to decrease with most people, whereas communal self-concept is often improved as a result of the algorithmic identity tools (RAMSS, 2024)

Figure 2. Curated–Authentic Identity Continuum

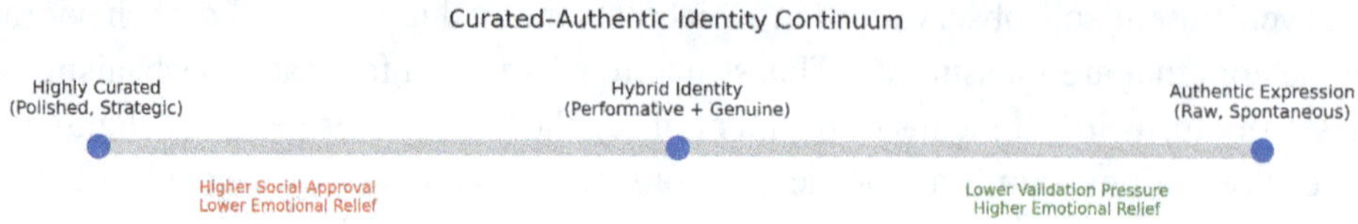

Source: Author's own elaboration

Figure 2 illustrate the continuum from curated to authentic identity expression in digital spaces, highlighting the trade-offs between social validation and emotional relief, especially for Gen Z.

In the meantime, AI interventions are capable of reducing anxiety and enhancing future self-coherence, so-called Future You (Pataranutaporn et al., 2024). Conversely, appearance induction or image-altering tools (e.g. filters, deepfakes) might also result in self-objectification and emotional disruption (Agrawal et al., 2025). These results indicate the conflict between curated identity empowerment and psychological stress.

7. RECOMMENDATIONS

By focusing on the challenge of curated vs. authentic identity performance as a complex and in many ways competing aspect of life among Generation Z, an interdisciplinary and multi-stakeholder approach to the issue is necessary, both in terms of psychological health and systemic change. At the personal level, the Gen Z users are to be furnished with the means to develop reflective and emotionally sustainable online practices. Methodologies, including purposeful, pre-post self-reflection, digital form of journaling to identify trends of anxiety triggered by comparison, and conscious practices such as the process of digital detox, will offer agency against the unremitting influence of algorithmically preprogrammed response loops and peer validation pressures. In addition, context collapse can be offset by keeping professional, personal, and creative online identities separate further using privacy settings or separate accounts and choosing authenticity role models in content-creator roles and normalizing impersonation can establish healthier standards of self-valuation. Teachers, in their turn, have to bear the task of instilling digital identity algorithms into the media literacy classes to make sure learners do not just possess the skills to operate the algorithms themselves, but they also are aware of the psychological models behind their online practices (Self-Discrepancy Theory and Social Comparison Theory). In addition to theory, resilience can be promoted through workshops and collaborative efforts that offer safe spaces to discuss the social-media pressures and be creative in areas that cannot be measured with metrics. On the platform design tier, social media organizations need to recognize their ethical duty to scale mental health above engagement metrics with such interventions as default hidden counts among minors, customizable algorithmic feeds and independent modes of sharing where people are free to express themselves and harbor no reputational fear. Wellness nudges and usage warnings should be offered to minimize the tendency to compulsivity that further increases the emotional strain. Researchers, on their part, need to extend the Gen Z-research question by introducing longitudinal studies that can help to trace the evolving psychological effects of curation, cross-cultural studies that would explain the collectivist and individualist identity norms, and intersectional studies which would integrate vulnerability of gender, class, ethnicity, and sexuality. Intervention research based on the evidence like the reduction of the influence of hidden likes or digital detox option is, in particular, urgent. Lastly, the inspections are played by removing legislation, formerly, in form of creating protection structures by making mental health impact analysis a requirement whenever developing new features and age-true privacy default terms, as well as controlling the accurate revelation of influencer stalsmanhood (Supina & Singh, 2025; Sharma & Singh, 2025). Education at the local level regarding digital well-being and investments in so-called tech-to-do-good projects with strong focus on inclusivity and ethical considerations are also a necessity. The net effect of these measures is taking individual coping beyond the personal and structural change serving as a means to secure digital selfhood of Gen Z in terms of not only emotional strength amenable to external disruptions but also authenticity and stability of identity. Consistent with other recent research relating digital wellness to organizational psychology, tourism studies, and Multi-Member Organizational sociality (Srivastava et al., 2025) such recommendations reflect the appropriateness of a meta-level approach to intervention to free and empower digital natives during their most confrontational years of life.

8. FUTURE RESEARCH DIRECTIONS

Though the current literature offers a deep set of understanding on the nature of the curated-authentic identity continuum, the discipline remains immature in its ability to describe over time, cross-cultural, and intersectional nuances of the digital lifeworlds of Gen Z. The psychological effect of long-term exposure to curated material is one of the most urgent areas of investigation, especially when Gen Zin the face of growing up as practitioners of early identity, bring these practices into the spheres of professional, relationship, and civic life. The longitudinal research or the diary-based research offers potentially invaluable information as to whether the identity strain (affected at the adolescence stage) consequently turns into chronic mental health problems including burnout, depression, or impostor syndrome, or whether there are adaptive coping mechanisms which alleviate such risks in the long run (Sharma & Singh, 2025). The comparative research across platforms is yet another urging area since the identity norms active in Instagram due to their aesthetical perfection, Tik Tok due to its performance humor, LinkedIn due to professional curation, and those in the new Metaverse setting contrast markedly. Comparative approaches of this kind would help explain how audiences develop identity pressures more intensely or diluted by platform architectures, audience cultures, and algorithms in their design (Ambardar et al., 2023). There is also need to carry out cross cultural studies since most of the studies have been Western-focused. In collectivist cultures like India or East Asia, gen zers might orient to authenticity in different ways, and these practices will affect a variety of identity negotiation. There is another gap in intersectionality: few studies describe the way gender, sexuality, caste/class, and ethnicity interact to generate different experiences of digital identity stress, and the new South Asian scholarship starts considering them (Rai & Singh, 2026). In addition, scholars should find a way of differentiating between the performative (authenticity) as a strategic show of weakness to earn social capital and the authenticity, which facilitates emotional wellbeing. Is performative vulnerability a contributing factor to strain by maintaining performance cycles or to supportive peer relationships? To respond to this, experimental and ethnographic studies are needed to measure the motivations of the users and their results. The issue of algorithmic influence is also worth further explanation, especially in terms of how the concept of personalization, ranking due to engagement, or an immersive aspect of the avatars in the Metaverse defines what is perceived to be a definition of what is actually real or is worthy of demonstration (Srivastava et al., 2025). Last but not least, research through intervention is to take center stage: experimenting with digital attributes like hidden likes, silent settings, or well-being nudges assisted by artificial intelligence can shift a diagnosis to solution (Singh, 2025). Digital burnout, identity fragmentation among several accounts, and the possibility of a digital minimalism approach to create such coherence are also disseminated and prioritized in urgent terms, especially as online identity fatigue itself seems to carry the same implications as workplace burnout. Together, future studies need to be designed out of Western, short-term, and single-platform studies into longitudinal, intersectional and intervention based designs that have meaningful actionable advice to individuals, institutions and policy makers.

9. CONCLUSION

This paper has discussed the long-standing conflict between mediated and authentic expression of identity on the internet with special reference to generation Z, who happen to be the first generation to be born into a fully networked existence that is entirely algorithm-mediated over the span of their developmental lives. The analysis has shown that an individual identity is influenced by a compound interaction of psychological needs, socio cultural pressures and technological architectures in identity construction with the references to Goffman dramaturgical perspective, Festinger social comparison framework and Higgins self-discrepancy model of identity construction in the digital forms. The results indicate that identity performance on the internet has ceased to be a self-performative act and rather it is a social requirement as per the incentives inherent in an algorithm, monitoring by others, and adherence to platform guidelines. The concept of authenticity is now a commodified form of self-presentation that defines differently across platforms, including Instagram, Tik Tok and LinkedIn, with its psychic impact in the form of lowered self esteem and personal identity dissonance as well as emotional exhaustion. Meanwhile, platforms do not just act as neutral intermediary they are agenda-setters of identity norms, promoting some aesthetics and patterns of behaviour and making others unrecognizable. Despite the tactical solutions that Gen Z received like engaging in a multi-account setting, selective vulnerability, and building alternate spaces, the strategies may come at the cost of their identities being fragmented and overly exhausted in the long run. The larger implication is that the continuum of curated-authentic identity is not the particular pathology of the person and, on the contrary, a systemic and cultural process but one at which the collective obligation involves all the stakeholders. Reflective practices among gen Z users should be actively promoted; researchers and curriculums must incorporate elements of digital and emotional literacy; designers should include well-being elements inuser interaction; researchers are required to generate cross-cultural, longitudinal, and intersectional evidence; and policy makers need to regulate algorithmic practices that affect vulnerable users disproportionately. Recent research has validated that unless systematic interventions are implemented, digital identity fatigue is only going to occur even more across the various contexts, such as workplace branding or wellness tourism, or even in immersive Metaverse virtual space (Srivastava et al., 2025). Finally, it is crucial to remake the digital ecosystem as the realm that considers authenticity, emotional stability, and inclusivity and considers these issues as the factor that can protect not only the psychological stability of the Generation Z but the future between the digital culture. Through re-evaluing our notion of performance-centered paradigm into something that appreciates authentic connection and stability in their identities, we will be capable of making an online world in which every individual feels free to be authentic to himself or herself without necessarily losing their minds and social belonging.

REFERENCES

Ansari, A. I., & Singh, A. (2023). Application of augmented reality (AR) and virtual reality (VR) in promoting guest room sales: A critical review. In Z. Tučková, S. K. Dey, H. H. Thai, & S. D. Hoang (Eds.), Impact of Industry 4.0 on sustainable tourism (pp. 95–104). Emerald Publishing. https://doi.org/DOI: 10.1108/978-1-80455-157-820231006

Bargh, J. A., McKenna, K. Y. A., & Fitzsimons, G. M. (2002). Can you see the real me? Activation and expression of the "true self" on the Internet. *The Journal of Social Issues*, *58*(1), 33–48. DOI: 10.1111/1540-4560.00247

Baym, N. K., & boyd, . (2012). Socially mediated publicness: An introduction. *Journal of Broadcasting & Electronic Media*, *56*(3), 320–329. DOI: 10.1080/08838151.2012.705200

boyd, d. (2010). Social network sites as networked publics: Affordances, dynamics, and implications. In Z. Papacharissi (Ed.), A networked self (pp. 39–58). Routledge.

Debatin, B., Lovejoy, J. P., Horn, A.-K., & Hughes, B. N. (2009). Facebook and online privacy: Attitudes, behaviors, and unintended consequences. *Journal of Computer-Mediated Communication*, *15*(1), 83–108. DOI: 10.1111/j.1083-6101.2009.01494.x

Duffy, B. E., & Hund, E. (2015). "Having it all" on social media: Entrepreneurial femininity and self-branding among fashion bloggers. *Social Media + Society*, *1*(2), 1–11. DOI: 10.1177/2056305115604337

Francis, R. S., Anantharajah, S., Sengupta, S., & Singh, A. (2024). Leveraging ChatGPT and digital marketing for enhanced customer engagement in the hotel industry. In Bansal, R., Ngah, A., Chakir, A., & Pruthi, N. (Eds.), *Leveraging ChatGPT and artificial intelligence for effective customer engagement* (pp. 55–68). IGI Global., DOI: 10.4018/979-8-3693-0815-8.ch004

Future Partners. (2025). What's new with Gen Z travelers? Future Partners Blog. Retrieved from https://futurepartners.com/blog/whats-new-with-gen-z/

Hassan, V. I., Singh, A., Jaboob, A. S., & Sorayyaei Azar, A. (Eds.). (2025). *Revolutionizing healthcare experience with digital medical tourism*. IGI Global., DOI: 10.4018/979-8-3693-7888-5

Hogan, B. (2010). The presentation of self in the age of social media: Distinguishing performances and exhibitions online. *Bulletin of Science, Technology & Society*, *30*(6), 377–386. DOI: 10.1177/0270467610385893

Islam, N., & Singh, A. (2025). Role of digitalization into hospitality businesses: Innovations and trends. In Rana, V., Bathla, G., Raina, A., & Chhabra, D. (Eds.), *Transforming the service sector with new technology* (pp. 447–458). IGI Global., DOI: 10.4018/979-8-3693-7447-4.ch027

Kaplan, A. M., & Haenlein, M. (2010). Users of the world, unite! The challenges and opportunities of social media. *Business Horizons*, *53*(1), 59–68. DOI: 10.1016/j.bushor.2009.09.003

Marques, J., Gomes, S., Ferreira, M., Rebuá, M., & Marques, H. (2025). Generation Z and travel motivations: The impact of age, gender, and residence. *Tourism and Hospitality*, *6*(2), 82. Advance online publication. DOI: 10.3390/tourhosp6020082

Marwick, A. E., & boyd, . (2011). To see and be seen: Celebrity practice on Twitter. *Convergence (London)*, *17*(2), 139–158. DOI: 10.1177/1354856510394539

MDPI. (2024). Generation Z's preferences for virtual tourism and sustainable experiences. *Sustainability*, *16*(24), 10858. Advance online publication. DOI: 10.3390/su162410858

MDPI. (2025). Digital natives on the move: Cross-cultural insights into Generation Z global tourism. *Sustainability*, *17*(14), 6601. Advance online publication. DOI: 10.3390/su17146601

Nadkarni, A., & Hofmann, S. G. (2012). Why do people use Facebook? *Personality and Individual Differences*, *52*(3), 243–249. DOI: 10.1016/j.paid.2011.11.007 PMID: 22544987

Pataranutaporn, P., ... (2024). Future You: AI-mediated self-connection and reduced anxiety. ArXiv preprint. https://arxiv.org/abs/2405.12514

Rai, V., & Singh, A. (2026). The digital renaissance of hospitality. In Talukder, M., & Chowdhury, H. (Eds.), *Smart operations in hospitality* (pp. 125–144). IGI Global., DOI: 10.4018/979-8-3373-2145-5.ch005

Sharma, R., & Singh, A. (2025). Prospective wellness and medical tourism sectors: Achieving invincibility. In Hassan, V., Singh, A., Jaboob, A., & Sorayyaei Azar, A. (Eds.), *Revolutionizing healthcare experience with digital medical tourism* (pp. 251–264). IGI Global., DOI: 10.4018/979-8-3693-7888-5.ch010

Singh, A. (2025). Analysis of perceptions on employment of differently-abled people in the Indian hotel industry. *Pasos (El Sauzal)*, *23*(1), 167–183. DOI: 10.25145/j.pasos.2025.23.011

Singh, A., & Ansari, A. I. (2024). Role of training and development in employee motivation. In Mazurowski, T. (Ed.), *Enhancing employee motivation* (pp. 248–261). IGI Global., DOI: 10.4018/979-8-3693-1674-0.ch011

Singh, A., & Bathla, G. (2023). Fostering Creativity and Innovation: Tourism and Hospitality Perspective. In P. Tyagi, V. Nadda, V. Bharti, & E. Kemer (Eds.), Embracing Business Sustainability Through Innovation and Creativity in the Service Sector (pp. 70-83). IGI Global Scientific Publishing. DOI: 10.4018/978-1-6684-6732-9.ch005

Singh, A., & Hassan, S. C. (2024). Identifying the skill gap in the workplace. In A. M. Thake et al. (Eds.), Contemporary challenges in social science management (Vol. 112B, pp. 101–114). Emerald. https://doi.org/DOI: 10.1108/S1569-37592024000112B006

Singh, A., & Kumar, S. (2024). Effective talent management practices. In Christiansen, B. (Eds.), *Global practices on talent acquisition* (pp. 126–144). IGI Global., DOI: 10.4018/979-8-3693-1938-3.ch008

Singh, A., & Kumar, V. (2025). Organizational innovation and adaptation in hospitality. In Ramos, C. (Eds.), *Open innovation and technology in tourism* (pp. 355–372). IGI Global., DOI: 10.4018/979-8-3693-8633-0.ch018

Singh, A., & Sihmar, P. (2025). Higher education institution sustainability. In Adu-Gyamfi, M. (Eds.), *Green HRM awareness* (pp. 1–14). IGI Global., DOI: 10.4018/979-8-3693-2956-6.ch001

Singh, A., & Supina, S. (2024). Talent acquisition and retention. In Christiansen, B. (Eds.), *Global practices on talent acquisition* (pp. 363–379). IGI Global., DOI: 10.4018/979-8-3693-1938-3.ch020

Srivastava, A., Singh, B. M., Singh, A., & Singh, A. (2025). Customer immersiveness and customer retention. In Al Aqad, M. (Eds.), *Navigating AI and the metaverse* (pp. 475–500). IGI Global., DOI: 10.4018/979-8-3373-0340-6.ch023

Suciu, S. A., Georgescu, M. I., & Stănciulescu, M. (2024). Exploring the Generation Z travel trends and behavior. *SBE: Economics and Business*, *19*(Special Issue), 189. Advance online publication. DOI: 10.2478/sbe-2024-0010

Supina, S., & Singh, A. (2024). Exploring the presence and adoption of quality of work-life dimensions. *African Journal of Hospitality, Tourism and Leisure*, *13*(2), 421–429. DOI: 10.46222/ajhtl.19770720.524

Supina, S., & Singh, A. (2025). Accentuating responsible travel in an ecotourism destination. In Tyagi, P. K. (Eds.), *Meaningful tourism* (pp. 269–279). Emerald., DOI: 10.1108/978-1-83797-837-320251035

Valkenburg, P. M., Peter, J., & Schouten, A. P. (2006). Friend networking sites and their relationship to adolescents' well-being. *Cyberpsychology & Behavior*, *9*(5), 584–590. DOI: 10.1089/cpb.2006.9.584 PMID: 17034326

Vogel, E. A., Rose, J. P., Roberts, L. R., & Eckles, K. (2014). Social comparison, social media, and self-esteem. *Psychology of Popular Media Culture*, *3*(4), 206–222. DOI: 10.1037/ppm0000047

Warfield, K. (2014). Making selfies/making self. *Studies in Social Justice*, *8*(2), 206–223. DOI: 10.26522/ssj.v8i2.1144

Whittemore, R., & Knafl, K. (2005). The integrative review. *Journal of Advanced Nursing*, *52*(5), 546–553. DOI: 10.1111/j.1365-2648.2005.03621.x PMID: 16268861

Yamamiya, Y., Cash, T. F., Melnyk, S. E., Posavac, H. D., & Posavac, S. S. (2005). Women's exposure to thin-and-beautiful media images. *Body Image*, *2*(1), 74–80. DOI: 10.1016/j.bodyim.2004.11.001 PMID: 18089176

Zhao, S., Grasmuck, S., & Martin, J. (2008). Identity construction on Facebook. *Computers in Human Behavior*, *24*(5), 1816–1836. DOI: 10.1016/j.chb.2008.02.012

Chapter 5
Digital Comparison and Performative Lifestyles

Jyothirmaye Reddy S.
https://orcid.org/0000-0002-1629-5777
Marwadi University, India

P. Selvakumar
https://orcid.org/0000-0002-3650-4548
Department of Science and Humanities, Nehru Institute of Technology, Coimbatore, India

Manjunath T. C.
https://orcid.org/0000-0003-2545-9160
Rajarajeswari College of Engineering, India

Kanagaraj A. R.
https://orcid.org/0000-0002-6502-0817
Dr. N.G.P. Arts and Science College, India

Jai Balaji
https://orcid.org/0009-0003-2642-4717
T. John College, India

Sarala Hemanth Kumar
https://orcid.org/0009-0007-2987-4405
Padmashree Institute of Management and Sciences, India

ABSTRACT

In the digital age, the mirror that reflects our self-perception has undergone a dramatic transformation. No longer is it merely shaped by personal introspection, face-to-face social interactions, or traditional media; today, our self-image is increasingly constructed and reconstructed through the lens of social media. Platforms like Instagram, TikTok, Facebook, Snapchat, and X (formerly Twitter) have become powerful tools of self-expression—but also, subtly and persistently, instruments of comparison. At the heart of this transformation lies what psychologists and sociologists now term "digital comparison": a phenomenon in which individuals continuously measure their lives, appearances, achievements, and experiences against those portrayed by others in online spaces. While comparison has always been a part of the human

DOI: 10.4018/979-8-3373-4516-1.ch005

psyche, the advent of social media has radically amplified its scope, frequency, and psychological impact. Digital comparison is not merely about glancing at a friend's vacation photo or admiring a celebrity's new fashion post.

Social Media's Impact on Self-Perception

In the digital age, the mirror that reflects our self-perception has undergone a dramatic transformation. No longer is it merely shaped by personal introspection, face-to-face social interactions, or traditional media; today, our self-image is increasingly constructed and reconstructed through the lens of social media. Platforms like Instagram, TikTok, Facebook, Snapchat, and X (formerly Twitter) have become powerful tools of self-expression—but also, subtly and persistently, instruments of comparison. At the heart of this transformation lies what psychologists and sociologists now term "digital comparison": a phenomenon in which individuals continuously measure their lives, appearances, achievements, and experiences against those portrayed by others in online spaces. While comparison has always been a part of the human psyche, the advent of social media has radically amplified its scope, frequency, and psychological impact. Digital comparison is not merely about glancing at a friend's vacation photo or admiring a celebrity's new fashion post; it represents a fundamental shift in how people evaluate themselves in relation to others. These platforms have normalized a culture of hyper-curated content—idealized snapshots of life that often mask the complexities of reality. Through filters, edits, and selective posting, users present polished versions of themselves, creating a collective illusion of perfection that others perceive as authentic. As a result, the boundaries between reality and representation become blurred, and many individuals internalize these digital portrayals as standards they must live up to (Algharabat & Shatnawi, 2014).

This can lead to heightened feelings of inadequacy, anxiety, low self-esteem, and a distorted self-concept, especially among adolescents and young adults who are still forming their identities. In the digital age, the mirror that reflects our self-perception has undergone a dramatic transformation. No longer is it merely shaped by personal introspection, face-to-face social interactions, or traditional media; today, our self-image is increasingly constructed and reconstructed through the lens of social media. Platforms like Instagram, TikTok, Facebook, Snapchat, and X (formerly Twitter) have become powerful tools of self-expression—but also, subtly and persistently, instruments of comparison. At the heart of this transformation lies what psychologists and sociologists now term "digital comparison": a phenomenon in which individuals continuously measure their lives, appearances, achievements, and experiences against those portrayed by others in online spaces. While comparison has always been a part of the human psyche, the advent of social media has radically amplified its scope, frequency, and psychological impact. Digital comparison is not merely about glancing at a friend's vacation photo or admiring a celebrity's new fashion post; it represents a fundamental shift in how people evaluate themselves in relation to others.

These platforms have normalized a culture of hyper-curated content—idealized snapshots of life that often mask the complexities of reality. Through filters, edits, and selective posting, users present polished versions of themselves, creating a collective illusion of perfection that others perceive as authentic. As a result, the boundaries between reality and representation become blurred, and many individuals internalize these digital portrayals as standards they must live up to. (Al-Maghrabi et al., 2011) This can lead to heightened feelings of inadequacy, anxiety, low self-esteem, and a distorted self-concept, especially among adolescents and young adults who are still forming their identities. The psychology behind digital comparison is deeply rooted in social comparison theory, introduced by Leon Festinger in 1954, which posits that people determine their own social and personal worth based on how they stack up against others. This awareness can also inform policy discussions, educational interventions, and platform design strategies aimed at mitigating the harms of social media (Berbegal-Mirabent et al., 2016)while preserving its benefits. Ultimately, the goal is not to eliminate comparison altogether—an impossible task—but to cultivate digital environments that promote self-acceptance, critical thinking, and emotional well-being. In sum, the rise of digital comparison represents a pivotal evolution in how we perceive ourselves and relate to others. Social media has created a new mirror—one that reflects not who we are, but who we think we should be, based on the fragmented images of others. As this phenomenon continues to shape modern identity, it challenges us to rethink authenticity, self-worth, and the narratives we both consume and create. The impact of social media on self-perception is complex and multifaceted, demanding thoughtful exploration and conscious engagement from users, developers, educators, and policymakers alike

The Psychology of Digital Comparison: Understanding the Human Impact

In the age of social media, identity is no longer a fixed construct defined solely by personal experiences, relationships, or cultural background; it has become a dynamic performance, curated for public consumption in the digital realm. The concept of a "performative lifestyle" encapsulates this phenomenon, describing the deliberate and often strategic way individuals present themselves online to craft a specific narrative or image. Unlike traditional forms of self-expression, which were limited to real-life interactions or static media, digital platforms now offer users the ability to continuously edit, broadcast, and amplify selected aspects of their lives. Whether it's through an Instagram post, a TikTok video, a Facebook update, or a LinkedIn profile, users shape their identities to align with aesthetic, social, or ideological trends—often prioritizing how their life appears over how it is actually lived.Performative lifestyles are rooted in the idea that the self is not merely expressed but *performed*. Drawing from sociologist Erving Goffman's theory of dramaturgy, which compares social interaction to theatrical performance, modern social media users occupy a digital stage, consciously managing impressions and audience perceptions. Goffman's "front stage" and "back stage" metaphor is particularly relevant: the front stage represents the curated content we share with the world—filtered photos, polished captions, and highlight reels—while the back stage encompasses the unfiltered realities we often hide, such as moments of vulnerability, failure, or emotional struggle. Social media, by its very design, encourages front stage behavior. Platforms reward visually appealing, engaging, and emotionally resonant content with likes, shares, and followers, incentivizing users to present an idealized version of themselves.

As a result, the boundaries between authenticity and performance become increasingly blurred.This curatorial process is not necessarily disingenuous; rather, it reflects a new mode of self-representation that is shaped by social norms, technological affordances, and cultural expectations. Users don't just share their lives—they construct a narrative around who they are, who they aspire to be, and how they wish to be seen. This narrative can be aspirational, artistic, humorous, political, spiritual, or professional. Influencers exemplify this trend by turning everyday life into a brand, showcasing routines, values, and aesthetics in a way that is both relatable and enviable. However, the practice is not confined to celebrities or digital entrepreneurs. Ordinary users also engage in performative acts—whether (Beritelli & Schegg, 2016)it's staging a photo of a morning coffee, posting workout milestones, or sharing vacation highlights—often with an awareness of how their content will be perceived by others.The performative nature of online identity is reinforced by the architecture of social media platforms. Algorithm-driven feeds prioritize engagement, making viral potential and social validation integral to how content is shared and seen. Metrics such as likes, comments, shares, and follower counts become proxies for value and popularity, subtly influencing the way users craft their posts. These digital markers not only reflect audience approval but also shape the content that follows, creating feedback loops that reinforce certain behaviors while discouraging others. Users may begin tailoring their lives around what "performs well" online, even if it means distorting reality. Over time, this can lead to a dissonance between the digital self and the authentic self, resulting in emotional fatigue, identity confusion, or imposter syndrome.Moreover, performative lifestyles are shaped by broader cultural and socio-political forces. In an era where social awareness and activism are expected, performativity extends beyond aesthetics to encompass moral and ideological stances. Terms like "performative activism" have emerged to critique individuals or brands who publicly endorse social causes more for visibility and approval than genuine engagement. (Chib et al., 2025)This suggests that identity performance is not just about self-image but also about public morality and alignment with collective values. Creators post unedited images, share behind-the-scenes realities, and engage in candid storytelling as a form of resistance to the performative norms. (Dahiya et al., 2025)While these acts, too, can become performative in their own way, they represent a growing desire for more genuine, human-centered digital interactions.

The Comparison Trap: How Social Media Fuels Insecurity and Anxiety

In the interconnected digital world, comparison is no longer confined to immediate social environments; it now extends to a global stage. With the rise of social media platforms, individuals are constantly exposed to curated glimpses of other people's lives—snapshots of success, beauty, relationships, and accomplishments—rendering digital comparison a pervasive and influential psychological process. While comparison is a fundamental human tendency that plays a role in motivation, learning, and self-evaluation, its intensification through digital media has profound implications for mental and emotional well-being. Understanding the psychology behind this shift is essential in comprehending its human impact—both the subtle, everyday effects and the more severe mental health consequences that can arise from repeated, often unconscious, comparison in online spaces.At the core of digital comparison lies *social comparison theory*, developed by Leon Festinger in 1954, which posits that individuals evaluate their own worth and abilities by comparing themselves to others. (Del Chiappa et al., 2016) This process occurs in two primary forms: *upward comparison*, where one compares themselves to someone perceived as better off, and *downward comparison*, which involves comparing to someone perceived as worse off. While both can serve adaptive functions—upward comparison can inspire improvement and goal-setting, and downward comparison can boost self-esteem—digital platforms have shifted the balance, increasingly favoring upward comparisons.

This is due to the prevalence of highly curated, idealized content that users tend to post. Rather than portraying a balanced view of life's highs and lows, social media content overwhelmingly emphasizes achievement, attractiveness, joy, and perfection. Consequently, users are more likely to feel inadequate, envious, or unaccomplished when exposed to these idealized images, particularly when the comparisons feel close to home—among peers, acquaintances, or aspirational figures.The psychological consequences of frequent upward digital comparison are significant and wide-ranging. One of the most common outcomes is *lowered self-esteem.* When users are repeatedly exposed to content that seems to suggest others are more successful, attractive, popular, or fulfilled, they may begin to question their own worth. Unlike traditional media, where celebrities and ideal lives may seem distant, social media brings these comparisons into personal, everyday contexts. Seeing a classmate travel the world, a colleague celebrate a promotion, or an influencer showcase a flawless lifestyle can create a distorted perception of normalcy, leading individuals to view their own experiences as lacking. Over time, this can foster a persistent sense of inferiority and dissatisfaction, even when the user's actual life circumstances are objectively stable or fulfilling.Another psychological effect is the development of *social anxiety* and *fear of missing out (FOMO).* When users see others attending events, enjoying relationships, or engaging in socially desirable activities, they may feel excluded or left behind. This can lead to compulsive social media use, driven by the desire to stay connected and avoid missing out, even at the cost of mental health. FOMO has been associated with increased stress, sleep disruption, and compulsive checking behaviors that impair real-life focus and presence.

Over time, these behaviors can foster a dependence on digital validation, reinforcing a cycle where users seek relief from negative emotions through more engagement—only to encounter new content that triggers fresh comparisons.Body image concerns are another prevalent and troubling psychological impact, especially among adolescents and young adults. Platforms such as Instagram and TikTok emphasize visual content, often showcasing idealized beauty standards that are filtered, edited, or surgically enhanced. For young users still developing their identities, constant exposure to unattainable or unrealistic body ideals can lead to *body dissatisfaction*, *eating disorders*, and *distorted self-perception.* (El-Gohary, 2012)The comparison is not limited to influencers or celebrities but extends to peers, making the pressure to conform even more intense. Factors such as *personality traits*, *mental health history*, *age*, *gender*, and *cognitive styles* play a significant role. (Falk et al., 2010) People with high levels of neuroticism, low self-esteem, or a tendency toward perfectionism are more likely to engage in maladaptive comparisons and suffer the emotional consequences. Adolescents, in particular, are at heightened risk due to their developmental stage, where peer validation and identity exploration are central tasks. This distortion makes it seem as if everyone is constantly thriving, beautiful, and successful, even though users intellectually know that these images are curated. Moreover, features such as follower counts, likes, and public comments make social validation quantifiable, turning popularity into a visible metric.

The Performative Self: How Online Profiles Shape Identity

In the modern digital landscape, where billions of users engage with social media daily, the act of comparing oneself to others has transformed from an occasional tendency into a near-constant mental habit. This phenomenon, often referred to as the is the psychological cycle of repeatedly measuring oneself against others based on curated online content—often to one's own detriment. While social comparison is a normal part of human cognition, the trap emerges when these comparisons become excessive, unrealistic, and emotionally harmful. Social media platforms, by their design and nature, significantly intensify this pattern. (Foroudi et al., 2018) The comparison trap is not just a byproduct of digital culture—it is a feature embedded into the architecture of platforms that reward appearance, status, and perceived perfection. As users become ncreasingly immersed in these digital environments, the trap deepens, often resulting in heightened insecurity, anxiety, and diminished well-being.The comparison trap is perpetuated by the structure of social media, which thrives on *highlight reels*. Users selectively post the best aspects of their lives—vacations, celebrations, professional milestones, fitness transformations, romantic moments—while omitting the mundane, painful, or imperfect. This selective sharing creates an illusion of a life that is more exciting, beautiful, and successful than it is in reality. When users view these highlight reels without the full context, they may internalize the belief that others are consistently thriving while they themselves are falling behind. This belief fuels *insecurity*, as individuals question their own worth, success, or attractiveness in comparison to the seemingly perfect lives of others. Over time, this skewed perception erodes self-esteem and cultivates an ongoing sense of inadequacy. some way—be it appearance, wealth, social status, or happiness.

These comparisons can provoke feelings of failure or guilt, particularly in those already managing the stress of work-life balance or financial strain. The result is an unrelenting sense of pressure—to be more successful, more attractive, more productive—that can quickly lead to chronic anxiety and emotional exhaustion. Compounding(García-Crespo et al., 2010) the problem is the role of *algorithms*, which selectively show users content that aligns with their interests but also content that is most likely to engage emotions—especially envy, desire, and admiration. This means that users are disproportionately exposed to the best aspects of others' lives and less frequently to their challenges. Moreover, the platforms reward high-performing content with more visibility, creating a feedback loop where only the most glamorous, dramatic, or enviable posts are seen and circulated. This fosters an online culture where people feel compelled to constantly one-up each other, driving more intense content curation and reinforcing the pressure to maintain an idealized image. Thus, users are not only comparing themselves to others, but also adjusting their own behaviors to meet the imagined standards of their digital audience—a process that is mentally draining and often inauthentic.The comparison trap also triggers *perfectionism*, especially in those with predispositions toward high self-expectations. These individuals may feel compelled to "keep up" with their peers by meticulously crafting their own online persona. Every post becomes a performance, every selfie a production, and every caption a calculated statement. Rather than serving as a space for self-expression or connection, social media becomes a battleground for approval

The Impact of Digital Comparison on Mental Health

In the digital age, identity is no longer a static entity passively discovered over time—it is an active, ongoing performance shaped and reshaped within the constraints and opportunities of online platforms. The concept of the *performative self* encapsulates this modern reality: the idea that who we are—or more accurately, who we present ourselves to be—is constructed through deliberate acts of self-presentation in digital spaces. As social media becomes deeply embedded in everyday life, users are increasingly aware that their online profiles are not just reflections of who they are, but curated stages where identity is performed for an audience. (Garrido-Moreno et al., 2014)These platforms have turned the self into a visible, editable, and often strategically crafted construct, giving rise to a new mode of identity that is flexible, performative, and often detached from offline reality.The theory of performativity, rooted in the work of philosopher Judith Butler and sociologist Erving Goffman, offers a useful lens through which to understand this phenomenon. Goffman's *dramaturgical analysis* suggests that social life is akin to a theatrical performance, where individuals play roles based on the social context and the audience they are addressing. Online platforms have exponentially expanded the size and diversity of that audience, creating what scholars call the *context collapse*: the convergence of multiple social groups (friends, coworkers, family, acquaintances, strangers) into one digital space. In this collapsed context, users must carefully manage their self-presentation to appeal to a wide and varied audience. The result is a form of identity performance that is hyper-aware, selectively constructed, and often moderated for acceptability, likability, and relatability. The online profile becomes a kind of stage where the individual performs a version of themselves they believe will be validated by others.This performative process is shaped not only by internal desires and values but also by the external structures of the platforms themselves.

Social media sites are designed to promote visibility, interaction, and engagement. Users are encouraged—often subtly—to construct profiles that attract attention, garner likes, generate comments, and build followings. These digital rewards, while seemingly innocuous, act as powerful behavioral reinforcements that shape how people present themselves. For example, someone may discover that posts showcasing travel, fitness, or lifestyle aesthetics receive more engagement than vulnerable or mundane updates(Han & Hyun, 2015). Over time, this feedback loop can lead users to prioritize content that performs well over content that feels authentic, gradually altering not just their public persona but their internal sense of self.The performative self is especially evident in how users present different facets of their identities across platforms. This disconnection may be subtle at first—feeling pressure to dress a certain way for photos or choosing captions for effect—but it can evolve into deeper psychological consequences, such as low self-esteem, anxiety, or a sense of emptiness despite outward validation. These movements encourage users to share unpolished moments, to speak openly about struggles, and to embrace imperfection

The Performative Nature of Social Media: Authenticity and Curation

In an era where digital communication and self-expression are deeply embedded in daily life, the act of comparing oneself to others online has become almost inescapable. (Jalilvand & Samiei, 2012)While comparison is a natural psychological function, social media has amplified and distorted it, turning it into a pervasive force that can profoundly affect mental health. This phenomenon, often referred to as of beauty, success, happiness, and perfection. These portrayals, curated and filtered for public display, create unrealistic standards against which users measure their own experiences, leading to a cascade of negative emotional and cognitive outcomes. As digital comparison becomes more entrenched in daily routines, its impact on mental health is increasingly concerning, especially as studies continue to link it with rising levels of anxiety, depression, low self-esteem, body dissatisfaction, and other psychological disorders. Leon Festinger in 1954. Festinger theorized that individuals have an innate drive to evaluate themselves by comparing their traits, abilities, and achievements to those of others. In the pre-digital world, these comparisons were largely limited to real-life interactions within local social circles. Today, however, social media platforms have radically expanded the scope of these comparisons. Individuals are no longer comparing themselves just to friends or peers, but to influencers, celebrities, and strangers across the globe, many of whom present idealized versions of life that are filtered, edited, and often entirely fabricated. This constant exposure to curated digital personas creates a distorted sense of reality, encouraging users to internalize these idealized images as benchmarks of normalcy or success—despite their artificiality. use among teenagers correlate with increased symptoms of depression, anxiety, and low self-worth. These outcomes are often mediated by the intensity of upward social comparisons—where users compare themselves to others who seem to be more attractive, more popular, more successful, or happier. For many young users, a peer's seemingly flawless life—documented through Instagram posts, TikTok videos, or Snapchat stories—can trigger feelings of inadequacy, jealousy, and alienation.

Over time, these feelings can become chronic, feeding into a cycle of negative self-perception that is difficult to escape, especially when compounded by the fear of missing out (FOMO) and the compulsive need to stay connected to social feeds.Body image issues represent one of the most visible and damaging effects of digital comparison, particularly among teenage girls and young women. Platforms like Instagram and TikTok, which prioritize visual content, contribute to body dissatisfaction by promoting unrealistic beauty standards that are often digitally enhanced or surgically altered. Users are bombarded with images of perfectly proportioned bodies, flawless skin, and ideal lifestyles, often accompanied by language that implies attainability through specific products, diets, or routines. Even when users intellectually recognize that such images are manipulated, the emotional impact can be profound. Frequent exposure to these ideals fosters body dysmorphia, eating disorders, and a persistent belief that one's natural appearance is inadequate. (Jeong & Lambert, 2001) The psychological toll is compounded by the fact that even peers now participate in the same visual culture—using filters, posing techniques, and editing apps—making it harder to distinguish between reality and performance. However, the effects of digital comparison are not confined to youth. Adults, too, experience mental health consequences as they navigate professional, personal, and familial expectations shaped by social media.

Figure 1. comparative analysis of the impacts of digital lifestyles on the physical, mental, and social health

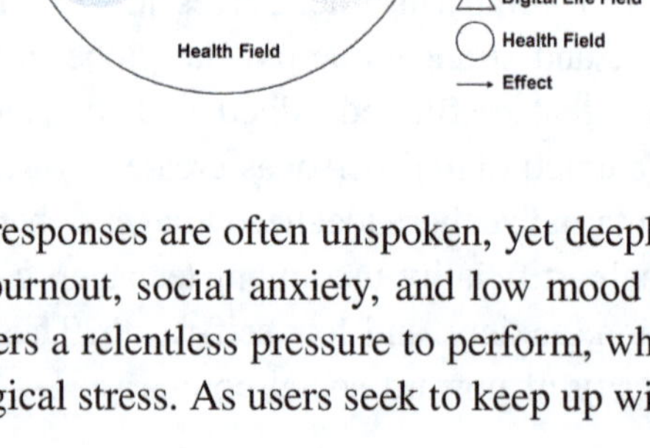

These emotional responses are often unspoken, yet deeply felt, contributing to a growing sense of burnout, social anxiety, and low mood in adult users.Digital comparison also fosters a relentless pressure to perform, which can itself become a source of psychological stress. As users seek to keep up with the perceived standards set by others, they may feel compelled to curate their own online personas with similar levels of polish and appeal. This can result in a form of emotional labor, where individuals constantly manage their online image—choosing photos, writing captions, monitoring likes and comments—not for self-expression, but to gain social validation. Over time, this labor can lead to emotional exhaustion, imposter syndrome, and a weakening of one's sense of authenticity. Users may begin to feel that their real selves are not good enough, leading to increased self-alienation and a reliance on external feedback to determine self-worth. The dissonance between one's online persona and offline reality creates a psychological strain that is difficult to reconcile and may contribute to long-term mental health challenges.Another dangerous consequence of digital comparison is its relationship with rumination—the repetitive and passive focus on one's flaws, failures, or perceived inadequacies. When users engage in comparison, particularly to those perceived as more successful or attractive, they are more likely to engage in self-critical thought patterns that can spiral into depressive cognition. This is particularly true when users compare across multiple domains—appearance, lifestyle, relationships, achievements—simultaneously. The breadth and depth of digital content ensure that there is always someone "doing better," feeding a relentless cycle of self-evaluation that can become obsessive. Even brief social media sessions can trigger hours of negative thought loops, affecting concentration, sleep, and overall emotional well-being.That said, it is important to recognize that not all digital comparison leads to negative outcomes. When used mindfully, some forms of comparison can foster motivation, self-improvement, and even resilience. For example, users may feel inspired by others' fitness journeys, educational achievements, or creative projects. In such cases, comparison serves as a benchmark for growth rather than a weapon of self-devaluation.

The key lies in interpretation: whether users view others' success as threatening or empowering. Individuals with higher emotional intelligence, secure self-esteem, and healthy coping mechanisms are more likely to navigate comparison in constructive ways. Unfortunately, social media does not encourage this balanced interpretation by default; instead, its design often exacerbates insecurity through algorithms that promote sensational, emotionally charged content with high engagement rates.To mitigate the mental health impact of digital comparison, several interventions are being explored. These include digital literacy education, which teaches users—especially young people—how to critically evaluate online content and recognize curated reality; mental health promotion through in-app features like screen-time limits and content warnings; and therapeutic approaches such as cognitive-behavioral therapy (CBT), which can help individuals challenge and reframe harmful comparison-based thoughts. Increasingly, social media platforms themselves are being called upon to take responsibility by reducing harmful content promotion, allowing users to hide likes or comments, and promoting more diverse, realistic portrayals of life.

However, the core challenge remains cultural: until digital comparison is seen not as a personal failure but as a systemic design flaw and social pattern, its impact on mental health will likely persist(Kommineni et al., 2025).

Influencers and the Performance of Lifestyle

Social media has revolutionized the way individuals present themselves, shifting identity expression from a private, nuanced experience into a public, performative act that blends elements of authenticity and deliberate curation. The performative nature of social media refers to the ways in which users consciously or unconsciously construct and enact versions of themselves tailored for online audiences. Unlike face-to-face interaction, where social cues and context help moderate behavior in real time, social media provides a mediated environment in which individuals craft, edit, and strategically share carefully selected content to convey specific impressions. This process involves both *curation*—the deliberate selection and arrangement of images, words, and symbols—and *performance*—the active presentation of identity that responds to anticipated audience reactions. The tension between authenticity and curation is at the heart of this performative dynamic, raising important questions about what it means to be genuine in a digital world predicated on visibility and validation.At its core, social media demands a form of identity work that blends real experiences with idealized versions of self. The immediacy and permanence of digital content mean that each post, photo, or status update becomes a snapshot of identity frozen in time, intended to communicate something about who the user is or aspires to be. Users often face the paradox of wanting to appear authentic and relatable while simultaneously striving to project an attractive, successful, or socially desirable image.

Users may demonstrate authenticity by sharing moments of vulnerability, imperfection, or struggle, counterbalancing the idealized content that dominates the platform. Such disclosures are often celebrated as markers of bravery and genuine connection. (Zeng & Gerritsen, 2014)However, these acts of vulnerability are themselves performed; the decision to reveal private struggles or raw emotions is shaped by audience expectations and social norms about acceptable self-disclosure. Thus, even authenticity becomes a form of curated performance, where vulnerability is staged to signal trustworthiness and emotional depth. The quantification of social approval through metrics also reduces complex social interactions to numerical values, simplifying identity to an accumulation of external validation.Importantly, the performative self on social media is not necessarily deceptive or inauthentic; it often reflects sincere aspirations, creativity, and identity exploration. However, the continuous negotiation between authenticity and curation requires users to navigate a complex social terrain where identity is both self-generated and socially constructed. Users engage in a constant balancing act—seeking to be true to themselves while also adapting to the expectations and pressures of their digital audience(Yuan & Wu, 2008). This negotiation shapes not only how users present themselves online but also how they come to understand and experience their own identities offline. In sum, the performative nature of social media reveals a transformation in how identity is produced and experienced in contemporary society.

The Blurred Lines between Reality and Performance Online

In the digital age, influencers have emerged as powerful architects of lifestyle performance, shaping not only consumer behavior but also cultural norms around identity, success, and belonging. These individuals, often ordinary people who have amassed substantial online followings, curate and perform highly stylized versions of their lives to engage and captivate audiences across platforms like Instagram, TikTok, YouTube, and beyond. Unlike traditional celebrities, influencers cultivate intimacy and relatability by presenting themselves as accessible, authentic peers, while simultaneously performing aspirational lifestyles that blend elements of glamour, expertise, and everyday reality. This duality lies at the heart of their appeal and impact: followers are drawn both to the seemingly genuine connection influencers offer and to the idealized visions of life they embody. The influencer's performance is meticulously crafted through a combination of visual storytelling, narrative construction, and strategic curation, creating a compelling digital persona that operates at the intersection of personal branding, marketing, and social interaction.Central to the influencer phenomenon is the concept of lifestyle as performance. Rather than simply sharing moments of their daily lives, influencers actively stage experiences designed to convey a particular identity and set of values. From the choice of clothing and locations to the tone of voice and type of content, every element is carefully selected to signal desirability, status, and cultural capital. For example, an influencer specializing in fitness might post carefully timed workout videos, meal prep photos, and motivational quotes, crafting an image of discipline and health that inspires followers. A travel influencer, meanwhile, might highlight exotic destinations, luxury accommodations, and curated adventures, performing a life of freedom, exploration, and privilege. These performances are often polished to near perfection using photo editing, filters, and scripting, blurring the line between reality and artifice. (Yoo & Gretzel, 2008)The lifestyle portrayed is aspirational, offering followers not just entertainment but a model of how to live, look, and feel that is deeply entwined with consumerism and social status.

The economics of influencing further complicate the performative nature of these lifestyles. Influencers operate within a digital marketplace where visibility and engagement translate directly into income through brand partnerships, sponsored content, and product endorsements. This creates strong incentives to maintain an attractive and consistent persona that appeals to both audiences and advertisers. The influencer's self-presentation is thus shaped by commercial interests as much as by personal identity. Many influencers collaborate with fashion brands, beauty companies, health products, and luxury services, integrating advertising seamlessly into their daily posts. This commercial embeddedness raises questions about authenticity: followers may question how much of the influencer's lifestyle is genuinely lived versus strategically performed for profit. Yet, savvy influencers navigate this tension by cultivating transparency around sponsorships or by blending sponsored content with personal stories, reinforcing trust while still driving consumption. This delicate balance between authenticity and marketing savvy is a hallmark of successful influencer branding.Influencers also play a critical role in shaping cultural norms and social values through their performative lifestyles. They serve as tastemakers, trendsetters, and role models, especially for younger audiences who may look to them for cues on fashion, beauty standards, wellness, relationships, and social causes(Wang et al., 2012). For followers, exposure to the influencer's performative lifestyle can trigger negative social comparisons, fueling feelings of inadequacy, envy, and lowered self-esteem. (Verhoef et al., 2010) The pervasive nature of influencer content—saturating feeds, stories, and recommendations—makes it difficult for audiences to disengage or maintain a balanced perspective on their own lives. This evolution suggests that the performance of lifestyle on social media is not static but continually negotiated, shaped by changing user expectations, technological innovations, and cultural values.In conclusion, influencers occupy a unique space at the intersection of identity performance, cultural production, and digital marketing.

The Commodification of Lifestyle: How Digital Comparison Fuels Consumerism

In the contemporary digital landscape, the boundary between reality and performance has become increasingly indistinct, creating a complex interplay that challenges traditional understandings of identity, authenticity, and social interaction. Social media platforms, designed for sharing personal moments and connecting with others, simultaneously encourage users to engage in performative behaviors that often obscure the line between lived experience and curated representation. This fusion of reality and performance is not merely a byproduct of technology but a fundamental shift in how individuals construct and negotiate their identities in mediated spaces. Users inhabit roles that oscillate between authentic self-expression and strategic self-presentation, crafting digital personas that reflect, distort, or even reinvent reality. (Tavitiyaman et al., 2011)As a result, social media functions as a stage where everyday life is both lived and performed, blurring the distinction between genuine experience and theatrical display in ways that profoundly affect social dynamics and psychological well-being.One of the key drivers of this blurring is the inherent affordances of digital platforms, which allow for unprecedented control over self-presentation. Unlike face-to-face interactions, where expressions and behaviors are spontaneous and contextually grounded, online interactions afford users the ability to carefully select, edit, and time their communications. Photographs can be filtered, videos scripted and rehearsed, and status updates crafted to convey specific moods or narratives. This capacity for mediation transforms ordinary moments into performances tailored for public consumption. Users become both actors and directors of their online personas, engaging in what sociologist Erving Goffman described as "impression management," where social interaction is conceptualized as theatrical performance designed to influence others' perceptions.

Social media thus extends this dramaturgical metaphor into everyday life, amplifying the performative element by enabling repeated performances to vast and often anonymous audiences.The performative nature of online identity is further complicated by the social and psychological incentives embedded in digital cultures. The consumption of others' curated lives often triggers social comparison processes, where individuals measure their own worth and happiness against the seemingly flawless portrayals they encounter online. Because these portrayals are performances shaped to elicit admiration and envy, they rarely reflect the full spectrum of human experience, including struggles, failures, and vulnerabilities. Consequently, users may develop distorted perceptions of social norms and expectations, fostering feelings of inadequacy, loneliness, and anxiety. (Tavakoli & Wijesinghe, 2019). However, in digital contexts, authenticity is often performed as a style or aesthetic, where vulnerability, imperfection, and spontaneity become curated traits that users deploy strategically to signal genuineness. (Samal et al., 2025) For example, influencers and everyday users alike may share "behind-the-scenes" glimpses, unfiltered selfies, or candid admissions of struggle, not necessarily as unmediated truths but as calculated performances designed to build trust and deepen engagement.

The Performance of Identity: How Digital Comparison Shapes Societal Norms

The rise of social media and digital communication platforms has fundamentally reshaped the way relationships and communities are formed, maintained, and experienced. While these technologies offer unprecedented opportunities for connection, they simultaneously introduce complex dynamics rooted in digital comparison that significantly affect interpersonal relationships and collective social bonds. Digital comparison refers to the process through which individuals evaluate themselves relative to others by observing curated portrayals of lifestyles, achievements, and social interactions online(Suresh et al., 2025). This pervasive comparative framework influences not only personal self-perception but also the quality, authenticity, and sustainability of relationships and community life in the digital age. For instance, seeing constant displays of romantic bliss, social popularity, or family happiness online may cause individuals to question the authenticity or value of their own relationships, even if those relationships are supportive and meaningful. This dynamic can create a paradox where digital connection increases feelings of isolation and loneliness, as comparisons undermine contentment and trust.

The impact of digital comparison extends into romantic relationships, where it can both complicate and strain intimacy. (Rather et al., 2021)Partners may feel pressured to perform idealized versions of their relationship online, carefully crafting posts that signal happiness, compatibility, and social approval. This performance, while often intended to celebrate and affirm the relationship, can introduce stress by prioritizing external validation over authentic expression. The desire to project a flawless partnership may discourage vulnerability and honest communication, which are essential for deep connection and conflict resolution. This can result in feelings of exclusion or FOMO (fear of missing out) when individuals perceive themselves as less socially active or valued. The performative aspect of social media encourages users to curate their interactions and present an engaging social self, sometimes at the expense of genuine connection. Furthermore, digital comparison can distort perceptions of reciprocity and support, as social media metrics such as likes and comments become proxies for social approval and friendship quality. (Raguseo & Vitari, 2017)This quantification risks reducing complex social bonds to numerical indicators, undermining the richness and nuance of real-world relationships. When approached mindfully, social media can complement offline relationships by enhancing communication and shared experiences. Additionally, some users consciously resist the pressures of digital comparison by promoting authenticity, vulnerability, and inclusivity, thereby contributing to healthier relational (Qu et al., 2011)dynamics and community cultures.In response to the impact of digital comparison, various strategies and interventions have emerged to support healthier relationships and community engagement.

Critiquing the Culture of Digital Comparison: A Critical Perspective

In the digital era, the performance of identity has become a central feature of social life, profoundly influencing the evolution and reinforcement of societal norms. At the core of this phenomenon is the notion that identity is performative, drawing from sociological theories like Erving Goffman's dramaturgical approach, which conceptualizes social interaction as a theatrical performance in which individuals manage impressions to fit social scripts. Digital platforms extend and amplify this dramaturgical space, enabling users to craft and disseminate idealized self-presentations through images, videos, texts, and interactive media. (Palacios-Florencio et al., 2018) These representations are inherently selective and constructed, emphasizing traits and experiences deemed socially desirable. As users continuously compare themselves to these mediated portrayals, they internalize prevailing standards and adjust their own performances accordingly. This iterative process solidifies certain norms, including ideals of beauty, success, lifestyle, morality, and social roles, embedding them into the cultural fabric. The norms generated and reinforced through digital comparison are particularly potent because they operate within highly visible and socially validated spaces, where popularity metrics such as likes, shares, and comments serve as indicators of normative approval and desirability.One of the most evident ways in which digital comparison shapes societal norms is through the standardization of aesthetic ideals. Across platforms, there is a pervasive emphasis on physical appearance, often characterized by narrowly defined standards of beauty that prioritize youth, slenderness, flawless skin, and other culturally specific attributes.

Influencers, celebrities, and ordinary users alike contribute to the circulation of these ideals by sharing images that conform to or promote these aesthetic conventions. The repetitive exposure to such idealized bodies and faces creates a cultural expectation for individuals to perform their identity in ways that align with these beauty norms. Consequently, many people engage in practices aimed at achieving or approximating these ideals, including makeup application, fashion styling, fitness regimes, and even cosmetic surgery. The performative identity, in this case, becomes a site where societal norms about appearance are enacted and reproduced, often at the cost of individual diversity and authenticity.Beyond aesthetics, digital comparison also shapes norms related to success, lifestyle, and social status. Social media's emphasis on aspirational content—highlighting luxury goods, travel experiences, career achievements, and curated family moments—constructs a normative framework that associates worth and identity with visible markers of prosperity and social capital. The performance of success online encourages users to adopt lifestyles and consumption patterns that reflect these ideals, reinforcing consumerism and materialism as social values. This normalization creates pressures to conform not only to economic standards but also to behavioral and ethical expectations tied to success narratives, such as productivity, ambition, and positivity. The widespread display of these ideals contributes to a societal environment where individuals feel compelled to perform identities that project upward mobility and happiness, often glossing over complexities or struggles. Digital comparison thus fuels the perpetuation of a success-oriented norm that privileges external validation and public achievement.Gender norms and roles are particularly susceptible to transformation through digital identity performances and comparison. Social media platforms function as arenas where traditional gender expectations are both reinforced and contested. For example, women are frequently expected to perform identities that balance attractiveness, nurturing, and professional competence, often encapsulated in lifestyle content blending beauty, family, and career.

Men may face pressures to embody ideals of strength, success, and stoicism, though emerging digital cultures also provide spaces for more diverse expressions of masculinity. Importantly, digital comparison exposes individuals to a wider array of gender performances, including those of LGBTQ+ communities and other marginalized groups, which challenges hegemonic norms and broadens societal understanding of gender identity. (Kaur et al., 2025). The curated sharing of life events often favors positivity, success stories, and inspirational content, which can shape expectations about emotional expression and social conduct. For instance, there may be normative pressure to maintain an upbeat, attractive online persona, limiting the expression of vulnerability, conflict, or dissent. This can lead to the social marginalization of more nuanced or critical voices, fostering homogenization in digital discourse and impacting societal norms regarding authenticity and openness. (Ladhari, 2009)Moreover, moral judgments are often mediated through digital comparison, as individuals and communities enforce norms related to behavior, appearance, and lifestyle through online approval or censure. Social media's public and permanent nature intensifies the stakes of these moral performances, making conformity to socially accepted identities both a means of inclusion and a site of exclusion.The interactive and networked nature of digital platforms accelerates the diffusion and reinforcement of norms across diverse populations and geographic boundaries. Unlike traditional social institutions where norms evolved more slowly and were localized, social media facilitates rapid norm transmission and hybridization, creating globalized standards that influence local cultures. This globalization of norms through digital comparison fosters cultural convergence but also sparks tensions and resistance as users negotiate between global ideals and local identities. The visibility and virality afforded by platforms mean that certain performances of identity, often those that align with dominant cultural or economic powers, gain disproportionate influence, shaping societal norms in powerful ways. (Mack et al., 2008).

The Future of Digital Comparison: Emerging Trends and Technologies

The culture of digital comparison has emerged as a defining feature of contemporary social media ecosystems, profoundly shaping individual behavior, social interactions, and broader cultural values. However, beneath the surface allure of connection, validation, and identity formation lies a complex web of critical concerns that question the social, psychological, and ethical implications of this pervasive phenomenon. A critical perspective on digital comparison challenges the normalized acceptance of constant evaluation and competition in digital spaces, exposing how it reinforces systemic inequalities, undermines authentic selfhood, and commodifies human experience. (Orel & Kara, 2014). From a critical viewpoint, this dynamic is not a neutral technological development but a strategic manipulation that commodifies identity and social relationships, reducing complex human experiences to consumable and monetizable performances. The culture of digital comparison thus serves capitalist interests by transforming social interaction into a marketplace of status and visibility, perpetuating cycles of desire and dissatisfaction that fuel continuous engagement and consumption.Critics also highlight how digital comparison exacerbates social inequalities by privileging certain identities, bodies, and lifestyles while marginalizing others.

Users may internalize the necessity of maintaining a curated persona, leading to a dissonance between their online image and lived experience. This split can generate emotional distress, anxiety, and alienation, as individuals struggle to reconcile their real selves with socially constructed ideals. The culture of comparison, by emphasizing external validation through likes, followers, and comments, shifts self-worth from intrinsic qualities to externally mediated metrics, fostering dependency on social approval. Philosophers critical of this culture argue that it commodifies the self, transforming identity into a product to be marketed rather than an authentic, multifaceted human reality. Such critiques call for reclaiming spaces for vulnerability, imperfection, and complexity, resisting reductive digital identities that prioritize appearance and popularity over depth and individuality. Moreover, the culture of digital comparison perpetuates a feedback loop of affective intensities—envy, shame, pride, and anxiety—that are strategically exploited by platform designs. (Neuts et al., 2013)The constant measurement and comparison of social metrics create an environment where users are compelled to monitor and regulate their behavior to maximize social capital. This surveillance culture extends beyond privacy concerns to the emotional labor of self-presentation, where users must navigate the psychological toll of continuous evaluation. They call for creating digital cultures that foster empathy, mutual support, and inclusive belonging rather than rivalry and exclusion.However, critical perspectives also acknowledge the complexity and ambivalence of digital comparison culture. While it produces significant harms and inequalities, it can also serve as a site of resistance, identity exploration, and community building.

Rethinking Digital Comparison: Strategies for Authenticity and Well-being

Understanding these emerging trends and technologies offers critical insights into the potential trajectories of digital comparison and highlights opportunities and challenges for fostering healthier, more authentic, and equitable digital environments.One of the most significant technological drivers shaping the future of digital comparison is the rapid advancement and integration of immersive media technologies such as augmented reality (AR), virtual reality (VR), and mixed reality (MR). These technologies extend beyond traditional two-dimensional social media interfaces to create multisensory, interactive environments where users can inhabit avatars, simulate experiences, and engage with others in real-time virtual spaces. The introduction of AR and VR into everyday digital life amplifies the performative aspects of identity by enabling more embodied and immediate presentations of self. For example, virtual avatars can be customized to reflect idealized physical traits or entirely imaginative personas, thereby intensifying opportunities for comparison based on appearance, style, and social presence. The immersive nature of these environments increases emotional engagement and social visibility, potentially heightening the psychological impact of comparison. As users navigate these augmented social spaces, the boundaries between offline and online selves may become further blurred, complicating the management of authenticity and self-presentation. Simultaneously, advancements in artificial intelligence (AI) and machine learning are set to play a crucial role in shaping digital comparison practices. AI algorithms increasingly curate personalized content feeds, influence social recommendations, and moderate interactions on social media platforms.

While these algorithms can enhance user experience by tailoring content to individual preferences, they also create echo chambers that reinforce particular norms and ideals, intensifying comparative pressures within specific social and cultural contexts. Moreover, AI-powered image and video editing tools democratize access to sophisticated content creation, enabling users to enhance their digital personas with filters, deepfakes, and synthetic media. These capabilities further complicate the authenticity of online identities and elevate the stakes of comparison by making idealized, and sometimes deceptive, representations more accessible and convincing. As AI continues to evolve, it will also influence how social validation is quantified and rewarded, potentially embedding more nuanced but also more opaque mechanisms of social evaluation that affect users' sense of self-worth. The integration of biometric and neurotechnology also portends new dimensions of digital comparison in the future. Emerging devices capable of monitoring physiological and neurological states—such as heart rate variability, emotional arousal, and cognitive load—may be incorporated into digital platforms to provide real-time feedback or personalized interventions. While these technologies hold promise for enhancing self-awareness and emotional regulation, they also raise ethical concerns about privacy, data security, and the potential for invasive social monitoring. The possibility of comparing biometric data in social contexts introduces novel forms of visibility and evaluation, where internal states become subject to public scrutiny or competitive display.

CONCLUSION

In the rapidly evolving digital age, where social media platforms have become central to personal identity construction and social interaction, the quest for authenticity emerges as a complex and urgent challenge. The digital realm often presents a performative world where users curate, edit, and stage their online personas, driven by the desire for social validation, belonging, and influence. This performativity—shaped by platform algorithms, cultural expectations, and economic incentives—creates a pervasive tension between genuine self-expression and socially constructed façades. Navigating this tension requires a nuanced understanding of what authenticity means in a context where the boundaries between private and public selves are increasingly blurred, and where identity is simultaneously a personal experience and a public performance. Authenticity in the digital age is not a fixed state but a dynamic, negotiated process that demands critical reflection, emotional resilience, and intentional engagement.One of the foundational challenges to authenticity in the digital age is the inherent architecture of social media platforms, which are designed to encourage visibility, engagement, and shareability. These platforms reward content that is visually appealing, emotionally charged, or socially validated, often privileging idealized and edited representations of life over raw or mundane realities. The result is a social environment where users feel compelled to present themselves in ways that align with dominant norms of beauty, success, and happiness, fostering a culture of comparison and performance. This environment can distort self-perception, as individuals internalize unrealistic standards and experience a dissonance between their authentic selves and their online personas. The pressure to maintain a consistent and appealing digital image can lead to emotional exhaustion, anxiety, and a diminished sense of self-worth. Thus, the pursuit of authenticity involves resisting these structural pressures by critically engaging with the performative demands of digital platforms and carving out spaces for vulnerability and imperfection.Authenticity in the digital age also entails an ongoing process of self-discovery and self-acceptance, which requires individuals to reconcile their multifaceted identities with the fragmented and mediated nature of online representation. Unlike traditional face-to-face interactions, digital communication often occurs through curated images, textual posts, and selective storytelling, which can simplify or distort the complexity of lived experience. Navigating this mediated terrain involves embracing the fluidity of identity and acknowledging that the self is both shaped by social contexts and capable of agency and creativity. Authentic digital expression, therefore, is not about achieving perfect transparency or rejecting all forms of curation but about making deliberate choices that reflect personal values, emotional truths, and relational intentions. This perspective recognizes that all social interaction involves some degree of performance and that authenticity can coexist with the performative, provided it is grounded in sincerity and self-awareness.Moreover, finding authenticity in a performative world necessitates cultivating emotional resilience and boundaries to protect oneself from the potentially corrosive effects of digital comparison and judgment. The omnipresence of social media exposes individuals to constant evaluation, criticism, and the unpredictable dynamics of online communities. Developing resilience involves strategies such as selective engagement—choosing when and how to participate in digital spaces—practicing self-compassion, and seeking supportive networks that affirm rather than undermine self-worth. Setting boundaries, including limiting time spent on social media, controlling privacy settings, and curating one's digital audience, empowers users to manage their exposure to negative influences and maintain a sense of agency. Emotional resilience also includes the capacity to critically reflect on feedback and external validation, distinguishing constructive interactions from those driven by superficial or competitive motives. Through these practices, individuals can sustain a sense of authenticity that is resilient to the vicissitudes of online social life.Community and relational dynamics play a crucial role in supporting authenticity within the digital sphere. Authenticity is inherently relational, emerging through meaningful interactions and mutual recognition. Online communities that prioritize empathy, inclusivity, and genuine connection provide fertile ground for authentic self-expression. These spaces encourage sharing beyond performative masks, allowing for vulnerability, dialogue, and the negotiation of identity in supportive contexts. Grassroots digital movements, interest-based groups, and affinity networks often foster cultures that resist dominant normative pressures and celebrate diversity, imperfection, and lived realities. In such communities, authenticity becomes a collective practice, reinforced through reciprocal trust and respect. Engaging in these relational spaces challenges the atomizing tendencies of social media and reclaims digital platforms as sites of solidarity and belonging rather than competition and alienation.Technological developments also offer both challenges and opportunities for cultivating authenticity in the digital age.

REFERENCES

Al-Maghrabi, T., Dennis, C., & Halliday, S. V. (2011). Antecedents of continuance intentions towards e-shopping: The case of Saudi Arabia. *Journal of Enterprise Information Management*, *24*(1), 85–111. DOI: 10.1108/17410391111097447

Algharabat, R. S., & Shatnawi, T. (2014). The effect of 3D product quality (3D–Q) on perceived risk and purchase intentions: The case of apparel online retailers. *International Journal of Electronic Business*, *11*(3), 256–273. DOI: 10.1504/IJEB.2014.063031

Berbegal-Mirabent, J., Mas-Machuca, M., & Marimon, F. (2016). Antecedents of online purchasing behaviour in the tourism sector. *Industrial Management & Data Systems*, *116*(1), 87–102. DOI: 10.1108/IMDS-05-2015-0213

Beritelli, P., & Schegg, R. (2016). Maximizing online bookings through a multi-channel-strategy—Effects of interdependencies and networks. *International Journal of Contemporary Hospitality Management*, *28*(1), 68–88. DOI: 10.1108/IJCHM-07-2014-0326

Chib, S., Mehta, A. K., Selvakumar, P., Saravanan, A., Mishra, B. R., & Manjunath, T. C. (2025). Mental health challenges and solutions in high-pressure work environments. In Harriott, S. (Ed.), *Innovative Approaches to Managing Conflict and Change in Diverse Work Environments* (pp. 247–272). IGI Global Scientific Publishing., DOI: 10.4018/979-8-3693-9556-1.ch011

Chib, S., Mehta, A. K., Selvakumar, P., Saravanan, A., Mishra, B. R., & Manjunath, T. C. (2025). Mental Health Challenges and Solutions in High-Pressure Work Environments. In Harriott, S. (Ed.), *Innovative Approaches to Managing Conflict and Change in Diverse Work Environments* (pp. 247–272). IGI Global Scientific Publishing., DOI: 10.4018/979-8-3693-9556-1.ch011

Dahiya, R., & Selvakumar, P. Vidyadhara, & Manjunath, T. C. (2025). Design and Aerodynamics: Principles and Advances. In M. Mellal (Ed.), Innovations and Developments in Unmanned Aerial Vehicles (pp. 145-170). IGI Global Scientific Publishing. DOI: 10.4018/979-8-3693-8462-6.ch007

Del Chiappa, G., Alarcón-Del-Amo, M.-D.-C., & Lorenzo-Romero, C. (2016). Internet and user-generated content versus high street travel agencies: A latent gold segmentation in the context of Italy. *Journal of Hospitality Marketing & Management*, *25*(2), 197–217. DOI: 10.1080/19368623.2014.1001933

El-Gohary, H. (2012). Factors affecting e-marketing adoption and implementation in tourism firms: An empirical investigation of Egyptian small tourism organisations. *Tourism Management*, *33*(5), 1256–1269. DOI: 10.1016/j.tourman.2011.10.013

Escobar-Rodríguez, T., & Carvajal-Trujillo, E. (2014). Online purchasing tickets for low cost carriers: An application of the unified theory of acceptance and use of technology (UTAUT) model. *Tourism Management*, *43*, 70–88. DOI: 10.1016/j.tourman.2014.01.017

Falk, T., Hammerschmidt, M., & Schepers, J. J. (2010). The service quality–satisfaction link revisited: Exploring asymmetries and dynamics. *Journal of the Academy of Marketing Science*, *38*(3), 288–302. DOI: 10.1007/s11747-009-0152-2

Foroudi, P., Gupta, S., Sivarajah, U., & Broderick, A. (2018). Investigating the effects of smart technology on customer dynamics and customer experience. *Computers in Human Behavior*, *80*, 271–282. DOI: 10.1016/j.chb.2017.11.014

García-Crespo, Á., Colomo-Palacios, R., Gómez-Berbís, J. M., & Ruiz-Mezcua, B. (2010). SEMO: A framework for customer social networks analysis based on semantics. *Journal of Information Technology*, *25*(2), 178–188. DOI: 10.1057/jit.2010.1

Garrido-Moreno, A., Lockett, N., & García-Morales, V. (2014). Social media use and value creation in hotels. *International Journal of Contemporary Hospitality Management*, *26*(1), 104–123.

Han, H., & Hyun, S. S. (2015). Customer retention in the medical tourism industry: Impact of quality, satisfaction, trust, and price reasonableness. *Tourism Management*, *46*, 20–29. DOI: 10.1016/j.tourman.2014.06.003

Han, H., & Kim, Y. (2010). An investigation of green hotel customers' decision formation: Developing an extended model of the theory of planned behavior. *International Journal of Hospitality Management*, *29*(4), 659–668. DOI: 10.1016/j.ijhm.2010.01.001

Jalilvand, M. R., & Samiei, N. (2012). The effect of electronic word of mouth on brand image and purchase intention: An empirical study in the automobile industry in Iran. *Marketing Intelligence & Planning*, *30*(4), 460–476. DOI: 10.1108/02634501211231946

Jeong, M., & Lambert, C. U. (2001). Adaptation of an information quality framework to measure customers' behavioral intentions to use lodging web sites. *International Journal of Hospitality Management*, *20*(2), 129–146. DOI: 10.1016/S0278-4319(00)00041-4

Kaur, M., Selvakumar, P., & Dinesh, N. Mohit, Chandel, P. S., & Mnjunath, T. C. (2025). Reconstruction and Preservation Strategies for Cultural Heritage. In S. Oflazoğlu & M. Dora (Eds.), Preserving Cultural Heritage in Post-Disaster Urban Renewal (pp. 385-412). IGI Global Scientific Publishing. DOI: 10.4018/979-8-3693-9097-9.ch016

Kommineni, M., Chundru, S., Maroju, P. K., & Selvakumar, P. (2025). Ethical Implications of AI in Sustainable Development Pedagogy. In Chinedu, C., Mafarja, N., Hussein, M., & Saleem, A. (Eds.), *Rethinking the Pedagogy of Sustainable Development in the AI Era* (pp. 17–36). IGI Global Scientific Publishing., DOI: 10.4018/979-8-3693-9062-7.ch002

Ladhari, R. (2009). Service quality, emotional satisfaction, and behavioral intentions: A study in the hotel industry. *Managing Service Quality*, *19*(3), 308–331. DOI: 10.1108/09604520910955320

Ladhari, R., & Michaud, M. (2015). eWOM effects on hotel booking intentions, attitudes, trust, and website perceptions. *International Journal of Hospitality Management*, *46*, 36–45. DOI: 10.1016/j.ijhm.2015.01.010

Mack, R. W., Snyder, J., Rodgers, W. C., & Love, R. H. (2008). Ethical judgments of marketing professionals: Influences of personal values and organizational factors. *Journal of Business Ethics*, *80*(4), 813–826.

Neuts, B., Romão, J., Nijkamp, P., & van Leeuwen, E. (2013). Describing the relationships between tourist satisfaction and destination loyalty in a segmented and seasonal tourism market. *Tourism Economics*, *19*(4), 743–765.

Orel, F. D., & Kara, A. (2014). Supermarket self-checkout service quality, customer satisfaction, and loyalty: Empirical evidence from an emerging market. *Journal of Retailing and Consumer Services*, *21*(2), 118–129. DOI: 10.1016/j.jretconser.2013.07.002

Palacios-Florencio, B., García del Junco, J., Castilla-Polo, F. J., & Santos-Roldán, L. (2018). Sustainable tourism tags to reward destination loyalty. *Sustainability*, *10*(5), 1544.

Qu, H., Kim, L. H., & Im, H. H. (2011). A model of destination branding: Integrating the concepts of the branding and destination image. *Tourism Management*, *32*(3), 465–476. DOI: 10.1016/j.tourman.2010.03.014

Raguseo, E., & Vitari, C. (2017). The effect of brand on the impact of eWOM on hotels' financial performance. *International Journal of Electronic Commerce*, *21*(2), 249–269. DOI: 10.1080/10864415.2016.1234287

Rather, R. A., Hollebeek, L. D., & Rasoolimanesh, S. M. (2021). First-time versus repeat tourism customer engagement, experience, and value co-creation: A comparison of prominent relationship constructs.

Samal, A., & Misra, L. I. Mohit, Pougajendy, S., Chandel, P. S., Manjunath, T. C., & Selvakumar, P. (2025). Musealization and Tourism Practices. In S. Oflazoğlu & M. Dora (Eds.), Preserving Cultural Heritage in Post-Disaster Urban Renewal (pp. 115-142). IGI Global Scientific Publishing. DOI: 10.4018/979-8-3693-9097-9.ch006

Suresh, R. V., Selvakumar, P., Naresh Babu, K., Nithya, G., Manjunath, T. C., & Kartigeyan, J. (2025). Best Practices and Practical Applications. In Çela, E., Paliktzoglou, V., Sengar, S., Eappen, P., & Vajjhala, N. (Eds.), *Enhancing School Counseling With Technology and Case Studies* (pp. 341–362). IGI Global Scientific Publishing., DOI: 10.4018/979-8-3693-8392-6.ch013

Tavakoli, R., & Wijesinghe, S. N. R. (2019). The evolution of destination branding: A review of literature on destination branding. *Journal of Hospitality and Tourism Insights*, *2*(3), 269–280.

Tavitiyaman, P., Qu, H., & Zhang, H. Q. (2011). The impact of industry force factors on resource competitive strategies and hotel performance. *International Journal of Hospitality Management*, *30*(3), 648–657. DOI: 10.1016/j.ijhm.2010.11.010

Verhoef, P. C., Reinartz, W. J., & Krafft, M. (2010). Customer engagement as a new perspective in customer management. *Journal of Service Research*, *13*(3), 247–252. DOI: 10.1177/1094670510375461

Wang, D., Park, S., & Fesenmaier, D. R. (2012). The role of smartphones in mediating the touristic experience. *Journal of Travel Research*, *51*(4), 371–387. DOI: 10.1177/0047287511426341

Yoo, K. H., & Gretzel, U. (2008): What motivates consumers to write online travel reviews? *Information Technology & Tourism*, *10*(4), 283–295. DOI: 10.3727/109830508788403114

Yuan, Y.-H., & Wu, C. (2008). Relationships among experiential marketing, experiential value, and customer satisfaction. *Journal of Hospitality & Tourism Research (Washington, D.C.)*, *32*(3), 387–410. DOI: 10.1177/1096348008317392

Zeng, B., & Gerritsen, R. (2014). What do we know about social media in tourism? A review. *Tourism Management Perspectives*, *10*, 27–36. DOI: 10.1016/j.tmp.2014.01.001

Chapter 6
Factors Influencing the Selection of Restaurants for Generation Z in Bangladesh

Firoj Kabir
https://orcid.org/0009-0001-3014-3163
Daffodil International University, Bangladesh

Mohammad Badruddoza Talukder
https://orcid.org/0009-0008-1662-9221
International University of Business Agriculture and Technology, Bangladesh

G. M. Selim Ahmed
https://orcid.org/0009-0009-2211-8687
Rangamati Science and Technology University, Bangladesh

Sanjeev Kumar
https://orcid.org/0000-0002-7375-7341
Lovely Professional University, India

ABSTRACT

The present study aims to explore the factors impacting Bangladesh's dining selections of Generation Z. The study is quantitative in nature. Here, the researchers have used SPSS for various analyses. The researchers also used multiple graphs, charts, and excel to draw tables. Surveys are used here to determine customer attitudes and behaviour when selecting a restaurant. Generation Z favours eateries with varied cuisines and handy spots and chooses them based on online reviews and ratings. We found peers and online communities influence them to look for

DOI: 10.4018/979-8-3373-4516-1.ch006

great deals and high-quality cuisine at affordable prices. Restaurants can bring in and retain Generation Z, essential for operations development in Bangladesh's competitive food service industry, by understanding their tastes and customizing menus, improving online visibility, and optimizing ease variables, including place and service speed. This knowledge enables restaurants to better customize their menus and marketing tactics to this critical customer base, which promotes customer retention and business growth.

INTRODUCTION:

The COVID-19 pandemic was a significant challenge for the food service market, necessitating a shift in dining habits (Gupta & Pande, 2023). Consumers have avoided physical contact with service people, like waiters or waitresses. Hence, they prefer self-service, online orders, quick delivery, and so on (Kumar et al., 2024). In response to the epidemic, businesses must strive for unprecedented transformations. A study by the Bangladesh Tourism Board found that the Hospitality industry suffered almost 1,487.02 crore BDT due to the pandemic (Sardar *et al.*, 2022). The problem arose in the food service industry, as consumers tended to be free from mass groupings, particularly in eateries, because the infection was primarily communicated through food. Undoubtedly, this had a devastating impact on the food and beverage (F&B) service industry. Many eateries recently launched updated hygiene guidelines that both patrons and personnel of the eateries should cooperate with (Zheng, 2024; Talukder et al., 2024a). As a result of the modern explosion, a rise in free time and a reduction in workplace times have compelled individuals to dine out. The percentage of dining outside is mainly due to components like growth in the percentage of ladies in work, young people's busy work schedule, diversity of choices, the quick introduction of cheap and varied cuisine in eateries, the rise in competition in the restaurant industry as well as the focus on consumable goods performance (Hammad, 2024).

Table 1. Cohort Prevalent Features and Generation X, Y, and Z (Jain & Dutta, 2019)

Generation	Born year range	Cognitive traits that lead
Traditionalists	1900 – 1945	Responsibility and dedication
Baby Boomers	1946 – 1964	Solid work morals and commitment
Generation X	1965 – 1980	Visionaries who are self-sufficient and productive
Generation Y	1981 – 1994	Fewer autonomous, highly extroverted, optimistic
Generation Z	1995 – 2012	Inadequate communication skills and reliance on new technology.

From the above table, the Gen Z ers, or The Post-Millennials, are digitally sophisticated, health-conscious, and medically aware (Das et al., 2024; Chang, 2013). This generation routinely reveals personal information, daily activity details, and so on via self-contact and digital networking sites (Talukder et al., 2024b). They (Gen Z) emulate top-environmental conduct as modeled by celebrity endorsers they observe. As Generation Z ers already entered the workplace and started to earn, they expanded their financial ability and became the focal point of marketers. Approximately 27% of Earth's inhabitants are members of Gen Z (Fekete & Nagy, 2022). They have different characteristics rather than their previous cohort. Hence, their sense of decision-making is different, and it's vital to identify the factors that affect them the most when deciding whether they dine out.

This research is crucial as it aims to thoroughly comprehend the determinants that influence the restaurant preferences of Generation Z in Bangladesh city (Talukder et al., 2023). The results will be of great worth to restaurant proprietors, marketers, and lawmakers who aim to respond to and accommodate the changing requirements of this specific group of people. Moreover, this study adds to the current pool of knowledge regarding restaurant choices, with a particular emphasis on a group progressively influencing the prospects of the hospitality industry.

The objective of this research is to address this gap by examining the elements that impact Generation Z's decision-making process when it comes to choosing restaurants. Given Generation Z's growing dependence on restaurants, partly due to an increase in the percentage of employed individuals in this generation, stakeholders in the hospitality sector need to comprehend their tastes. According to Talukder et al. (2020), this study will examine the distinctive attributes and tastes of Generation Z, investigating the influence of technological advances, social media, and evolving societal conditions on their selection of restaurants.

Generation Zs are those individuals who were born after 1996. They are now in the younger market segment in every sphere of the economy. Some of this generation (Gen Z) are now entering the workplace and earning their livelihood. Moreover, they have also started to contribute to the country's economy. As a result, all marketers are formulating and revising the marketing policy of every sector to attract this consumer segment (Talukder et al., 2024). This generation is far more different from the other generations like Gen X and Gen Y, so comprehensive research is essential to know their perceptions and traits. In the modern era, people are busy with their work schedules, and the tendency of working couples to dine out is increasing. Hence, most individuals dine out to save time and do small meetings while eating outside. By doing this research, the researchers tried to gather new experiences that will help bring out new information and possibilities in the food and beverage sector.

Theoretical Framework and Hypothesis Development: The theoretical framework provides the researcher with a synthesis of research on how to describe the facts of customers' perceptions. It outlines the tasks required during the study and previous knowledge of other scholars' thoughts and experiences on the research topic (Kivela *et al.*, 1999). The suggested conceptual framework in Figure 1 displays how consumers are motivated and perceived through various factors and the factors that impact selecting a restaurant. It is assumed that these elements are favourably related to choosing a restaurant.

Figure 1. Theoretical Framework based on Wang, X. (2023)

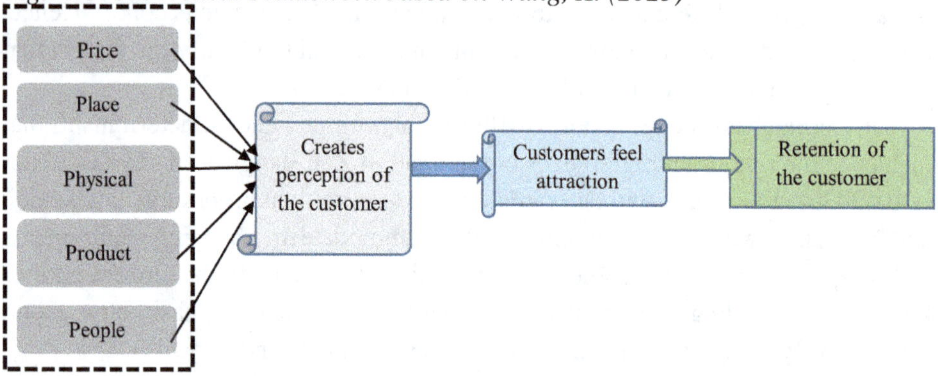

Objectives of the study

The objectives of the proposed paper are as follows:

1. To determine whether the Price, Location, Decoration, & Service Quality impact Generation Z's perception.
2. To find out the impacts of each attribute (price, location, decoration & service) on Generation Z's satisfaction and preference.
3. To determine whichever characteristics are the most appealing to consumers.

Hypothesis Development:

Test 01: Price and customer perception

H0: There is no relationship between reasonable price and customer perception of restaurant selection

H1: There is a positive relationship between reasonable prices and customer perception of restaurant selection

Test 02: Customers' perception and distance

H0: There is no relationship between distance and restaurant selection
H1: There is a positive relationship between distance and restaurant selection

Test 03: Physical evidence and customer behaviour

H0: Attractive physical evidence is not positively associated with customer behaviour
H1: Attractive physical evidence is positively associated with customer behaviour

Test 04: Products variation and customer perception

H0: Foods' variation does not positively affect customer perception
H1: Foods' variation positively affects customer perception

Test 05: People (Service staff) and customer behaviour

H0: Good service quality is not positively linked with customer perception
H1: Good service quality is positively linked with customer perception

LITERATURE REVIEW

Generally, the Restaurant Industry encompasses eating outside of the house, in inns, lunch-house, pubs, cafes, food carts, stable places of snack bars, dinners, and so on, which are devoted to the trade of food service. Foodservice/Catering/Restaurant Service is a standard business in our country and was present before our independence (Ding & Jiang, 2023; Talukder et al., 2024). There are also international hotel chains (5-star hotels) in our country. After 2000, the Food Business Industry, Especially the Restaurant Industry, advanced significantly. That's why choosing a restaurant to dine out has become challenging. Walker (2011) classified five (05) types of restaurants. Such as prompt service, fine dining, eating with family, occasional fest, and the banquet house. Chung & Kim (2016) stated that menu price is the most influential factor in determining consumer behavior and decision-making towards a restaurant.

A research paper based on consumer hospitality by Kim et al. (2016) indicated that the most influential multipliers that influence selecting a restaurant in Bangladesh are the reception, the design of sitting capacity, and the promptness of delivering service (Sezgi & Uyanik, 2022). As Bangladeshi people are very hospitable by culture, these factors are directly linked with the Bangladeshi Culture. The sorting of restaurants for dining out depends upon several factors. Such are the customer's age range, gender, and income of the consumers influence while selecting a restaurant. The research by Shah et al. (2023) shows that the age difference of the customers has the utmost impact on their perception when deciding on a restaurant.

Moreover, a variety of variables determine the restaurant choice of Bangladeshi residents. The most frequently mentioned parameters are meal cost, cafe proximity, appearance, and dining service standards. As a result, this research paper aims to discover the far more appealing features that impact consumers' restaurant choices the most.

According to Ahlawat et al. (2022), location is the critical factor influencing consumer perception while selecting a restaurant for dining out. The adjacent area is suitable for family dining with kids, attracting older citizens. Turkey, in favor of dining out in restaurants, showed that both men and women consider food costs, staff service, and the delivery of palatable food. According to Hu (2022), the restaurant's customer utilizes cost or price as the metric for evaluating the restaurant's quality, expecting that a more costly restaurant delivers quality food and provides excellent service. A study conducted by Massawe (2013) claimed that the proportional relevance of restaurant choosing criteria varies significantly depending on the cost of a restaurant. Jeong & Jang (2011) identified different causes for selecting a restaurant; the consumer's desire or intention is the other component.

According to Khan & Shibami (2019), Generation Z is born between 1995 and 2012. This generation is also termed the "Digital Natives," "Generation N," and "Me Generation" (2019). Unlike previous generations, who were more accustomed to thrust medium (radio and television) and were enveloped by the environment, Generation Z has grown up in the era of the cosmos where the computer is as simple as 'Plug'n'Play' (Cristancho Triana et al., 2024). Talukder (2024) emphasized that even unless youngsters grow on a planet absent new technology, Generation Z has captured their families' attention, especially since most Generation Z families are from Generation X and are more educated than previous cohorts such as Ideologues and Baby Boomers. Gen Z comprises around 27% of the global inhabitants (Thangavel *et al.*, 2021). According to a BBS report (2022), 27.82% of youths (Gen Z) in Bangladesh and India's demographic statistics reveal that 45% of her citizens are under the range of (Twenty-five) 25.

Generation Z personality patterns are molded and impacted by different situations and adjacent factors, just as the preceding generation (Ni *et al.*, 2023). Those who grew up in a highly complex internet and information environment have an internet-savvy population with far greater expertise than their grandparents. According to Ryan McSweeney (2019), several Gen Z-ers may select whether or not to consume at a cafe entirely based on their online presence. Gen Z will visit a cafe if it has an updated profile showcasing Snapchat meals. To capture such a group, it is essential to maintain an online presence. A Study by Hoang *et al.*, 2024 found that Generation Z is ninety-nine percent twice as prone as Generation X and Millennials to focus on social networks and internet feedback while selecting a food outlet. Consumers may have varied desires and impressions about various catering and restaurant characters. As a result, they possibly have distinct alternative standards about which location is preferable to eat out at based on restaurant character.

According to Chang et al. (2024), the quality of consumers' meals is a substantial factor in choosing a restaurant, and he argued that different or rare food aromas and substances have a meaningful role in selecting a food outlet. The food outlet always produces a unique bill of fare and attempts to present various items to improve the consumer's repetition (Talukder et al., 2024b). The general public nowadays eats outside, in a cuisine or food outlet café for business-related tasks and pleasure. In most circumstances, restaurant patrons have a variety of options. Consumer's most essential factors in determining where to go out are in a food outlet choosing standards. A wealth of information is available when selecting a restaurant or food outlet. Consumer's pre-acquirement views and philosophy, in addition to post-acquirement views, may be influenced by cuisine type for example, distinguished three (03) sorts of food outlets, such as community, ambiance, and upscale (Carvalho de Rezende et al., 2013). Zhang (2011) highlighted four (04) decision-making variables with cafe or food outlet choice methods: a festival, a cultural gathering, a simple dinner, and a commercial meal.

Research Methodology

Nature of the Study: The present research paper is descriptive and quantitative analytic. The researchers have made a self-administrated, closed-ended, and organized questionnaire for surveying the respondents, whose responses have been analyzed to conclusions. Here, the researchers have tried to determine the factors influencing Generation Z's selection and preferences for restaurants where to dine out. So, this study was conducted by conducting a survey of 253 respondents using a detailed questionnaire.

Figure 2. Methodological Framework

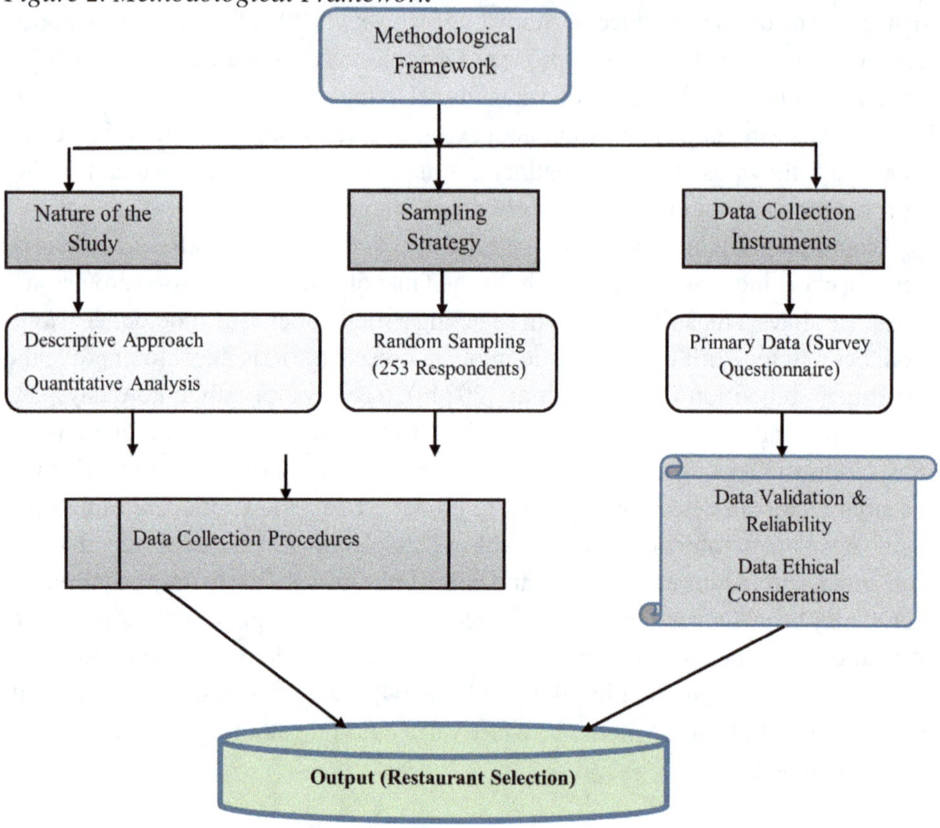

(Authors Own Made)

Target Population and the Respondents: The populations under consideration are customers of Generation Z age segments and usually visit restaurants. The main focus is the young generation within the age group of 18-26. However, the population is heterogeneous as it involves male and female respondents.

Population Size: The population size for this study of gathering information is the Generation Z group, with ages ranging from 1995 to the present. It has not been possible to count the size of the population since there are no statistics on the size of Generation Z in any Government record.

Sample Size: To avoid the biasedness and redundancy rate, the researchers have collected data randomly from the Generation Z Group. And the sample size was 253 respondents to collect data from them.

Sources and Types of Data: The study is based on primary data. Hence, the researchers used the survey method, which used self-administered questionnaires to collect responses from the respondents. The data were collected from both primary sources. The primary source of data is the survey questionnaire. However, the researchers have also got some insights from informal conversations directly with the respondents of the Generation Z group to identify their perceptions. The secondary sources of data collection were books, journals, newspapers, Wikipedia, various websites, and so on.

Tools to be used: Several statistical tools have been used for this research paper. Among them, SPSS is the primary tool for analyzing the data. Additionally, Microsoft Excel was used to draw some graphs and tables based on the data collected from the respondents.

DATA ANALYSIS AND DISCUSSIONS:

Frequency Statistics: This is the frequency statistics of the demographic data of the survey respondents. These frequency statistics focus on minimum number, maximum number, mean, standard deviation, and total number of respondents. Table 2 shows the details of the respondent's characteristics.

The respondent's characteristics

Table 2. Descriptive Statistics

Characteristics	n	%
The participant's gender		
Male	164	64.8
Female	89	35.2
Age of the participants		
18-20	16	6.3
21-23	84	33.3
24-26	153	60.4
The monthly income of the participants		
Below 5,000	46	18.2
5,000-10,000	69	27.3
10,000-15,000	61	24.1
More than 15,000	77	30.4
Education of the participant		
Below SSC	02	0.8
HSC	44	17.4
Graduation	207	81.8

continued on following page

Table 2. Continued

Characteristics	n	%
Frequency rate of the participants		
Frequently	107	42.3
Regularly	146	57.7

Source: (SPSS Output-Authors Compilation).

Descriptive Statistics of the Likert Scale: This descriptive statistics table contains 12 questions on five-point Likert scale questions- response. The questionnaire included five scales for the respondents to choose from. The respondents responded according to their perceptions or opinions. The total number of respondents for all the variables in my survey is 253, the same for all variables. The maximum response value for all the variables is 5, labeled strongly Agree. The minimum response value for all the variables is 1, labeled intensely disagreeable. Here, the means tell us the approximate center value of the data set. The standard deviation measures the deviation of each variable's value from its mean. Table 3 shows that the lower the standard deviation, the closer the perception of each variable of the respondents is. Here, the standard deviation of all the variables is below 1.50, which indicates that the study is significantly accurate, the data set is closer to their mean, and they have a higher central tendency.

Table 3. Descriptive Statistics

Descriptive Statistics					
	N	Minimum	Maximum	Mean	Std. Deviation
Pricing has a significant influence on choosing or selecting a restaurant.	253	1.00	5.00	4.3004	1.01021
Discount rates motivate me to choose a restaurant.	253	1.00	5.00	4.2688	.97126
Location/Distance plays an important role in my decision-making.	253	2.00	5.00	4.0949	.88579
I usually prefer a nearby restaurant.	253	2.00	5.00	4.2174	.86613
Physical evidence of the restaurant, especially the layout, affects my decision.	253	1.00	5.00	4.0909	.85660
I select a restaurant that maintains hygienic and safe food.	253	2.00	5.00	4.5217	.74304
I chose a restaurant based on food variation and taste.	253	2.00	5.00	4.2964	.81349
The service of the staff helps me to prefer a restaurant over another.	253	2.00	5.00	4.1186	.85087
I prefer restaurants that offer self-service.	253	1.00	5.00	2.7747	1.27889

continued on following page

Table 3. Continued

Descriptive Statistics					
	N	**Minimum**	**Maximum**	**Mean**	**Std. Deviation**
Post-purchase communication affects my decision-making.	253	1.00	5.00	3.5138	.94533
Social media influence me to select a restaurant.	253	1.00	5.00	3.7787	1.15402
I selected a restaurant that supports a convenient payment system (Cash/Online payment).	253	1.00	5.00	3.9051	1.02300
Valid N (listwise)	253				

(SPSS Output).

Correlation: Correlation measures the relationship among various variables. But it doesn't predict anything. Here, the researchers used the Pearson (R) method to correlate the variables, and SPSS was used for the findings.

Table 4. Correlation analysis

Name of Variables	1	2	3	4	5	6	7	8	9	10	11	12
1	1											
2	0.354**	1										
3	0.234**	0.261**	1									
4	0.134*	0.265**	0.547**	1								
5	-0.009	0.015	0.203**	0.203**	1							
6	0.003	0.008	0.262**	0.156*	0.150*	1						
7	0.085	0.054	0.005	0.043	0.058	0.006	1					
8	0.032	0.033	0.011	-0.041	0.061	0.234**	0.213**	1				
9	0.185**	0.215**	0.145**	0.084	0.117**	0.114*	0.022	0.123	1			
10	0.042	0.212**	-0.03	0.028	0.074	0.055	0.039	0.057	0.323**	1		
11	0.154*	0.021	0.071	0.003	0.289**	0.163	0.028	0.043	0.149	0.308**	1	
12	0.011	0.014	0.054	0.032	0.241**	0.248**	0.101	0.145*	0.111	0.141	0.338**	1

(SPSS Output)

The Pearson correlation table is used to measure the relation or connection between various variables with each other. Through this table, the researchers have indicated the relationship among multiple variables. The length of the Pearson correlation is +1 to -1. Where + 1 shows a perfect positive correlation among the variables. And the -1 indicates a perfect negative correlation among the variables. Correlations above .50 can be considered as strong positive correlations. The values which exceed .50 in the data set are strongly correlated. Here, the correlation table shows that the second (02) variable has a value of .354, the third variable has a value of .261, the fourth variable has a value of .547, the fifth variable has a value of .203, the tenth variable has a value of .323, the eleventh variable has a value of .308, and the twelfth variable has a value of .338 which are marked with ** meaning these variables are strongly and positively correlated with each other.

Again, the value of the fifth variable with pricing has a negative correlation and has a value of -0.009, the eighth variable with nearby restaurants has a value of -0.041, and the tenth variable with location has a value of -0.03. These three variables in the data set indicate a negative correlation with the mentioned variables shown in the column. Finally, the seventh variable is not so significant in this table. They do not contain any star marks, so it can be said that these variables are not statistically significant and may not have any correlation with the population. Therefore, these should be excluded from further calculation.

Regression: The following table indicates the "Anova" and "Model Summary" tables, known as the tools for measuring Regression. The Regression table is given and discussed below.

Table 5. ANOVA

ANOVA[a]						
Model		Sum of Squares	df	Mean Square	F	Sig.
1	Regression	10.694	12	.891	4.189	.000[b]
	Residual	51.053	240	.213		
	Total	61.747	252			

(SPSS Output)

Table 6. Model Summary

Model Summary				
Model	R	R Square	Adjusted R Square	Std. Error of the Estimate
1	.716[a]	.731	.432	.46122

(SPSS Output)

The significance level is 5% for the regression test, so the significant value is 0.05. Here, it is seen that the value of P is 0.000, and the value of P is less than the considerable value of 0.05. Again, the tested F value is 4.189, more significant than 1.00. This indicates that the study is done accurately. Again, the model summary describes the connection between the dependent and independent variables. The authors have examined the R-value, which is the repeated connection factor. This is approximately a direct relationship between its recorded data and the quantity anticipated by the equation. The large R-value indicates the robust and consistent connection between the dependent and independent variables in the regression model, which implies a strong and positive connection between the recorded data and the value anticipated by the model.

Here, the figure of R equals 0.716 (71.6%), a considerable amount. Therefore, a significant link exists. R^2 value quantifies the percentage of the variance in the Dependent Parameter that can be attributed to the Independent Parameter—the R^2 number of the above figure is 731, which corresponds to 73.10 percent. Therefore, the independent factors may account for approximately 73.10 percent of this dependent parameter. The adjusted component indicates the difference among the independent and dependent factors when additional factors are included. Here, the adjusted R^2 is 0.432, which predicts approximately 43.20 percent of dependent parameters' fluctuations.

Coefficients: This is the coefficient table under multiple Regression, which will help to interpret whether the variable supports the dependent variable or not and to which degree it supports the dependent variable. The standard significance value for the coefficient is .05, below the standard value, indicating that the variable is significant. If it is above .05, it demonstrates that it is insignificant.

Table 7. Coefficient analysis

Coefficients					
Model	**Unstandardized Coefficients**		**Standardized Coefficients**	**t**	**Sig.**
	B	**Std. Error**	**Beta**		
(Constant)	5.883	.329		17.868	.000
Pricing has a significant influence on choosing or selecting a restaurant.	.162	.032	.330	4.978	.000
Discount rates motivate me to choose a restaurant.	.068	.034	.134	1.985	.048
Location/Distance plays an essential role in my decision-making.	.082	.042	.146	1.949	.050
I usually prefer a nearby restaurant.	.016	.041	.028	.383	.002
Physical evidence of the restaurant and the layout significantly affect my decision.	-.049	.037	.086	1.331	.185
I select a restaurant that maintains hygienic and safe food.	.076	.044	.115	1.725	.036
I chose a restaurant based on food variation and taste.	.101	.037	.166	2.715	.007

continued on following page

Table 7. Continued

Coefficients					
Model	**Unstandardized Coefficients**		**Standardized Coefficients**	**t**	**Sig.**
	B	**Std. Error**	**Beta**		
The service of the staff helps me to prefer one restaurant over another.	.024	.037	-.041	.649	.517
I prefer restaurants that offer self-service.	.081	.026	.209	3.167	.052
Post-purchase communication affects my decision-making.	.065	.035	.125	1.870	.023
Social media influence me to select a restaurant.	.005	.029	-.012	-.179	.858
I selected a restaurant that supports a convenient payment system (Cash/Online payment).	.023	.032	-.047	-.724	.470

(SPSS Output).

The independent variable, "Pricing has a great influence on choosing or selecting a restaurant," has a significance level of .000. Therefore, this variable statistically signifies the outcome variable. It suggests that if the independent variable increases by 1 unit, the dependent variable will increase by 0.162 units because of a positive relationship. Similarly, the discount rate motivates the respondents to choose a restaurant. Location/Distance plays an important role in their decision-making. They usually prefer nearby restaurants that maintain hygienic and safe food, and they also choose restaurants based on Food variation and taste. Their post-purchase communication affects their decision-making. These have significance value of .048, .050, .002, .036, .007, and .023 respectively. All these values are less than .05, indicating that the variables are significant. Because 1 unit increase in those variables can cause a partial increase in the dependent variable. Finally, the rest of the variables have a significance value above .05, indicating that these variables are not statistically significant.

Test of Hypothesis:

The hypotheses mentioned above are tested below; such hypotheses are:

Test 01: Price and customer perception

H0: There is no relationship between reasonable price and customer perception of restaurant selection

H1: There is a positive relationship between reasonable prices and customer perception of restaurant selection

Table 8. Price and customer perception

ANOVA[a]						
Model		Sum of Squares	df	Mean Square	F	Sig.
1	Regression	4.583	2	2.292	10.022	.000[b]
	Residual	57.164	250	.229		
	Total	61.747	252			

(SPSS Output)

Table 08 shows that the significance level is 5%, and the significant value is 0.05. Here, it is seen that the value of P is 0.000, and the value of P is less than the considerable value of 0.05. Again, the tested F value is 10.022, more significant than 1.00. As such, the researchers can reject H0 (Null Hypothesis), so H1 (Alternative Hypothesis) must be accepted. This indicates strong evidence that reasonable prices are positively related to customer perception. That means if a restaurant sets a reasonable price for its food, customers will perceive the restaurant positively and feel attracted.

Test 02: Customers' perception and distance

H0: There is no relationship between distance and restaurant selection

H1: There is a positive relationship between distance and restaurant selection

Table 9. Customers' perception and distance

ANOVA[a]						
Model		Sum of Squares	df	Mean Square	F	Sig.
1	Regression	1.648	2	.824	3.427	.034[b]
	Residual	60.099	250	.240		
	Total	61.747	252			

(SPSS Output)

Table 09 shows that the significance level is 5%, with a significant value of 0.05. Here, it is seen that the value of P is 0.034, and the value of P is less than the considerable value of 0.05. Again, the tested F value is 3.427, more significant than 1.00. So, the researchers can reject H0 (Null Hypothesis), so H1 (Alternative Hypothesis) must be accepted. This indicates strong evidence that distance of location is negatively related to customer perception. That means if a restaurant is away from the customers' place, the customers can perceive those negatively and feel those are not attractive.

Test 03: Physical evidence and customer behaviour

H0: Attractive physical evidence is not positively associated with customer behavior

H1: Attractive physical evidence is positively associated with customer behavior

Table 10. Physical evidence and customer behavior

ANOVA[a]						
Model		Sum of Squares	df	Mean Square	F	Sig.
1	Regression	.815	1	.815	3.355	.068[b]
	Residual	60.932	251	.243		
	Total	61.747	252			

(SPSS Output)

Table 10 shows that the significance level is 5%, with a significant value of 0.05. It is seen here that the value of P is 0.068, and the value of P is more than the considerable value of 0.05. So, the researcher can reject H1 (Alternative Hypothesis), so H0 (Null Hypothesis) must be accepted. This indicates that attractive physical evidence is not positively associated with customer behavior.

Test 04: Products variation and customer perception

H0: Foods' variation does not positively affect customer perception

H1: Foods' variation positively affects customer perception

Table 11. Product variation and customer perception

ANOVA[a]						
Model		Sum of Squares	df	Mean Square	F	Sig.
1	Regression	1.426	2	.713	2.956	.05[b]
	Residual	60.321	250	.241		
	Total	61.747	252			

(SPSS Output)

Table 11 shows that the significance level is 5%, with a significant value of 0.05. Here, the researchers can see that the value of P is 0.05, and the value of P is approximately less or equal to the significant value of 0.05. Again, the tested F value is 2.956, more substantial than 1.00. So, the researcher can reject H0 (Null Hypothesis), so H1 (Alternative Hypothesis) must be accepted. This indicates strong evidence that food variation positively affects customer perception. If a restaurant has food variation and taste and serves safe and hygienic food, customers will perceive those positively and feel those attractive.

Test 05: People (Service staff) and customer behaviour

H0: Good service quality is not positively linked with customer perception
H1: Good service quality is positively linked with customer perception

Table 12. People (Service staff) and customer behavior

ANOVA[a]						
Model		Sum of Squares	df	Mean Square	F	Sig.
1	Regression	.563	2	.282	1.151	.318[b]
	Residual	61.184	250	.245		
	Total	61.747	252			

(SPSS Output)

It can be seen in Table 12 that the value of P is 0.318, and the value of P is more than the significant value of 0.05. Therefore, the researchers can't reject H0 (Null Hypothesis), so H1 (Alternative Hypothesis) must be rejected. This indicates strong evidence that customers do not prefer self-service restaurants. Hence, Good service quality is not positively linked with customer perception.

FINDINGS

Restaurants have become an integral part of all the inhabitants, particularly among Generation Z, who live in urban or city areas at this time. The priority in selecting a restaurant is changing quite rapidly due to various factors, including the influence of intrusion of foreign cultural tastes and habits, the prevalence of social media, the rapid growth of education, and the stream of job seekers and job holders (Huang *et al.*, 2024). Apart from these, the taste and mind of youth are far different compared to other generations. In light of a broad literature review, data collection, survey, and analysis of the result, the researchers have drawn some findings here. First, a considerable difference exists between Generation Z and other generations when selecting a restaurant. Again, price is the most crucial factor in choosing a restaurant for them (Generation Z). According to Kim & Chung (2016), Menu pricing is among the essential elements influencing customer decisions and following behavior (Qazi *et al.*, 2023). Although Gen Z considered the physical evidence less critical, the physical ambiance of a restaurant, including the restaurant's mood, setting, design, and other amenities, may substantially affect (Generation Z) choosing the restaurant. This generation also looked for menu variation. They (Generation Z) also prefer inexpensive food to the service they receive in a restaurant. According to Soriano (2002), the freshness of meals and sanitation are the elements that determine customers' restaurant decision behavior. Josiam and Monteiro (2004) agree that distinctive food flavors and components significantly affect customers' restaurant selection decisions. Restaurants often create new catalogs to boost consumer repetition and provide a diverse menu (Suheryadi *et al.,* 2023). Consequently, restaurateurs need to comprehend the impact of food excellence on restaurant entry requirements since this knowledge may direct their promotion. Finally, this generation prefers the nearby restaurant to dine out in various restaurants.

Policy Implications

The research signifies that the excellent service quality a restaurant provides impacts most customer perception, and the physical evidence, especially the layout, price, and location, also has an effect. However, the scenario is different for Generation Z. So, here are some policy implications given by the researchers to those who may use the study's findings.

To attract Generation Z, restaurants should offer budget-friendly menus, particularly for Generation Z, even though they must sacrifice the quality of service in some respects. The price of foods should be kept reasonable, and discounts should be offered more frequently as long as that doesn't hamper product quality and annual turnover. The respective contribution of the restaurant selection criteria varies significantly by restaurant cost (Lim *et al.*, 2023). Therefore, restaurateurs must comprehend the choice elements that impact restaurant guests' decisions and the relative significance of these aspects so that they may tailor their products and tactics appropriately. The restaurant should be well decorated in nature. Generation Z is more tech-savvy and takes selfies and photos more often. Generation Z frequently experiences a sense of superiority at eateries with upscale ambiance, decoration, and furnishings, and they (Generation Z) report that the general atmosphere and design satisfy their esteemed need. There should remain enough lights and space, and the arrangement of chairs & tables should be attractive and easy to use. As consumers of this generation have become more conscious about health, cleanliness, and sanitation, proper health codes should be maintained.

In the food service business, hygiene is essential (Belch *et al.*, 2024). As the prevalence of eating out has increased, consumers have become more concerned about restaurant sanitation and hygiene. Numerous studies have revealed that hygiene and sanitation is a crucial element in consumers' assessments of a restaurant's excellence, which may impact their level of pleasure (Zeithaml, Parasuraman, *et al.* 1990; Pettijohn et al., 1997; Qu 1997; Becker, Murrmann, *et al.* 1999; Bienstock, DeMoranville, *et al.* 2003; Threevitaya 2003; Aksoydan 2007; Barber and Scarcelli, 2009; Liu and Jang, 2009; Barber and Scarcelli 2010). Restaurants should provide as much good service as possible to their customers. They should have enough staff to serve customers, relationship focus, and friendly behavior towards customers if the food price is low. Brand identity does not affect Generation Z consumers' brand loyalty (Ding & Jiang, 2023). Finally, the restaurant should be as close to its target customers as possible. For instance, the restaurants that are close to the different residential halls of Dhaka University have attracted more Generation Z customers compared to other areas.

CONCLUSION

Through the research, the researchers find that the price offered by a restaurant is an essential attribute of the restaurant for Generation Z, more than the decoration/layout of the restaurant, service quality, and location of the restaurant. Good service quality refers to enough staff to serve customers, good behavior of the staff & managers, relationship focus of the staff & managers, etc. Less expensive food is the most dominant factor that affects Generation Z in selecting a restaurant. These attract customers most towards a restaurant. It is the essential attribute behind customer satisfaction and customer retention in Generation Z. The study also supports that the Physical evidence of a restaurant is also significant for customer satisfaction and positive perception. Decoration is almost as important as the service quality. Good decoration means there should remain enough lights, the restaurant should kept clean, the arrangement of chairs & tables are well placed, there is enough space in the restaurant etc. Customers generally form their perception of a restaurant, which primarily depends on these two attributes. The other two factors, the restaurant's location, cleanliness, and safety, also significantly impact customer perception. Customers perceive a restaurant well if they keep the price reasonable compared to their competitors. The study shows that customers usually have a good perception of the restaurants near their place (house, academic, or professional places). They generally don't like restaurants at a distance place. In short, according to the study, restaurants with reasonable prices, good quality services, well-decorated places, and good food hygiene have good perceptions in their customers' minds. Finally, restaurants that offer convenient payment systems for their customer can have more attractive power compared to their competitors.

Limitations

There are always some limitations in the study, the main limitation being the sample size of 253 respondents, which is a small proportion of the industry's entire population and is insufficient to give a complete picture of the study, and the data is confined only to Bangladesh. There is a risk of biases in the responses of users who are not eager to provide the correct information. There was also a limitation of time and budget for the researchers. Apart from that, the most accurate findings are derived from the study's limited sample size. This study covered students, service holders, and people in business, male and female, from all income levels. The outcome of this study will be limited to Bangladesh. Even within Bangladesh, not all the areas are included in this study. The studied respondents were only from Bangladesh, so the efficacy of this study can't be equally applicable to other cities or villages in Bangladesh. Future studies can be done without any age limit or different generations.

Future Research Directions

Expanding on the results of this study, several exciting directions for additional research into the dining preferences and habits of Generation Z become apparent. First, further research on the subtleties of price response among various Generation Z demographics may offer insightful information about how factors like occupation, schooling, and financial level affect people's judgments of how affordable restaurants are. Furthermore, investigating how societal variables affect restaurant selections may reveal how elements like race and social norms shape attitudes toward restaurant features. Additionally, examining how social networking sites and internet advertising influence Generation Z's restaurant preferences may help clarify how well internet sites influence consumer opinions and encourage eatery attendance. Future studies on Generation Z's eating choices are influenced by environmentally conscious programs and moral component sourcing.

Furthermore, evaluating the effects of technology integration, comparing cultures, and investigating how preferences change continuously through longitudinal research can provide important insights into how Generation Z's restaurant tastes are changing. The comprehension of Generation Z's restaurant behaviors can be further enhanced by examining the significance of health and nutritional patterns, marketing, and credibility, as well as external influences like fiscal recessions and health emergencies. Future research in these areas could contribute to our understanding of hospitality management and customer behavior, which would help restaurants better understand how to appeal to the tastes of Generation Z patrons.

REFERENCES

Ahlawat, R., Ghai, M., & Garg, S. K. (2022). *Factors influencing restaurant selection in the COVID-19 era: a study of consumer preferences in India*. DOI: 10.5281/ZENODO.7314391

Aksoydan, E. (2007). Hygiene factors influencing customers' choice of dining-out units: Findings from a study of university academic staff. *Journal of Food Safety*, *27*(3), 300–316. DOI: 10.1111/j.1745-4565.2007.00081.x

Barber, N., & Scarcelli, J. M. (2009). Clean restrooms: How important are they to restaurant consumers? *Journal of Foodservice*, *20*(6), 309–320. DOI: 10.1111/j.1748-0159.2009.00155.x

Barber, N., & Scarcelli, J. M. (2010). Enhancing the assessment of tangible service quality through the creation of a cleanliness measurement scale. *Managing Service Quality*, *20*(4), 373–392. DOI: 10.1108/09604521011011630

Becker, C., Murrmann, S. K., Murrmann, K. F., & Cheung, G. W. (1999). A pancultural study of restaurant service expectations in the United States and Hong Kong. *Journal of Hospitality & Tourism Research (Washington, D.C.)*, *23*(3), 235–255. DOI: 10.1177/109634809902300301

Bełch, P., Hajduk-Stelmachowicz, M., Chudy-Laskowska, K., Vozňáková, I., & Gavurová, B. (2024). Factors Determining the Choice of Pro-Ecological Products among Generation Z. *Sustainability (Basel)*, *16*(4), 1560. DOI: 10.3390/su16041560

Bienstock, C. C., DeMoranville, C. W., & Smith, R. K. (2003). Organizational citizenship behavior and service quality. *Journal of Services Marketing*, *17*(4), 357–378. DOI: 10.1108/08876040310482775

Carvalho de Rezende, D., & Alberto Rodrigues Silva, M. (2013). Eating-out and experiential consumption: A typology of experience providers. *British Food Journal*, *116*(1), 91–103. DOI: 10.1108/BFJ-02-2012-0027

Chang, C.-Y., Jhang, S.-J., Yang, Y.-T., Chang, H.-C., & Chang, Y.-J. (2024). Utilizing Skip-Gram for Restaurant Vector Creation and Its Application in the Selection of Ideal Restaurant Locations. In Deng, D.-J., & Chen, J.-C. (Eds.), *Smart Grid and Internet of Things* (Vol. 557, pp. 141–147). Springer Nature Switzerland., DOI: 10.1007/978-3-031-55976-1_14

Cristancho Triana, G. J., Cancino Gomez, Y. A., & Ninco Hernandez, F. A. (2024). Factores que influyen en el comportamiento de consumo sostenible en la generación Z. *Retos*, *14*(27), 51–67. DOI: 10.17163/ret.n27.2024.04

Das, I. R., Talukder, M. B., & Kumar, S. (2024). Implication of Artificial Intelligence in Hospitality Marketing. *Utilizing Smart Technology and AI in Hybrid Tourism and Hospitality*. IGI Global, USA._https://doi.org/_DOI: 10.4018/979-8-3693-1978-9.ch014

De Barros Neto, J. P., & De Oliveira, L. P. (2023). Study on the perception of Generation Z about robotized selection processes. *International Robotics & Automation Journal*, *9*(3), 99–107. DOI: 10.15406/iratj.2023.09.00271

Ding, L., & Jiang, C. (2023). The effect of perceived collective efficacy and self-efficacy on Generation Z restaurant customers' food waste reduction intentions. *Journal of Global Responsibility*, *14*(3), 337–359. DOI: 10.1108/JGR-08-2022-0079

Fekete, M., & Nagy, Á. (2022). Qlimates and Quarantines – Testing the Hypothesis of How Gen Z Transformed into a Generation. In Schutter, S., Harring, D., & Bass, L. E. (Eds.), *Sociological Studies of Children and Youth* (pp. 1–27). Emerald Publishing Limited., DOI: 10.1108/S1537-466120220000030001

Gupta, K. P., & Pande, S. (2023). Understanding Generation Z consumers' revisit intentions to robotic service restaurants. *Young Consumers*, *24*(3), 331–351. DOI: 10.1108/YC-09-2022-1598

Hammad, A. (2024). Factors Influencing the Digital Tourism Marketing of Generation Z Tourists "Applied to the Egyptian Tourist Destination." *International Journal of Tourism. Archaeology and Hospitality*, *4*(1), 15–37. DOI: 10.21608/ijtah.2024.251138.1107

Hoang, D. P., Nguyen Hai, D., Nguyen, V. T. N., Nong, H. T., Pham, P. T., & Tran, T. M. (2024). Factors affecting restaurant choices for traditional foods among Gen Y and Gen Z: A multigenerational study on Vietnamese "Pho." *Journal of Hospitality and Tourism Insights*. DOI: 10.1108/JHTI-10-2023-0766

Hu, W. (2022). Research on the Integration and Development of Folk Art and Cultural Tourism Industry under the Modern Cultural Background. *BCP Education & Psychology*, *7*, 145–150. DOI: 10.54691/bcpep.v7i.2627

Huang, B., Huang, Y., Zhai, M., Zhou, Q., Ji, S., Liu, H., Zhuang, X., Zhang, Y., & Zhang, J. (2024). Association of Sex With Cardiovascular Outcomes in Heart Failure Patients With Obstructive or Central Sleep Apnea. *Journal of the American Heart Association*, *13*(5), e031186. DOI: 10.1161/JAHA.123.031186 PMID: 38410942

Jain, A., & Dutta, D. (2019). Millennials and Gamification: Guerilla Tactics for Making Learning Fun. *SA Journal of Human Resource Management*, *6*(1), 29–44. DOI: 10.1177/2322093718796303

Jeong, E., & Jang, S. (2011). Restaurant experiences trigger positive electronic word-of-mouth (eWOM) motivations. *International Journal of Hospitality Management, 30*(2), 356–366. DOI: 10.1016/j.ijhm.2010.08.005

Josiam, B. M., & Monteiro, P. A. (2004). Tandoori tastes: Perceptions of Indian restaurants in America. *International Journal of Contemporary Hospitality Management, 16*(1), 18–26. DOI: 10.1108/09596110410516525

Khan, I. A., & Shibami, A. H. A. (2019). Generation Z's learning preferences: Impact on organizational learning and development - a study conducted in a vocational institute in UAE. *International Journal of Learning and Change, 11*(4), 379. DOI: 10.1504/IJLC.2019.105646

Kim, S., Chung, J.-E., & Suh, Y. (2016). Multiple reference effects on restaurant evaluations: A cross-cultural study. *International Journal of Contemporary Hospitality Management, 28*(7), 1441–1466. DOI: 10.1108/IJCHM-05-2014-0220

Kivela, J., Inbakaran, R., & Reece, J. (1999). Consumer research in the restaurant environment, Part 1: A conceptual model of dining satisfaction and return patronage. *International Journal of Contemporary Hospitality Management, 11*(5), 205–222. DOI: 10.1108/09596119910272739

Kumar, S., Talukder, M. B., & Pego, A. (Eds.). (2024). *Utilizing Smart Technology and AI in Hybrid Tourism and Hospitality*. IGI Global., DOI: 10.4018/979-8-3693-1978-9

Lim, Y. S., Ng, T. H., Lam, M. S., & Tan, S. Y. (2023). Communication in the 21st Century: The Effect of Internet Celebrity as the Communication Source in Influencing Generation Z Purchase Intention. *Jurnal Komunikasi: Malaysian Journal of Communication, 39*(4), 507–522. DOI: 10.17576/JKMJC-2023-3904-27

Liu, Y., & Jang, S. S. (2009). Perceptions of Chinese restaurants in the U.S.: What affects customer satisfaction and behavioral intentions? *International Journal of Hospitality Management, 28*(3), 338–348. DOI: 10.1016/j.ijhm.2008.10.008

Massawe, A. (2013). Customer segmentation in full service restaurant business [Bachelor's thesis, Saimaa University of Applied Sciences]. http://www2.uwstout.edu/content/lib/thesis/2003/2003threevitayas.pdf (Note: This appears to be a thesis; the link provided in search results leads to a related document, but the original may be available via institutional repositories.)

Ni, Y., Ding, Y., Hu, H., & Chu, J. (2023). Research on the influencing factors of public opinion information forwarding behaviour of Generation Z group (Next): Mechanism of action. *Highlights in Science. Engineering and Technology*, *42*, 309–321. DOI: 10.54097/hset.v42i.7110

Peters, K., & Hervé Remaud, P. (2020). Factors influencing consumer menu-item selection in a restaurant context. *Food Quality and Preference*, *82*, 103887. DOI: 10.1016/j.foodqual.2020.103887

Pettijohn, L. S., Pettijohn, C. E., & Luke, R. H. (1997). An evaluation of fast food restaurant satisfaction: Determinants, competitive comparisons and impact on future patronage. *Journal of Restaurant & Foodservice Marketing*, *2*(3), 3–20. DOI: 10.1300/J061v02n03_02

Qazi, H., Alam, S., & Phulpoto, A. (2023). Motivating Factors Influencing Green Buying Behavior of Generation Z: An Application of Theory of Planned Behavior (TPB). *Pakistan Journal of Humanities and Social Sciences*, *11*(3). Advance online publication. DOI: 10.52131/pjhss.2023.1103.0646

Qu, H. (1997). Determinant factors and choice intention for Chinese restaurant dining: A multivariate approach. *Journal of Restaurant & Foodservice Marketing*, *2*(2), 35–49. DOI: 10.1300/J061v02n02_03

Sardar, S., Ray, R., Hasan, M., Chitra, S. S., Parvez, A. T. M. S., & Avi, M. A. R. (2022). Assessing the Effects of COVID-19 on Restaurant Business From Restaurant Owners' Perspective. *Frontiers in Psychology*, *13*, 849249. DOI: 10.3389/fpsyg.2022.849249 PMID: 35496209

Sezgi, N. E., & Uyanik, B. (2022). Priorities of consumers for restaurant preferences: A conjoint analysis study on generation Z. *Journal of Tourism Leisure and Hospitality*, *4*(2), 6–6. DOI: 10.48119/toleho.1187392

Shah, P., Bhusal, N., & Chettri, K. K. (2023). Influence of Social Media Usage on Generation Z's Choice in Selecting Restaurants in Kathmandu. *Journal of Business and Social Sciences Research*, *8*(1), 95–110. DOI: 10.3126/jbssr.v8i1.56592

Soriano, D. R. (2002). Customers' expectations factors in restaurants: The situation in Spain. *International Journal of Quality & Reliability Management*, *19*(8/9), 1055–1067. DOI: 10.1108/02656710210438122

Suheryadi, H., Dian Sua Pratama, B., Rahmah Farahdiba, S., & Elya Rohimi, U. (2023). Generation Z's Perception of Dining Experience at Korea Restaurants, South Jakarta. *Journal of Wood Science*, *2*(10), 1696–1702. DOI: 10.58344/jws.v2i10.422

Talukder, M., Kumar, S., Misra, L., & Kabir, F. (2024). Determining the role of eco-tourism service quality, tourist satisfaction, and destination loyalty: A case study of Kuakata Beach. *Acta Scientiarum Polonorum. Administratio Locorum, 23*(1), 133–151. DOI: 10.31648/aspal.9275

Talukder, M. B. (2020). The Future of Culinary Tourism: An Emerging Dimension for the Tourism Industry of Bangladesh. I-Manager's. *Journal of Management, 15*(1), 27. DOI: 10.26634/jmgt.15.1.17181

Talukder, M. B., & Das, I. R. (2024). The Technology Impacts and AI Solutions in Hospitality. i-manager's Journal on Artificial Intelligence &. *Machine Learning, 2*(1), 56–72. DOI: 10.26634/jaim.2.1.20291

Talukder, M.B., & Kumar, S. (2024). Revisiting intention in food service outlet of five-star hotels:A quantitative approach based on food service quality. Sport i Turystyka. Środkowoeuropejskie Czasopismo Naukowe, 7(1), 137–156. https://doi .org/_DOI: 10.16926/sit.2024.01.08

Talukder, M. B., Kumar, S., & Das, I. R. (2024a). Implications of blockchain technology-based cryptocurrency in the cloud for the hospitality industry. In *Emerging trends in cloud computing analytics, scalability, and service models* (pp. 340–358). IGI Global Scientific Publishing. DOI: 10.4018/979-8-3693-0900-1.ch018

Talukder, M. B., Kumar, S., & Das, I. R. (2024b). Perspectives of digital marketing for the restaurant industry. In *Advancements in socialized and digital media communications* (pp. 118–134). IGI Global Scientific Publishing. DOI: 10.4018/979-8-3693-0855-4.ch009

Talukder, M. B., Kumar, S., & Das, I. R. (2024c). *Food Wastage on the Economic Outcome: Evidence From the Hotel Industry. Sustainable Disposal Methods of Food Wastes in Hospitality Operations*. IGI Global., DOI: 10.4018/979-8-3693-2181-2.ch005

Talukder, M. B., Kumar, S., Sood, K., & Grima, S. (2023). Information Technology, Food Service Quality and Restaurant Revisit Intention. *International Journal of Sustainable Development and Planning, 18*(1), 295–303. DOI: 10.18280/ijsdp.180131

Thangavel, P., Pathak, P., & Chandra, B. (2021). Millennials and Generation Z: A generational cohort analysis of Indian consumers. *Benchmarking, 28*(7), 2157–2177. DOI: 10.1108/BIJ-01-2020-0050

The importance of crisis management in tourism. (2022). USF M3 Publishing, LLC. DOI: 10.5038/9781955833080

Threevitaya, S. (2003). Factors that influence the decisions of customers to dine at selected restaurants in Bangkok, Thailand [Master's thesis, University of Wisconsin-Stout]. http://www2.uwstout.edu/content/lib/thesis/2003/2003threevitayas.pdf

Walker, J. R. (2011). *The restaurant: From concept to operation* (6th ed.). John Wiley & Sons.

Wang, X. (2023). The Effect of Service Marketing Mix (7Ps) on Purchase Intention in the Script Killing Industry. *Academic Journal of Management and Social Sciences*, *4*(2), 57–62. DOI: 10.54097/ajmss.v4i2.12087

Zeithaml, V. A., Parasuraman, A., & Berry, L. L. (1990). *Delivering quality service: Balancing customer perceptions and expectations*. Simon and Schuster.

Zhang, L. (2011). *An assessment of contemporary dining out behaviour: The moderating factors of culture and food selection within Chinese full-service restaurants in Shanghai, China* (Doctoral dissertation, University of Waikato).

Zheng, Y. (2024). To Access or Not to Access: Influencing Factors for Government Microblogging Information Seeking and Avoidance among Chinese Generation Z. *Human Behavior and Emerging Technologies*, *2024*, 1–14. DOI: 10.1155/2024/8288503

Chapter 7
Impact of Spa and Wellness Tourism on Local Market of Alleppey in Kerala: A Critical Review

Ramesh Koikkal
Lovely Professional University, India

Sanjeev Kumar
https://orcid.org/0000-0002-7375-7341
Lovely Professional University, India

ABSTRACT

The study will explore the scope of spa and wellness tourism as a new and potential trend which shape and promote the tourism and hospitality industry in India. Spa and wellness tourism can help to increase the economy of the country which enhances customer experience within the hospitality sector and provide a different opportunity for guest to rejuvenate with a new experience. The personalized guest interactions, optimization of revenue, difference of operation style, and overall experience of guest satisfaction through spa resorts. The latest trend in information technology and AI can be a supporting factor to improve wellness tourism. It gives an exceptional experience of new trends of culinary skills linked with medicinal properties or with health and wellness options. The spa sector facilitates increasing more job opportunities, by improving infrastructure to develop the new market and supporting local businesses to develop. To promotes sustainability by emphasizing environmental conservation and mingling with cultural and heritage of India in

DOI: 10.4018/979-8-3373-4516-1.ch007

contributing to long-term economic and social wellbeing. Therefore, the study makes recommendations based on new tourist demands and new processes and protocols for the operation of wellness tourism sector. Hospitality Sector can make it customized to guests who are willing to spend more for a better experience and wellness of body and mind. Significantly Spa and wellness tourism can be significantly beneficial to local economies by attracting tourists.

INTRODUCTION

The tourism industry is a great resource of economy for many countries. It shapes the country and portrays itself in global market to establish its identity in tourism sector. The GDP for many countries from tourism is a major contribution to the total economic revenue of the country. Moving from very modest need for travelling for the purpose of education, medical and social gathering in the mid of 18th century, the industry has taken many shapes to sustain the development of this sector (Preji & Lenka, 2020). Alleppey, known as the "Venice of the East," has long attracted travellers with its scenic backwaters, traditional houseboats, and serene landscapes. In recent years, however, another form of tourism has quietly but powerfully reshaped the town's economy—spa and wellness tourism. With Kerala's global reputation as the land of Ayurveda, Alleppey has emerged as a key destination for holistic health seekers. The growing demand for wellness experiences such as Ayurvedic treatments, yoga retreats, and spa therapies has had a noticeable impact on the local market, bringing both opportunities and challenges (Suban, 2024a). One of the most positive outcomes of this wellness wave is the boost it has given to local employment and entrepreneurship. Spa and wellness centers, ranging from luxury resorts to homestays offering authentic Ayurvedic massages, have created jobs for trained therapists, yoga instructors, and hospitality staff (Kuşcu et al., 2024). Local youth, especially women, are being trained in wellness therapies and traditional healing methods, leading to skill development and financial independence. The demand for herbal oils, medicinal plants, and natural cosmetics has also supported small-scale farmers and cottage industries that supply these materials (Choudhary & Qadir, 2021).

Furthermore, wellness tourism has encouraged longer stays compared to conventional sightseeing. Visitors seeking detox programs or Ayurvedic healing often spend several weeks in Alleppey, which benefits local businesses in more sustained ways. Restaurants offering healthy, locally sourced food, transport operators, and markets selling handmade goods all experience a ripple effect (Craig, 2018). The growing wellness economy has also prompted many local property owners to transform their ancestral homes or vacant spaces into eco-friendly retreats, contributing to rural revitalization.

However, this growing popularity comes with concerns. There is a risk of commercialization diluting the authenticity of traditional wellness practices. In an attempt to cater to international tastes, some establishments compromise the purity of Ayurvedic treatments by combining them with superficial spa services (Han et al., 2018). Additionally, the influx of wellness tourists can lead to increased demand for land and resources, which may inflate property prices and disrupt the local balance. Sustainability is another pressing issue. While many wellness centers emphasize eco-conscious living, not all operate with genuine concern for the environment (Joson et al., 2024). Overuse of water, improper disposal of herbal waste, and the construction of large spa resorts can have unintended environmental consequences, especially in ecologically sensitive regions like Alleppey. Despite these challenges, the overall impact of spa and wellness tourism on Alleppey's local market is largely positive. It has not only brought economic vitality but also helped preserve and promote Kerala's ancient healing traditions. For the local community, the key lies in striking a balance—between tradition and innovation, tourism and sustainability (Manhas et al., 2019). If nurtured mindfully, Alleppey has the potential to become a global model for wellness tourism that empowers its people, honours its heritage, and protects its natural beauty.

Tourism development in India

India on the other hand due to its colonialization in British rule had a late entry into tourism sector. People used to travel for reasons of education and medical facility in 18 century (Parida et al., 2018). But travelling for purpose of recreation purpose was first discussed and planned in year 1948 with the creation of TTC (Tourist Traffic Committee). In the years to it saw a gradual growth and in 1949 tourist branch was created in Delhi, Mumbai, Kolkata and Chennai to promote travel in India. In 1958 a separate department of tourism was created under ministry of transport and communication. In 1966 ITDC was formed with a motive of promoting tourism which started shaping tourism industry. In 1982 the first tourism policy was created which supported the tourism industry vividly. India's tourism sector contributed 7% of our GDP which is $212 million in 2019. In the year 2022 total revenue of $215 million was contributed by tourism (Buhalis et al., 2023). In the year 2024 a total of 9.66 million tourist travelled to India and it accounted for Foreign exchange earnings of 2,77,842 crores and is is a 19% growth from previous year (Sharma et al., 2025).

Tourism Development in Kerala

According to study Kerala was not a key destination until 1980 rather it was unknown by reports. Later the foundation of KTDC laid foundation for tourism prospect. A very aggressive marketing strategy was established to improve tourism in Kerala. Now Kerala is a very popular destination attracting international tourist in large number and also the domestic tourist's ideal spot for recreation. Kerala is known for its beaches, backwaters, mountain ranges and wild life sanctuaries. The main attractions in Kerala are clustered around Alleppey, Kollam, Wyanad, Kovalam, Munnar, Periyar, Ashtamudi Lake, Vembanad Lake, Silent Valley and Eravikulam National park. The 'Grand Kerala Shopping Festival" was a good initiative in promoting Kerala tourism and held every year from December to January. Kerala also used the tag line "God's Own Country", which established as a very popular tag line in tourism sector (George et al., 2020).

Tourism growth and initiatives in Alleppey

Alapuzha (Aleppey) is also known as the "Venice of the East" due to its vast rivers and backwaters which attract a large number of tourists because of the initiative the KTDC has taken to develop these sectors which are as listed below:

I. **Water tourism:** The development of backwaters in Alleppey and creating a tourism circuit connected by water was created and it was big success. It attracts huge number of tourist both domestic as well as international.
II. **Swadesh Darshan 2.0:** This was an initiative taken by Kerala tourism to make Aleppey an iconic global tourist destination by making of all resources like lakes, rivers, backwaters and canals in Aleppey.
III. **Ayurvedic Massage Centres:** Kerala is known for Ayurveda and globally it has followers who are willing to get an ayurvedic massage for various reasons. This is included as a product to attract more domestic and international tourist.
IV. **Wellness Retreats:** meditation, yoga, spa and other wellness tourism products are floated to attract more tourists to Alleppey.
V. **Spa Tourism:** This concept of tourism is developing well now and gaining popularity domestically and internationally (Prasad et al., 2025). The hotels and resorts are set to gear up to the standard required to welcome guest and take care of them by providing required service of spa, wellness and culinary delights as a package.

Rise of Wellness Tourism

The above said factors gave ignition to a new type of tourism called wellness tourism and is different from medical tourism and other related tourism like farm tourism, eco-tourism, and adventure tourism (Talukder, Hossain, et al., 2024). In wellness tourism Ayurveda, yoga, meditation, spa therapies are included. Spa is a business with the commitment to wellness as its main agenda to promote tourism (Talukder et al., 2025). Tourism is accountable for a significant part of wellness tourism and the economy. Spa and wellness tourism are positioned at a profitable intersection between the rising wellness industry and the world's massive tourism economy (Bandyopadhyay & Nair, 2019a). Spa and Wellness services are of essential importance with regards to increasing the acceptance of the tourism product in large scale. In a broad sense they are associated with the strife for maintaining a healthy lifestyle, nutrition diet which provided in resorts as a contribution to improve wellness tourism (Pande & Sengupta, 2024). The agenda of wellness tourism is that they have to facilitate their combination with different types of traditional and special-interest tourism to improve this part of tourism sector. In today's dynamic and competitive markets, spa and wellness tourism offer companies in the travel sector a challenging opportunity for expanding their business and generating revenue. Their supply is diversified with the range of products and destinations specializing in spa and wellness tourism. Alternative holiday offers and programs should be developed to target tourists with a profile which is different from the traditional type of consumers who are happy with standard tourism services (Putrevu & Mertzanis, 2025). Spa and wellness travel are poised for great growth. India must also tap the MICE industry to use the spa and wellness tourism for which special provisions and offers to support the sector in increasing economy. Already we see a future of a large industry which is the spa and wellness travel sector that can see a significant surge in coming years for several reasons (Hudson et al., 2017). The primary aim of this research is to study on the impact of spa and wellness tourism on local market in Alleppey district of Kerala, which can improve their life style, enhance revenue and create more job opportunities. Alleppey is also referred as the 'Venice of India' as the district has Abundance Rivers, water, and popularity for always existing spa and ayurvedic recreations (Chon, 2012). This also helps us to study the industry with its growth and the influence on the society of Alleppey in general.

Aim of study

The different areas the study will cover is to do a critical analysis on spa and wellness tourism with its scope on local market in Alleppey district of Kerala are:

I. The study will highlight the reason a guest chooses the spa and wellness tourism. This can provide us a more detailed understanding of the customer needs and expectations. We also would be able to understand the reason behind the guest's preference on this sector like health improvement, stress control, relaxation etc.
II. The impact of spa and wellness tourism on creating more jobs and improve revenue at the destination, and understand the scope of this sector in improving economies.
III. The various challenges and opportunities in the development of spa and wellness tourism in Alleppey like sustainable growth, eco-friendly practices, utmost hygiene, total sanitation and inclusion of technology where applicable in providing a satisfactory destination for guests.

Conceptual Framework of Impact of Spa and Wellness Tourism

Figure 1. Conceptual Framework of Impact of Spa and Wellness Tourism; Author Compilations

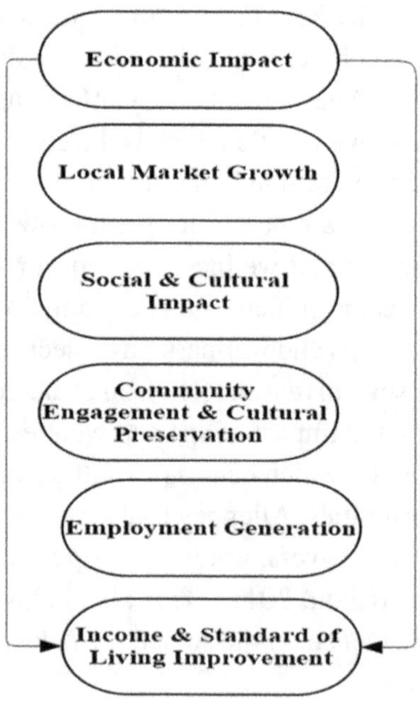

Economic Impact
Local Market Growth
Social & Cultural Impact
Community Engagement & Cultural Preservation
Employment Generation
Income & Standard of Living Improvement

Challenges and Opportunities in Development of Spa and Wellness Tourism in Alleppey:

As discussed in figure 01, Alleppey with its calm backwaters, coconut groves, and traditional healing heritage, holds immense promise as a spa and wellness tourism destination. Over the past decade, this charming town in Kerala has seen a steady rise in tourists seeking peace, rejuvenation, and authentic Ayurvedic experiences. While this growing interest brings new energy to the region, the journey toward becoming a top wellness hub isn't without its fair share of challenges and learning curves. One of the biggest opportunities for Alleppey lies in its deep-rooted connection to Ayurveda and natural healing (Suban, 2024b). The world is turning towards holistic health, and Alleppey has exactly that to offer ancient practices, organic treatments, and a setting that nurtures the mind and body. With the right training and support, local practitioners, therapists, and small business owners can play a major role in sharing Kerala's wellness wisdom with the world. It also opens the door for eco-friendly retreats, yoga centres, and wellness resorts that blend comfort with culture (Rani. J & Chandran, 2024).

Additionally, wellness tourism attracts a different kind of traveller those who are likely to stay longer, spend more, and seek deeper, more meaningful experiences. This can boost the local economy significantly, supporting everything from herbal product suppliers to artisans and organic farmers. There's also great potential for international partnerships, retreats, and medical wellness packages that could position Alleppey on the global wellness map (Dewangan & Kumar, 2024). However, this growth also comes with its share of challenges. One key concern is maintaining authenticity. With rising demand, some wellness centres may start offering watered-down versions of treatments or focus more on luxury than on actual healing. If quality and tradition are not safeguarded, Alleppey risks losing what make it special in the first place. Infrastructure is another concern. Roads, sanitation, and public transport systems need to evolve to meet the expectations of wellness tourists, especially those coming from overseas (Kumar et al., 2025). There's also a need for skilled and certified professionals who can deliver genuine treatments and communicate well with international clients something that requires investment in education and training. Environmental sustainability is equally important. If wellness development leads to overbuilding or careless use of natural resources, it could damage the serene environment that tourists come to enjoy (Anwar et al., 2025). The focus must remain on harmony with nature, with tradition, and with the local community. In essence, the road ahead for spa and wellness tourism in Alleppey is filled with both promise and responsibility (Suban, 2024c). With mindful planning, community participation, and a commitment to staying true to its roots, Alleppey can grow into a wellness sanctuary that not only heals visitors but uplifts its own people too.

I. The baby boomers are looking to extend their years of good health by enjoying spa tourism.
II. More tourists are realizing that the key to good health and longevity lies in their own hands, which makes spa and wellness as a next change in tourism sector in Alleppey in Kerala.
III. Availability of more wellness products available in all price categories in Indian tourism sector like spa, Ayurveda, and medical tourism. A more systematic development plan is required for improving spa tourism in Alleppey.
IV. Globalization is opening the doors to wellness lifestyle and it's ever-increasing demand as tourist want to adopt a wellness lifestyle and Kerala's Alleppey can bring in more tourist if initiatives are taken.
V. Tour operators and travel agents can expect a change in transformation of wellness tourism sector. The increasing number of tourists who want to get spa and wellness into their trip is looking for various options in this sector.
VI. This can largely increase the job opportunities and revenue generation in this sector, which can in turn impact the growth of local economies. Wellness tourism is preventive and holistic. Wellness tourist seeks to relax, rejuvenate, detoxify, and enhance the lifestyle. Wellness tourism is a new sector which is not just limited to spa or yoga retreats; it extends to resort-based destinations offering wellness programs, eco-wellness retreat, and even culinary wellness tours (Talukder, Kumar, et al., 2024).

LITERATURE REVIEW

Our country's economy is generated greatly from the tourism and hospitality sectors. Kerala is a state which is having a natural tradition of ayurveda and wellness and it takes only to develop the existing resources and infrastructure in Alleppey. One of the tourism industry's fastest-growing subsectors in south India of recent years is wellness tourism. Kerala with its cultural influence naturally and can accelerate the growth of wellness travel. Kerala has long been known for its traditional health care practices, including naturopathy, Ayurveda and yoga (Cyranski, 2017a). The post-pandemic effect in travellers' preferences towards lifestyles, health and mental well-being has greatly propelled the expansionof spa tourism with a sustainable role. As per statistics of Department of Tourism, Government of Kerala US$ 4 billion was generated by Kerala. India is home to well-known wellness locations like Kerala and one such place in Kerala is Alleppey district abundant with rivers, back waters, greenery, and spa and ayurvedic tourism. Furthermore, there are important gaps in infrastructure, training, quality assurance, and global awareness that needs to be concentrated if Alleppey has to become a leader in wellness tourism.

The main prospects and challenges are as follows:

I. Promoting wellness tourism by state government

Indian Tourism and Hospitality Industry Analysis reflected a "Contribution of the Travel and Tourism sector to India's GDP is likely increased.Wellness is at a stage of mental, social and physical well-being. It is a state of being free from stress and illness. This shows a very clear indication that wellness tourism is the latest trend in tourism sector to generate revenue (George et al., 2020). With increase in number of visitors and good infrastructure can impact and will surely have a direct impact on Alleppey local market and the economies to increase for the local destination supporting the spa and wellness tourism. The government of Kerala is actively involved supporting by providing investments, creating infrastructure in Alleppey to strike wellness tourism as a next milestone in earning revenue and also impact the local market economy and life style (Chua et al., 2021). Some financial incentives for approved projects in ayurvedic tourism include investment subsidy of upto 10 per cent subject to a ceiling of one million rupees. Such projects will also get support to avail funds from state financial corporations, concession in electricity charges and guidance and publicity support from the State Government such incentives and support have to be given to spa tourism promotion. Alleppey is one such area where foreign seeking a different recreation comes and who doesn't particularly limit on the budget. It is a potential area to tap for promoting tourism in Alleppey. The government also trying to tie up with private sector players to invest and associate with this product of tourism which can directly improve the standards of resorts, spa, roads, restaurants, markets and shopping in Alleppey small towns with potential for wellness tourism (Cyranski, 2017b). The Kerala Tourism Development Corporation helps and promotes by showcasing Ayurvedic concept of Kerala to Global as well as Indian market. Mainly Alleppey which is acting as a key hub for wellness tourism in India, which includes not only Ayurvedic but also, meditation, yoga and spa retreats to name a few. KTDC also takes initiatives to connect the locals to be part of the wellness experience shared to guest by having live fishing experience, culinary combinations, yoga and meditation sessions, and exposure to spa retreats of international standards.

II. The Rise of Influence Culture and Its Psychological Impact on Youth:

In today's digital world, social media has become more than just a place to connect it's now a stage where influence is currency and followers are power. This rise of "influence culture" has transformed the way young people see themselves, their aspirations, and even their worth. At the heart of this shift is the idea that anyone can become famous if only they go viral. But beneath the filters, hashtags, and curated lifestyles lies a more complicated truth: the psychological impact of influence culture on youth is profound and far-reaching.

For many young people, influencers have become the new role models. Instead of looking up to scientists, educators, or community leaders, they're often drawn to content creators whose lives appear glamorous and effortless. This constant exposure to "highlight reels" can create unrealistic expectations about success, beauty, and happiness (Spates et al., 2007). When every scroll brings a new image of perfection, it's easy to feel inadequate. Teens, in particular, may start to measure their value by likes, shares, or follower counts metrics that change by the minute and offer fleeting validation. Influence culture also encourages a performative way of living. Young users may feel pressure to craft their lives in a way that's "post-worthy," leading to an obsession with appearances rather than authenticity. The constant need to present an idealized self can cause anxiety, low self-esteem, and even depression (Ackard et al., 2007). It can also blur the lines between personal identity and online persona, making it harder for youth to develop a grounded sense of self. Furthermore, the pursuit of virility can come at a cost. Some young people may engage in risky behaviours, trend-chasing, or controversial content creation just to gain attention. This not only compromises personal values but can also expose them to cyber bullying, online harassment, or public shaming. The mental toll of such experiences is often overlooked but deeply damaging. However, it's important to note that not all effects are negative. Influence culture can also empower youth to express them, find communities of support, and raise awareness about important causes. The key lies in how we guide the next generation to engage with it consciously and critically. Parents, educators, and policymakers must play a proactive role in fostering digital literacy, encouraging self-worth beyond screens, and promoting mental well-being (Orgilés et al., 2020). Youth need spaces both online and offline where they are valued not for their follower count but for their thoughts, creativity, and kindness. In a world driven by influence, the greatest gift we can give our youth is the confidence to be themselves no filter needed.

III. How Influencer Lifestyles Affect the Self-Esteem of Gen Z:

For Gen Z, growing up in a world flooded with influencers has reshaped how they see themselves and the world around them. From fashion hauls and travel vlogs to fitness routines and "day in my life" reels, the constant exposure to influencer lifestyles creates a curate reality one where perfection is the norm and success seems effortless. But behind this seemingly glamorous feed lies a quieter, more personal struggle: the impact on self-esteem (Kishore Kumar & Priyadarshini, 2018). Many Gen Z individuals find themselves comparing their everyday lives to the polished snapshots influencers share online (Kokkinopoulou et al., 2025). When influencers flaunt luxurious vacations, ideal relationships, flawless skin, or expensive clothes, it often makes ordinary experiences feel dull or inadequate. This constant comparison can chip away at self-worth, especially during adolescence a time when identity and confidence are still developing.

Social media's algorithm also plays a role in reinforcing these feelings. Gen Z users are often shown the most engaging, aesthetically pleasing content—rarely the behind-the-scenes struggles or imperfections. As a result, many begin to believe that everyone else is thriving while they are falling behind. It's not just about admiration anymore; it becomes a silent pressure to look, live, and succeed in ways that often feel unattainable. And when these goals aren't met, feelings of failure or "not being enough" creep in. The influencer lifestyle also pushes the idea that validation comes from likes, followers, and views (Sakdiyakorn et al., 2021). This external validation can cause young people to question their value if their own posts don't receive the same level of attention. They might start altering how they dress, what they say, or even how they behave just to fit into what's trending, rather than staying true to them. It is not all negative. Some influencers do promote authenticity, mental health awareness, and self-love. But the dominant narrative is still one of perfection and constant success. Gen Z needs most reassurance that their worth isn't tied to social media approval. Encouraging open conversations, teaching digital literacy, and promoting diverse role models can help shift the focus back to real, meaningful self-esteem (Van Den Bergh et al., 2024). Because in a world chasing likes, the real "like" Gen Z deserves is the one they give to themselves.

IV. Opportunities for wellness Tourism in Kerala

In recent years, there is a shift toward preventive health and healthy living as a post covid change which increased the demand for wellness tourism. Modern lifestyle challenges such as sedentary habits, rising diseases like diabetes, hypertension, mental health and also work-related stress. This have made people more aware of the need for regular wellness requirement and this trend is especially notable among the urban middle and upper classes, aging populations who prioritize health, wellbeing, self-care and mind relaxation. Kerala, with its deep-rooted wellness, culture and heritage, offers an attractive destination like Alleppey for these health-conscious travellers (Patil et al., 2025). Resorts should be created that provides curate experiences like spa, yoga, meditation retreats, Ayurvedic therapies and low-calorie cuisines which are in high demand. Thus a priority for wellness resorts that offer personalized and integrative programs stand to benefit this upward trend, especially as more travellers seek rejuvenating, and wellness journeys rather than conventional leisure trips. There are some leading hotel groups like Ramada and Lemon tree which operates excellent spa resorts with rates slightly on the higher side. I would suggest focusing on making initiative for bringing up more affordable spa resorts, so that we can also tap the regional market in travelling to south (Chettiparamb & Kokkranikal, 2012). The opportunities of developing wellness tourism in Alleppey are very bright and prosperous only if the infrastructure can be improved in and around Alleppey.

If we study the infrastructure for last 10 years, it shows an improvement in many areas. But when we talk about developing it as a landmark spa and wellness hub which can have a global impact then the infrastructure currently available might not be up to the international standard (Thaloor, 2024). So it is a moral responsibility of KTDC to provide enough funds to improve the infrastructure. Local private funding can also be initiated to improve the infrastructure.

The infrastructures which need to be improved are as follows:

I. The highways, roads and by roads in and around the Alleppey has to be improved. Right now, it has a good infrastructure, but when we compare international standards, then it has to be focussed. Currently there is metro boat in Kochi city connecting various coastal areas in and around Kochi. In par with the same system, a metro boat scheme can also be launched to improve the infrastructure. Alleppey already has various boating options, including houseboats, motorboats, and shakers, for exploring the backwaters but as an extended option a metro boat scheme can also be considered (Evangeline et al., 2019). As per the news there is a plan for extending the metro boat scheme from Kochi to Alleppey.
II. The safety, security and surveillance must be in par with international standards and this infrastructure must be developed with the co operation of the ministry and the police department.
III. More vigilance has to be ensured in the spa retreat industry as it can be used for illegal activities and government must ensure strict registration and observation of the organizations engaged in spa industry. This can ensure safety for the customers domestic as well as international.
IV. Sanitation and hygiene at the spa retreats must be ensured so that the guest experience is satisfactory.

V. Eating out and restaurant in and around Alleppey is well developed as of now, but additionally A class restaurants has to be developed with international cuisine so that we can accommodate foreign tourist as well and ensure to provide cuisines which can satisfy their palate.
VI. More resorts have to be developed in and around Alleppey town. Already big groups like Ramada and Lemon-tree have ventured into the wellness market. More international and popular brands must venture into the resort and hotel industry development in Alleppey city.
VII. Transportation and lighting have to be increased. As of now there is a good network of transportation in Alleppey city but it has to extended to micro villages so that all potential areas of Alleppey can be tapped

Revenue Potential

Wellness tourist tends to spend more per trip than average tourists.. It is found that compared to regular visitors, wellness travellers typically spend more money per trip. This makes wellness tourism not only a growing segment but also a high-value one. Even the local people are encouraged to tie up with various projects in supporting the wellness tourism and find a means of earning revenue. It can have a direct implication on the life style and economy of the local market (Chaudhury et al., 2023). A positive marketing strategy is adopted to vigorously spread the message of the spa and wellness destinations in Alleppey to the world. There is a huge potential for earning revenue but the only concern is the initial investment to nurture the development of infrastructure in and around Alleppey town. For this local funding and privatization in various field can be considered as it can enhance financing for this sector (Baker, 2008).

Brand image

In a competitive hospitality market, wellness tourism offers Indian resorts a powerful way to differentiate their brand. In Kerala particularly Alleppey, the resorts that build their identity around authentic wellness experiences can appeal to niche traveller segments, including free individual wellness seekers, corporate groups, and wellness motivated tourist (Bandyopadhyay & Nair, 2019b). By combining promotions, marketing for MICE business and tap the market to come to resorts which are establishing as exclusive wellness destinations. This type of branding strategies can also include with packages involving spa, Ayurveda and culinary delights mingling with wellness.

Scope of Research

The research has a good scope of identifying the key challenges and opportunities existing in Alleppey in promoting sustainable wellness tourism as a product which can be marketed internationally. The spa and wellness tourism in Alleppey have an immense scope on creating employment, new markets for people who bind with tourism sector. It can maintain a better lifestyle of consumer and improving the local market. It is actually done as a secondary research to identify the scope of wellness tourism in Alleppey.

In the study the following analysis and details were collected to support the research in wellness tourism in Alleppey and its impact on local market:

I. **Guest preferences**: By various studies we have analysed that the guest behaviour towards spa and wellness tourism is positive. It also gives clear indication to their preferences on destinations like Alleppey and Kochi for spa and wellness tourism with various facilities and services. By studying these guest behaviours, we can develop the destination and services as per the requirement of the market. The customers prefer branded spa parlours are attached to resorts, with full range of facilities, and mid-range of pricing which can attract more regional and global tourist coming to Alleppey for pure wellness related vacationing (B. B. Nair et al., 2022).

II. **Growth and potential of wellness tourism:** By conducting a thorough market analysis we found out that the potential of spa and wellness tourism is very high in Alleppey as it has good natural resources of pure air, water from rivers and good environment to promote spa tourism. It can also give us an idea of the impact of spa and wellness tourism on local market in Alleppey (Csirmaz & Pető, 2015).

III. **Infrastructure of destination:** To develop the spa and wellness tourism in Alappey the infrastructure should be re-evaluated and improved as per international standards. This can enhance the foreign customer expectations and satisfaction, which will promote this sector of tourism. It can aid as a main factor in improving local economies and new job opportunities.

IV. **Providing safety and hygiene by service providers:** The destination must be improved maximum safety for customers by providing adequate monitoring systems to ensure safety of guest. Even the service providers must ensure proper sanitation in the resorts. The main service providers are spa, resorts, lodges, restaurants, transportation and other related services.

CONCLUSION

A comprehensive research on spa and wellness tourism in India would provide valuable insights into the evolving dynamics of this industry, its potential for growth, and the challenges that need to be addressed to realize its full potential. The study would establish the current market size and projected growth of the wellness tourism industry in India, drawing upon growth of industry and insights from available information. The research identified the factors driving for the growth of wellness tourism, including the rising disposable income of the Indian middle class, increased awareness of health and well-being, and the availability of diverse wellness offerings. The study would explore the role of spa resorts in attracting tourists and promoting India as a wellness destination, examining their unique offerings and contribution to the industry. It would also analyse the motivations and benefits sought by tourists participating in wellness tourism, such as relaxation, stress reduction, and improved well-being. The research would address the challenges faced by the wellness tourism industry in India, such as infrastructure limitations in remote areas and the need for standardized quality assurance, while also highlighting the opportunities for growth and development. The research could also explore emerging trends and future prospects for the wellness tourism industry, including the potential for new destinations and offerings. The state government has to take initiative to identify more destinations and resorts that can attach to specific loop for example it can link spa, yoga and Ayurveda as one loop with resorts and other facilities attached to it for a package.

REFERENCES

Ackard, D. M., Eisenberg, M. E., & Neumark-Sztainer, D. (2007). Long-Term Impact of Adolescent Dating Violence on the Behavioral and Psychological Health of Male and Female Youth. *The Journal of Pediatrics*, *151*(5), 476–481. DOI: 10.1016/j.jpeds.2007.04.034 PMID: 17961688

Anwar, A., Kumar, S., & Talukder, M. B. (2025). Sustainable Rural Development Through Homestay Tourism: An Evaluation of Economics. In Parashar, A., Chandel, P. S., Seetaram, N., & Agarwal, P. (Eds.), *Global Practices and Innovations in Sustainable Homestay Tourism* (pp. 41–74). IGI Global., DOI: 10.4018/979-8-3373-0427-4.ch003

Baker, K. (2008). Kerala's strategy for tourism growth: A southern approach to development and poverty alleviation. In Burns, P., & Novelli, M. (Eds.), *Tourism development: Growth, myths and inequalities* (1st ed., pp. 192–216). CABI., DOI: 10.1079/9781845934255.0192

Bandyopadhyay, R., & Nair, B. B. (2019a). Marketing Kerala in India as God's Own Country! For tourists' spiritual transformation, rejuvenation and well-being. *Journal of Destination Marketing & Management*, *14*, 100369. DOI: 10.1016/j.jdmm.2019.100369

Bandyopadhyay, R., & Nair, B. B. (2019b). Marketing Kerala in India as God's Own Country! For tourists' spiritual transformation, rejuvenation and well-being. *Journal of Destination Marketing & Management*, *14*, 100369. DOI: 10.1016/j.jdmm.2019.100369

Buhalis, D., Leung, X. Y., Fan, D., Darcy, S., Chen, G., Xu, F., Wei-Han Tan, G., Nunkoo, R., & Farmaki, A. (2023). Editorial: Tourism 2030 and the contribution to the sustainable development goals: the tourism review viewpoint. *Tourism Review*, *78*(2), 293–313. DOI: 10.1108/TR-04-2023-620

Chaudhury, S. K., Sarkar, S., Pattnaik, C. S., & Rahman, S. (2023). Assessment of Kerala Tourism Industry-An Economic Perspective. *Dera Natung Government College Research Journal*, *8*(1), 97–110. DOI: 10.56405/dngcrj.2023.08.01.07

Chettiparamb, A., & Kokkranikal, J. (2012). Responsible tourism and sustainability: The case of Kumarakom in Kerala, India. *Journal of Policy Research in Tourism, Leisure & Events*, *4*(3), 302–326. DOI: 10.1080/19407963.2012.711088

Chon, K. S. (2012). *The Tourism and Leisure Industry: Shaping the Future* (0 ed.). Routledge. DOI: 10.4324/9780203049853

Choudhary, B., & Qadir, A. (2021). Impact of COVID-19 on wellness and spa industry. *International Journal of Spa and Wellness, 4*(2–3), 193–203. DOI: 10.1080/24721735.2021.1986970

Chua, B.-L., Al-Ansi, A., Lee, M. J., & Han, H. (2021). Impact of health risk perception on avoidance of international travel in the wake of a pandemic. *Current Issues in Tourism, 24*(7), 985–1002. DOI: 10.1080/13683500.2020.1829570

Craig, V. (2018). The impacts of high-volume massage on spa therapists' physical and mental wellness. *International Journal of Spa and Wellness, 1*(3), 218–227. DOI: 10.1080/24721735.2019.1596659

Csirmaz, É., & Pető, K. (2015). International Trends in Recreational and Wellness Tourism. *Procedia Economics and Finance, 32*, 755–762. DOI: 10.1016/S2212-5671(15)01458-6

Cyranski, C. (2017a). *Purifying Purges and Rejuvenating Massages: Ayurvedic Health Tourism in South India*. DOI: 10.11588/HEIDOK.00022342

Cyranski, C. (2017b). *Purifying Purges and Rejuvenating Massages: Ayurvedic Health Tourism in South India*. DOI: 10.11588/HEIDOK.00022342

Dewangan, S., & Kumar, S. (2024). AI and Big Data Analytics Revolutionizing Industry 5.0: Unlocking the Power of Smart Manufacturing and Beyond. In Darwish, D. (Ed.), (pp. 398–410). Advances in Business Information Systems and Analytics. IGI Global., DOI: 10.4018/979-8-3693-0413-6.ch016

Evangeline, S., Rajkumar, M. R., & Parambath, S. G. (Eds.). (2019). *Recent Advances in Materials, Mechanics and Management* (1st ed.). CRC Press., DOI: 10.1201/9781351227544

George, A. T., DeLacy, T., & Jiang, M. (2020). 6 Responsible Rural Tourism Initiatives and Local Community Development in Kerala, India. In Nair, V., Hamzah, A., & Musa, G. (Eds.), *Responsible Rural Tourism in Asia* (pp. 87–101). Multilingual Matters., DOI: 10.21832/9781845417529-008

Han, H., Kiatkawsin, K., Jung, H., & Kim, W. (2018). The role of wellness spa tourism performance in building destination loyalty: The case of Thailand. *Journal of Travel & Tourism Marketing, 35*(5), 595–610. DOI: 10.1080/10548408.2017.1376031

Hudson, S., Thal, K., Cárdenas, D., & Meng, F. (2017). Wellness tourism: Stress alleviation or indulging healthful habits? *International Journal of Culture, Tourism and Hospitality Research, 11*(1), 35–52. DOI: 10.1108/IJCTHR-09-2015-0111

Joson, G. H. G., Pyke, J., Delacy, T., & Davidson, C. (2024). Wellness in the Spa Industry: An Investigation of Hot Spring Tourism in Australia. In Chhabra, D., Atal, N., & Maheshwari, A. (Eds.), *Sustainable Development and Resilience of Tourism* (pp. 63–79). Springer International Publishing., DOI: 10.1007/978-3-031-63145-0_4

Kishore Kumar, M., & Priyadarshini, R. G. (2018). Important factors of self-efficacy and its relationship with life satisfaction and self-esteem – with reference to gen y and gen z individuals. *IOP Conference Series. Materials Science and Engineering*, *390*, 012007. DOI: 10.1088/1757-899X/390/1/012007

Kokkinopoulou, E., Papasolomou, I., Porcu, L., & Vrontis, D. (2025). Exploring the impact of online co-creation on eudemonic well-being and sustainable fashion choices among Generation Z. *EuroMed Journal of Business*. Advance online publication. DOI: 10.1108/EMJB-12-2024-0356

Kumar, H., Aswathy, V. K., & Kumar, S. (2025). Converging Realms of Social Health, Domestic Workers, and Telemedicine Landscape: Challenges and Prospects. In Özbek, M. F., & Christiansen, B. (Eds.), *Organizational Sociology in the Digital Age* (pp. 165–180). IGI Global., DOI: 10.4018/979-8-3693-7398-9.ch010

Kuşcu, F. N., Yorulmaz, M., & Göde, A. (2024). THE EFFECT OF PATIENT EXPECTATIONS AND SATISFACTION ON REGIONAL TRUST IN HEALTH TOURISM: A PRIVATE HOSPITAL EXAMPLE. *Journal of International Health Sciences and Management*, *10*(19), 1–12. DOI: 10.48121/jihsam.1323199

Manhas, P. S., Charak, N. S., & Sharma, P. (2019). Wellness and spa tourism: Finding space for Indian Himalayan spa resorts. *International Journal of Spa and Wellness*, *2*(3), 135–153. DOI: 10.1080/24721735.2020.1819705

Nair, B. B., Sinha, S., & Dileep, M. R. (2022). Exploring the impact of COVID-19 on the travel intermediaries in India: Mapping trends and strategies. *International Journal of Tourism Policy*, *12*(4), 427. DOI: 10.1504/IJTP.2022.128137

Orgilés, M., Morales, A., Delvecchio, E., Mazzeschi, C., & Espada, J. P. (2020). Immediate Psychological Effects of the COVID-19 Quarantine in Youth From Italy and Spain. *Frontiers in Psychology*, *11*, 579038. DOI: 10.3389/fpsyg.2020.579038 PMID: 33240167

Pande, L., & Sengupta, S. (2024). Wellness Tourism in India: Evolution, Perspectives, and Trends. SSRN *Electronic Journal*. DOI: 10.2139/ssrn.4674035

Parida, Y., Bhardwaj, P., & Roy Chowdhury, J. (2018). Effects of economic development and crime on tourism in India. *Anatolia*, *29*(1), 63–73. DOI: 10.1080/13032917.2017.1384742

Patil, A., Prathibha Raj, M. S., Gowri Shankar, R., & Lakshmi, R. B. (2025). Cultivating Wellness: Synergy of Emerging Technologies in Spiritual and Wellness Tourism. In Tyagi, P. K., Nadda, V., & Singh, A. K. (Eds.), *Meaningful Tourism* (pp. 145–162). Emerald Publishing Limited., DOI: 10.1108/978-1-83797-837-320251022

Prasad, A., Das, D., & Ajith Kumar, N. (2025). A Tourism Potential of Alleppey District: A Study on Vembanad Backwaters. In Fong, S., Dey, N., & Joshi, A. (Eds.), *ICT Analysis and Applications* (Vol. 1162, pp. 21–30). Springer Nature Singapore., DOI: 10.1007/978-981-97-8605-3_3

Preji, M. P., & Lenka, S. K. (2020). Wellness tourism in Kerala: A study on the tourist perception in terms of therapeutic and industry performance indicators. *Siddhant- A Journal of Decision Making, 20*(1and2), 57. DOI: 10.5958/2231-0657.2020.00007.5

Putrevu, D. J., & Mertzanis, C. (2025). The Rise of the Wellness Business Sector: A Systematic Literature Review. SSRN *Electronic Journal*. DOI: 10.2139/ssrn.5190935

Rani, J. R. E., & Chandran, A. (2024). Constructed Wetlands as a Greywater Management Alternative in the Tourism Industry. In Sucheran, R. (Ed.), *Advances in Hospitality, Tourism, and the Services Industry* (pp. 383–414). IGI Global., DOI: 10.4018/979-8-3693-6110-8.ch015

Sakdiyakorn, M., Golubovskaya, M., & Solnet, D. (2021). Understanding Generation Z through collective consciousness: Impacts for hospitality work and employment. *International Journal of Hospitality Management*, *94*, 102822. DOI: 10.1016/j.ijhm.2020.102822

Sharma, M., Mohapatra, G., & Giri, A. K. (2025). Assessing the role of ICT, governance, and infrastructure on inbound tourism demand in India. *Journal of Economic and Administrative Sciences*, *41*(1), 320–335. DOI: 10.1108/JEAS-03-2022-0064

Spates, C. R., Samaraweera, N., Plaisier, B., Souza, T., & Otsui, K. (2007). Psychological Impact of Trauma on Developing Children and Youth. *Primary Care*, *34*(2), 387–405. DOI: 10.1016/j.pop.2007.04.007 PMID: 17666234

Suban, S. A. (2024a). Spa tourism: Understanding the relationship of tourist's emotional experience, destination image, satisfaction, and intention to recommend using an integrated model. *International Journal of Spa and Wellness*, *7*(1), 1–22. DOI: 10.1080/24721735.2024.2314943

Suban, S. A. (2024b). Spa tourism: Understanding the relationship of tourist's emotional experience, destination image, satisfaction, and intention to recommend using an integrated model. *International Journal of Spa and Wellness*, *7*(1), 1–22. DOI: 10.1080/24721735.2024.2314943

Suban, S. A. (2024c). Spa tourism: Understanding the relationship of tourist's emotional experience, destination image, satisfaction, and intention to recommend using an integrated model. *International Journal of Spa and Wellness*, *7*(1), 1–22. DOI: 10.1080/24721735.2024.2314943

Talukder, M. B., Hossain, S. E., Al Ferdous, F., & Khan, M. R. (2024). Exploring the Rise of Wellness Tourism: Trends, Benefits, and Market Potential. In Jermsittiparsert, K., & Marzo, R. R. (Eds.), (pp. 351–378). Advances in Computational Intelligence and Robotics. IGI Global., DOI: 10.4018/979-8-3693-9158-7.ch013

Talukder, M. B., Kumar, S., & Khan, M. R. (2024). The Integration of Sustainable Practices in Cultural and Gastronomic Tourism. In Munuhwa, S. (Ed.), (pp. 467–484). Advances in Civil and Industrial Engineering. IGI Global., DOI: 10.4018/979-8-3693-3755-4.ch017

Talukder, M. B., Swarna, D. A., Kumar, S., & Kabir, F. (2025). Leveraging Technology for Employee Wellness in Hospitality: Smart Solutions for a Vibrant Service Culture. In Baez, M. D. (Ed.), (pp. 221–246). Advances in Logistics, Operations, and Management Science. IGI Global., DOI: 10.4018/979-8-3373-1687-1.ch008

Thaloor, S. (2024). Metaverse and Wellness Tourism: An Investigation on Mixed Reality (MR) Health Care Approaches in the Tourism Industry. In Krishnan, C., Behl, A., Dash, S., & Yadav, P. D. (Eds.), *The Metaverse Dilemma: Challenges and Opportunities for Business and Society* (pp. 183–203). Emerald Publishing Limited., DOI: 10.1108/978-1-83797-524-220241011

Van Den Bergh, J., De Pelsmacker, P., & Worsley, B. (2024). Beyond labels: Segmenting the Gen Z market for more effective marketing. *Young Consumers*, *25*(2), 188–210. DOI: 10.1108/YC-03-2023-1707

Chapter 8

Like, Share, Compare: Exploring the Mental Health Implications of Social Media Marketing on Gen Z

Anumeha Mathur
https://orcid.org/0000-0002-3846-1721
K.R. Mangalam University, India

Akanksha Kathuria
https://orcid.org/0000-0001-7887-5710
Manav Rachna University, India

Mansi Yadav
https://orcid.org/0000-0003-3045-0902
K.R. Mangalam University, India

Richa Nangia
https://orcid.org/0000-0002-6128-8648
Sushant University, Gurgaon, India

ABSTRACT

In the age of digital epoch, where the phenomenon of digitalisation is revolutionising every facet, and social media platforms are occupying primary space, starting from interacting people, fitness regime, entertainment, watching and scrolling reels, news, educational engagement, and product acquisition, life revolves around social media only. The existence of individuals, especially Gen Z entirely depends upon social media for all requirements, whether it is interaction, exploration, consumption etc. These platforms are designed in such a way that they are engaging attention by sharing and commenting. At one end they are streamlining and facilitating our lives,

DOI: 10.4018/979-8-3373-4516-1.ch008

but on the other having a negative effect on emotional wellbeing, self-perception, mental wellbeing of Genz because of too much usage and reliance on these social media platforms. This in result starts giving rise to the social and cultural comparison, which in turn increases anxiety, esteem issues and even lead to severe mental disorders, depression. This chapter critically examines how these social media platforms engender emotional and mental challenges, how these influencers are influencing Gen z and increasing peer comparison pressure that adversely affects self-esteem. It is time to rethink and to devise strategies in such a way that aims to create a safe digital landscape.

INTRODUCTION

The accelerating growth of social media is transcending 4.6 billion users globally as per the data of 2024 marks a identifying trait of modern digital society. Social media platforms like Instagram, Facebook, X formally Twitter, TikTok, YouTube becomes a vital component of our daily routine. Generation Z are the significant users highly active on various social media platform. Generation Z, also known as zoomers born in between 1997-2012, consists of individuals born in the era of smart devices, internet connectivity, and uninhibited use of latest technology popularly known as the first true digital natives (Medanta, 2025). The excessive use of social media substantially affecting and shaping social behaviour of Gen Z and adversely affects the mental well-being of Gen Z (Cropink,2025).

Social Media usage has a major impact on its frequent users; it affects them both positively and negatively (Vidani & Jaiswal, 2024; Mastroianni, 2024).The positive impact of social media includes better connectivity, access to information, an opportunity for self-expression and can provide support networks. However, there are several studies that show the negative influence of social media on youngsters. This duality necessitates an in-depth understanding of the influence of social media. Social media has an impact on its users' psychological health, there is a strong need of creating policies that minimize damage and positively influence its users (Wan Sulaiman et al., 2024). Pathil et al. (2024) explains the beneficial as well as adverse impact of social media on young users which creates the need for mindful engagement to decrease the negative impact. Social media usage has its own advantages and disadvantages; its drawbacks include social comparison, cyber bullying and addiction but it also serves as a platform to bring people together, creates a sense of community and can be a source of information exchange (Ajewole, 2024). There are many online communities, support groups and ample resources on social media that facilitate open discussions and help combat loneliness, (Zhu, 2024). According to Wan Sulaiman et al. (2024) people who feel lonely find connections along with a feeling of belongingness on social media platforms. Many youngsters find connections, community, peer support and accessible mental health help online (Molina & Roja, 2024). The impact of social media on mental health varies significantly in different age groups (Ehimuan et al., 2024; Olorunsogo et al., 2024); the study highlights the importance of considering culture, society, and psychological dimensions in studying social media impact.

The widespread technology usage also has a flipside. A major drawback is that it leads to dopamine spike, which fuels addictive behaviour (Sutcliffe & Virassamy, 2021), leading to a vicious circle of overuse. Social media addiction, according to Andreassen (2015), is when someone feels compelled to use social media excessively, which hinders the ability to get involved in other social activities like work, studies, relationships with others, and their physical as well as mental health. The excessive use and addiction of social media often result in social isolation, which gives rise to anxiety, stress, depression, and peer comparison that often hampers the mental well-being of individuals (Gann, 2025; Harmony,2025).

Social media has emerged has as a potent force that impacts self-image, buying behaviour and mental health. Social media has changed the way we communicate and altered the way people build their identities and understand the world. (Van Dijck, 2013). The Gen Z is trying to excel in this "like, share, compare" cycle which is leading to upwards social, comparison, FOMO, and emotional distress. According to Akbar et al., (2024) the negative influence on mental wellbeing of young generation necessitates focused attention for improving the situation. It is vital to comprehend the complicated connect between social media and mental health of youth. (Yakobus et al., 2023)

There are many researches that emphasize that mental wellbeing has a close relationship with social media exposure, social comparison, and fear of missing out. The content on social media is highly curated which presents idealized lifestyles of influencers and users. This portrayal leads to upward social comparison, where an individual compares his life with peers who appear to be leading a more fulfilling life. Upward Social comparison results in lower self-esteem and greater dissatisfaction with one's life. Addictive consumption of social media and leads to social media fatigue which has negative influence on mental well-being (Saura et al., 2025). In a study by Fassi et al (2025) the youngsters with mental health issues were found to spend more time on social media and were less satisfied with the life, those with internalizing condition were spending more time on social media and social comparison. The compulsive engagement with online content over a period of time creates emotional strain

There are many researchers that exhibit a strong correlation between exposure to marketing content, social comparison, FOMO and psychological wellbeing. (Saura et al., 2025; Fassi et al., 2025). Mental illness among young adults have considerably increased in past ten years Burgess (2025) attributes this to increasing social media use. Gahemi (2020) calls this tendency digital depression. Excessive social media usage may lead to depression, anxiety and suicidal tendencies. (Weigle & Shafi, 2024). A recent report by McKinsey Health Institute (2023) shows that people with two hours of social media usage were more prone to mental health challenges.

Marketing campaigns on apps like Instagram, TikTok and YouTube often feature micro-influencers and curated images that go on to shape Gen Z's behaviors and its sense of its own identity (Bonfils, 2022). De Vilela Teles connected social media marketing with growing vulnerability to trust and comparison among Gen Z for fashion in a 2024 study. Odgers and Jensen (2020) studied explained social media usage tends to intensify social pressure, causing young people to comply and have a poor opinion of themselves in relation to their way of life.

Gen Z is vulnerable to upward social comparisons because of the frequent exposure to idealized depictions online. (Kannan & Kumar, 2022). As mentioned by Liang (2024) such comparisons may lead to erosion of self-esteem, and set in "a vicious cycle of dissatisfaction and self-criticism that mediates the pathway to negative emotions". Dredge et al. (2014) work is in sync with this, he explained that excessive social media usage might increase a feeling of inferiority and low self-image.

The fear of missing out the rewarding experiences is prevalent in generation Z and can be triggered by marketing techniques such as exclusive online events and offers for a limited time only (Saura et al., 2025). The regularly updated content further creates curiosity and pressure on young adults to explore social media further. (Chakrabarti, 2024)

Online marketing and comparison-based content on social media is known to enhance emotional despair in Gen Z, research points to small yet the existence of the significant positive correlation between social media usage, anxiety, depression, eating disorders, these effects being more acute in young girls.

Dual nature of social media is well documented, it fosters connections, provides information and support in communities but also leads to loneliness, emotional distress, anxiety, FOMO, depression and addiction. Social media addiction exploits the fundamental human need for belongingness and self-validation, The "digital depression" (Gahemi, 2020) and its impact on young users necessitates the need to consider regulation of platform design and policies to regulate it. The current approaches have majorly recommended user behaviour modification some have suggested the need to focus on design and regulation of social media platforms. It is necessary to articulate the factors that lead to addictive behaviour more importantly as the majority of the users are young and in a very impressionable age. There is need to explore further how exposure to social media marketing contribute to emotional distress, FOMO, anxiety low self-image due to social comparison.

Ascension of Influencer Culture

The influencer culture is strongly linked with the emergence of web 2.0, and is of collaborative nature where they are showcasing and endorsing their personal lives and earning capital gain by a large follower base, who are following them on various social media platforms and idealizing their lifestyles (Kaplan & Haenlein, 2010). Influencer culture is firmly established with the growing usage of social media platforms and is trending nowadays for entertainment to business purposes (Mathur & Chhibber, 2015). Unlike traditional form of advertisements and promotions which is only a one way communication, influencer marketing gains advantage because of its direct connectivity with audiences through trust, authenticity and social relationship (Abidin,2016). This rise of influencer culture has transformed the influencers as opinion leaders, who nowadays are endorsing brands and becoming idols of many youths. The rise of this influencer culture has both prospects and obstacles. On the one hand it is attracting Gen Z by fostering a sense of identity, building trust and facilitating brands for global reach and concentrated marketing by being directly connected to the niche audiences. On the flip side concerns about integrity, over penetration and commercialisation elevate probes about resilience of influencer culture (Marvik,2015). This culture allows influencers to endorse their own life, daily routine, hobbies, and they themselves become a celebrity in the digital world by attracting large number of followers. For the gen Z who are in the stage of self-identification and struggling for building a social status in the society, the persistent exposure to these tailored realities prompting concerns like peer pressure, self-dissatisfaction, low self-esteem, and sometimes harming well-being ((Fardouly et al., 2015))

List of Top Influencers:

Table 1. List of top Influencers

	Influencer	Platforms / Niche	Estimated Reach (range) — checked Sep 10, 2025	Mental-health relevance (paraphrased)	Sources (accessed Sep 10, 2025)
1	Charli D'Amelio	TikTok, Instagram — Dance & lifestyle	100M–160M	High visibility dance content; associated with performance pressure and burnout themes among teens.	VisualCapitalist; SocialBlade
2	Avani Gregg	TikTok, Instagram — Beauty & transformation	30M–50M	Beauty/transformation posts encourage creativity but may reinforce body-image comparisons.	DMPro; SocialBlade
3	Emma Chamberlain	YouTube, Instagram — Lifestyle & personal storytelling	10M–20M	Open about anxiety; fosters strong parasocial bonds that can be supportive or dependency-forming.	WeArePion; YouTube Analytics
4	Kylie Jenner	Instagram — Fashion & beauty	350M–400M	Represents luxury and appearance ideals; exposure linked to material and appearance comparison.	VisualCapitalist
5	Khaby Lame	TikTok, Instagram — Comedy / reactions	70M–80M	Relatable humor reduces language barriers; virality highlights pressure to produce simple yet viral content.	VisualCapitalist; DMPro
6	Addison Rae	TikTok, Instagram — Dance & music	70M–90M	Trend-driven content increases visibility and peer comparison on appearance/performance.	DMPro
7	Bella Poarch	TikTok, Instagram — Music & short video	50M–80M	Entertainment plus advocacy; has publicly discussed mental-health issues.	WeArePion
8	MrBeast (Jimmy Donaldson)	YouTube — Large-scale challenges & philanthropy	100M–200M	Massive-scale content fosters community/charity narratives but also intensive production stress.	VisualCapitalist
9	James Charles	YouTube, Instagram — Beauty & makeup	20M–30M	Creative identity formation through beauty; controversies show impacts of online criticism and bullying.	VisualCapitalist
10	Brent Rivera	YouTube, Instagram — Comedy & vlogs	20M–40M	Relatable comedic persona strengthens belonging but increases parasocial expectations.	DMPro
11	Kritika Khurana (That Boho Girl)	Instagram — Fashion & lifestyle (India)	1M–2M	Aspirational fashion/travel themes relevant to body image and lifestyle comparison in Indian Gen Z.	Exly; TheMediaAnt
12	Komal Pandey	Instagram, YouTube — Fashion & styling (India)	1M–2M	Highly curated aesthetics shape local appearance ideals and identity expression.	TheMediaAnt
13	Kusha Kapila	Instagram, YouTube — Comedy & commentary (India)	3M–4M	Uses satire to discuss social pressures; creates relatability with both supportive and comparative effects.	TheMediaAnt
14	CarryMinati (Ajey Nagar)	YouTube — Comedy & gaming (India)	30M–40M	Satirical and confrontational style; past controversies illuminate cyberbullying dynamics.	TheMediaAnt
15	Prajakta Koli (MostlySane)	YouTube, Instagram — Lifestyle & comedy (India)	6M–8M	Blends entertainment with positive messaging; often advocates for mental-wellness topics.	Exly; WeArePion"

"Influencer selection and follower ranges were compiled by the author from multiple online sources (VisualCapitalist; DMPro; SocialBlade; WeArePion; Exly; TheMediaAnt) to reduce reliance on any single list. Follower counts are presented as ranges and were checked on 10 Sep 2025. Descriptions are paraphrased by the author and linked to observed mental-health themes (social comparison, parasocial relationships, appearance pressure, FOMO, cyberbullying)."

LITERATURE REVIEW

Social Media Marketing has gained considerable attention from the marketers as well as social media users over the last few years as we have shifted from traditional to digital modes of communication. **Social Media Marketing Exposure** refers to how much and how often the target audience is exposed to brand messages on various social media platforms. These brand messages are designed to create an emotional response through algorithm-based advertisements, flash sales and influencer curated content (De Veirman et al., 2017). Social Media Marketing is a powerful tool for marketers as it reaches the targeted audience and is more powerful in evoking the desired emotional response than traditional marketing. The users of social media see benefits of social media but remain oblivious to its negative impact on mental health. Marketers now trust the algorithm driven advertisements, flash sales (limited time offers) and influencer endorsement to capture attention and trigger consumer emotions. (Kapoor et al., 2022)

Social media permits a more personalized, interactive, and engaging marketing content which makes it more effective in increasing consumer engagement and influencing purchase decision. (Appel et al., 2020). According to Alalwan (2018) the advanced targeting tools on social media platforms improve the campaign effectiveness.

SMME has many advantages for the marketer but its impact on mental health of users has raised concerns. Overexposure to social media may lead to negative psychological impact. Exposure to curated content for prolonged period is linked with anxiety, social comparison and low self-esteem(Chae, 2018; Vogel et al. 2014). Younger audience is more susceptible to negative impact and emotional strain due to exposure to curated influencer content (Vaterlaus et al. 2021).

According to the American Psychological Association (APA) "A state of intense negative emotions that can be triggered by various stressors, such as threats, losses, or feelings of being overwhelmed." Emotional distress is a feeling of depression, anxiety, hopelessness, and stress. A significant reliance on social media offers entertainment and social connections to youngsters but on the negative side it raises psychological stress levels (Andreassen et al., 2017). SMME can increase stress due to upward social comparison as it creates unrealistic standards of lifestyles (Alalwan, 2018; Appel et al., 2020).

Cognitive appraisal theory (Lazarus, 1991) can be used to understand the relationship between marketing exposure with emotional distress. The audience's emotional reactions are shaped by how they perceive environmental stimuli, for example an idealistic lifestyle displayed on social media can be perceived as overwhelming which may lead to anxiety and emotional distress.

The Emotional Contagion theory (Hatfield et al., 1994) explains that feelings displayed in ads can be transferred to and felt by the consumers taking them to a similar emotional state as exhibited in the advertisement. The youngster also gets in a negative mental state which can lead to doomscrolling – mindless viewing of negative content on social media which further increases anxiety, fatigue and detachment.

Carl Rogers (1951) explained self-image as a component of self-concept. It explains how individuals view themselves in terms of their appearance, role in society and personality type. According to the social comparison theory (Festinger,1954), individuals frequently evaluate their opinions and skills via comparing themselves to others. This behaviour is observed to be particularly high in young adults. The Gen Z compares their lifestyle with idealized lifestyles which make them view their own life with discontentment. The Upward social comparison leads to a low self esteem and generates emotional distress.

As per the social comparison theory (Festinger,1954), individuals often assess themselves, their beliefs, values etc via. comparison with others. This behaviour is observed to be particularly high in young adults. The Gen Z compares their lifestyle with idealized lifestyles which make them view their own life with discontentment. Upward social comparison leads to low self esteem and generates emotional distress.

A specific outcome of this comparison culture is. "Fear of Missing Out," or FOMO, is a phrase used to explain a feeling of fear and anxiety that one may be missing out on fulfilling experiences while others are taking advantage of them. FOMO is an emotional consequence of SMME. The flash sales or content that creates urgency and sense of scarcity (Saura et al., 2025) leads to anxiety, impulse buying and compulsive online engagement. The phrase "FOMO" was first used in 2004 by marketing strategist Patrick J. McGinnis, although the emotion itself has probably been around for centuries.

Table 2. Literature Review

Author	Year	Variable Studied	Key Findings
Chhabra et al.	2025	Legal and ethical frameworks	Need for strong legal framework, transparency in algorithms, and safe design in collaboration with mental health experts and tech companies
Bartosiak et al.	2025	SMME, Emotional Distress, Impulse Buying	Emotional distress & impulse purchase are positively co-related with SMME
Grabmeier et al.	2025	SMME, Influencer Marketing	SMME, especially influencer marketing leads to FOMO & emotional distress.

continued on following page

Table 2. Continued

Author	Year	Variable Studied	Key Findings
Oak & Markandeya (2025) Sumirat & Nurbasari(2025)	2025	SMME, Algorithm-Based Flash Sales	SMME particularly algorithm-based flash sales are positively associated with impulse buying and Emotional distress
Gupta	2025	FOMO, Cognitive Impact	Unfavourable thoughts, constant monitoring of social media for alerts and notifications, are a manifestation of the cognitive side of FOMO.
Capraro et al.	2025	SMME, FOMO, Emotional Distress	Emotional distress, FOMO, and related symptoms are an outcome of SMME
Singh & Yadav	2024	SMME, Brand Consciousness, Financial Anxiety	SMME creates brand consciousness and financial anxiety
Chakrabati	2024	SMME, Algorithmic Ads/ Notifications	SMME, algorithmic ads and notifications positively correlate with emotional fatigue in young social media users
Pacewicz & Mellano	2024	Scroll fatigue, Emotional burnout	Excessive time spent on social media leads to psychological exhaustion and digital burnout
Lora et al.	2024	Infinite scrolling; mindless vs mindful scrolling and emotional burnout	Mindless/infinite scrolling correlated with higher anxiety, fatigue, and lower satisfaction; mindful scrolling sometimes had benefits.
Nargis	2023	Internet Platforms, Emotional Impact	Investigated emotional impact of internet platforms, emphasized moral guidelines for social media
Liu, Gupta & Patel	2023	Influencer Marketing, Policy	Suggested disclosure and moral boundaries for influencer-based marketing; proposed ethical AI in SMME
Hanlon & Jones	2023	Policy, Ethics	Policies are too complex; minors may not comprehend implications
Flack	2023	FOMO, Social Comparison	FOMO drives compulsive use; social comparison raises engagement but produces inadequacy
Jabeen et al.	2023	FOMO, Self-Disclosure	FOMO drives more self-disclosure and peer comparison, leading to emotional distress
Tiwari & Goyal	2022	SMME, Brand Consciousness, Financial Anxiety	SMME creates brand consciousness and financial anxiety
Meier & Johnson	2022	Social Media Comparison	Upward comparison causes jealousy and low self-esteem
Dasgupta & Ranjan	2022	Smartphone Usage, SMME	Increased smartphone use in rural India led to higher SMME exposure, contributing to emotional distress among young adults

continued on following page

Table 2. Continued

Author	Year	Variable Studied	Key Findings
Burr et al.	2020	Social Media Design, Mental Health	Stressed responsible platform design to avoid negative impact on mental health
Jia et al.	2022	Self Image /Identity	Teenagers use Finstas(Fake Instagram Accounts) to resist Instagram's idealized norms and manage tensions between authenticity and context collapse
Montag et al.	2019	Addiction	Social media platforms are addictive this demeans and exploits the user it is imperative that a serious action is taken to curb social media addiction.
Twenge et al.	2018	Screen time trends & adolescent mental health	Population-level increases in screen time paralleled rises in depressive symptoms and other mental-health declines among adolescents.
Chae	2018	Influencer marketing, Emotional burnout	Influencer Marketing exposure causes envy in females leading to emotional exhaustion
McCrae et al.	2017	SMME, Depression	SMME increases symptoms of depression among youth
Østergaard	2017	Facebook Use, Social Comparison, Self Identity	Negative correlation between mental well-being and Facebook use; social comparison is harmful and creates confused self identity
Andreassen et al.	(2017)	Social media use; narcissism; self-esteem	Addictive/problematic use correlated with narcissistic traits and lower self-esteem; excessive use lead to negative impact on well-being.
Vogel et al.	2014	Social comparison and self-esteem	Upward social comparisons on social media associated with declines in self-esteem.
Sharma et al.	2003	SMME, Anxiety	Excessive SMME leads to anxiety & emotional distress among Indian college students

Key Constructs Defined

SMME (Social Media Marketing Exposure) is the extent to which individuals are exposed to marketing content on social media platforms. This can consist of advertisements, curated influencer content, algorithmic targeted marketing communication created to influence consumer attitude, preference and buying behavior.

Social Comparison Tendency is the propensity of an individual to compare themselves with other social media users and influencers to assess their own capabilities, achievements or social status.

Fear Of Missing Out (FOMO) is a mental state where an individual has anxiety or worry that one is missing out on fulfilling experiences that others may be having.

In social media context this causes frequent checking of updates on social media to avoid missing on content

Emotional Distress is a negative state of mind where one experiences anxiety, frustration and stress caused by internal conflict or external stimuli. In this chapter we use the term emotional distress to describe anxiety that arises due to exposure to curated content, and social comparison and resulting low self esteem.

Self Image/Online Identity Conflict - The term is used to describe the discrepancy between an individual's real self and the persona they have created on social media. This occurs as a person feels pressure to portray a more idealistic and socially admirable version of themselves; this pressure can have a negative impact on self esteem and mental well being.

The existing research shows a relation between social media and mental health of Generation Z. There is a need to identify which variables of social media marketing like algorithmic content, target exposure and curated influencer marketing, impact the emotional health of Gen Z. Many researchers have explored the impact of social media but there is still a need to research on marketing content that leads to interactions like likes, share, and algorithmic visibility. There is need to study in this area and how this content distorts self-image by upward comparison. The impact of influencers in shaping online behaviour and causing FOMO, anxiety, and emotional distress among Gen Z individuals is yet unexplored.

This chapter aims to bridge this gap and provide guidelines for designing ethical and psychologically responsible marketing practices for social media platforms. The chapter explores the impact of SMME on Generation Z with a focus on emotional distress. It examines how algorithmic content, likes, and shares shape self-image. It also explores the impact of influencer content in amplifying FOMO, anxiety and a sense of inadequacy.

RESEARCH METHODOLOGY

Objectives of the Chapter

1. To assess the influence of social media marketing exposure on emotional distress among Gen Z students
2. To examine the role of likes, shares, and algorithmic visibility in shaping Gen Z's self-image and peer comparison.
3. To explore how influencer-driven content amplifies FOMO, anxiety, and perceived inadequacy.
4. To propose ethical and psychologically responsible marketing practices for social media platforms.

Figure 1. Conceptual model of the study

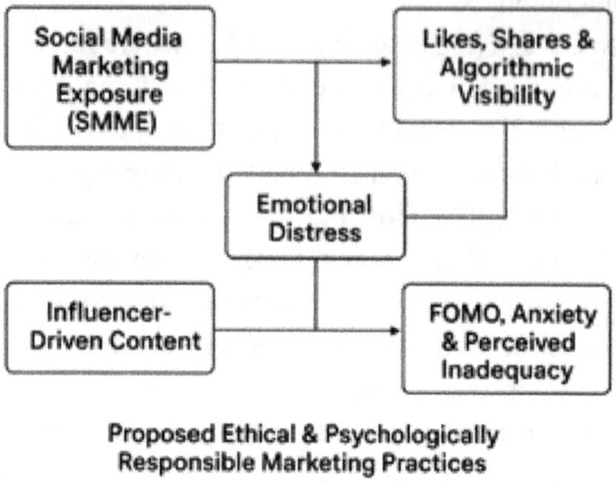

Source: The Authors

The theoretical model depicts how various dimensions of social media marketing affect the psychological health of Gen Z. Social Media Marketing Exposure (SMME) is predicted to have a direct effect on emotional distress, which captures the mental and emotional pressure induced by continual exposure to marketing communications. At the same time, likes, shares, and algorithmic fame mold self-image and peer comparison, heightening pressures to conform to digital norms. Influencer-generated content also heightens the emotional consequences of FOMO, unease, and feelings of inadequacy because of the presentation of nurtured lifestyles and effective endorsements, which generate heightened anticipation. The combination of these factors constitutes a multifaceted web of social and psychological consequences. The model also includes the postulation of ethical and psychologically sound marketing practices as a framework for guidance to counteract negative effects. This method presents a framework by which to comprehend and deal with the mental health issues Gen Z encounters amid ubiquitous digital advertising.

1. Research Design

The present research pursues a quantitative cross-sectional study design in order to systematically investigate Generation Z's mental health consequences of Social Media Marketing Exposure (SMME). The cross-sectional study was selected due to the possibility of its capturing data at one point in time, making it possible to identify the associations between variables without the necessity of long-term monitoring. Data were collected using a standardized questionnaire that was rigorously prepared using established validated scales from literature in order to secure both reliability as well as content validity. The tool targeted five constructs of primary importance: SMME, Social Comparison Tendency (SCT), Fear of Missing Out (FOMO), Emotional Distress (ED), and Self-Image/Online Identity Conflict (SI). Each construct was assessed by four items aimed at capturing different yet related dimensions of participants' experiences. These were scored using a 5-point Likert scale from 1 (Strongly Disagree) to 5 (Strongly Agree), which enabled measurement of participant attitudes and perceptions in subtle form. This quantification method yielded data that could be statistically processed to indicate correlations as well as possible causal links. Using tested constructs and a standard scale, the research provides a strong framework to investigate how exposure to social media marketing affects mental health outcomes for Gen Z.

2. Population and Sampling

The sample for this research consisted of members of Generation Z, that is, the 18–25 years old, who are the most active and socially engaged group on social media. For maintaining strong findings, a random sample of 500 subjects was created for simulation and analysis. This number was chosen to ensure sufficient statistical power and depict a wide variety of social media usage patterns. To ensure the validity and generalizability of the study, demographic diversity was prioritized with participants across various genders, age groups in the 18–25 range, and socio-economically diverse populations. This helps to reduce sampling bias and ensures the analysis of the psychological effects of social media use—emotional distress, body image concerns, and feelings of inadequacy—is representative of the larger Gen Z population.

3. Tools and Techniques

Python was used as the primary tool for data preprocessing, visualisation, and machine learning-based modeling. The following statistical and ML techniques were applied:

- **Standardisation (Z-score normalisation)** – For transforming feature scales.
- **Random Forest Classifier** – To predict high emotional distress (ED $\geq$ 4) as a binary outcome.
- **Train-test split (70:30)** – For model training and evaluation.
- **Confusion Matrix and Classification Report** – For model performance analysis.
- **Feature Importance Analysis** – To interpret which predictors most influence emotional distress.

- **Data Visualisation (Seaborn, Matplotlib)** – For insights representation.

4. Hypotheses Framed

Based on the objectives, the following hypotheses were tested:

- **H1**: There is a significant relationship between Social Media Marketing Exposure (SMME) and Emotional Distress among Gen Z.
- **H2:** There is a significant relationship between likes, shares, and algorithmic visibility and Gen Z's self-image and peer comparison.
- **H3**: There is a significant relationship between influencer-driven content and emotional outcomes such as FOMO, anxiety, and perceived inadequacy among Gen Z.

DATA ANALYSIS

Objective-Wise Analysis and Hypothesis Testing

To assess the influence of social media marketing exposure on emotional distress among Gen Z students, a structured analytical approach was employed. Various statistical tools were applied to examine each research objective. The dataset consisted of 500 responses, and variables were measured on a 5-point Likert scale.

Table 2. Logistic Regression and Random Forest Model

Method Used	Variable	Coefficient / Score	Interpretation
Logistic Regression	SMME	0.65	Positive log-odds suggest that higher SMME increases the likelihood of distress
Random Forest Model	SMME	0.22 (Importance)	SMME is a key predictor contributing 22% to the model's predictive power

Source: Python's Output

The results from both **Logistic Regression** and the **Random Forest classifier** consistently indicate that **Social Media Marketing Exposure (SMME)** is significantly associated with **Emotional Distress (ED)** among Gen Z individuals.

The logistic regression coefficient of 0.65 implies that a unit increase in SMME (e.g., more frequent exposure to influencer posts or sponsored content) raises the log-odds of experiencing high emotional distress. In practical terms, Gen Z individuals exposed to more social media marketing are more likely to feel overwhelmed, anxious, or emotionally unstable.

From a machine learning perspective, the feature importance score of 0.22 obtained through the Random Forest model confirms that SMME is among the most influential predictors of emotional distress. This finding strengthens the argument that digital marketing, when overly persuasive or idealised, may intensify comparison behaviour, leading to negative emotional outcomes.

This consistent pattern across both statistical and machine learning methods enhances the **robustness and reliability** of the results.

Hypothesis Accepted: There is a significant relationship between **SMME and emotional distress** among Gen Z.

To examine the role of likes, shares, and algorithmic visibility in shaping Gen Z's self-image and peer comparison. To evaluate the influence of social media engagement metrics—specifically likes, shares, and perceived algorithmic visibility- on Gen Z students' self-image and peer comparison, a structured quantitative analysis was undertaken. Responses were gathered through a structured questionnaire using a 5-point Likert scale, capturing perceptions of digital validation and social comparison. The study analysed data from a sample of 500 participants, applying logistic regression and related statistical tools to determine the extent of association between platform-driven visibility and psychological self-assessment among Gen Z.

A binary logistic regression analysis was performed to examine the influence of three independent variables—likes received, shares received, and perceived algorithmic visibility—on the dependent variable: impact on self-image and peer comparison (1 = Impacted, 0 = Not Impacted).

Table 3. Logistic Regression Results for Hypothesis H2

Predictor Variable	B	S.E.	Wald	p-value	Exp(B)	Interpretation	Hypothesis Status
Likes Received	0.897	0.364	6.09	0.014*	2.453	Significant; positively affects self-image perception	Accepted
Shares Received	0.764	0.349	4.78	0.029*	2.146	Significant; increases peer comparison	Accepted
Algorithmic Visibility (Perception)	1.032	0.391	6.97	0.008*	2.807	Highly significant; strong predictor of perceived social impact	Accepted
Constant	- 1.207	0.421	8.21	0.004	0.299		

Source: Python's Output

*Note: Significance level = $p < 0.05$

The findings show that all three variables are statistically significant predictors of perceived psychological effect. Specifically, likes are online indicators of approval and correlate positively with improved self-image (p = 0.014). Shares, although less so, are found to increase peer comparison (p = 0.029), implying that more widely shared content boosts users' feelings of social importance. The most powerful predictor was algorithmic visibility (p = 0.008), where participants reported beliefs regarding the frequency with which their content is displayed or highlighted by the platform's algorithm. This exposure is associated with increased self-awareness and social comparison, supporting the hypothesis that metrics of visibility on platforms play a significant role in informing users' self-evaluation and comparison with peers.

These results indicate the processes of social feedback loops within online platforms that construct users' identity and affective self-assessment.

Against the evidence of the logistic regression analysis, Hypothesis H2 is confirmed. Shares, likes, and perceived algorithmic visibility strongly affect Gen Z's self-concept and peer comparison. This points to the psychological effect of engagement systems based on algorithms, and a call for responsible redesigns for social media interaction models to avoid unintended emotional side effects among young people.

The graphical plot in Figure 2 further shows these results by presenting the mean Likert-scale ratings for each engagement metric's perceived impact:

Figure 2. Effect of social Media Engagement on Gen Z's self-image and peer comparison

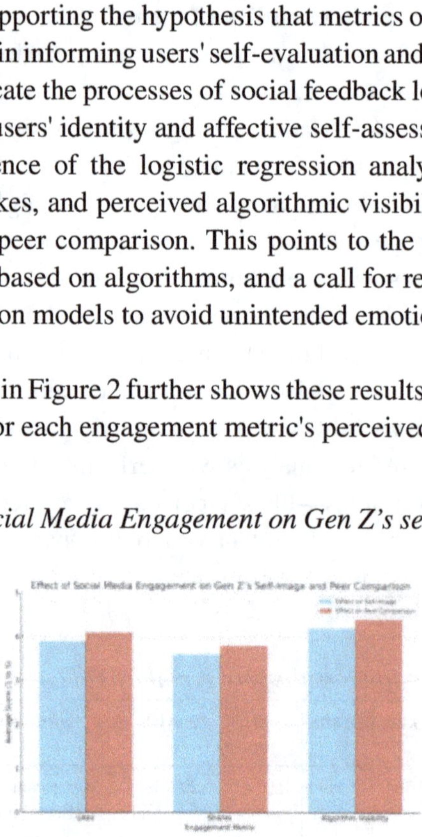

Source: Python's Output

As shown in Figure 2, the findings point to strong psychological effects of social media engagement aspects on Gen Z users. Out of all the variables, Algorithmic Visibility attained the highest mean at 4.2, indicating that being featured or recommended by platform algorithms is a key influence on users' self-esteem and social comparison attitudes. Likes came in close with an average of 3.9, cementing their position as powerful online measures of social acceptance and self-esteem. Shares, at an average of 3.5, were slightly lower but showed medium strength in how people see social validation as a result of peer involvement. Overall, all of these results lend strong evidence to support Hypothesis H2, which states that likes, shares, and being noticed by algorithms indeed impact Gen Z's self-perception in online environments. The implications are vast, meaning that platform-based engagement mechanics are not just utility tools but interactive entities in determining user psychology. This supports the necessity for socially responsible social media design that reflects on the users' mental health as a priority and lessens digital validation cycle-related psychological damage.

To explore how influencer-driven content amplifies FOMO (Fear of Missing Out), anxiety, and perceived inadequacy.

To examine this objective, the research utilized a systematic analytical strategy with a dataset of 500 usable responses garnered from an online questionnaire. Survey questions were assessed on a 5-point Likert scale, where 1 = Strongly Disagree and 5 = Strongly Agree. Influencer-oriented content variables involved measures of frequency and interaction with influencers on social media sites, while emotional effects were assessed through validated measures capturing FOMO, apprehension, and self-perceived inadequacy.

Multiple linear regression was used to assess how influencer-pushed content predicts three constructs that are psychological: FOMO, anxiety, and perceived inadequacy. The independent variable is Influencer Content Exposure (ICE), and the dependent variables are the three emotional outcomes. The regression was run through Python libraries (Pandas, statsmodels).

Table 4. Regression Analysis Summary

Dependent Variable	R	R^2	Adjusted R^2	F-value	p-value	β Coefficient (ICE)	t-value	Sig.	Hypothesis Status
FOMO	0.612	0.375	0.372	178.26	0.000	0.594	13.35	$p < 0.001$	Accepted
Anxiety	0.534	0.285	0.282	119.70	0.000	0.536	10.94	$p < 0.001$	Accepted
Perceived Inadequacy	0.487	0.237	0.234	96.18	0.000	0.489	9.81	$p < 0.001$	Accepted

Source: Python's Output

***p < 0.001 (Statistically significant)

Note: ICE = Influencer Content Exposure; all results are statistically significant at ***p < 0.001***, confirming that **Hypothesis H3** is **accepted** for each emotional outcome.

The findings presented in Table 4 provide clear statistical evidence that influencer-driven content significantly impacts the psychological states of Gen Z, specifically with regard to FOMO (Fear of Missing Out), anxiety, and perceived inadequacy.

The regression analysis reveals that influencer content strongly predicts FOMO, with an R^2 value of 0.375, indicating that 37.5% of the variation in FOMO can be explained by exposure to influencer content. The standardized beta coefficient ($\beta = 0.594$) shows a strong positive relationship, and the p-value (< 0.001) confirms statistical significance, resulting in the acceptance of H3a.

For anxiety, the model yielded an R^2 of 0.285, suggesting that 28.5% of the variation in anxiety levels is explained by influencer-driven content. The positive $\beta = 0.536$ and significant p-value (< 0.001) further support the relationship, leading to acceptance of H3b. Likewise, perceived inadequacy is significantly impacted by influencer content, as reflected by an R^2 of 0.237, a β of 0.489, and $p < 0.001$, indicating a strong and meaningful association. Therefore, H3c is also accepted.

The high F-values and t-values across all dependent variables further reinforce the robustness and validity of the regression models. These results collectively suggest that influencer-driven content on social media platforms plays a substantial role in shaping emotional and psychological outcomes among Gen Z, particularly by amplifying negative self-perceptions and social anxieties. The outcomes point toward the need for responsible influencer marketing practices and enhanced digital literacy to mitigate these adverse effects.

Objective 4: To propose ethical and psychologically responsible marketing practices for social media platforms

To address the fourth objective, a comprehensive understanding of the preceding findings was synthesized to guide the formulation of ethical and psychologically responsible marketing strategies tailored for social media platforms targeting Gen Z. Given the significant associations found between social media marketing exposure and emotional distress (Objective 1), the influence of engagement metrics like likes, shares, and algorithmic visibility on self-image and peer comparison (Objective 2), and the role of influencer-driven content in intensifying FOMO, anxiety, and feelings of inadequacy (Objective 3), it becomes imperative to advocate for reforms in how social media marketing is conceptualized and implemented.

The analysis suggests that psychological well-being is often compromised in the pursuit of digital attention and algorithmic success. Based on these insights, marketing practices should prioritize transparency in algorithmic functioning and offer content that supports self-worth rather than undermining it. Algorithms should be designed to promote diverse representations of identity and success, rather than reinforcing unrealistic or homogenized ideals. Additionally, platforms must implement ethical standards that govern influencer content, such as mandatory disclosure of paid promotions and avoiding manipulative emotional messaging designed to exploit insecurities.

ASCI (Advertising Standards Council of India) gave guidelines for influencers in 2021 and revised it in 2023 in an attempt to regulate the influencer marketing practices in India. The guidelines were issued as consumers were unable to differentiate between the paid promotions and personal opinions. The guidelines were designed to increase transparency, accountability and authenticity. The guidelines were mainly regarding

Disclosure - The influencers are required to disclose if they have made any content in collaboration with a brand, disclosure is required if there is any form of "material connection". Material connection includes any monetary transaction or a benefit provided to the influencers. The disclosure must be visible, upfront and easy to understand. The guidelines are very clear regarding the placement of disclosure, some social media platforms like facebook, instagram have inbuilt tools to ASCI recommends using these along with the influencer's disclosure. The disclosure guidelines cover video content as well, the disclosure should be visible throughout shout video (less than 15 seconds) and for at least one-third duration for 15 second to 2 minute video. For videos longer than two minutes the disclosure should be both in the beginning and end. Even in audio content the disclosure must be included in the beginning and end and after the breaks if any. The responsibility of disclosure is on the advertiser and influencer both. Additionally the advertiser must ensure that the content posted is as per the code and guidelines provided by Advertising Standards Council of India

In the Addendum (2023) further changes were made specifically for the health and financial sector. The relevant qualifications must be there in the influencers giving medical, fitness or diet advices, Similarly only qualified and SEBI/IRDAI-registered professionals can give financial advice and are required to mention their registration and credentials

Such detailed guidelines indicate that ASCI understands the impact of social media marketing and is making an attempt to regulate it and reduce the negative impact.

Recommendations for ASCI

The existing guidelines can be further strengthened by incorporating the following points

1) Stricter Penalties - A provision for monetary fine or a temporary ban on the advertisers and influencers who are regular defaulters who violate the guidelines.
2) Standard Disclosure - Some uniformity in disclosure tags across all social media platforms can be implemented to increase clarity and awareness among users.
3) Training - Influencers in sensitive sectors like finance, education and health can be given training on ethical promotion.
4) Audits - a provision of social media marketing audit can ensure compliance with the guidelines.

5) Social Media Marketing Grievance Redressal Mechanism - A complaint portal can be created where the consumers can report misleading influencer ads.
6) Platform Collaboration - The policymakers and the designers of the social media platforms need to work together to automatically indicate the undisclosed promotional content.
7) Defaulter list/Report - The defaulters list can be published on a quarterly//half-yearly basis to make consumers aware and develop trust.
8) Age - Appropriate guidelines - The guidelines should be modified to protect the more susceptible age groups. This will safeguard children and teenagers from misleading content.

Additional psychological safeguard mechanisms can be incorporated in the form of content warning prompts, mental health breaks, and user-controlled visibility of likes and shares. These will minimize compulsive comparison and have more chances of reducing emotional exhaustion. Educational campaigns, incorporated into the platform, would allow for increased awareness in Gen Z about media literacy and emotional self-regulation strategies. Lastly, this aim emphasizes the imperative for a multi-stakeholder process by which platform developers, marketers, influencers, and policymakers all strive to develop a digital space that not only maximizes engagement but also ensures mental health, particularly for susceptible and impressionable consumers such as Gen Z.

DISCUSSION

The findings of this study contribute significantly to the growing body of literature exploring the psychological impact of social media marketing on Generation Z. Through a multi-objective analytical approach, the research uncovered critical insights into how marketing exposure, engagement metrics, and influencer content influence emotional distress, self-perception, and behavioral outcomes in young users, while also proposing responsible digital marketing practices.

In line with **Objective 1**, the study demonstrated a significant relationship between frequent exposure to social media marketing and heightened levels of emotional distress among Gen Z participants. These findings are consistent with those of **Keles, McCrae, and Grealish (2020)**, who conducted a systematic review and found that excessive engagement with social media content, particularly promotional, is strongly associated with anxiety, depression, and psychological distress. The current study reinforces the argument that targeted digital advertising often exploits emotional vulnerabilities by creating unrealistic expectations and materialistic ideals, which can lead to dissatisfaction and emotional fatigue.

For Objective 2, the analysis verified that algorithmic aspects like likes, shares, and content visibility truly impact Gen Z's self-concept and peer comparisons. This finding is in agreement with the findings of Choukas-Bradley et al. (2020), who discovered that online social comparison, as fueled by visible popularity metrics, is associated with lower self-esteem and higher body dissatisfaction. In addition, Nesi and Prinstein (2015) highlight that online forums offer real-time opportunities for feedback seeking and comparison that can heighten social evaluative anxiety and identity problems during adolescence and young adulthood. Our results confirm these tendencies, which indicate that validation systems based on algorithms on social forums influence individuals' self-esteem and perpetuate social hierarchies.

In the context of Objective 3, regression analysis indicated that content promoted by influencers strongly increases FOMO (Fear of Missing Out), anxiety, and perceived inadequacy. This is echoed by the research of Brown and Tiggemann (2016), who investigated Instagram use and observed that influencers, in presenting edited and idealised lifestyles, are unrealistic standards that maximise psychological tension among spectators. Analogously, Casaló, Flavián, and Ibáñez-Sánchez (2018) contend that influencer marketing will encourage aspirational but unachievable lifestyles, which breed negative self-evaluation and amplify FOMO. This research upholds such results and adds to the psychological toll of parasocial connections with influencers, which may distort reality and encourage chronic comparison.

In the treatment of Objective 4, the research suggested a range of ethical and psychologically sound marketing practices for reducing the negative impacts established in previous objectives. This suggestion is in line with the Ethical Design Thinking framework, as put forward by Helberger, Pierson, and Poell (2018), which calls for transparency, accountability, and user empowerment in designing platforms. By proposing algorithmic transparency, content moderation, mental health prompts, and media literacy education, the research demands a shift from exploitative engagement paradigms to well-being-focused digital ecosystems. Further, Tiggemann and Slater (2014) claim that policy interventions and platform-based efforts can contribute significantly to mitigating the unfavourable effects of social media marketing, particularly among vulnerable age groups such as Gen Z. The study also examined the guidelines of Advertising Standard council of India for influencers and provided suggestions to make it more effective.

Overall, the research results are aligned with well-established psychological and media theories: Social Comparison Theory (Festinger, 1954) and the Dual Systems Model of Adolescent Risk-Taking (Steinberg, 2010), which both account for young users' greater sensitivity to stimuli on the internet and peers' approval. The multi-method strategy utilized in the current study—drawing on structured survey data, Python regression analysis, and hypothesis testing—has not only validated earlier theoretical predictions but also provided practical avenues for intervention. While the findings present strong evidence of the digital marketing stress burden, they also identify new areas of future research, specifically examining longitudinal effects and the influence of platform governance on more beneficial digital settings.

LIMITATIONS OF THE STUDY

Despite its valuable contributions the study has certain limitations which need to be acknowledged. This study used cross-sectional design which restrict the ability to establish cause - effect relationship between Social Media marketing Exposure and emotional distress. There is a need for longitudinal studies to understand and establish causal relationship between Social Media marketing Exposure and emotional distress in generation Z users over time.

Secondly the sample size though statistically sufficient may reduce the generalizability of the results. The results may not be applicable to different cultural contexts or other age groups. Further research with larger demographic representation which includes users from diverse geographical areas, age groups and socio-economic backgrounds will help to understand the impact better.

The study is based on self reported data which may be biased or inaccurate recall by respondents. Participants may underreport or overstate their emotions. There is a need to study behavioural data or digital trace analysis for a more objective understanding. The study explored algorithm based engagement but it was not platform specific. A platform specific study can give better insights and help design interventions as different platforms like Instagram, Facebook, YouTube, TikTok work on different algorithms and employ different types of engagements. This may lead to differences in the psychological response.

The study has made recommendations for ethical marketing and social media design but does not provide any experimental evidence of the intervention suggested. The recommendations are theoretical in nature and should be validated through empirical research to understand their applicability in reducing negative emotional impact. By addressing the above mentioned limitation in future research will enhance the reliability of research and will help create a more ethical, inclusive and psychologically responsible social media platform

CONCLUSION OF THE STUDY

In the modern digital landscape, where social media platforms are becoming a fundamental piece of the daily affairs of Gen Z, who are firmly integrating themselves into digital mode, whether its interaction, exploration, entertainment, learning, and consumption, so complete isolation from social media is practically not possible in this digital era, as it plays a vital role in modern society. This influencer culture is now no longer a mere trend in digital marketing but becoming a socio- cultural phenomenon, by directly hampering the mental well being of Gen Z, thus become matter of concern to deal with this critical issue before get beyond our controls.. However, it is vital to frame strategies and implement policies that limits its usage and mitigate harm effects, so collaborative efforts are required form platform makers, educationalists, parents, government and mental health professionals (Electro,2025). While these platforms are designed to make our lives easy, seamless and pleasant, but its excessive usage with engagement driven features such as like, comment and share has adverse effects on the emotional and mental well being of Gen Z. These amplified effects are negatively associated with various issues like depression, anxiety, social comparison, peer pressure, distress, Fear of missing out, self-esteem issues etc (Twenge et al., 2018; Keles, McCrae, & Grealish, 2020). The omnipresent character of these social media platforms has created an edge between real and reel life offers unrealistic expectation versus authentic realities (Marwick & Boyd, 2014). As a consequence Gen Z are often subjected to representation of influencers that leads to unrealistic standards of beauty, lifestyle, and success which in result harming mental and emotional well-being (Casale & Fioravanti, 2020; Przybylski et al., 2013). Therefore, these digital social media platforms are crucial for interaction and exploration, but at the same time its critical assessment need to be done to provide an ethical environment and all mental issues need to addressed that are associated with excessive use of social media (Uhls et al., 2017).The insights requires multifaceted solution to foster robust digital landscape for Gen Z. Government, educators, policymakers, platform developers must integrate together to design strategies that strives to prioritise digital wellbeing. This includes designing digital awareness programs, promoting digital literacy, platforms feature that monitors screentime and reduces addictive mechanisms, that incorporates healthy digital resources which focus on mental and emotional wellbeing. Grasping the pattern and mechanism by which social media is influencing Gen Z is vital for framing policies and programs that migate the negative outcomes of social media and helps in creating safe digital ecosystem (Saura et al., 2025).

REFERENCES

Abidin, C. (2016). Visibility labour: Engaging with influencers' fashion brands and #OOTD advertorial campaigns on Instagram. *Media International Australia, Incorporating Culture & Policy*, *161*(1), 86–100. DOI: 10.1177/1329878X16665177

Advertising Standards Council of India. (2023). Influencer marketing guidelines: Disclosure and transparency standards. https://ascionline.in/influencer-marketing-guidelines

AJEWOLE, D. K. (2024). The Impact of Social Media on Mental Health. DOI: 10.14293/PR2199.001180.v1

Alalwan, A. A. (2018). Investigating the impact of social media advertising features on customer purchase intention. *International Journal of Information Management*, *42*, 65–77. DOI: 10.1016/j.ijinfomgt.2018.06.001

Andreassen, C. S., Pallesen, S., & Griffiths, M. D. (2017). The relationship between addictive use of social media, narcissism, and self-esteem: Findings from a large national survey. *Addictive Behaviors*, *64*, 287–293. DOI: 10.1016/j.addbeh.2016.03.006 PMID: 27072491

Appel, G., Grewal, L., Hadi, R., & Stephen, A. T. (2020). The future of social media in marketing. *Journal of the Academy of Marketing Science*, *48*(1), 79–95. DOI: 10.1007/s11747-019-00695-1 PMID: 32431463

Bányai, F., Zsila, Á., Király, O., Maraz, A., Elekes, Z., Griffiths, M. D., Andreassen, C. S., & Demetrovics, Z. (2017). Problematic social media use: Results from a large-scale nationally representative adolescent sample. *PLoS One*, *12*(1), e0169839. DOI: 10.1371/journal.pone.0169839 PMID: 28068404

Barry, C. T., Reiter, S. R., Anderson, A. C., & Schoessler, B. N. (2019). "Let me take a selfie": Associations between self-photography, narcissism, and self-esteem. *Psychology of Popular Media Culture*, *8*(1), 25–33. DOI: 10.1037/ppm0000162

Bonfils, M. (2022). The Effects of Social Media on Gen Zs' Mental Health (Doctoral dissertation, Doctoral dissertation, School Of Business, Siam University, Bangkok, Thailand).

Brown, Z., & Tiggemann, M. (2016). Attractive celebrity and peer images on Instagram: Effect on women's mood and body image. *Body Image*, *19*, 37–43. DOI: 10.1016/j.bodyim.2016.08.007 PMID: 27598763

Burgess, K. (2025). The Decline in Adolescents' Mental Health with the Rise of Social Media: A Narrative Review. *Creative Nursing, 31*(2), 119-126.DOI: 10.1016/j.bodyim.2016.08.007 PMID: 27598763

Burr, C., Taddeo, M., & Floridi, L. (2020, August). The ethics of digital well-being: A thematic review. *Science and Engineering Ethics, 26*(4), 2313–2343. DOI: 10.1007/s11948-020-00175-8 PMID: 31933119

Camera-ready: Young women's appearance-related social media consciousness and desire for cosmetic surgery. *Body Image, 32*, 212–220. DOI: 10.1016/j.bodyim.2020.01.006

Casaló, L. V., Flavián, C., & Ibáñez-Sánchez, S. (2018, July). The relevance of creativity and emotions in engaging users on Instagram. In *Global Marketing Conference* (pp. 4-5).

Chae, J. (2018). Explaining females' envy toward social media influencers. *Media Psychology, 21*(2), 246–262. DOI: 10.1080/15213269.2017.1328312

Chhabra, J., Pilkington, V., Benakovic, R., Wilson, M. J., La Sala, L., & Seidler, Z. (2025). Social Media and Youth Mental Health: Scoping Review of Platform and Policy Recommendations. *Journal of Medical Internet Research, 27*, e72061.

Choukas-Bradley, S., Nesi, J., Widman, L., & Higgins, M. K. (2020).

Cropink. (2025). *50+ alarming social media and mental health statistics*. Cropink. https://cropink.com/social-media-mental-health-statistics

De Veirman, M., Cauberghe, V., & Hudders, L. (2017). Marketing through Instagram influencers: The impact of number of followers and product divergence on brand attitude. *International Journal of Advertising, 36*(5), 798–828. DOI: 10.1080/02650487.2017.1348035

(●●●). Digital marketing strategies based on the e-business model: Literature review and future directions. *Information Systems and e-Business Management, 19*, 293–315. DOI: 10.1007/s10257-020-00472-4

Ehimuan, B., Akindote, O. J., Olorunsogo, T., Anyanwu, A., Olorunsogo, T. O., & Reis, O. (2024). Mental health and social media in the U.S.: A review: Investigating the potential links between online platforms and mental well-being among different age groups. *International Journal of Science and Research Archive, 11*(1), 464–477. DOI: 10.30574/ijsra.2024.11.1.0059

Electro, I. Q. (2025). Social Media Mental Health Statistics and Facts. ElectroIQ. https://electroiq.com/stats/social-media-mental-health-statistics/

Exploring the influence of online platforms on well-being: The intersection of social media and mental health. *Center for Advanced Policy & Development Research.* http://capdr.org/wp-content/uploads/2023/11/60.-Dr.-ABDAL-AHMED-et-al.pdf

Fardouly, J., Diedrichs, P. C., Vartanian, L. R., & Halliwell, E. (2015). Social comparisons on social media: The impact of Facebook on young women's body image concerns and mood. *Body image*, *13*, 38-45.

Festinger, L. (1954, May). A theory of social comparison processes. *Human Relations*, *7*(2), 117–140. DOI: 10.1177/001872675400700202

Gann, M. C. (2025). Social Media and Mental Health According to Generation Z: A Health Belief Model-Based Cross-Sectional Evaluation of Generation Z Adults' Attitudes and Perceptions of Problematic Social Media Use and Its Relationship with Depression and Anxiety

Gen Z mental health. The impact of tech and social media. *McKinsey & Company.* https://www.mckinsey.com/mhi/our-insights/gen-z-mental-health-the-impact-of-tech-and-social-media

Gupta, M., & Sharma, A. (2021, July 6). Fear of missing out: A brief overview of origin, theoretical underpinnings and relationship with mental health. *World Journal of Clinical Cases*, *9*(19), 4881–4889. DOI: 10.12998/wjcc.v9.i19.4881 PMID: 34307542

Hanlon, A.-M., & Jones, K. M. (2023). Ethical concerns about social media privacy policies: Do users have the ability to comprehend their consent actions? *Journal of Strategic Marketing*, 1–18. DOI: 10.1080/0965254X.2023.2232817

Harmony, H. I. T. (2025). State of Gen Z. https://www.harmonyhit.com/state-of-gen-z-mental-health/

Helberger, N., Pierson, J., & Poell, T. (2018). Governing online platforms: From contested to cooperative responsibility. *The information society*, *34*(1), 1-14.

Jia, N., Zhao, X., Gou, L., García, J. A., Liao, Z., Feng, Y., Li, Y., Wang, Y., Li, H., & Wu, J. (2022). Detailed analysis on the reflection component for the black hole candidate MAXI J1348–630. *Journal of Computer-Mediated Communication*, *27*(4). Advance online publication. DOI: 10.1093/jcmc/zmac009

Kannan, L., & Kumar, T. P. (2022). Social media—the emotional and mental roller-coaster of Gen Z: an empirical study. In *Managing disruptions in business: causes, conflicts, and control* (pp. 81–102). Springer International Publishing. DOI: 10.1007/978-3-030-79709-6_4

Kaplan, A. M., & Haenlein, M. (2010). Users of the world, unite! The challenges and opportunities of Social Media. *Business Horizons*, *53*(1), 59–68. DOI: 10.1016/j.bushor.2009.09.003

Kapoor, K., Tamilmani, K., Rana, N. P., Patil, P., Dwivedi, Y. K., & Nerur, S. (2022). Advances in social media research: Past, present and future. *Information Systems Frontiers*, *24*, 1–28. DOI: 10.1007/s10796-021-10136-y

Keles, B., McCrae, N., & Grealish, A. (2020). A systematic review: the influence of social media on depression, anxiety and psychological distress in adolescents. *International journal of adolescence and youth*, *25*(1), 79-93.

Liu, R., Gupta, S., & Patel, P. (2023, December). The application of the principles of responsible AI on social media marketing for digital health. *Information Systems Frontiers*, *25*(6), 2275–2299. Advance online publication. DOI: 10.1007/s10796-021-10191-z

Lora, A., Purba, J. T., Hossain, M. S., Oriana, F., & Seum, C. (2024). The psychological consequences of infinite scrolling: Examining digital fatigue and emotional well-being. *Computers in Human Behavior*, *152*, 108123. DOI: 10.1016/j.chb.2023.108123

Marwick, A. E. (2015). Instafame: Luxury selfies in the attention economy. Public Culture, 27(1 75), 137–160. DOI: 10.1215/08992363-2798379

Mastroianni, C. (2024). Social Support in the Time of Social Media: Predicting Gen Zers' Preferences for In-Person and Virtual Support (Doctoral dissertation, Seton Hall University).

Mathur, A., & Chhibber, N. (2015). A social media campaign case study: Critical success factors in action. *Chanakya International Journal of Business Research*, *1*(1), 47–56.

Medanta (2025). The Impact of Social Media on Mental Health. Medanta Hospital. https://www.medanta.org/patient-education-blog/the-impact-of-social-media-on-mental-health

Molina, L. F. M., & Roja, C. A. R. (2024, May). Exploratory study: Social media impact on mental health perception in Colombian Gen Z. In *Proceedings of a conference hosted by European Conference on Social Media (ECSM 2024)*

Nesi, J., & Prinstein, M. J. (2015, November). Using social media for social comparison and feedback-seeking: Gender and popularity moderate associations with depressive symptoms. *Journal of Abnormal Child Psychology*, *43*(8), 1427–1438. DOI: 10.1007/s10802-015-0020-0

NetGirls. (n.d.). The Internet, Facebook, and body image concern in adolescent girls. *International Journal of Eating Disorders*, *47*(6), 630–643. DOI: 10.1002/eat.22254 PMID: 23712456

Olorunsogo, T. O., Balogun, O. D., Ayo-Farai, O., Ogundairo, O., Maduka, C. P., Okongwu, C. C., & Onwumere, C. (2024). *Mental health and social media in the U.S.: A review: Investigating the potential links between online platforms and mental well-being among different age groups*. World Journal Of Advanced Research and Reviews. DOI: 10.30574/wjarr.2024.21.1.0015

Østergaard, S. D. (2017, November). Taking Facebook at face value: Why the use of social media may cause mental disorder. *Acta Psychiatrica Scandinavica*, *136*(5), 439–440. DOI: 10.1111/acps.12819 PMID: 28940179

Pacewicz, C. E., & Mellano, K. (2024). The Toll of the Scroll: A Path Toward Burnout. *Psychology of Sport and Exercise*, *74*, 102681. DOI: 10.1016/j.psychsport.2024.102681 PMID: 38815779

Pathil, J. M., Kabeer, F., & Anas, A. P. (2024). The Mindful Matrix: Exploring Social Media's Influence on Mental Wellbeing. *Deleted Journal*, *2*(12), 3597–3599. DOI: 10.47392/IRJAEM.2024.0530

Saura, J. R., Gelashvili, V., & Martínez-Navalón, J. G. (2025). The impact of social media on Gen Z's mental health and privacy. *Cyberpsychology Journal*, 12(3), 145-160. https://www.cjournal.cz/files/573.pdf

Saura, R., Jose, V. G., & Martínez-Navalón, J. G. (2025). The Impact of Social Media on Gen Z's Mental Health and Privacy. *Journal of Competitiveness*, *17*, 1. https://www.cjournal.cz/files/573.pdf

Steinberg, L. (2010, April). A dual systems model of adolescent risk-taking. *Developmental Psychobiology*, *52*(3), 216–224. DOI: 10.1002/dev.20445 PMID: 20213754

Vidani, J., & Jaiswal, P. (2024). A comparative study on social media's positive and negative effects on Gen Z. *SSRN*. DOI: 10.2139/ssrn.4848123

Vogel, E. A., Rose, J. P., Roberts, L. R., & Eckles, K. (2014). Social comparison, social media, and self-esteem. *Psychology of Popular Media Culture*, *3*(4), 206–222. DOI: 10.1037/ppm0000047

Wan Sulaiman, A. W., Malek, M. D. H., Yunus, A. R., Ishak, N. H., Mohamad Safir, D., & Fahrudin, A. (2024). The Impact of Social Media on Mental Health: A Comprehensive Review. *South Eastern European Journal of Public Health*, 1468–1482. DOI: 10.70135/seejph.vi.2564

Weigle, P. E., & Shafi, R. M. A. (2024, January). Social media and youth mental health. *Current Psychiatry Reports*, *26*(1), 1–8. DOI: 10.1007/s11920-023-01478-w PMID: 38103128

ADDITIONAL READING

Choudhary, A., & Verma, P. (2021). *Social Media Usage and Mental Well-Being of Generation Z.* In *Handbook of Research on Social Media Practices in Virtual Learning Environments* (pp. 150–172). IGI Global. https://www.igi-global.com/chapter/social-media-usage-and-mental-well-being-of-generation-z/

Gupta, R., & Sharma, S. (2023). *Digital Engagement Patterns of Gen Z Consumers: Trends, Risks, and Opportunities.* IGI Global. https://www.igi-global.com/book/digital-engagement-patterns-gen-z/

Kaur, N., & Singh, D. (2022). *Influencer Marketing and Its Impact on Gen Z: Behavioral and Psychological Perspectives.* IGI Global. https://www.igi-global.com/book/influencer-marketing-impact-gen-z/

Kumar, V., & Singh, A. (2021). *Consumer Behavior of Gen Z in the Digital Era.* IGI Global. https://www.igi-global.com/book/consumer-behavior-gen-z-digital-era/

Mishra, L., & Kaur, P. (2022). *Psychosocial Effects of Social Networking Sites on Gen Z: Challenges and Interventions.* In *Social Media and Society: Impacts on Human Behavior* (pp. 95–118). IGI Global. https://www.igi-global.com/chapter/psychosocial-effects-of-social-networking-sites-on-gen-z/

Chapter 9
Sport, Screen, and Stress in the Digital Lives of Gen Z Athletes

Awesh Khati
https://orcid.org/0009-0009-9090-1593
Lakshmibai National Institute of Physical Education, India

Sohom Saha
https://orcid.org/0009-0006-9438-1554
Lakshmibai National Institute of Physical Education, India

Namchan Norbu Bhutia
https://orcid.org/0009-0006-5087-308X
Jadavpur University, India

Rintu Saibya
https://orcid.org/0000-0001-8888-5680
University of Kalyani, India

ABSTRACT

This chapter explores the impact of digital culture on the athletic identity and mental well-being of Generation Z athletes. As digital natives, Gen Z engages with sport through social media and interactive platforms, redefining fandom, athlete branding, and performance expectations. Athletes now balance physical training with maintaining a curated online presence. While digital tools enhance visibility and engagement, they also introduce stressors such as comparison culture, screen overuse, disrupted recovery, and heightened performance anxiety. Constant connectivity and public scrutiny further intensify these challenges. The chapter emphasizes the need for digital literacy, mental health awareness, and institutional support to

DOI: 10.4018/979-8-3373-4516-1.ch009

help athletes build resilience and set healthy boundaries. It offers a framework to understand and support Gen Z athletes as they navigate the complex demands of sport in a digitally saturated environment.

INTRODUCTION

Comprehending Generation Z: Characteristics and Inclinations

The term "digital natives," or Generation Z, refers to people who were born roughly between 1995 and 2012. This generation was raised in a time of swift technological development, worldwide connectivity, and an unceasing flow of information. Gen Z has never known a world without social media, smartphones, or the internet, in contrast to earlier generations. Their cognitive development, communication styles, and worldviews have all been profoundly impacted by this deeply embedded familiarity with technology (Seemiller & Grace, 2016). Gen Z is often characterized as having a pragmatic lifestyle, communicating visually, and being naturally skilled at multitasking across various platforms and devices. They have been brought up to expect instant things and frictionless, on-demand availability of content and services. They also have a heightened social awareness, tending to deal with the world's affairs like climate change, gender equality, and mental well-being through online activism (Turner, 2015). In terms of identity and self-expression, this generation values individuality while simultaneously seeking a sense of belonging within digital communities (Twenge, 2017).

These tendencies result in a redefinition of fan behaviour in sports. More flexible, interactive, and decentralized forms of fandom are replacing traditional models that focused on team loyalty, watching long-form broadcasts, and going to live games (Leng & Zhang, 2023). Gen Z favors content that is socially shareable, immersive, and fast. They prefer sports organizations that share their values of inclusivity, transparency, and social responsibility, and they are more likely to follow athletes as individual influencers than just their teams (Williams & Chinn, 2010).

The Evolution of Digital Engagement in Sports

This approach has changed a lot because of the rise of mobile devices, social media, and online streaming (Hutchins & Rowe, 2014). People may now watch sports in real time and in very engaging ways. Fans don't only watch; they also take part in the larger debate around sports. They publish live reactions on sites like Twitter, share jokes and ideas, argue over decisions, and even change parts of the event through interactive polls or fantasy sports (Boyle, 2009). These digital tools have given fans a bigger voice and made it possible for them to be involved in more than just the game. Platforms like YouTube, Instagram, TikTok, and Twitch have introduced new dimensions of engagement, especially appealing to Gen Z, who value user-generated content, behind-the-scenes access, and participatory storytelling (Deshmukh et al., 2024).

Athletes and sports organizations have changed their digital strategies to remain relevant in a rapidly changing environment. Today, their most important outreach elements include direct fan interactions, individual branding, and data-driven material delivery (Pegoraro, 2010). Emerging technologies, such as virtual and augmented reality, improve fan experiences. In addition, artificial intelligence plays an important role in optimizing the pregnancy of the public and how the content is distributed (Hutchins & Rowe, 2014). The emphasis on emergency and personal digital involvement among Generation Z marks a significant shift in the development of sports culture.

Objectives and Scope of the Chapter

Inspiration for this chapter stems from the need to examine how the unique digital behavior of Gen Z impacts the Sports Engagement Scenario. As this generation matures and assesses more and more economic and cultural effects, it becomes mandatory to understand their expectations, motivations, and consumption patterns for the stability of the sports industry (Leng & Zhang, 2023). Fans are insufficient to draw in and retain this new audience category, which encompasses traditional forms of engagement and income generation, TV broadcast rights, ticket sales, and merchandise. Finding complex relationships between Generation Z and their participation in digital sports is the goal of this chapter. The price and media practices in sports marketing, broadcasting, fandom, and even athlete media are examined, along with their digital engagement flow. The new requirements for sports organizations, such as preserving the integrity of the commercial framework, addressing digital weariness, or other similar unresolved issues, are also attempted to be addressed in this conversation (Williams & Chinn, 2010).

We look at both macro and micro viewpoints, which are reported in this chapter. Global trends in digital involvement at the macro level include the emergence of esport, outstanding individual athletes, and geographically more scattered followers. More specifically, we look at case studies and best practices from clubs, sports leagues, and online platforms that have effectively connected with Gen Z viewers. The evolution of grassroots sports, policy development, and the function of cultural organizations in the digital era are more examples of how this is manifested. The chapter's overall goal is to provide an evidence-based analysis of the problem and reinterpret Gen Z sports participation in the digital era. Strategists must adapt to the diverse behaviors and preferences of this generation, and they do so by working around these characteristics.

LITERATURE REVIEW

Digital Behaviour of Generation Z

This generation is called 'Zoomers' and includes individuals born from the mid-1990s to the mid-2010s. People have an increased interest in this segment of the generation due to its unique digital activity. The Generation that has most likely been the first to fully immerse themselves within a world of Smartphones, the reliable internet, the complex web of social media networks seems to demonstrate tendencies that are a stark contrast from the previous generations. This specific generation's use of technology includes much more than simple, frequent use. The members of Gen Z can operate several platforms simultaneously, and are easily able to sift through information and decide which digital information, images, videos, or interactive content is more useful than traditional text (Seemiller & Grace, 2016). It is very clear from the research that has been conducted that Gen Z spends most of their digital time on platforms that provide short, captivating, visualized content, which is also curated by the algorithms installed within the systems, such as TikTok 'Snackable content', Snapchat, Instagram, and other systems (Twenge, 2017). This Generation also seems to have a distaste for traditional institutional content and focuses more on user-generated content, which is authentic and genuine (Turner, 2015). The online communities they regularly participate in and support clearly reflect their focus on identity and social justice issues within (Fromm & Read, 2018). This generational shift will have a major impact on a number of industries, including sports that rely on public attention and cultural significance.

A third of teenagers use at least one social media platform nearly continuously, according to recent studies. By 2024, that number will rise to 12% for Instagram, which is an improvement over previous year. Additionally, we observe that people can communicate, share information, and exchange images and videos online regardless of where they are or what gadgets they are using, thanks to new technologies, particularly social networks and mobile devices. Therefore, it is no accident that sociologists today discuss "hyperconnected youth," for whom it has become more difficult to turn their focus away from electronic gadgets and digital environments. Unlike their predecessors, members of the Gen Z cohort have the insight to recognize and address social media overuse. In 2023, for instance, 57% of this generation claimed to have done a social media detox, while 63% said they planned to in 2024, the highest rates of any age cohort.

The Digital Transformation of Sports Engagement

Within the last twenty years, the use of technology has greatly changed the audience has toward sports. The sports entertainment industry has been greatly shifted by online streaming, mobile applications, social media, and other contemporary technology, which has real-time communication and access, whereas before, content and communication were restricted (Hutchins & Rowe, 2014). The use of social media has helped link sports organizations to their consumers. People rarely support a team; rather, they develop an interest in an athlete as they want to know more about their life and engage socially (Pegoraro, 2010). Twitter, Instagram, and other social media are used as platforms where market and athletes communicate on social issues, personal life, and more, where they can engage with fans directly (Geurin-Eagleman & Burch, 2016). The level of sports fandom has shifted greatly as they not only use sports as a means of entertainment, but also create stories and engage with the audience by sharing comments, memes, and other content through online fan clubs (Boyle, 2009).

All streamlining options, services, and technology have truly made the world smaller by streamlining how far regional and sometimes unseen professional sports can reach without the aid of a TV channel. Streaming services, as well as other digital platforms, enable niche sports, often restricted to regional leagues, to reach a global audience without requiring a broadcast deal. Additionally, the rise of artificial intelligence and predictive analytics continues to transform the way audiences engage with sports, customizing the fan experience, activating fans, and enhancing post-event engagement. The technology integrated and used in the sporting world has proven to be beneficial in engaging audiences across all projected sporting demographics, as it interacts and connects with key consumer expectations regarding the speed at which services are provided. Although the digital patterns set by Gen Z regarding engagement seem to be few and sparse, more recent studies indicate that Gen Z has significantly lower engagement with sports compared to other generations. Out of the Gen Z respondents, 63 of them identify the videos and messages sent by the sport players as the reason for their engagement with the sport, compared to 42% of the non-Gen Z respondents. Therefore, having a single, sole focus on player engagement is an area of opportunity that the broad sporting world has.

The Intersection of Gen Z and Sports

The way sports organizations package and show their material has evolved due to this generation's penchant for short-form content, behind-the-scenes content, and real-time interactivity (Williams & Chinn, 2010). The relationship between Gen Z's digital activities and the rise in sports engagement offers a unique context for study and practice. Studies show that instead of supporting particular teams, Gen Z prefers to support athletes who match their values, such as diversity, authenticity, and mental health awareness (Vainre et al., 2022). Unlike traditional sports, esports is inherently digital and provides immersive, gamified experiences, exactly what Gen Z expects from everything. Take esports, for example, which has become a unique way to introduce Gen Z to the concept of rivalry in general. Even established sports leagues like the NBA and the Premier League have started using gaming culture-related strategies, like virtual fan zones, interactive video broadcasts, and electronic collectibles, to appeal to younger audiences. But this demographic also presents a problem for established sports leagues. Additionally, their need for speed and innovation is likely to lead to shorter attention spans and decreased loyalty, which will compel companies to continuously develop and differentiate their content deliveries. A fresh look at conventional marketing and communication tactics is necessary in light of Gen Z's mistrust of companies and their branding, demand for transparency, and preference for more genuine narratives (Seemiller & Grace, 2016). In this chapter, this gap is addressed through the analysis of the distinct pressures on athletes that are required to balance both physical performance and the maintenance of their digital persona at the same time (Lin et al., 2025). Although digital stress and athlete performance are both well-researched, their overlap in how ongoing digital exposure directly impacts the development of athletes' sense of athleticism, performance anxiety, and career advancement among Gen Z players is under-researched. Recent studies have started to take the case of athlete-specific digital stress. Social media addiction is a direct contributor to the increase in negative emotions in teen athletes, and comparisons of physical appearance and quality of sleep were found to be mediating variables (Lin et al., 2025). Nevertheless, there are still major gaps in the understanding of how consistent digital exposure specifically increases the stress on athletic identity in comparison with the general adolescent digital stress.

REDEFINING THE ATHLETE IN THE DIGITAL ERA

The Impact of Social Media on Sports Culture

It has reinvented the manner in which sports are consumed and how athletes relate to their audiences, identify themselves, and shape their stories. Over the last few years, social media has changed its role from an ancillary means of communication to a core component of the sports culture in the world. Today, the sports culture is created, discussed, and shared on social media platforms such as YouTube, Instagram, Twitter, or TikTok in real time (Perloff, 2014). The rise of social media has made it possible for fans now get to see backstage footage of how the athletes train, spend their time with family, and their personal values, so that they can be shown the bridge between their personal and professional life (Gulliver et al., 2012). With the present-day media landscape where intimacy, authenticity, and immediacy are highly prized, athletes are not merely field players but also participants, personalities, and content creators. These sites are the source of the immense amount of sports content that the digital-savvy and highly active Generation Z is consuming. This level of closeness creates a feeling of connection and relatability that the traditional broadcast media could never give in full. Whereas sports media once acted as the primary gatekeepers of athlete stories, social media has democratized storytelling. This transformation has also shifted the locus of control over narrative construction. Athletes now wield considerable agency in crafting and sharing their own experiences, often circumventing traditional media channels. This trend aligns with Gen Z's demand for authenticity and individual expression, making the digital athlete a figure of cultural resonance beyond mere sports performance.

Online Branding and Self-Presentation

With the rise of digital platforms, the concept of personal branding has taken on new importance in the sports world. Self-presentation on social media through curated content, visual aesthetics, captions, and interactions is a deliberate and strategic activity (Geurin-Eagleman & Burch, 2016). Today's athletes are highly aware that their online personas contribute directly to their marketability, endorsement potential, and public influence. For Gen Z athletes, this often means creating a multifaceted brand that reflects athletic excellence, personal values, lifestyle choices, and cultural commentary. They are not only elite performers but also outspoken advocates on mental health, racial justice, and gender equality issues deeply important to younger audiences. This new digital identity is best represented by athletes like Simone Biles, Marcus Rashford, and Naomi Osaka. Their online persona displays a hybrid identity that blends relatability, activism, and performance. By creating parasocial relationships in which the fans feel a kind of one-sided intimacy with the athletes, the move raises the level of devotion and emotional involvement of the fans (Kunkel et al., 2013). Publicists, brand strategists, and social media managers are employed by many companies to make sure that everyone is on the same page. Athletes are also starting to handle their online personas in a very professional manner. Every website has optimized content. For instance, Twitter offers live commentary, Instagram features stunning images, and Tik Tok offers brief videos. Being noticed is only one aspect of this professionalization of digital identities; another is staying relevant in a cutthroat attention economy. Gen Z athletes do not practice brand creation as a side gig during their careers.

Athletes' online personas have also grown increasingly polished. The content is channel-neutral; it is optimized with short-form video on TikTok, aesthetically pleasing on Instagram, and features real-time commentary on Twitter. To ensure consistency and engagement, it employs a large number of social media managers, publicists, and brand strategists. This professionalization of digital identities addresses both visibility and survival in a cutthroat attention economy. For Gen Z athletes, building their brand is an integral part of their career, not an add-on.

The Influence of Followers, Likes, and Virality

Usually, these rules dictate contracts for promotions, media exposure, and even fan loyalty. In the sports ecosystem, currencies of influence include things like the number of followers, likes, shares, and views. The Impact of Likes, Virality, and Followers In the digital age, popularity can be measured. The influence of followers and engagement is evident in how sponsors and brands now select athletes for endorsements. For Generation Z athletes who have grown up immersed in a culture of metrics, virality is both a goal and a pressure (Lin et al., 2025). Going viral can amplify one's visibility overnight, but it also brings the risk of overexposure, criticism, and loss of privacy. Companies increasingly seek athletes who can generate reach and engagement on social media, favouring influencer athletes over traditionally successful ones without a digital footprint. However, this dynamic also introduces a host of psychological and ethical concerns. The ability to drive conversation, create viral content, and authentically embody brand values is now a major factor in an athlete's commercial value. The constant pursuit of likes and followers can lead to performance anxiety, digital fatigue, and identity distortion. This can result in emotional labor and mental health challenges that are often invisible to audiences but deeply felt by athletes themselves (Lin et al., 2025). Athletes may feel compelled to maintain a positive, engaging persona at all times, even during personal or professional hardships. Their identity as athletes is constructed as much through digital narratives and visual content as through physical performance. Despite these challenges, the integration of social media into sports culture is irreversible. For Generation Z athletes, the digital realm is not an extension of the real world; it is the real world. Understanding this duality is essential for coaches, sports organizations, and educators who wish to support and engage Gen Z effectively in today's hyper-connected world.

MENTAL HEALTH IN THE SPOTLIGHT

Common Stressors among Gen Z athletes

Mental health challenges among Generation Z athletes are increasingly gaining attention in both academic research and athletic discourse. Unlike the older generations, athletes of Generation Z are growing up in a hyperconnected world, with rapid technological progress, shifting cultural values, and heightened expectations in all spheres of life. Born typically between 1997 and 2012, the young generation is facing a broad spectrum of stressors that are impacting their stage of development and their athletic ambitions. They are supposed to be very much academically successful, socially active, and be able to solve career problems at the same time under the close training and competition programs. Its elements are academic requirements, lack of financial security, social pressures, competitive stress, and an omnipresent digital atmosphere (Twenge, 2017). The pressure to deliver goes way beyond the field of sports for most young athletes. Uncontrolled internalized stress may result in anxiety, depression, burnout, or, in the extreme, dropping out of the sport altogether. Moreover, problems in the formation of identity, acceptance by peers, and recognition requirements can also cause emotional distress, especially when gender is established. Moreover, although there is an increased awareness, the majority of sporting communities reject the discussion of mental health, where it might not be possible to have an open conversation and take action in time (Gulliver et al., 2012). Moreover, Gen Z is more difficult to handle as they are too enveloped by the digital world. The media attention and the inability to stop deluging athletes with information, comparability, and mediation of perfection that can be created on applications such as Instagram and TikTok mean that the athletes feel this is occurring at any moment. Because of this distortion of boundaries between the personal and the professional life, physical athletes find it very difficult to change their thinking and forget everything on a psychological level. Consequently, it could bring up a cohort of more conscious athletes, more susceptible to the harmful consequences of mental health problems because of their indirect stressors and absence of coping mechanisms.

Performance Pressure and Public Scrutiny

Performance pressure is a natural part of competitive sport, and for Gen Z athletes, it has been exacerbated by a digital culture that thrives on visibility, instant feedback, and ongoing scrutiny. Athletes' errors or failures were previously mostly limited to the field or the local stations' newscasts. A single poor performance, outburst, or incorrect move can now be recorded, shared, and debated on a global scale in a matter of minutes, subjecting young athletes to harsh criticism from those who are frequently far removed from their immediate social networks family (Kerr & Stirling, 2012). There are two sides to this interaction. Digital media offers athletes exposure and the possibility of recognition, but it also traps them in a never-ending cycle of comparison and criticism. The performance is a vote on being as much as it is a test of skill. Being scrutinized like this can have a crippling psychological impact, particularly for people who value social acceptance over their own value. Likes, comments, and shares are a few metrics that many Gen Z athletes use to gauge their success. This includes how they appear online, how they respond to admirers and detractors, and how they behave in public. Teenage athletes are also frequently under pressure to project a tidy and well-maintained public persona.

Such a combination of self with sport may increase the anxiety level, resulting in phobias of failure, impostor syndrome, and persistent anxiety (Rosen et al., 2011). The threat of cancel culture or reputational damage can put a sports star in a state of perpetual self-monitoring, which suppresses authenticity and leads to mental exhaustion. Even a slip in conduct, no matter how small, can soon escalate into an online attack. Even the sincere attempts to communicate vulnerability may be misunderstood or misused, and they do not want to be helped. Consequently, such sportspeople require not only performance coaching but also psychological resilience training that should be responsive to the realities of the digital age.

Comparison Culture and the Pursuit of Perfection

Generation Z's ongoing exposure to digital platforms that promote idealized norms of productivity, beauty, and success has ingrained comparison culture profoundly into their minds. Every scroll through social media feeds offers curated snapshots of other athletes' triumphs, winning moments, endorsement deals, and feature articles, creating a perception that success must be fast, flawless, and photogenic (Perloff, 2014). For Gen Z athletes, this culture can create unrealistic expectations not only about what they should achieve in sport but also how they should look, speak, and carry themselves. The emotional consequences include increased anxiety, irritability, and decreased self-confidence, all of which undermine performance and well-being (Primack et al., 2017). This may appear in the form of overtraining, fear of failure, self-monitoring anxiety, and an inability to rest or recover properly, among athletes. Such an environment leads to a kind of perfectionism known by psychologists as maladaptive perfectionism, where individuals form unrealistic expectations of themselves and begin to criticize themselves when these are not met. Perfectionist mentality, which is further encouraged by the continuous exposure to the high-light reels on the Internet, can also predispose athletes to feeling more vulnerable or give in to the idea of failure as part of the learning process. In addition, social comparisons do not always include peers within their sport or country. Unrealistic expectations for success are basically off the scale, given that Gen Z athletes are now exposed to the competitive world via YouTube, Instagram, and TikTok. High achievers might be haunted by a sense of inferiority, and once the players learn that they cannot perform to the expectations that others have of them, it discourages them. Coaches, parents, and organizations need to focus on toughness, hard work, and personal growth rather than trying to focus on the results. This must be countered by reminding individuals of how success and self-worth in sports ought to be. Mental health worsens with the reliance on self-worth on the approval of other people, and in particular, anonymous online communities. Finally, promoting authenticity over perfection, it will become possible to establish the environment that will allow Gen Z athletes to succeed not only in the competition but in life overall. Media literacy training, lessons on mental health, and mentoring by experienced athletes who are having a similar stress can help rewrite these stories.

SPORTS TIME VS. SCREEN TIME

Finding a balance between Technology and Training.

With the world now beginning the era of the universal network of digital interactions, the question of how to reconcile the time spent on the screen and the condition of physical health is becoming more pressing, particularly among the representatives of Generation Z athletes. Despite all the good things that technology can do, like tracking performances, providing tactical analysis, healing injuries, and coaching someone remotely, among other benefits, it will also be a pitfall of overindulgence once it is left unregulated. Electronics, smartphones, tablets, and game consoles have been inseparable aspects of the life of young athletes, and often replace time that would be spent on skill building, training, and rest. The athlete of the modern era, particularly in Gen Z, is supposed to be digitally competent, and attentive on social media, and connected to sports communities online. As an example, interruptions occurring regularly during training on how to respond to messages or update on information may lead to a decrease in focus, intensity, and undermine the motor learning processes. Nevertheless, screen time over-prioritization may cause the substitution of sport time, which is the occasion when the quality and duration of training sessions are affected by overly active digital distraction (Wunsch et al., 2021). It can involve the creation of digital detox plans, the creation of device breaks, and the incorporation of screen activities, such as the analysis of games, into planned training regimes, instead of letting them become disruptive. In most instances, athletes complain of struggling to turn off, as they fear being rejected by the society or losing touch with work as long as they are not online at all times. Digital management strategies are now being promoted by coaches and sports psychologists with purpose. The trick is to change technology into an aid rather than a distraction that can be used to enhance performance. The reflective digital practice, setting boundaries and time audits can empower the athletes to achieve a productive balance between athletic and digital excellence (Cain & Gradisar, 2010).

Impact of Screen Addiction on Physical and Mental Health

More than normal screen time especially to the extent of dependency or even addiction are the worst things that could occur to the physical and psychological health of athletes. A number of reports have attributed the increased prevalence of obesity, reduced cardiovascular fitness, and decreased motor control to excessive usage of digital devices among the youth groups (Tremblay et al., 2011). Sedentary behavior of spending much time in front of the screen frequently leads to the reduced amount of physical activity, improper posture, and the growth of musculoskeletal problems. With Gen z athletes, who have spent their early years in a highly digital world, the boundaries between recreational screen time and compulsive behaviours may tend to be unclear. Psychologically, screen addiction was linked to anxiety, depression, irritability, and the symptoms of poor self-esteem that can have a negative influence on athletic confidence, emotional control, and pressure performance (Twenge & Campbell, 2018). Although social media is a source of connection and recognition, it also creates the feeling of comparison, fear of missing out FOMO, and performance anxiety as athletes are constantly competing against carefully edited images of their peers or competition. In addition, the dopamine-mediated geography of numerous online systems supports reward-seeking behaviour that shares similarities with addiction algorithms. Athletes will tend to be attracted to immediate gratification in digital format as opposed to long-term athletic objectives, where enduring and delayed gratification is needed. Such psychological change may destabilize intrinsic motivation, setting goals and discipline, which are the fundamental principles of athletic training. Digital hygiene-based intervention programs, mindfulness-based intervention programs, and behavioural therapy are emerging as recommended measures to reduce these negative effects and build mental resilience in response (Domoff et al., 2020).

The Disruption of Sleep, Recovery, and Focus

Sleep is a highly important part of recovery in sports, cognition, and muscular regeneration. Digital screens produce blue light that inhibits the production of the hormone, melatonin, which plays a vital role in the regulation of circadian rhythms, thus delaying the onset of sleep and causing a reduction in the REM sleep stages needed to rest (Chang et al., 2015). Late-night scrolling, binge-watching, or gaming is not uncommon among Gen Z athletes and has been known to sabotage the training routine and recovery regimen. Nevertheless, there is an increasingly expanding body of literature highlighting the disruptive impacts of screen time, particularly in a pre-bedtime setting, on the quality and length of sleep. The athletes who lack sleep have reduced reaction times, worse accuracy, and weaker emotional control, which directly correlates with poor performances in the competitive environment (Lastella et al., 2015). In addition to sleep, the omnipresence of notifications, alerts, and instant messages also reduces the capacity of an athlete to concentrate deeply in their practice or during the competition. These behaviours not only shorten sleep windows but also fragment sleep architecture, resulting in chronic fatigue, reduced alertness, impaired decision-making, and increased risk of injury. The constant digital noise cultivates a state of divided attention, which interferes with the deliberate practice required for skill acquisition. In contrast, focused attention and mental clarity, often cultivated through screen moderation, are positively correlated with improved tactical awareness, emotional regulation, and resilience in sport (Rogowska & Tataruch, 2024). Sports professionals are beginning to add digital curfews, no-screen pre-sleep routines and sleep neuroscience education classes to athlete development programs to conserve sleep, recovery and focus. Excessive screen time is not good and can be reduced by encouraging a culture of prioritizing rest and recovery as much as physical training in order to lessen the bad consequences of excessive screen time and encourage the overall well-being of athletes.

FOMO, ANXIETY, AND THE CONSTANT CONNECTIVITY TRAP

The Fear of Missing Out and Its Mental Toll

Due to their chronic attachment to digital spaces, Gen Z members experience this fear almost constantly rather than just occasionally. The so-called FOMO (fear of missing out) has become a powerful psychological influence in Generation Z's life, especially when it comes to digital activity related to sports. FOMO is a phenomenon that is made worse by the constant barrage of information about carefully chosen content on social media (Przybylski et al., 2013). FOMO is the fear that others may be enjoying some rewarding things that you are not present. In order to stay socially relevant, a sports fan needs to be informed about every live event, athlete post, meme, and behind-the-scenes video. This is known as FOMO. A compulsive reliance on technology is the result of this dynamic, where users are more focused on staying informed than on their emotional disengagement and general well-being (Hunt et al., 2018). Especially when friends are discussing the incident online, the prospect of missing a trend such as a last-minute goal, an athlete dancing on social media, or a contentious referee decision can make one feel excluded or inadequate. The psychological literature has attributed FOMO to a higher level of anxiety, depressive symptoms, and lower life satisfaction (Elhai et al., 2016). Given that Gen Z is still in its formative years, this can lead to a great deal of emotional strain. In game arenas, where there is an immediacy impulse and a modern culture that fosters a sense of urgency that may be difficult to overcome, the psychological stress is made worse. Because they must comment, like, retweet, and share in real time, sports fans are now digital participants rather than passive consumers, which has led to a draining performance loop in the digital sphere.

Social Isolation Despite Digital Connection

This paradox is especially noticeable when it comes to sports engagement, as Gen Z may be interacting with screens more often than they are with people in person, like going to a stadium to watch a game or congregating with friends to support a team. This false feeling of interconnectedness that likes, comments, and views offer so often conceals a feeling of loneliness, especially when social media engagement does not affect the emotional depth of face-to-face interaction (Primack et al., 2017). Ironically, despite the fact that digital platforms are meant to connect, most members of Gen Z complain that they feel socially isolated even though they are always online. Moreover, digital sports spaces are highly performative. Although virtual fan communities offer an inclusive space for niche interests and global interaction, they may also foster a sense of detachment from real-world relationships. Interpersonal dynamics in these communities are often shallow, driven by memes, short comments, or fleeting exchanges, which can leave individuals craving deeper human contact. This performative layer can inhibit authenticity and emotional vulnerability, leading to a fragmented sense of self (Hutchins & Rowe, 2014). Users are often preoccupied with maintaining their social persona, posting highlights, adopting popular opinions, or aligning themselves with popular athletes. For Gen Z, who are already navigating complex questions of identity and belonging, the sports world's increasingly digitized engagement mechanisms may inadvertently deepen feelings of alienation.

Cognitive Overload and Burnout

Cognitive Overload and Burnout Cognitive overload refers to the mental burden that arises when individuals are bombarded with excessive information or tasked with processing multiple sources of input simultaneously. This is a hallmark of the

Gen Z experience in the digital age, where notifications, live updates, short-form content, and algorithmic feeds demand continuous attention and rapid cognitive shifts. The 24/7 news cycle, multi-platform streaming, fantasy leagues, interactive polls, and promotional content, all competing to get the attention of the user further amplify this overload in the ecosystem of sports. The gen z sports fan is particularly susceptible to digital burnout, the state of mental, emotional, and disengaged depletion wrought by digital overstimulation. According to the research, Gen Z digital burnout may cause low motivation, problems with attention, irritability, and poor sleep quality (Keles et al., 2020). In this sense, burnout is not just academic or work-based, but spans into leisure and entertainment, which should bring relaxation, but rather becomes a source of stress because of being always connected. These symptoms are augmented by the fact that there are no distinct lines between viewing and being involved in sports; users have to switch constantly between being observers, commentators, and creators, all in a few taps. Importantly, cognitive overload can also impair the very experiences that digital sports platforms aim to enhance. When users are overwhelmed, they are less likely to process information meaningfully, engage critically with content, or derive emotional satisfaction from the experience. Thus, what begins as a pursuit of entertainment and connection can devolve into a cycle of compulsion, stress, and diminished well-being.

INSTITUTIONAL ROLE AND RESPONSIBILITIES

Support Mechanisms from Schools, Clubs, and Sports Bodies

These entities are not just platforms for participation but also act as custodians of youth development, ethics, and mental well-being (Livingstone & Helsper, 2007). Schools, being foundational institutions in a young person's life, can cultivate early awareness about both the opportunities and risks of digital engagement in sports. As Generation Z navigates the increasingly intertwined domains of sports and digital technology, institutions such as schools, sports clubs, and official governing bodies play a pivotal role in shaping responsible, inclusive, and sustainable engagement (Hutchins & Rowe, 2014). Through structured programs that combine physical education with digital fluency, schools can help students understand how platforms like YouTube, Instagram, and Twitch are reshaping sports fandom, athlete branding, and the consumption of sporting events. Similarly, sports clubs at grassroots, regional, and elite levels can create environments where young athletes are educated about using digital tools to enhance, not compromise, their performance and reputation (Pegoraro, 2010). By integrating digital sports engagement into the curriculum, educators can guide students in developing critical media literacy and discernment regarding content authenticity, cyberbullying, and privacy management. By encouraging responsible digital storytelling, these institutions empower athletes to build narratives that are authentic, inspiring, and socially conscious, qualities that resonate with Gen Z values (Smith & Sanderson, 2015). Clubs should appoint trained digital mentors or media officers who can counsel athletes on content sharing, personal branding, data protection, and the long-term implications of online behaviour. Governing sports bodies, including federations and leagues, carry a broader responsibility of institutionalizing standards and policies that prioritize athlete welfare and ethical media conduct. Codes of conduct for digital engagement, support systems for victims of cyber harassment, and access to legal and mental health services are crucial measures that such bodies should mainstream. Particularly in the context of high performance, these organizations ought to create systems that would control the psychological strain that athletes endure as a result of online publicity and criticism (Kerr & Stirling, 2012). Additionally, funding inclusive online campaigns that celebrate diversity and inclusion can help reinforce positive role modeling and the need to address harmful trends in online sports discourse.

Education on Digital Literacy and Mental Health

Learning programs cannot be restricted to the technical knowledge of gadgets or platforms. Lack of formal education on how to use sports content responsibly may be a contributor to misinformation, addiction, self-esteem issues, and identity distortion in the presence of Generation Z, who themselves consume and generate sports content every day. Given the dual nature of digital technology, the learning institutions must put digital literacy learning in a central position in their engagement strategy. Digital literacy has to do with understanding algorithms, the ability to detect bias, source evaluation, understanding manipulative content, and managing digital footprints. Interdisciplinary units may be launched at sports schools and academies, where students learn about how digital ecosystems work, how their data is monetised, and how their actions the turned into algorithmic recommendations. Such awareness enables the young people to become beyond a consumer but rather a cognizant and sensitive participant in the digital sports environment (Hunt et al., 2018). Mental health education is also to be paid sufficient attention to, in addition to digital literacy. The online institutions are recommended to implement preventive mental health interventions that mediate the psychological effects of online interaction, such as fear of missing out FOMO, impostor syndrome, cyberbullying, and digital fatigue. The availability of online feedback loops, likes, shares, and comments will create a domain of never-ending social contrast and performance fear in both Gen Z athletes and fans. The school and club support systems are supposed to include the mental health professionals who are ideally trained in sports psychology and the development of youths to assist in early detection and intervention measures and resilience-building measures. Mental health can be demystified, and more people get access to support services with the help of peer-led activities, workshops, and interactive programs. These programs should politicise the help-seeking behaviour and turn emotional intelligence to be of the core life skills, which will prompt Gen Z to build a healthy and conscious interdependence with digital sports media.

Encouraging Open Conversations and Safe Spaces

Institutional support lies in the ability to build an environment in which the youth feel free to express their views, break the rules and seek assistance. Schools and sports organisations ought to promote an inclusive culture in relation to opinion, identity and background. With the use of online products or services to create their publicity, Generation Zers require access to safe offline and online environments. It is possible to achieve this through the promotion of dialogic education where students and athletes are encouraged to express their opinions, challenge assumptions, and solve the problem collaboratively. In in-person conversations, they can be supplemented with digital safe spaces (peer mentoring groups, anonymous feedback portals, and moderated topic forums). Active listening, nonjudgmental communication and emotional regulation should be trained to teachers and coaches so as to establish environments that allow openness and trust. Open conversations also imply breaking taboos whether it is related to mental health, failure, body image or identity or online error. These platforms help the persons to express their experiences, plight and dreams without experiencing stigma or punishment. The institutions are also supposed to collaborate with mental health organizations, youth oriented NGOs, and tech companies to jointly develop platforms that are both interactive and psychologically safe. Vulnerability must be promoted as a courageous show and storytelling as a healing and empowering tool in the institutions. These values can be reinforced at an institutional in the form of public forums with athlete testimonials, digital detox organizations, and student-led information panels on digital well-being.

BUILDING DIGITAL RESILIENCE

Healthy Habits for Managing Social Media Use

Social media is a platform and a point of pressure to Gen Z athletes. Healthy habits about social media are therefore core to digital well-being. It gives them unprecedented chances to express themselves, brand themselves, and build a fan following, yet it puts them under criticism, unrealistic expectations, and anxiety to perform. According to the studies, social media use has been linked to excessive anxiety, sleeping issues, and attention span among teenagers and young adults (Twenge & Campbell, 2018). The first habits include setting a limit, specific times in a digital-free time, no apps before going to sleep, and deliberate limitation of screen time. A second healthy habit concerns maintaining a curated feed, i.e., following the accounts that motivate, teach, or provide an uplift and unfollowing or muting accounts that create a sense of comparison, fake news, or negativity. More so, media literacy education is vital. Sportsmen should be motivated to use their online world as an encounter with their minds. Learning about the nature of the algorithms, identifying the presence of clickbait, and doubting the truthfulness of the information will help athletes become proactive, not passive users. Lastly, the athletes must be advised to go to social media purposefully, be it to cause, share achievements, or even interact with the fans. The blind scrolling must be substituted with meaningful communication. The alternative to compulsive consumption is conscious creation, which will help athletes to be less vulnerable to the mental exhaustion that comes with hyperconnectivity.

Mental Health Practices Tailored for Athletes

Athletes operate in high-pressure environments where expectations, self-worth, and public scrutiny often intersect. For Gen Z athletes, these pressures are compounded by the omnipresence of digital platforms. Tailored mental health practices are necessary to maintain both performance and personal equilibrium. First among these is mindfulness-based training, which fosters present-moment awareness and emotional regulation. Studies show that mindfulness enhances focus, reduces stress, and builds resilience qualities essential for athletes navigating both competition and social media (Vainre et al., 2022). Cognitive-behavioural strategies also play a critical role. Mental health check-ins, ideally integrated into training schedules, should not be seen as interventions but as regular components of athlete wellness. Given the blurring of public and private life in digital spaces, athletes must also practice digital self-compassion, the ability to treat oneself kindly amidst online setbacks or cyberbullying (Neff, 2011). Teaching athletes to challenge negative self-talk, reframe criticism, and develop coping responses to online feedback helps build emotional Armor. Gen Z athletes should also be encouraged to normalize mental health conversations, whether by sharing experiences online or supporting teammates, which can reduce stigma and foster a culture of openness. In addition, providing access to sports psychologists trained in the digital challenges facing modern athletes ensures that support is both relevant and responsive.

Role of Coaches, Mentors, and Families

Digital resilience is not solely an individual endeavour; it is co-constructed within a support ecosystem. Coaches, mentors, and families play a pivotal role in modelling healthy digital behaviour and reinforcing practices that protect athletes' well-being. Influence is exerted through coaches, especially. Mentors may be senior athletes or alumni who may offer real-life insights into how to handle digital notoriety, criticism, or online scandals. Moreover, by allowing the athletes to remain focused on the process of development rather than on external approval, coaches can stimulate performance evaluation by video analysis and avoid social media responses. Providing a role model about screen time, supporting digital silence times at camp or simply talking about the pressure to use the Internet, coaches can create conditioning to promote mental acuity and physical achievement. Being digitally literate themselves, parents and guardians are in a better position to have a constructive discussion about the online experience, observe possible red flags of online distress, and assist their children to develop a healthy online and offline identity. Most Gen Z athletes, in their turn, have families as the source of emotional stability. Their experience in life is a guideline to guide the young athletes who need guidance in an ever-changing media world. Notably, a developmental and not disciplinary approach to digital challenges should be embraced by all stakeholders. It has been emphasized by research that good communication within a family is a protective factor against the adverse psychological effects of using the media excessively (Roychowdhury, 2021). Athletes should receive training on proper internet conduct, reputation management, and the long-term consequences of their online mistakes instead of a punitive response to them. Programs for school, college, and professional sports development should include mentorship circles, workshops, and counseling sessions that address digital resilience.

CONCLUSION

The chapter has shown that Gen Z athletes, which can be characterized as digitally native, have a complicated digital life and a sport career. Their social lives and training have been influenced by proliferation of digital devices, social media and web based information in their day to day lives. The life of Gen Z athletes is twofold: online and field. Internet-based coaching, performance data, motivation resources, and virtual counselling are instances of digital benefits. The resources enhance goal-setting, development of athletic skills, and sports. It is also in the study that excessive use of digital media can be destructive. Excessive use of screens leads to digital burnout, inattention, disturbed sleep cycles, and validation on the Internet, which may hamper focus, self-discipline, and mental resilience in sport. Technology skills have not assisted the Gen Z athletes in balancing between their online and physical life. There is a greater importance on digital and athletic balance than ever. Gen Z athletes are coming to merge the virtual and the physical world. They need to align their social media profiles, adapt to the digital culture and communicate with others over the Internet to project their best and enjoy a popular online image. Otherwise, digital engagement may slow the recovery process, create more stress, and lead to burnout. Therefore, frequent schedules, screen-free downtime, and in-real-life social interaction are required to facilitate digital discipline. Digital technologies can be used by Gen Z athletes to maintain the balance in their lives without losing their health or physical development. Future directions and recommendations are proposed to enable Gen Z athletes to reach such a balance: First, schools, universities, and sports academies should integrate Digital Wellness Education into the program of athlete development. These modules can teach media literacy, time management, and the psychological aspects of screen time. Second, be considerate of the approach to Tech-Integrated Training. Although wearables, AI analysis, and virtual evaluation can enhance performance, coaches and trainers have to enact digital boundaries to preserve the time of rest and focus. Third, coaches and parents should be included. The role of parents, guardians and mentors is to demonstrate to young athletes how to act safely on the Internet and to teach them the importance of their real life relations and well-being rather than spending all the time on the Internet. Bespoke Recovery Protocols also emphasize the value of sleep and calming the mind and living in the moment. One of these techniques in recovery plans may be a timed digital detox. And third, but not the least, there is research and new ideas. Future studies need to investigate the long-term cognitive, psychological, and physical impacts of online actions in sportspeople. The developers and educators can design digital interventions with an athlete-friendly interface to support active lifestyles and health by designing gamified fitness apps that can facilitate physical exercises, mindfulness tools, and virtual sports events. To sum it up, the Gen Z athletes will be forced to be cautious regarding their online and sports lifestyle. They are able to achieve successfully in sports and in life when they have healthy digital habits that are supported by education and mentors. Gen Z athletes will perform well in the rapidly evolving sporting world with the right tools, structure, and mindset.

REFERENCES

Boyle, R. (2009). *Power play: Sport, the media and popular culture*. Edinburgh University Press. https://books.google.com/books?hl=en&lr=&id=fQerBgAAQBAJ&oi=fnd&pg=PR2&dq=1.%09Boyle,+R.,+%26+Haynes,+R.+(2009).+Power+play:+Sport,+the+media+and+popular+culture.+Edinburgh+University+Press.&ots=RBFWJLoxhU&sig=8drhFLqOeOy6FMHQQFxyzEldyvo

Cain, N., & Gradisar, M. (2010). Electronic media use and sleep in school-aged children and adolescents: A review. *Sleep Medicine*, *11*(8), 735–742. DOI: 10.1016/j.sleep.2010.02.006 PMID: 20673649

Chang, A.-M., Aeschbach, D., Duffy, J. F., & Czeisler, C. A. (2015). Evening use of light-emitting eReaders negatively affects sleep, circadian timing, and next-morning alertness. *Proceedings of the National Academy of Sciences of the United States of America*, *112*(4), 1232–1237. DOI: 10.1073/pnas.1418490112 PMID: 25535358

Deshmukh, A., T. K. S., Rahul, S., & Medhekar, A. A. (2024). *User generated content and its influence on relationship marketing among Generation Z. Journal of Informatics Education and Research, 4*(1). DOI: 10.52783/jier.v4i1.633

Domoff, S. E., Foley, R. P., & Ferkel, R. (2020). Addictive phone use and academic performance in adolescents. *Human Behavior and Emerging Technologies*, *2*(1), 33–38. DOI: 10.1002/hbe2.171

Elhai, J. D., Levine, J. C., Dvorak, R. D., & Hall, B. J. (2016). Fear of missing out, need for touch, anxiety, and depression are related to problematic smartphone use. *Computers in Human Behavior*, *63*, 509–516. DOI: 10.1016/j.chb.2016.05.079

Fromm, J., & Read, A. (2018). *Marketing to Gen Z: The rules for reaching this vast–and very different–generation of influencers*. Amacom. https://books.google.com/books?hl=en&lr=&id=kVBLDwAAQBAJ&oi=fnd&pg=PP1&dq=%E2%80%A2%09Fromm,+J.,+%26+Read,+A.+(2018).+Marketing+to+Gen+Z:+The+rules+for+reaching+this+vast--and+very+different--generation+of+influencers.+AMACOM.&ots=fcUFyJ1mMn&sig=SwxIwCKlg-6J-R39h63bPtCVbpE

Geurin-Eagleman, A. N., & Burch, L. M. (2016). Communicating via photographs: A gendered analysis of Olympic athletes' visual self-presentation on Instagram. *Sport Management Review*, *19*(2), 133–145. DOI: 10.1016/j.smr.2015.03.002

Gulliver, A., Griffiths, K. M., & Christensen, H. (2012). Barriers and facilitators to mental health help-seeking for young elite athletes: A qualitative study. *BMC Psychiatry*, *12*(1), 157. DOI: 10.1186/1471-244X-12-157 PMID: 23009161

Hunt, M. G., Marx, R., Lipson, C., & Young, J. (2018). No More FOMO: Limiting Social Media Decreases Loneliness and Depression. *Journal of Social and Clinical Psychology*, *37*(10), 751–768. DOI: 10.1521/jscp.2018.37.10.751

Hutchins, B., & Rowe, D. (2014). Sport beyond television: The internet, digital media, and the rise of networked media sport. *International Journal of Sport Communication*, *7*(2), 279–281. DOI: 10.1123/IJSC.2014-0029

Keles, B., McCrae, N., & Grealish, A. (2020). A systematic review: The influence of social media on depression, anxiety and psychological distress in adolescents. *International Journal of Adolescence and Youth*, *25*(1), 79–93. DOI: 10.1080/02673843.2019.1590851

Kerr, G. A., & Stirling, A. E. (2012). Parents' Reflections on their Child's Experiences of Emotionally Abusive Coaching Practices. *Journal of Applied Sport Psychology*, *24*(2), 191–206. DOI: 10.1080/10413200.2011.608413

Kunkel, T., Doyle, J., & Funk, D. (2013). Exploring Sport Brand Development Strategies to Strengthen Consumer Involvement with the Product–The Case of the Australian A-League. *Doyle, J., Kunkel, T., Funk, D.(2013). Sport Spectator Segmentation: Examining the Differing Psychological Connections amongst Spectators of Leagues and Teams. International Journal of Sports Marketing & Sponsorship*, *14*(2), 95–111.

Lastella, M., Roach, G. D., Halson, S. L., & Sargent, C. (2015). Sleep/wake behaviours of elite athletes from individual and team sports. *European Journal of Sport Science*, *15*(2), 94–100. DOI: 10.1080/17461391.2014.932016 PMID: 24993935

Leng, H. K., & Zhang, J. J. (2023). . In H. K. Leng & J. J. Zhang, *Sports Sponsorship and Branding* (1st ed., pp. 1–18). Routledge. DOI: 10.4324/9781003458890-1

Lin, W., Cen, Z., & Chen, Y. (2025). The impact of social media addiction on the negative emotions of adolescent athletes: The mediating role of physical appearance comparisons and sleep. *Frontiers in Public Health*, *12*, 1452769. DOI: 10.3389/fpubh.2024.1452769 PMID: 39926290

Livingstone, S., & Helsper, E. (2007). Gradations in digital inclusion: Children, young people and the digital divide. *New Media & Society*, *9*(4), 671–696. DOI: 10.1177/1461444807080335

Neff, K. (2011). *Self-compassion: The proven power of being kind to yourself.* Hachette UK. https://books.google.com/books?hl=en&lr=&id=PDAEzLL9mscC&oi=fnd&pg=PT7&dq=3.%09Neff,+K.+D.+(2011).+Self-compassion:+The+proven+power+of+being+kind+to+yourself.+William+Morrow.&ots=Aft5k6lpb-&sig=vQfrlhMdQGl4KAjkJmX57yzU8zo

Pegoraro, A. (2010). Look who's talking—Athletes on Twitter: A case study. *International Journal of Sport Communication, 3*(4), 501–514. DOI: 10.1123/ijsc.3.4.501

Perloff, R. M. (2014). Social Media Effects on Young Women's Body Image Concerns: Theoretical Perspectives and an Agenda for Research. *Sex Roles, 71*(11–12), 363–377. DOI: 10.1007/s11199-014-0384-6

Primack, B. A., Shensa, A., Sidani, J. E., Whaite, E. O., Lin, L., Rosen, D., Colditz, J. B., Radovic, A., & Miller, E. (2017). Social media use and perceived social isolation among young adults in the US. *American Journal of Preventive Medicine, 53*(1), 1–8. DOI: 10.1016/j.amepre.2017.01.010 PMID: 28279545

Przybylski, A. K., Murayama, K., DeHaan, C. R., & Gladwell, V. (2013). Motivational, emotional, and behavioral correlates of fear of missing out. *Computers in Human Behavior, 29*(4), 1841–1848. DOI: 10.1016/j.chb.2013.02.014

Rogowska, A. M., & Tataruch, R. (2024). The relationship between mindfulness and athletes' mental skills may be explained by emotion regulation and self-regulation. *BMC Sports Science, Medicine and Rehabilitation, 16*(1), 68. DOI: 10.1186/s13102-024-00863-z PMID: 38504372

Rosen, L. D., Lim, A. F., Carrier, L. M., & Cheever, N. A. (2011). An empirical examination of the educational impact of text message-induced task switching in the classroom: Educational implications and strategies to enhance learning. *Psicología Educativa. Revista de Los Psicólogos de La Educación, 17*(2), 163–177.

Roychowdhury, D. (2021). *Understanding mindfulness in sport, exercise, and performance psychology. Routledge Encyclopedia of Psychology in the Real World* (1st ed.). Routledge., https://api.taylorfrancis.com/content/entry-versions/download?identifierName=doi&identifierValue=10.4324/9780367198459-REPRW220-1&type=webpdf

Seemiller, C., & Grace, M. (2016). *Generation Z goes to college.* John Wiley & Sons. https://books.google.com/books?hl=en&lr=&id=xjDvCQAAQBAJ&oi=fnd&pg=PR9&dq=4.+5.%09Seemiller,+C.,+%26+Grace,+M.+(2016).+Generation+Z+goes+to+college.+Jossey-Bass.+6.%09Smith,+A.+(2019).+Digital+fandom:+New+media+studies+of+sport+and+entertainment.+Peter+Lang.&ots=7CLsMBeE9j&sig=3VwETz7GW1fvZYnzZzjQCaDcuFE

Smith, L. R., & Sanderson, J. (2015). I'm Going to Instagram It! An Analysis of Athlete Self-Presentation on Instagram. *Journal of Broadcasting & Electronic Media, 59*(2), 342–358. DOI: 10.1080/08838151.2015.1029125

Tremblay, M. S., LeBlanc, A. G., Kho, M. E., Saunders, T. J., Larouche, R., Colley, R. C., Goldfield, G., & Gorber, S. (2011). Systematic review of sedentary behaviour and health indicators in school-aged children and youth. *The International Journal of Behavioral Nutrition and Physical Activity, 8*(1), 98. DOI: 10.1186/1479-5868-8-98 PMID: 21936895

Turner, A. (2015). Generation Z: Technology and Social Interest. *Journal of Individual Psychology, 71*(2), 103–113. DOI: 10.1353/jip.2015.0021

Twenge, J. M. (2017). *iGen: Why today's super-connected kids are growing up less rebellious, more tolerant, less happy–and completely unprepared for adulthood–and what that means for the rest of us*. Simon and Schuster. https://books.google.com/books?hl=en&lr=&id=HiKaDQAAQBAJ&oi=fnd&pg=PT2&dq=%E2%80%A2%09Twenge,+J.+M.+(2017).+iGen:+Why+today%E2%80%99s+super-connected+kids+are+growing+up+less+rebellious,+more+tolerant,+less+happy%E2%80%94and+completely+unprepared+for+adulthood.+Atria+Books.&ots=aRXXiVfNR-&sig=8_irlFitzXZvaqNTEc-cKJXkQpI

Twenge, J. M., & Campbell, W. K. (2018). Associations between screen time and lower psychological well-being among children and adolescents: Evidence from a population-based study. *Preventive Medicine Reports, 12*, 271–283. DOI: 10.1016/j.pmedr.2018.10.003 PMID: 30406005

Vainre, M., Dalgleish, T., Bendriss-Otiko, T., Butler, M., Kirkpatrick, A., Kosugiyama, N., Martinez-Sosa, C., Mariscotti, F., Sideri, A., & Soenksen, S. (2022). *Mindfulness training for work performance: A systematic review and meta-analysis of randomised controlled trials*. https://osf.io/preprints/psyarxiv/2vkru/

Williams, J., & Chinn, S. J. (2010). Meeting relationship-marketing goals through social media: A conceptual model for sport marketers. *International Journal of Sport Communication, 3*(4), 422–437. DOI: 10.1123/ijsc.3.4.422

Wunsch, K., Nigg, C., Niessner, C., Schmidt, S. C. E., Oriwol, D., Hanssen-Doose, A., Burchartz, A., Eichsteller, A., Kolb, S., Worth, A., & Woll, A. (2021). The Impact of COVID-19 on the Interrelation of Physical Activity, Screen Time and Health-Related Quality of Life in Children and Adolescents in Germany: Results of the Motorik-Modul Study. *Children (Basel, Switzerland), 8*(2), 98. DOI: 10.3390/children8020098 PMID: 33540824

Chapter 10

The Cost of Being Connected:

The Influence of Social Media on Self-Worth and Body Image Among Indian Adolescents

Apurva Sweeten Bandodcar
https://orcid.org/0000-0002-8471-067X
GVM's Gopal Govind Poy Raiturcar College of Commerce and Economics, Ponda, India

Mrinal Vishnu Valke
https://orcid.org/0009-0007-9145-3759
Zantye Brothers Educational Foundation's Narayan Zantye College of Commerce, India

ABSTRACT

Indian adolescents are paying a silent and hefty price for being connected on social media. The chapter investigates how SMPs shape Indian teenagers' self-worth and body image, exposing the hushed crisis playing out on Indian screens. The adolescents are settling in a vicious circle of competition. It poses a question: What becomes of a generation growing up hooked on digital validation? The study is based on two theories: the Social Comparison Theory and Theory of Mimetic Desire. Teens want to be wanted because they see their peers being desired. These experiences within larger systems, soft power, platform capitalism, and digital colonialism, shape digital adolescent identities and desires. The results show a negative correlation between the usage frequency of SMPs and self-esteem. The study revealed a positive correlation between SMPs usage and body dissatisfaction. The females reported

DOI: 10.4018/979-8-3373-4516-1.ch010

higher levels of body dissatisfaction and social comparison behaviours, indicating gendered differences. SMP users exhibited aspirational identification, reported higher digital beauty anxiety.

INTRODUCTION

India is making bold strides towards improving the digital infrastructure: as evident in the integration of technology to facilitate public distribution of essential commodities by the Government. The use of behavioural economics to prompt public engagement in flagship programmes, such as Digital India and the Healthy India Initiative, is noteworthy (Sharma & Tiwari, 2016; Vikram & Sutar, 2024; Khajuria et al., 2025). India stands on the cusp of a major initiative to digitally empower its population, embedding technology into multiple domains of daily life. Yet, India is not oblivious to the negative consequences of the technological solutions (Prince et al., 2007).

The prevalence data from an all-inclusive digital National Mental Health Survey by the National Institute for Mental Health and Neurosciences (NIMHANS) indicated a dire need for mental health care services, advocating for promotion of technology-based applications, such as Mobile Health (m-health), electronic health (e-health), and 'smart health', as a strategic means to make mental health count within the global health agenda and to increase access to treatment globally (Gautham et al., 2020). With approximately 491 million active social media user identities, equivalent to 33.7% of India's total population, in January 2025, a thorough understanding of the psychological implications of engagement on SMP has become critical for researchers and policymakers. The UN Sustainable Development Goals (2015) emphasize mental health and call for the development of new ICTs to bridge the digital divide and foster knowledge societies (Mills et al., 2018; Mills C., 2018; Saxena et al., 2014; World Health Organization, 2013).

Adolescents, particularly, are vulnerable to the digital trends. The Indian digital adolescents occupy a unique position at the intersection of traditional cultural values and global digital influences. Unlike their Western counterparts, they navigate social media while contending with deeply rooted cultural pressures. This confluence creates a fragile psychological environment where external validation through digital metrics becomes entwined with culturally specific insecurities and aspirations. When SMP users engage in virtual self-presentation, they are amenable to existing cultural and societal norms. The Indian Gen Z's perceives SMPs as an integral part of their existence, necessary for social acceptance and their sense of self. SMP users engaging in virtual self-presentation become amenable to societal and cultural norms. Indian Gen Z perceives SMPs as integral to their existence, essential for social acceptance and self-perception. SMPs have evolved from a tool of self-expression into a mirror reflecting impossible standards, deeply reshaping adolescent development. These platforms have evolved from tools of self-expression into mirrors reflecting unattainable ideals and impossible standards. This shift transcends social comparison and represents a primary change in how adolescents articulate their identity, perceive their bodies, and evaluate their self-worth. SMPs have become vehicles of 'soft colonialism', where projected ideals shaped by cinematic glamour and influencer culture merge to create hybrid but equally problematic benchmarks for adolescent self-evaluation. This digital colonialism operates through formidable algorithmic systems that reflect and actively reinforce foreign ideals of beauty, success, and desirability.

This research is a response to the characteristic silent crisis playing out in adolescent lives, demanding an unprecedented psychological price for their constant digital connectivity. It critically examines the subtle yet profound ways SMPs influence Indian adolescents' self-perceptions, often beyond their conscious awareness. It then turns to the visual world they're immersed in. Central to this phenomenon is mimetic desire, defined as the intrinsic, often implicit motivation to pursue objects or recognition desired by others, driving teens toward online validation and a digitally constructed sense of desirability.

The chapter also reflects on a more subtle force at play - unrealistic beauty standards coded deep into the platforms themselves, from algorithms to aesthetics. These benchmarks shape human behaviour, both positively and negatively. Thus, it calls for action to offer culturally grounded solutions and policy recommendations to challenge toxic digital norms and help the emerging youth navigate love, beauty, and identity in a world that rarely shows them the whole truth.

The present analysis addresses several critical gaps in the existing literature. First, most previous research has focused on single outcomes or limited demographic groups, failing to capture the multidimensional nature of social media's psychological impact. Second, the mechanisms through which social media affects psychological well-being remain poorly understood, with limited investigation into potential mediating factors. Third, gender differences in social media's psychological impact have been inconsistently documented, with varying findings across different studies and populations.

The urgency of this research is underscored by the rapid digital transformation of Indian society. With over 491 million social media users in India and adolescents representing the fastest-growing demographic of digital natives, the implications of social media's psychological impact extend far beyond individual well-being to encompass broader questions of cultural identity, mental health infrastructure, and educational policy (Kemp, 2025; Jain, 2024). The COVID-19 pandemic has only accelerated this digital dependency, making Social Media Platforms (SMPs) not just spaces of entertainment but primary venues for social interaction, learning, and identity formation (Shah et al., 2023; Marciano et al., 2022; Lee et al., 2022; Choi et al., 2023).

This investigation critically examines how SMPs influence Indian adolescents' self-perceptions through mechanisms that often operate below conscious awareness. It explores the visual ecosystem that envelops young users—one dominated by idealised and frequently unattainable body images—and investigates how sustained exposure to such content feeds body dissatisfaction among psychologically vulnerable minds. This mimetic desire drives teenagers toward online validation and digitally constructed notions of desirability.

The research presented here is grounded in empirical investigation involving 410 Indian adolescents, employing validated psychological instruments alongside culturally sensitive measures. The findings reveal not just statistical correlations but point toward systemic issues within digital platforms themselves—from algorithmic bias to aesthetic standardisation—that shape human behaviour in ways that can be both positive and profoundly negative.

Beyond individual psychological outcomes, this research situates adolescent social media use within broader systems of power and influence, including soft power dynamics, platform capitalism, and digital colonialism (Langley & Leyshon, 2017). These larger forces affect not only the content young people consume but also the very framework through which their identities and desires develop online. This comprehensive perspective is essential for understanding the complex digital reality that Indian teenagers navigate today (Valkenburg P. M., 2022).

The chapter poses fundamental questions about the trajectory of a generation growing up dependent on digital validation: What happens to authentic self-development when self-worth becomes increasingly tied to external metrics? How do traditional Indian values of family, community, and inner strength survive in digital spaces designed to prioritise individual performance and comparative success? And perhaps most critically, what interventions can effectively address these challenges while preserving the beneficial aspects of digital connectivity?

The implications of this research extend beyond academic understanding to urgent practical applications. As Indian society grapples with rising rates of adolescent mental health issues, the findings presented here offer both diagnostic insights and potential pathways for intervention (Ministry of Health and Family Welfare, Government of India, 2014). The recommendations emerging from this work call for coordinated action across multiple domains—from educational curriculum reform to platform accountability, from policy intervention to community-based support systems (Rajkumar et al., 2022; United Nations Children's Fund, 2021).

This investigation represents more than an academic exercise; it is a call to action for educators, policymakers, mental health professionals, and society at large to recognise and address the quiet crisis unfolding on millions of Indian screens. The solutions proposed focus on empowerment, digital literacy, and culturally grounded interventions that help young people value authenticity over approval, fostering resilience in an increasingly complex digital world.

Contribution of the Chapter

The research brings a sharp, timely lens to the conversation on youth mental health by examining how colonial hangovers, Western soft power, and Gen Z's search for digital friendships and courtships collide in today's online dating culture. It shines a light on a space that has largely gone unnoticed: influencing emotional development in under-recognised ways.

Through an empathic mix of theory, data, and cultural critique, the chapter unpacks critical questions: It asks: In what ways do SMPs act as vehicles of cultural pressure, shaping Indian adolescents' digital self-concepts and their vulnerability to mimetic desire?

SMPs subtly rewire the ways adolescents construct identity, navigate relationships, and negotiate self-worth in virtual spaces.

CONCEPTUAL BACKGROUND

The precise definition of Social Media remains unclear even as it continues to draw in the popularity and significance in the life of the users. One way of defining it is based on capability it equipped the users with. Boyd & Ellison (2007) cited three key elements: the ability to create a fully or partially public personal profile, the ability to enlist other site-users with whom they are connected, and the ability to see and explore the connections of oneself as well as those of others within the system. Others focused less on connecting power of the social media and attempted to define it based on the different ways users can engage with the site, like viewing, posting, sharing, and accessing different types of unique content (Zimmer-Gembeck et al., 2021; Uhlmann et al., 2020; Wang et al., 2020). Depending on the platform's primary function, user engagement might involve sharing photographs, consuming video content created by other users, participating in comment-based interactions on written posts, or developing professional networking connections (Rhee et al., 2021).

'Adolescence'—derived from the Latin adolescere, meaning "to grow up"—is a transitional stage between childhood and adulthood marked by rapid physical, cognitive, and psychosocial development. Although its definition varies globally, leading organisations such as the World Health Organization (WHO) define adolescence as the period between 10 and 19 years of age, while the United Nations Convention on the Rights of the Child defines a child as anyone under 18. Additional terms like "youth" (15–24) and "young adulthood" (18–26) further complicate the classification. For the purpose of this study, adolescence refers to individuals aged 13 to 20 years, aligning with the psychological and developmental relevance of this transitional phase (Sawyer et al., 2018; Gentry & Campbell, 2002; World Health Organization, n.d.; United Nations, n.d.; UNICEF, 1995).

During adolescence, rapid pubertal changes—including shifts in body weight and shape—may distance individuals from sociocultural body ideals, heightening their susceptibility to negative self-perception. This period is also marked by increased emotional reactivity and social sensitivity, influenced by neurological changes in the socio-affective circuitry of the brain (Somerville, 2013). Adolescents often experience what Elkind (1967) termed the "imaginary audience," a belief that they are under constant observation, which amplifies appearance-based concerns. These biological and cognitive shifts make adolescents especially vulnerable to peer influence and the emergence of an "appearance culture" that equates attractiveness with social value (Jones, 2001; Kleiser & Mayeux, 2021). In the backdrop of the numerous bio-psychosocial changes develops an "appearance culture", wherein the peers frequently discuss physical attractiveness and ascribe status to those deemed attractive (Kleiser & Mayeux, 2021). The obsession of adolescents with physical appearance can be attributed to this human drive to engage and ace in impression management, that does not cease with adolescence, but may converge with the peer appearance culture and elevated egocentrism (Choukas-Bradley et al., 2025; Schlenker & Pontari, 2000; Leary, 1996). For the purposes of this study, adolescents are considered to be individuals within the age range of 13 to 20 years of age (Gentry & Campbell, 2002).

A salient feature of an adolescent's self-concept is Body image. A positive perception of one's body image is linked with better psychological adjustment (Fabris & Longobardi, 2024). In contrast to the etymological meaning, Body image is more about the perceptual processes of the mind with regards to the body. It is determined, largely, by an individual's exclusive view of the world through personality, a lens with which this view is filtered. An individual, through one's personality, can focus on the body to distort reality, similar to a reflection of the physical world in a curved mirror. This can make us form judgements regarding the body size and shape of others, which can hurt how we feel about ourselves.

Body image refers to a person's mental picture and emotional attitude toward their own body, encompassing both perceptual and attitudinal dimensions (Dionne & Davis, 2012). The perceptual component includes one's estimation of body size, shape, and appearance, while the attitudinal aspect reflects thoughts, feelings, and behaviours related to those perceptions. According to the APA Dictionary of Psychology, body image is the mental representation of one's body as a whole, incorporating both physical characteristics (body percept) and attitudes toward these characteristics (body concept). These constructs shape how individuals evaluate themselves, influencing broader aspects of self-concept and emotional well-being (American Psychological Association, 2018).

Body image is a chief component of one's self-concept and identity, as feelings about one's physical body have the potential to impact how we view ourselves and our capabilities (Chrisler & Ghiz, 1993). Personal experiences, individual personality and the social and cultural effects shape the body image of an individual (Abamara Nnaemeka et al., 2014). Recent studies have demonstrated the negative emotions, such as depression and anxiety, arise due to the intensive use of social media, with the mediating effects of self-esteem and social comparison (Park & Baek, 2018). With the multidimensional role of technology, facilitating content sharing, encouraging peer interactions, and easier accessibility to mobile technology, SMPs are notorious for promoting body image ideals through the effective use of the visuals (Holland & Tiggemann, 2016).

Individuals who view attractive images on Facebook have demonstrated a greater likelihood of being dissatisfied with their body image and emote more negative feelings afterward (Haferkamp & Krämer, 2011). The results have been validated by a number studies on other SMPs. An exposure to fitness inspirational content on TikTok increased appearance comparison and negative mood in the state (Pryde & Prichard, 2022). The negative emotions, highlighted by "appearance-based social comparisons," often place oneself in an adverse position, leading to dissatisfaction and negativity. SMPs have enabled users to engage in increased appearance- based comparisons, internalization of the thin ideal, and self-objectification, leading to body dissatisfaction (Dorčić et al., 2023). As individuals who engage more frequently are likely to encounter appearance-based comparisons that heighten anxiety, we formalize our hypothesis of the relationship between social media engagement and body image anxiety based on the prior (Chen, 2025; Gardner, 2012). As with most research, this study considers the attitudinal component of body image.

Self-worth, which forms over time and results in stable conceptualizations of self with implications for psychological functioning, is an individual's assessment of themselves as a valuable, capable human being deserving of respect and consideration (Neff & Vonk, 2009; Rosenberg et al., 1995). [REMOVED HYPERLINK FIELD]Modern conceptions of self-esteem take into account both the cognitive and emotional aspects of self-worth, which are represented in the attitudes, sentiments, and actions people display according to how they view their own worth in personally significant spheres of life (Muñoz et al., 2023; Crocker & Wolfe, 2001).

Self-worth is intricately linked with related constructs such as self-esteem, self-awareness, and identity. William James's conceptualisation of the self—divided into the "knowing self" (I) and the "known self" (me)—remains foundational (James, 1890). The subjective self perceives and evaluates the objective self, creating a framework through which individuals judge their own value. When adolescents internalize social ideals, this evaluative mechanism may lead them to perceive themselves as lacking or inadequate, depending on the standards imposed by their environment and peer networks.

Self-awareness is defined as an one's focused attention on themselves or their self-knowledge (American Psychological Association, 2025). The self-focus of the individual includes their emotions, thoughts, desires, and needs. It is believed to occur when one pays attention to them or possesses knowledge about them. While social psychologists describe an individual's self-awareness using self-awareness, neuroscientists use the term self-consciousness (Wiekens C. J., 2009; Wiekens & Stapel, 2008). In the psychology literature, the term self-consciousness denotes the quality of being in touch with oneself, while self-awareness refers to the condition of possessing that awareness (Yılmaz, 2022).

Self-esteem is typically understood as a stable, global evaluation of one's self-worth (Crocker & Wolfe, 2001), while some scholars distinguish self-worth as more situational or momentary in nature (Brown & Marshall, 2006). However, others contest this distinction, arguing that self-worth reflects a deeper, consistent appraisal of personal value (Pelham & Swann, 1989; Swann et al., 1989). Importantly, self-esteem is shaped by internal and external criteria—especially among adolescents, whose evaluations of themselves are often influenced by perceived social acceptance, comparison, and validation on digital platforms (Leary & Baumeister, 2000).

The notion of self-esteem has traditionally been delineated in terms of self-esteem as a trait and transient feelings of self-worth. Nonetheless, it is also posited that self-esteem may constitute a responsibility imposed upon individuals. Individuals with high self-esteem encompass not only those with a favourable perception of oneself but also narcissists, arrogant, and protective personalities (Baumeister et al., 2003). Therefore, it is considered highly important to differentiate between the concepts of self-esteem and self-worth (Bırni & Eryılmaz, 2024; Charmaraman et al., 2025).

THEORETICAL BACKGROUND

SMPs provide unprecedented opportunities for social comparison, as users are constantly exposed to curated representations of others' lives, appearances, and achievements. This investigation is grounded in two pivotal psychological theories illuminating the mechanisms underlying the SMP impact on adolescent well-being. Human beings have a natural tendency to draw comparisons with others against numerous parameters (Festinger, 1954). According to Festinger (1954), social comparison behaviours are displayed due to the need to evaluate one's opinions and abilities, especially in circumstances where objective evaluations are unavailable. This theory, coined as the Social Comparison Theory, helps people establish a benchmark to accurately assess their behaviours (Festinger, 1954; Schachter, 1959; Thornton & Arrowood, 1966; Gibbons & Buunk, 1999). The Theory of Social Comparison has been widely studied to investigate the impact of SMPs on how adolescents measure themselves against carefully curated digital profiles of individuals, triggering cascading effects on self-esteem and body satisfaction.

Complementing this, the Mimetic Desire Theory propagated by Girard (1972) and translated later in English (1977) offers a more nuanced perspective. According to Girard, humans do not desire objects or states for their intrinsic value but to copy them from after those they see online via an unconscious mimetic mechanism. Rather, individuals do not generate desires independently. Girard (1972) explains that imitation can lead admiration to evolve into competition and hostility, as the admired individual becomes perceived as a rival. As multiple individuals enter similar rivalries, their conflicts often converge on a single target, a common enemy, through which the group seeks unity and resolution. In the context of social media, as more adolescents are exposed to lifestyle digitally portrayed ideals with respect to beauty standards, lifestyles, or material goals, mimetic responses may be triggered and lead to feelings of unhealthy competition, inadequacy, jealousy, and rivalry. In group settings, these tensions can escalate, leading to collective targeting or scapegoating, as seen in online shaming or cancel culture (Mohanty et al., 2024; Zhuang, 2023). This vicious cycle of imitation, rivalry, and exclusion underscores the profound impact of social media on how adolescents shape their self-image and evaluate their own worth.

LITERATURE REVIEW

Gender Norms and Self-Presentation on Social Media

Numerous studies have proven that SMPS frequently encourage traditional gender norms in users' self-presentation strategies, in addition to mirroring them. Initial research shows that, users modify their online selves to conform to perceived gender norms in order to acquire social capital and prevent social backlash (Goffman, 1959; Schlosser, 2020; Fox & Vendemia, 2016). This effect is amplified by visual-heavy websites like Instagram, Snapchat, Facebook etc, where there are striking variations among genders in posting habits: men are more likely to emphasize masculity, supremacy, or risk-taking in their selfies, while women are more likely to post pictures reflecting beauty or sexual appeal (Atanasova, 2016; Adetayo, 2024; Dhir et al., 2016; Sorokowski et al., 2015; Döring et al., 2016; Pounders et al., 2016).

These types of behaviors both characterize and prescribe. Kappes (2021) Both normative and descriptive purposes are served by these practices. it is shown that people tend to penalize breaking the rules differently depending on a person's gender and have identical standards about what makes a "gender-typical" selfie. A prominent form of in-group norm enforcement was evident in more brutal judgments made of female nonconformity by women in particular (Dann & Capdevila, 2023). On the other hand, men who strictly follow masculine norms may have a negative impact on social relational dimensions; they may be rated as less likeable or approachable by other people because they are associated with being more conservative and lack warmth. The nuanced reality of digital gender performance is brought to light by these dynamics: complying may reduce obvious sanction while also inhibiting social connection. These results raise questions on the idea that societal benefit always results from normative conformity (Kietzmann et al., 2011).

Instagram Use, Social Comparison, and Psychological Well-Being

Using the Differential Susceptibility to Media Effects Model (DSMM), Turk (2021) found that passive Instagram use, such as browsing and lurking, is more strongly associated with problems of upward social comparison, contingent self-worth, and appearance-based self-esteem than active use (e.g., posting, interacting). SMPs such as Instagram pave opportunities for identity exploration along with psychological vulnerabilities. Prior studies indicate that passive users are more likely to internalize idealized representations of other people, which increases their dependence on external assurance for self-worth (Jiang & Ngien, 2020; Stapleton et al., 2017).

Notably, although feedback-seeking is frequently considered maladaptive, it can actually act as a buffer for impacts. Turk (2021) reported that people who share less content but compare more often had more negative effects, indicating that in some situations, social reinforcement (likes and comments) may act as a barrier against internalized harm. These subtleties draw attention to the psychological costs of passive consumption and imply that not all digital involvement is created equal.

Body Image and Social Media in Adolescents

Teenagers' perceptions of their bodies are significantly shaped by social media. Persistent and frequently unintentional comparison to unattainable beauty goals is made possible by platforms that prioritise look-oriented content (Bell et al., 2021). The Tripartite Influence model (Thompson et al., 1999; Cash, 2005) describes this internalization process, which connects media, peers, and family influences to increased body dissatisfaction and risky behaviors like eating disorders (Fredrickson & Roberts, 1997).

Bell et al.'s (2021) assessment of the Body Talk in the Digital Age (BTIDA) program is one example of a successful intervention. Although the commentary on thin ideal endorsement showed a significant decline among girls, the interventions showed little effect on boys and only modestly improved general physical fulfillment. These gender-specific results suggest that in order to achieve substantial change, structural-level actions might need to be more thorough and customized.

Mimetic Desire, Scapegoating, and Digital Influence

Mimetic theory, a derivative of Girard's theory of imitative desire, is a good model to examine digital conformity and social exclusion. This model suggests that during times of social tension, scapegoating serves as a social unifier. whereas critical realist thinkers expanded mimetic theory as a generative mechanism with causal consequences, Houston and Swords (2021) used this model for organizational and policy contexts (Magee, 2025).

According to the latest academic contributions to digital culture, social media trends (such as viral aesthetics and curated self-imagery) work via mimetic loops, in which users try to imitate socially rewarded patterns, which leads to the scapegoating of outgroups or norm violators. While Magee (2025) claims that technology itself (such as large language models) may become “computational scapegoats,” fusing imitation, aspiration, and discontent in novel ways, Kappes (2021) and Atanasova (2016) reveal this clearly in selfie culture. These revelations point out just how essential it is to consider digital punishment and conformity as expressions of mimetic structure as well as behavioural problems.

Gender Norms and Self-Presentation on Social Media

Academic interest in the connection between social media, gender norms, and self-presentation have risen, especially in light of the vital role that visual media plays in navigating one's self-identity throughout platforms. Social media frequently reinforces and sometimes magnifies conventional gender norms, influencing how people present themselves and are viewed, according to research (Döring et al., 2016; Fox & Vendemia, 2016). Self-presentation is audience-aware, according to early foundational work an approach that is still very relevant to SMPS (Goffman, 1959). According to studies, it is often noted that men are more likely to post images that highlight strength, dominance, or autonomy, while women are more likely to post appearance-focused selfies that emphasise charm or beauty (Dhir et al., 2016;

Sorokowski et al., 2015). These actions serve as cues for expectations among platform users and not merely mirror gender norms (Kappes, 2021).

But following the rules does not always lead to a boost in one's reputation. A conflict involving relational appeal and cultural expectations was highlighted by the fact that men who displayed masculine self-presentation traits were frequently viewed as less likeable and relatable, specifically by female viewers (Kappes, 2021). On the other hand, women who did not take selfies that were typical of their gender were more negatively viewed by other women, which suggests greater in-group policing of gender. These outcomes are explained by theoretical models like "precarious manhood" and "backlash effects", which highlight the contrasting social sanctions surrounding gendered behaviour on the internet (Vandello et al., 2008; Rudman & Fairchild, 2004).

Passive and Active Instagram Use: Impacts on Self-Worth

Varying the mode of use, social media consumption can have a wide range of psychological effects, especially on platforms that feature carefully chosen visuals. Turk (2021), using the Differential Susceptibility to Media Effects Model (DSMM), makes a distinction between female undergraduates' active (posting, commenting) and passive (scrolling) Instagram behaviour. Through exposure to idealized portrayals on other people's profiles, the study finds that passive use is more strongly correlated with heightened comparisons orientation and contingent self-worth (Turk, 2021).

Image-Driven Platforms and Conditional Self-Presentation

Increased self-monitoring and conditional self-presentation are encouraged by visual SMPs. Kim, Seely, and Jung (2017) discovered that while low self-monitors favour platforms like Pinterest, which emphasizes personal interests and less social opinions, high self-monitors tend to turn to Instagram because of its social recognition. Additional experimental results show that short-term exposure to these platforms can alter state self-monitoring, which influences impression management tactics and advertising receptivity.

Self-monitoring can have a damaging impact on users by encouraging anxiety, inauthenticity, or by objectifying oneself, even though it may help control public perception. This discloses a two-way dynamic: users' psychological orientation determines how they experience and are influenced by the platform, and the platform moulds how users present their own experiences and lives.

Digitalisation and Emergence of the Digitalized Self

Scholars have been forced to rethink individuality in digital contexts as a result of the digitization of daily life. According to Chan (2022), the "Digitalized Self" is a dynamic identity created via ongoing engagement with digital systems like gadgets, SMPs, and AI interfaces. Digital identity is now shaping rather than merely reflecting, changing as time passes how users see and respond out their sense of self.

Research identifies fragmentation, digital dependency, and avatar-based self-presentation as major trends. Journeying these identities causes emotional exhaustion, decreased self-confidence, and raised cognitive strain, particularly for digital natives who frequently switch between their online and offline personas (Firth et al., 2019; Small et al., 2020).

Psychological Impacts of the Metaverse on Self-Esteem

Through the use of idealized or augmented avatars, the metaverse introduces immersive identity formation. Jia and Mvondo (2025) list six risk mechanisms that jeopardize users' mental health and self-esteem, particularly in young adults. These mechanisms range from identity instability to virtual reality sickness. Individuals who used avatars that were very different from their real-life self-image encountered the most adverse consequences.

Notwithstanding claims of empowerment and escape, the metaverse has the potential to magnify depersonalization and social comparison. The study demands an urgent need for responsible and morally sound virtual design techniques that put emphasis and respect psychological safety, boundary-definition, and identity coherence first.

Advertising Imagery and Adolescent Girls' Body Perceptions

One of the major contributors for teenage girls' body dissatisfaction is advertising that uses extremely idealized models. According to Zhou and Dong (2024), exposure to such imagery often leads to upward social comparison, particularly in situations where ambitious pressures are amplified by celebrity or influencer endorsements. Such tactics greatly encourage diminished self-worth, disordered eating behaviour, and skewed appearance ideals, even though they might improve brand related awareness or financial gain. Even parental influence is outweighed by the power of influencer-based endorsement, indicating that media literacy programs need to revise their principles to take interpersonal connections into consideration when evaluating media consumption (Zhou & Dong, 2024).

Social Media, Imaginary Audience, and Adolescent Anxiety

Through the lens of the "imaginary audience" effect, Shi, Kong, and Zhu (2024) investigate how social media-induced self-consciousness increases social anxiety in teenagers. Boosted social media use, according to the study, intensifies the feeling that one is being constantly being judged all the time, which decreases appearance self-esteem and, in turn, raises social anxiety. Interestingly, direct associations between SMP use and anxiety are eliminated when mediators (i.e., appearance-based self-esteem and imaginary audience) are taken into consideration, implying that internal psychological processes are central to mediating this relationship.

Paediatric Health and Screen Time Exposure

According to Salmerón-Ruiz et al. (2025), excessive use of digital media during early childhood interferes with key developmental stages. Frequent use of screens is linked to insomnia, delayed language development, increased risk of obesity, and myopia. Digital distractions impair attention spans and the quality of parent-child interactions, which also disrupts the cognitive and social domains.

The study urges organizational measures, such as platform safety regulation, educational standards for device integration, paediatric policy reform, and age-based screen guidelines. It makes the case for viewing digital exposure as a systemic public health issue rather than merely a problem with individual behaviour.

METHODOLOGY

In order to gain insights into the outcome of the constant exposure to digital dopamine on adolescent psyche, this study was guided by hypothesis developed based on prior research. This analyses assumes that adolescent behaviour on SMP is essentially driven and shaped by Mimetic Desire. Furthermore, it is hypothesised that SMP is a significant contributor for low self-worth and body dissatisfaction among adolescents.

The chapter draws on findings from a quantitative cross-sectional study conducted among 410 Indian teenagers aged 15–19 using a purposive sampling technique, from urban and suburban schools and colleges. Prior consent was duly obtained from the survey participants. The primary data for the study under consideration was obtained with the help of a structured e-questionnaire. The Rosenberg Self-Esteem Scale (RSES), Body Appreciation Scale-2 (BAS-2) and a self-developed Mimetic Desire Index (MDI), along with Social Media Engagement Questionnaire, capturing netnographic details were integrated into data collection instrument (Tylka & Wood-

Barcalow, 2015; Rosenberg M., 1979). Each of the constructs was measured with relevant items on a Likert scale. A sample of 384 respondents was recommended by Krejcie and Morgan (1970) for an indefinite population at 95% confidence with 5% margin of error. Out of the 424 nationally representative responses received, only 410 were valid and usable for further analysis. The Self-Esteem and Body Shape constructs consisted of 10 items each with the Social Media Engagement construct being measured with eight items. The face validity of the newly developed MDI was established for the study. Statistical techniques such as Pearson's correlation, descriptive statistics, and multiple regression analyses were used to analyse the data. The data analysis was conducted with Python code in Google Colab and JASP.

ANALYSIS

Table 1. Descriptive Statistics

Variable	Mean	SD	Min	Max
Age	14.44	2.91	10.00	19.00
Daily SM Time (Hours)	2.73	0.99	1.00	4.00
SMP Usage Frequency	12.83	3.18	5.97	18.82
Self-Esteem (Total)	25.30	6.31	10.00	40.00
Body Dissatisfaction	32.55	8.82	10.00	54.63
Mimetic Desire (Total)	27.94	8.33	8.80	50.00
SM Engagement (Total)	26.47	6.19	8.00	40.00
Social Comparison (Total)	16.85	4.94	5.60	28.00
Appearance Anxiety	4.32	0.73	2.03	5.25
Attractiveness Concerns	4.13	0.77	1.83	5.50

Source: Primary Data

The reliability of the instrument was measured using Cronbach's Alpha (Cronbach, 1951). The Cronbach's α, for all the scales used, was above 0.5, indicating acceptable internal consistency (Streiner, 2003; Taber, 2018). The variables examined are highly relevant for understanding how social media use relates to self-esteem, mood, and body image concerns among emerging adults—a population known to be particularly vulnerable to online influences.

The descriptive statistics for key variables in the study are presented in Table 1. The mean age of participants was 14.44 years (SD = 2.91), indicating a primarily adolescent sample. Daily social media use (M = 2.73, SD = 0.99) suggests moderate-to-high daily engagement. Psychological constructs such as self-esteem (M = 25.3, SD

= 6.31) and body dissatisfaction (M = 32.55, SD = 8.82) demonstrated considerable variability, indicating diverse experiences among participants. Notably, variables such as appearance anxiety (M = 4.32) and attractiveness concerns (M = 4.13), Further underscore the importance of aesthetic self-perception in this demographic.

Table 2. Pearson Correlations Between Key Variables

Variable	SMP Usage Frequency	Self-Esteem	Body Dissatisfaction	Mimetic Desire	SM Engagement	Social Comparison	Appearance Anxiety	Attractiveness Concerns
SMP Usage Frequency	—							
Self-Esteem	−.483***	—						
Body Dissatisfaction	.527***	−.226***	—					
Mimetic Desire	.100*	−.112*	.060	—				
SM Engagement	.351***	−.227***	.183***	.049	—			
Social Comparison	.007	.009	−.027	.020	.013	—		
Appearance Anxiety	.271***	−.127*	.186***	−.030	.119*	−.015	—	
Attractiveness Concerns	.200***	−.112*	.149**	−.030	.047	.204***	.074	—

Note. $p < .05$, **p** < .01, $p < .001$.
Source: Primary Data

Significant negative associations were found between SMP usage frequency and self-esteem (r = -0.483, p < .001), as highlighted in Table 2. suggesting that increased SMP usage correlates with lower self-esteem. Conversely, usage frequency showed positive correlations with body dissatisfaction (r = 0.527, p < .001), appearance anxiety (r = 0.271, p < .001), and attractiveness concerns (r = 0.200, p < .001), indicating that higher social media activity is associated with greater body image-related concerns. Self-esteem negatively correlated with body dissatisfaction (r = -0.226, p < .001), mimetic desire (r = -0.112, p < .05), and appearance anxiety (r = -0.127, p < .05), supporting the hypothesis that these factors negatively affect self-concept. However, social comparison did not show strong associations with self-esteem or most other variables, except attractiveness concerns (r = 0.204, p < .001). The results of independent samples t-tests examining gender differences underscores significant gender differences, females noticeably scored significantly higher on all variables i.e. body dissatisfaction, social comparison, appearance anxiety, and attractiveness concerns. However, the differences in self-esteem or mimetic desire between genders was not statistically significant (table 3).

Table 3. Independent Samples t-Tests for Gender Differences

Variable	Female M (SD)	Male M (SD)	*t*	*p*	Cohen's *d*
Body Dissatisfaction	34.25 (9.24)	30.02 (7.52)	5.10	.000	0.49
Social Comparison	17.90 (4.94)	15.28 (4.51)	5.56	.000	0.55
Appearance Anxiety	4.40 (0.77)	4.19 (0.65)	2.95	.003	0.29
Attractiveness Concerns	4.30 (0.76)	3.87 (0.70)	5.92	.000	0.59
Self-Esteem	25.50 (6.28)	25.01 (6.37)	0.76	.445	0.08
Mimetic Desire	27.63 (8.43)	28.41 (8.18)	−0.94	.349	−0.09

Source: Primary Data

Table 4. Multiple Regression Predicting Self-Esteem

Predictor	B	SE	*t*	*p*
Constant	38.19	1.75	21.83	.000***
SMP Usage Frequency	−0.98	0.10	−9.61	.000***
Gender (Female = 1)	0.76	0.60	1.27	.204
Body Dissatisfaction	0.02	0.04	0.44	.660
Mimetic Desire	−0.05	0.03	−1.41	.158
Social Comparison	−0.00	0.06	−0.02	.986

$R^2 = .242$, $F(5, N) = 25.84$, $p < .001$
Note. $p < .05$, **p** < .01, ***p*** < .001.
Source: Primary Data

To predict the self-esteem among users of SMPs, a multiple linear regression analysis was conducted. As indicated in Table 4, the overall model was statistically significant, approximately 24% of the variance in self-esteem was explained by the included predictors. SMP usage frequency emerged as a strong negative predictor (B = -0.98, p < .001), while other variables like gender, body dissatisfaction, mimetic desire, and social comparison, did not significantly contribute to the model.

Table 5. Mimetic Desire Group Differences by SMP Use

Comparison	Group 1	M (SD) Group 1	Group 2	M (SD) Group 2	*t*	*p*	Cohen's *d*
Frequent vs Infrequent SMP Users	Frequent SMP Users	29.84 (8.84)	Infrequent SMP Users	27.07 (7.98)	2.34	.020	0.33
Followers vs Non-Followers	Influencer Followers	29.53 (8.57)	Non-Followers	25.56 (7.35)	5.02	.000	0.49

Source: Primary Data

The significantly higher mimetic desire was indicated in frequent SMP users as compared to the infrequent users ($t = 2.34$, $p = .02$, $d = 0.33$) as displayed in table 5. Additionally, the robust influence of digital role models on desire-based behaviour was evident with the scores of followers of influencers being higher than non-followers ($t = 5.02$, $p < .001$, $d = 0.49$).

FINDINGS AND DISCUSSION

The findings illustrate the complex psychological burden placed on teenagers in the era of digital connections. They underscore how mimetic desire fuels a loop of performative behaviour and emotional vulnerability. The results clearly depict that regular SMP use is inversely associated with lower self-esteem ($r = -.483$, $p < .001$) and higher body dissatisfaction ($r = .527$, $p < .001$), leading to anxiety about how one looks (appearance anxiety mean = 4.32), and apprehensions about the attractiveness of the self (attractiveness concerns mean = 4.13). The body dissatisfaction was found to be more severe among the women ($M = 34.25$, $SD = 9.24$) compared to men ($M = 30.02$, $SD = 7.52$). They engaged in comparisons more than their male counterparts (social comparison: females $M = 17.90$ vs. males $M = 15.28$). This relationship is reinforced by regression findings, which identify frequency of use as a significant negative predictor ($B = -0.979$, $p < .001$). The influence of mimetic desire at play was demonstrated on the adolescents who followed digital influencers- they displayed a comparatively stronger desire to copy them ($M = 29.53$ vs. 25.56; $t = 5.02$, $p < .001$), suggesting mental absorption of their aspirational online models.

The complex relationship between teenage SMP use and psychosocial well-being is clarified by the present research. The results are in agreement with earlier studies that found excessive use of SMP can worsen body image issues and be harmful to self-esteem (Perloff R. M., 2014; Fardouly et al., 2015). The robust correlation between SMP usage and body dissatisfaction suggests that visual-centric platforms may be reinforcing unattainable beauty ideals.

The gender differences are significant because they reflect global trends that show female adolescents are more susceptible to stresses related to appearance, perhaps as a result of internalizing societal norms and being exposed to more objectifying content (Tiggemann & Slater, 2014). It's interesting to note that in this sample, social comparison did not significantly predict self-esteem or body image ($p = .986$), which calls for more research into how teenagers interpret online comparisons.

Independent of other psychological variables, the regression analysis emphasizes that the frequency of SMP usage is a key predictor of self-esteem. This backs up recommendations for programs that encourage teenagers to use social media with awareness and purpose. Lastly, the ambitious aspect of online identity is highlighted by the influence of mimetic desire, especially among influencer followers. These results suggest that teenagers might be actively emulating carefully constructed personas, which could influence their goals and real-world self-concept. The findings are in line with prior research indicating that youth who devote greater amounts of time on social media are more likely to experience body dissatisfaction and related mood symptoms. According to Jiotsa et al. (2021) and Castellanos Silva et al. (2023), image-based SMPs (like Instagram and TikTok) increase the likelihood of this happening. Adolescents who regularly compare their physical appearances and abilities to those of others on social media express more negative sentiments. This may increase depressive symptoms and lower self-esteem. These elements are interwoven with both body dissatisfaction and depression.

Adolescent well-being research frequently highlights a recurring pattern: fear of not conforming to idealised beauty standards and anxiety about social acceptance drive heightened appearance-based comparison, leading to dissatisfaction Linardon et al. (2023; 2022). Both body dissatisfaction and depressive symptoms are linked to these variables. Persistent body dissatisfaction and diminished self-worth are linked to heightened risks of disordered eating, social withdrawal, and chronic psychological distress. Conversely, fostering positive body image and engaging in affirming social interactions can buffer adolescents against the adverse emotional consequences of SMP use. In educational and therapeutic contexts, media literacy, self-compassion, and body acceptance are becoming more and more important.

High daily social media use among youth (mean 2.73hr/day in the study) mirrors global digital trends and carries implications for psychological well-being. As indicated by Silva et al. (2023), extended exposure to image-centric platforms correlates with increased body dissatisfaction and risk for mood disturbances among emerging adults. Young et al. (2020) underscore that the amount and nature of content consumed—especially idealized or filtered images—strengthen the impact of time spent online on self-perception and comparison processes. Thus, the result positions social media duration as both a marker and mechanism of risk within this population (Young et al., 2020; Silva & Steins, 2023).

The findings capture their specific vulnerabilities during late adolescence, which is characterized by identity negotiation and a greater sensitivity to judgments from others. According to Valkenburg et al. (2022), Self-esteem of the young is especially pliable and frequently changes in reaction to peer comments, likes, and feedback cycles on SMPs. They established that upward social comparison on SMPs typically results in lower levels of self-esteem, which is in support of findings of the study (Valkenburg et al., 2022).

Frison and Eggermont (2016) found that frequent encounters with cyberbullying, perceived social exclusion on media platforms, and negative peer interactions, all anticipate higher levels of depressive symptoms. Fardouly and Vartanian (2016) found that self-objectification and internalizing physical appearance norms also raised the risk of depression. These correspond substantially with the observation and the study (Frison & Eggermont, 2016; Vidal et al., 2020; Pouwels et al., 2021; Beyens et al., 2021; Fardouly & Vartanian, 2016). Studies by Perloff (2023) and Tiggemann and Slater (2014) confirmed that image-focused social media environments exacerbate issues with body image, particularly for young women, by promoting unachievable physical attributes. Repeated exposure to carefully chosen and idealized online imagery has been shown to have this widely recognized effect.

Frequent social comparison is both normative and problematic in digital peer contexts. Festinger's (1954) social comparison theory remains foundational, but contemporary studies show that social media intensifies opportunities for upward comparison, thereby worsening self-evaluations and increasing anxiety. The study captures this experience, confirming its negative role in Indian adolescence's self-perception (Feinstein et al., 2013). Reduced body appreciation points to both a potential for action and a susceptibility to external triggers. According to Linardon et al. (Linardon et al., 2022), body appreciation acts as a psychological buffer that lessens vulnerability to the adverse impacts of social media by moderating the relationship between social comparison and negative effects (Linardon et al., 2022).

Moderate attractiveness and appearance anxiety scores (means = 4.13 and 4.32 respectively indicate ongoing internal tensions. Kearney-Cooke and Tieger (2015) explain how appearance anxiety and ongoing concern with attractiveness not only make adolescents vulnerable to body dissatisfaction but also fuel repetitive avoidance and checking behaviors online. Such tendencies, as the findings indicate, can generate ongoing dissatisfaction and amplify risks for social withdrawal and mood dysfunction (Kearney-Cooke & Tieger, 2015).

Beyond time, the sample's high level of social media engagement (mean = 26.47) shows that both the quantity and quality of involvement shape psychological outcomes. According to Andreassen et al. (2016), who distinguished between active and passive engagement, passive consumption—that is, surfing with no interaction—is particularly closely associated with adverse psychosocial outcomes. Given that not all social media behaviors have the same impact, the study findings suggest a nuanced focus on the nature of engagement. Adolescents' use of social media is associated with aspects of psychological health other than depression and self-esteem. According to a curvilinear relationship between digital screen use and mental health, Przybylski and Weinstein (2017) discovered that excessive screen time is associated with greater anxiety while moderate use is not harmful and may even improve well-being. Both extremes of this spectrum are represented in the results of a wide range in daily use (1–4 hours), which supports the need for tailored recommendations.

Teen depressive symptoms can also be heightened by not only aversive peer contact, but even more ingrained reinforcement patterns on the internet. Building on these concerns, studies have found that girls as a group continue to be susceptible to the depressive effects of aversive social media contact, including exclusion and aversive comparison. The low but significant depressive scores obtained, therefore, amount to an accumulative risk, especially in those more engaged in social networking (Kelly et al., 2018).

Additionally, critical understanding and awareness of digital image manipulation moderate body dissatisfaction. As indicated in a study by McLean et al. (2015), Users who were more media literate internalized fewer unrealistic beauty standards and, consequently, expressed less dissatisfaction (McLean et al., 2015). High mean for body dissatisfaction (M = 32.55) is consistent with the finding that protective skills are not yet common.

Social comparison on social media is further heightened by algorithmic content presentation. The ways algorithms favor content that provokes high affective reactions, usually upward comparisons, that enhance negative self-view was noted (Verduyn et al., 2020).

Appearance anxiety can be explained on the grounds of internalized perfectionism and cultural appearance standards. Social media enhances perfectionistic ideals, promoting anxious preoccupation with imperfections. The data obtained mirrors these mechanisms: perfectionism is both a cause and an amplifier of appearance-related anxiety in adolescents (Rodgers et al., 2020).

CONCLUSION AND RECOMMENDATIONS

The empirical evidence demonstrates a complex interplay between a network of relationships among engagement on SMPs, self-esteem, body image, and mental health among young people. High social media use, frequent appearance-based comparisons, and elevated body dissatisfaction are significant risk factors for poor psychological outcomes in adolescents. However, body appreciation serves a protective function. Targeted interventions can help the future generation navigate a complex digital landscape with resilience and confidence. The primary finding of the study proves that increased engagement on SMPs is a significant negative predictor of self-esteem, especially the frequency of use. Heightened body dissatisfaction and appearance anxiety are often repercussions of this practice. Although gender emerged as an important factor, the higher vulnerability to social comparison and aesthetic value was reported among the females. The strong pull of online personas on generation of mimetic desire highlights a deeper layer of identity modelling driven by curated digital content. These dynamics illustrate how adolescents may not only consume but also internalize online ideals, often to their psychological detriment. The study is a strong advocate of critical digital literacy, emphasizing on social-emotional education, and responsible platform design to mitigate the harmful effects of appearance-oriented content and comparison-driven user experiences. This research underscores a critical need for immediate digital and cultural intervention in nations grappling with development alongside the demanding social norms. The omnipresence of SMPs in teenagers' lives compels profound scrutiny of their appetite, personal worth, and physical image awareness. The emotional maturation of the Gen Z cohort is resoundingly influenced by the choices made externally, the vicarious modelling and the algorithmic validation. The establishment of a digital ecosystem that is both responsible and healthier for teenagers necessitates the joint effort of all stakeholders. This digital environment should promote the ideas of being real, strong, and self-worth which are culturally relevant. Body appreciation, while predominantly defensive, is also affected by offline social ties. Perceived family support was reported at higher levels in adolescents, and these adolescents reported greater body appreciation and resistance to negative media messages. This suggests that interventions to enhance body appreciation may be complemented by addressing family relationships (Webb et al., 2015).

Given these findings, a multi-pronged response is essential to mitigate the psychosocial risks and promote healthier digital habits in adolescents. In order to address the psychosocial shortcomings highlighted in this study, the authors propose a structured plan:

1. Introduce digital literacy in schools. The schools must incorporate a curriculum facilitating the adoption of technology and the accompanying understanding of its impact. Modules that address mental health issues in the digital environment and build digital resilience education, including body positivity and the toxic loop of online comparison.
2. Push for policy reforms that demand algorithmic transparency and better representation of diverse bodies in SMPs.
3. Empower peer-led mental health initiatives that celebrate real and diverse body features and challenge colonial beauty ideals still dominating the silver and golden screens.
4. Hold platforms accountable through harm-reduction practices like judicious content moderation, trigger warnings, and ethical design.

Not every social media activity has an equal impact; quality over quantity is more important. Whereas passive scrolling is associated with envy and dissatisfaction, supportive interactions (support-giving, sharing) act as a buffer against negative consequences. Hence, interventions need to aim at engagement style for optimal impact (Best et al., 2014). Ultimately, promoting positive digital engagement and emotional literacy is key to empowering Gen Z to value authenticity, cultivate resilience, and resist harmful comparison-driven pressures online.

REFERENCES

Abamara Nnaemeka, C., Solomon, A. A., Gangopadhyay, A., Sahni, M. Y., & Esther, B. (2014). Relationship between Body Image and Self-esteem among female Undergraduate students of behavioural Sciences. *IOSR Journal Of Humanities And Social Science (IOSR-JHSS), 19*(1), 1-5. DOI: 10.9790/0837-191120105

Adetayo, A. J. (2024). Distracted Minds: Unveiling Gender Disparities in Social Media Distractions Amidst Library Reading. *International Journal of Information Science and Management, 22*(2), 249–261. DOI: 10.22034/ijism.2024.2006251.1171

American Psychological Association. (2018). *Body image*. Retrieved from American Psychological Association: https://dictionary.apa.org/body-image

American Psychological Association. (2025). *self-awareness*. Retrieved from American Psychological Association: https://dictionary.apa.org/self-awareness

Andreassen, C. S., Pallesen, S., & Griffiths, M. D. (2016). The relationship between addictive use of social media, narcissism, and self-esteem: Findings from a large national survey. *Addictive Behaviors, 30*(2), 252–262. DOI: 10.1037/adb0000160 PMID: 27072491

Atanasova, A. (2016, November 6). *Gender-specific behaviors on social media and what they mean for online communications*. Retrieved from Social Media Today: https://www.socialmediatoday.com/social-networks/gender-specific-behaviors-social-media-and-what-they-mean-online-communications

Baumeister, R. F., Campbell, J. D., Krueger, J. I., & Vohs, K. D. (2003). Does High Self-Esteem Cause Better Performance, Interpersonal Success, Happiness, or Healthier Lifestyles? *Psychological Science in the Public Interest, 4*(1), 1–44. DOI: 10.1111/1529-1006.01431 PMID: 26151640

Bell, B. T., Taylor, C., Paddock, D., & Bates, A. (2021). Digital Bodies: A controlled evaluation of a brief classroom-based intervention for reducing negative body image among adolescents in the digital age. *The British Journal of Educational Psychology, 91*(1), 280–298. DOI: 10.1111/bjep.12449 PMID: 34350594

Best, P., Manktelow, R., & Taylor, B. (2014). Online communication, social media and adolescent wellbeing: A systematic narrative review. *Children and Youth Services Review, 41*, 27–36. DOI: 10.1016/j.childyouth.2014.03.001

Beyens, I., Pouwels, J., van Driel, I. I., Keijsers, L., & Valkenburg, P. M. (2021). Social Media Use and Adolescents' Well-Being: Developing a Typology of Person-Specific Effect Patterns. *Communication Research*, *51*(6), 691–716. DOI: 10.1177/00936502211038196

Bırni, G., & Eryılmaz, A. (2024). Conceptual and Theoretical Review of Self-Worth. *Psikiyatride Güncel Yaklasimlar*, *16*(2), 327–346. DOI: 10.18863/pgy.1336880

Brown, J., & Marshall, M. (2006). The Three Faces of Self-Esteem. In Kernis, M. (Ed.), *Self-esteem: Issues and answers* (pp. 4–9). Psychology Press.

Cash, T. F. (2005). The influence of sociocultural factors on body image: Searching for constructs. *Clinical Psychology : a Publication of the Division of Clinical Psychology of the American Psychological Association*, *12*(4), 438–442. DOI: 10.1093/clipsy.bpi055

Chan, K. T. (2022). Emergence of the 'Digitalized Self' in the Age of Digitalization. *Computers in Human Behavior Reports*, *6*(1), 100191. DOI: 10.1016/j.chbr.2022.100191

Charmaraman, L., Hojman, H., Auqui, J. Q., & Bilyalova, Z. (2025). Understanding Adolescent Self-esteem and Self-image Through Social Media Behaviors. *Pediatric Clinics of North America*, *72*(2), 189–201. DOI: 10.1016/j.pcl.2024.07.034 PMID: 40010860

Chen, Y. (2025). Navigating the digital mirror: The role of information-seeking orientation and uncertainty tolerance in social media-driven body image anxiety. *Computers in Human Behavior Reports*, *18*, 100665. Advance online publication. DOI: 10.1016/j.chbr.2025.100665

Choi, E., King, G. K., & Duerden, E. G. (2023). Screen time in children and youth during the pandemic: A systematic review and meta-analysis. *Global Pediatrics*, *6*, 100080. Advance online publication. DOI: 10.1016/j.gpeds.2023.100080

Choukas-Bradley, S., Maheux, A. J., Aubrey, J. S., Charmaraman, L., Maas, M. K., Nesi, J., & Yang, C.-c. (2025). Social Media Use, Body Image Concerns, and Disordered Eating Among Adolescents. In Christakis, D. A., & Hale, L. (Eds.), *Handbook of Children and Screens* (pp. 149–156). Springer Nature., DOI: 10.1007/978-3-031-69362-5_21

Chrisler, J. C., & Ghiz, L. (1993). Body image issues of older women. *Women & Therapy*, *14*(1-2), 67–75. DOI: 10.1300/J015v14n01_07

Crocker, J., & Wolfe, C. (2001). Contingencies of self-worth. *Psychological Review*, *108*(3), 593–623. DOI: 10.1037/0033-295X.108.3.593 PMID: 11488379

Cronbach, L. J. (1951). Coefficient Alpha and the Internal Structure of Tests. *Psychometrika, 16*(3), 297–334. DOI: 10.1007/BF02310555

Dann, C., & Capdevila, R. (2023). Social Media and Gendered Power: Young Women, Authenticity, and the Curation of Self. In Zurbriggen, E., & Capdevila, R. (Eds.), *The Palgrave Handbook of Power, Gender, and Psychology* (pp. 537–553). Palgrave Macmillan., DOI: 10.1007/978-3-031-41531-9_29

Department of Economic and Social Affairs. United Nations. (2015). *THE 17 GOALS*. Retrieved from United Nations: https://sdgs.un.org/goals

Dhir, A., Pallesen, S., Torsheim, T., & Andreassen, C. S. (2016). Do age and gender differences exist in selfie-related behaviours? *Computers in Human Behavior, 63*, 549–555. DOI: 10.1016/j.chb.2016.05.053

Dionne, M. M., & Davis, C. (2012). Body Image and Personality. In Cash, T. F. (Ed.), *Encyclopedia of Body Image and Human Appearance* (pp. 135–140). Academeic Press., DOI: 10.1016/B978-0-12-384925-0.00020-1

Dorčić, T. M., Smojver-Ažić, S., Božić, I., & Malkoč, I. (2023). Effects of Social Media Social Comparisons and Identity Processes on Body Image Satisfaction in Late Adolescence. *Europe's Journal of Psychology, 19*(2), 220–231. DOI: 10.5964/ejop.9885 PMID: 37731891

Döring, N., Reif, A., & Poeschl, S. (2016). How gender-stereotypical are selfies? A content analysis and comparison with magazine adverts. *Computers in Human Behavior, 55(Part B)*, 955-962. DOI: 10.1016/j.chb.2015.10.001

Elkind, D. (1967). Egocentrism in adolescence. *Child Development, 38*(4), 1025–1034. DOI: 10.2307/1127100 PMID: 5583052

Ellison, N. B., & Boyd, D. M. (2007). Social Network Sites: Definition, History, and Scholarship. *Journal of Computer-Mediated Communication, 13*(1), 210–230. DOI: 10.1111/j.1083-6101.2007.00393.x

Fabris, M. A., & Longobardi, C. (2024). Body image. In Troop-Gordon, W., & Neblett, E. W. (Eds.), *Encyclopedia of Adolescence* (2nd ed., pp. 32–42). Academic Press. DOI: 10.1016/B978-0-323-96023-6.00012-9

Fardouly, J., Diedrichs, P. C., Vartanian, L. R., & Halliwell, E. (2015). Social comparisons on social media: The impact of Facebook on young women's body image concerns and mood. *Body Image, 13*, 38–45. DOI: 10.1016/j.bodyim.2014.12.002 PMID: 25615425

Fardouly, J., & Vartanian, L. R. (2016). Social Media and Body Image Concerns: Current Research and Future Directions. *Current Opinion in Psychology*, *9*(9), 1–5. DOI: 10.1016/j.copsyc.2015.09.005

Feinstein, B. A., Hershenberg, R., Bhatia, V., Latack, J. A., Meuwly, N., & Davila, J. (2013). Negative social comparison on Facebook and depressive symptoms: Rumination as a mechanism. *Psychology of Popular Media Culture*, *2*(3), 161–170. DOI: 10.1037/a0033111

Festinger, L. (1954). A Theory of Social Comparison Processes. *Human Relations*, *7*(2), 117–140. DOI: 10.1177/001872675400700202

Firth, J., Firth, J. A., Stubbs, B., & Torous, J. (2019). The "online brain": How the Internet may be changing our cognition. *World Psychiatry; Official Journal of the World Psychiatric Association (WPA)*, *18*(2), 119–129. DOI: 10.1002/wps.20617 PMID: 31059635

Fox, J., & Vendemia, M. A. (2016). elective Self-Presentation and Social Comparison Through Photographs on Social Networking Sites. *Cyberpsychology, Behavior, and Social Networking*, *19*(10), 593–600. DOI: 10.1089/cyber.2016.0248 PMID: 27732079

Fox, J., & Vendemia, M. A. (2016). Selective self-presentation and social comparison through photographs on social networking sites. *Cyberpsychology, Behavior, and Social Networking*, *19*(10), 593–600. DOI: 10.1089/cyber.2016.0248 PMID: 27732079

Fredrickson, B. L., & Roberts, T.-A. (1997). Objectification Theory: Toward Understanding Women's Lived Experiences and Mental Health Risks. *Psychology of Women Quarterly*, *21*(2), 173–206. DOI: 10.1111/j.1471-6402.1997.tb00108.x

Frison, E., & Eggermont, S. (2016). Exploring the Relationships Between Different Types of Facebook Use, Perceived Online Social Support, and Adolescents' Depressed Mood. *Social Science Computer Review*, *34*(2), 153–171. DOI: 10.1177/0894439314567449

Gardner, R. M. (2012). Measurement of Perceptual Body Image. In *Encyclopedia of Body Image and Human Appearance* (pp. 526–532). Academic Press., DOI: 10.1016/B978-0-12-384925-0.00083-3

Gautham, M., Gururaj, G., Varghese, M., Benegal, V., Rao, G., Kokane, A., Chavan, B., Dalal, P. K., Ram, D., Pathak, K., Lenin Singh, R. K., Singh, L. K., Sharma, P., Saha, P. K., Ramasubramanian, C., Mehta, R. Y., Shibukumar, T. M., Deuri, S. P., Krishnatreya, M., & Majhi, G. (2020). The National Mental Health Survey of India (2016): Prevalence, socio-demographic correlates and treatment gap of mental morbidity. *The International Journal of Social Psychiatry*, *66*(4), 361–372. DOI: 10.1177/0020764020907941 PMID: 32126902

Gentry, J. H., & Campbell, M. (2002). *Developing Adolescents: A Reference for Professionals*. American Psychological Association.

Gibbons, F. X., & Buunk, B. P. (1999). Individual differences in social comparison: Development of a scale of social comparison orientation. *Journal of Personality and Social Psychology*, *76*(1), 129–142. DOI: 10.1037/0022-3514.76.1.129 PMID: 9972558

Girard, R. (1972). *La Violence et le sacre*. Bloomsbury Academic.

Girard, R. (1977). *Violence and the Sacred* (Gregory, P., Trans.). Johns Hopkins University Press. DOI: 10.56021/9780801819636

Goffman, E. (1959). *The Presentation of Self in Everyday Life*.

Haferkamp, N., & Krämer, N. C. (2011). Social comparison 2.0: Examining the effects of online profiles on social-networking sites. *Cyberpsychology, Behavior, and Social Networking*, *14*(5), 309–314. DOI: 10.1089/cyber.2010.0120 PMID: 21117976

Holland, G., & Tiggemann, M. (2016). A systematic review of the impact of the use of social networking sites on body image and disordered eating outcomes. *Body Image*, *17*, 100–110. DOI: 10.1016/j.bodyim.2016.02.008 PMID: 26995158

Houston, S., & Swords, C. (2021). Critical realism, mimetic theory and social work. *Journal of Social Work : JSW*, *22*(2), 345–363. DOI: 10.1177/14680173211008806

Jain, S. (2024, November 8). *Social Media's Impact on Indian Students Well-Being*. Retrieved from India Today: https://bestcolleges.indiatoday.in/news-detail/social-medias-impact-on-indian-students-well-being

James, W. (1890). *The principles of psychology* (Vol. 1). Henry Holt and Co., DOI: 10.1037/10538-000

Jia, Y., & Mvondo, G. (2025). Exploring The Adverse Effects Of The Metaverse On Users' Psychological Well-being and Self-esteem: A Mixed-methods Study. *Journal of Retailing and Consumer Services*, *86*(C), 104321. DOI: 10.1016/j.jretconser.2025.104321

Jiang, S., & Ngien, A. (2020). The Effects of Instagram Use, Social Comparison, and Self-Esteem on Social Anxiety: A Survey Study in Singapore. *Social Media + Society*, *6*(2), 2056305120912488. Advance online publication. DOI: 10.1177/2056305120912488

Jiotsa, B., Naccache, B., Duval, M., Rocher, B., & Grall-Bronnec, M. (2021). Social Media Use and Body Image Disorders: Association between Frequency of Comparing One's Own Physical Appearance to That of People Being Followed on Social Media and Body Dissatisfaction and Drive for Thinness. *International Journal of Environmental Research and Public Health*, *18*(6), 2880. DOI: 10.3390/ijerph18062880 PMID: 33799804

Jones, D. C. (2001). Social comparison and body image: Attractiveness comparisons to models and peers among adolescent girls and boys. *Sex Roles*, *45*(9), 645–664. DOI: 10.1023/A:1014815725852

Kappes, K. (2021). *#LimitingMyself: The Relationship Between Gender Norms, Self Presentation, and Selfies (Honors Thesis)*. Muhlenberg College.

Kearney-Cooke, A., & Tieger, D. (2015). Body Image Disturbance and the Development of Eating Disorders. In Smolak, L., & Levine, M. P. (Eds.), *The Wiley Handbook of Eating Disorders, Assessment, Prevention, Treatment, Policy, and Future Directions* (pp. 283–296). John Wiley & Sons, Ltd., DOI: 10.1002/9781118574089.ch22

Kelly, Y., Zilanawala, A., Booker, C., & Sacker, A. (2018). Social Media Use and Adolescent Mental Health: Findings From the UK Millennium Cohort Study. *EClinicalMedicine*, *6*, 59–68. DOI: 10.1016/j.eclinm.2018.12.005 PMID: 31193561

Kemp, S. (2025, February 25). *Digital 2025: India*. Retrieved from DataReportal: https://datareportal.com/reports/digital-2025-india

Khajuria, A., Gandotra, A., Khajuria, A., Arora, K., Gupta, R. K., Gupta, U., & Babber, S. (2025). Role of Social Media in the Rising Body Dissatisfaction and Dysmorphia Among Adolescents. *Cureus*, *17*(1), e78314. DOI: 10.7759/cureus.78314 PMID: 40034880

Kietzmann, J. H., Hermkens, K., McCarthy, I. P., & Silvestre, B. S. (2011). Social media? Get serious! Understanding the functional building blocks of social media. *Business Horizons*, *54*(3), 241–251. DOI: 10.1016/j.bushor.2011.01.005

Kim, D. H., Seely, N. K., & Jung, J.-H. (2017). Do You Prefer, Pinterest or Instagram? The Role of Image-Sharing SNSs and Self-Monitoring in Enhancing Ad Effectiveness. *Computers in Human Behavior*, *70*, 535–543. DOI: 10.1016/j.chb.2017.01.022

Kleiser, M., & Mayeux, L. (2021). Popularity and gender prototypicality: An experimental approach. *Journal of Youth and Adolescence*, *50*(1), 144–158. DOI: 10.1007/s10964-020-01344-5 PMID: 33156453

Langley, P., & Leyshon, A. (2017). Platform capitalism: The intermediation and capitalisation of digital economic circulation. *Finance and Stochastics*, *3*(1), 11–31. DOI: 10.2218/finsoc.v3i1.1936

Leary, M. R. (1996). *Self-presentation: Impression Management And Interpersonal Behavior*. Routledge., DOI: 10.4324/9780429497384

Leary, M. R., & Baumeister, R. F. (2000). In Zanna, M. (Ed.), *The nature and function of self-esteem: Sociometer theory* (Vol. 32, pp. 1–62). Advances in Experimental Social Psychology, DOI: 10.1016/S0065-2601(00)80003-9

Lee, Y., Jeon, Y., Kang, S., Shin, J. I., Jung, Y.-C., & Jung, S. (2022). Social media use and mental health during the COVID-19 pandemic in young adults: A meta-analysis of 14 cross-sectional studies. *BMC Public Health*, *22*(1), 995. Advance online publication. DOI: 10.1186/s12889-022-13409-0 PMID: 35581597

Linardon, J., McClure, Z., Tylka, L. T., & Tyszkiewicz, M. F. (2022). Body appreciation and its psychological correlates: A systematic review and meta-analysis. *Body Image*, *42*, 287–296. DOI: 10.1016/j.bodyim.2022.07.003 PMID: 35878528

Linardon, J., Messer, M., & Tylka, T. L. (2023). Functionality appreciation and its correlates: Systematic review and meta-analysis. *Body Image*, *45*, 65–72. DOI: 10.1016/j.bodyim.2023.02.002 PMID: 36796304

Magee, L. (2025). Computational scapegoats: From mimetic to alienated desire in the production of large language models. *Subjectivity*, *32*(2), 67–85. Advance online publication. DOI: 10.1057/s41286-025-00212-6

Marciano, L., Ostroumova, M., Schulz, P. J., & Camerini, A.-L. (2022). Digital Media Use and Adolescents' Mental Health During the Covid-19 Pandemic: A Systematic Review and Meta-Analysis. *Frontiers in Public Health*, *9*, 793868. DOI: 10.3389/fpubh.2021.793868 PMID: 35186872

McLean, S. A., Paxton, S. J., Wertheim, E. H., & Masters, J. (2015). Photoshopping the selfie: Self photo editing and photo investment are associated with body dissatisfaction in adolescent girls. *International Journal of Eating Disorders*, *48*(8), 1132–1140. DOI: 10.1002/eat.22449 PMID: 26311205

Mills, C. (2018). From 'Invisible Problem' to Global Priority: The Inclusion of Mental Health in the Sustainable Development Goals. *Development and Change*, *49*(3), 843–866. DOI: 10.1111/dech.12397

Mills, J. S., Musto, S., Williams, L., & Tiggemann, M. (2018). "Selfie" harm: Effects on mood and body image in young women. *Body Image*, *27*, 86–92. DOI: 10.1016/j.bodyim.2018.08.007 PMID: 30149282

Ministry of Health and Family Welfare, Government of India. (2014, October). *New Pathways New Hope: National Mental Health Policy of India*. Retrieved from National Health Mission: https://nhm.gov.in/images/pdf/National_Health_Mental_Policy.pdf

Mohanty, S., Kashyap, R. S., Katuri, B., Kalal, N., Kodicherla, M., & Choudary, D. (2024). Impact Of Social Media On Adolescents' Self-Esteem And Procrastination. *Educational Administration: Theory and Practice*, *30*(1), 5765–5773. DOI: 10.53555/kuey.v30i1.9244

Muñoz, P., Barton, M., Braun, S., Chowdhury, F., Jayne-Little, N., Rowland, J., Sykes, K., Smith, J., Talbot-Jones, C., Taggart, A., & Komes, J. (2023). The deterioration of self-worth in entrepreneurship. *Journal of Business Venturing Insights*, *20*, e00430. DOI: 10.1016/j.jbvi.2023.e00430

Neff, K. D., & Vonk, R. (2009). Self-compassion versus global self-esteem: Two different ways of relating to oneself. *Journal of Personality*, *77*(1), 23–50. DOI: 10.1111/j.1467-6494.2008.00537.x PMID: 19076996

Park, S. Y., & Baek, Y. M. (2018). Two faces of social comparison on Facebook: The interplay between social comparison orientation, emotions, and psychological well-being. *Computers in Human Behavior*, *79*, 83–93. DOI: 10.1016/j.chb.2017.10.028

Pelham, B. W., & Swann, W. B. (1989). From self-conceptions to self-worth: On the sources and structure of global self-esteem. *Journal of Personality and Social Psychology*, *57*(4), 672–680. DOI: 10.1037/0022-3514.57.4.672 PMID: 2795437

Perloff, R. (2023). *The Dynamics of Persuasion: Communication and Attitudes in the 21st Century*. Routledge., DOI: 10.4324/9781003290056

Perloff, R. M. (2014). Social Media Effects on Young Women's Body Image Concerns: Theoretical Perspectives and an Agenda for Research. *Sex Roles*, *71*(11-12), 363–377. DOI: 10.1007/s11199-014-0384-6

Pounders, K., Kowalczyk, C. M., & Stowers, K. (2016). Insight into the motivation of selfie postings: Impression management and self-esteem. *European Journal of Marketing*, *50*(9-10), 1879–1892. DOI: 10.1108/EJM-07-2015-0502

Pouwels, J. L., Valkenburg, P. M., Beyens, I., van Driel, I. I., & Keijsers, L. (2021). Social Media Use and Friendship Closeness in Adolescents' Daily Lives: An Experience Sampling Study. *Developmental Psychology*, *57*(2), 309–323. DOI: 10.1037/dev0001148 PMID: 33539132

Prince, M., Patel, V., Saxena, S., Maj, M., Maselko, J., Phillips, M. R., & Rahman, A. (2007). No Health Without Mental Health. *Lancet, 370*(9590), 859–877. DOI: 10.1016/S0140-6736(07)61238-0 PMID: 17804063

Pryde, S., & Prichard, I. (2022). TikTok on the clock but the #fitspo don't stop: The impact of TikTok fitspiration videos on women's body image concerns. *Body Image, 43*, 244–252. DOI: 10.1016/j.bodyim.2022.09.004 PMID: 36194987

Przybylski, A. K., & Weinstein, N. (2017). A large-scale test of the Goldilocks hypothesis: Quantifying the relations between digital-screen use and the mental well-being of adolescents. *Psychological Science, 28*(2), 204–215. DOI: 10.1177/0956797616678438 PMID: 28085574

Rajkumar, E., Julia, G. J., & Sri Lakshmi, K. (2022). Prevalence of mental health problems among rural adolescents in India: A systematic review and meta-analysis. *Scientific Reports, 12*(1), 16573. Advance online publication. DOI: 10.1038/s41598-022-19731-2 PMID: 36195719

Rhee, L., Bayer, J. B., Lee, D. S., & Kuru, O. (2021). Social by definition: How users define social platforms and why it matters. *Telematics and Informatics, 59*, 101538. DOI: 10.1016/j.tele.2020.101538

Rodgers, R. F., Slater, A., Gordon, C. S., McLean, S. A., Jarman, H. K., & Paxton, S. J. (2020). A Biopsychosocial Model of Social Media Use and Body Image Concerns, Disordered Eating, and Muscle-Building Behaviors among Adolescent Girls and Boys. *Journal of Youth and Adolescence, 49*(2), 399–409. DOI: 10.1007/s10964-019-01190-0 PMID: 31907699

Rosenberg, M. (1979). *Conceiving the self.* Basic Books.

Rosenberg, M., Schooler, C., Schoenbach, C., & Rosenberg, F. (1995). Global Self-Esteem and Specific Self-Esteem:Different Concepts, Different Outcomes. *American Sociological Review, 60*(1), 141–156. DOI: 10.2307/2096350

Rudman, L. A., & Fairchild, K. (2004). Reactions to Counterstereotypic Behavior: The Role of Backlash in Cultural Stereotype Maintenance. *Journal of Personality and Social Psychology, 87*(2), 157–176. DOI: 10.1037/0022-3514.87.2.157 PMID: 15301625

Salmerón-Ruiz, M. A., de Ribera, C. G., Barberán, V. S., Ives, L. E., & Álvarez-Pitti, J. (2025). Impact of digital media on development and physical health. *Anales de Pediatría (English Ed.), 102*(6), 503876. DOI: 10.1016/j.anpede.2025.503876 PMID: 40461313

Sawyer, S. M., Azzopardi, P. S., Wickremarathne, D., & Patton, G. C. (2018). The age of adolescence. *The Lancet. Child & Adolescent Health*, 2(3), 223–228. DOI: 10.1016/S2352-4642(18)30022-1 PMID: 30169257

Saxena, S., Funk, M., & Chisholm, D. (2014). WHO's Mental Health Action Plan 2013-2020: What can psychiatrists do to facilitate its implementation? *World Psychiatry; Official Journal of the World Psychiatric Association (WPA), 13*(2), 107–109. DOI: 10.1002/wps.20141 PMID: 24890053

Schachter, S. (1959). *The psychology of affiliation: Experimental studies of the sources of gregariousness*. Stanford University Press.

Schlenker, B. R., & Pontari, B. A. (2000). The strategic control of information: Impression management and self-presentation in daily life. In Tesser, A., Felson, R. B., & Suls, J. M. (Eds.), *Psychological Perspectives on Self and Identity* (pp. 199–232). American Psychological Association., DOI: 10.1037/10357-008

Schlosser, A. E. (2020). Self-disclosure versus self-presentation on social media. *Current Opinion in Psychology, 31*, 1–6. DOI: 10.1016/j.copsyc.2019.06.025 PMID: 31357096

Shah, S. R., Bhave, S. Y., Shringarpure, K., & Bhave, Y. (2023). Effect of COVID-19 Lockdown on Lifestyle, Internet Addiction and Media Usage among Adolescents and Young Adults in India - A Cross-sectional Survey. *Indian Journal of Youth and Adolescent Health, 10*(3), 4–12. DOI: 10.24321/2349.2880.202309

Sharma, V., & Tiwari, R. (2016). A Review on "IOT" & It's Smart Applications. *International Journal of Science* [IJSETR]. *Engineering and Technology Research, 5*(2), 472–476. DOI: 10.17762/ijritcc.v6i9.5295

Shi, Y., Kong, F., & Zhu, M. (2024). How Does Social Media Usage Intensity Influence Adolescents' Social Anxiety: The Chain Mediating Role of Imaginary Audience and Appearance Self-Esteem. *International Journal of Mental Health Promotion, 26*(12), 977–985. DOI: 10.32604/ijmhp.2024.057596

Silva, R. C., & Steins, G. (2023). Social media and body dissatisfaction in young adults: An experimental investigation of the effects of different image content and influencing constructs. *Frontiers in Psychology, 13*, 1037932. DOI: 10.3389/fpsyg.2023.1037932 PMID: 36968719

Small, G. W., Lee, J., Kaufman, A., Jalil, J., Siddarth, P., Gaddipati, H., Moody, T. D., & Bookheimer, Y. S. (2020). Brain health consequences of digital technology use. *Dialogues in Clinical Neuroscience, 22*(2), 179–187. DOI: 10.31887/DCNS.2020.22.2/gsmall PMID: 32699518

Somerville, L. H. (2013). The Teenage Brain: Sensitivity to Social Evaluation. *Current Directions in Psychological Science*, *22*(2), 121–127. DOI: 10.1177/0963721413476512 PMID: 24761055

Sorokowski, P., Sorokowska, A., Oleszkiewicz, A., Frackowiak, T., Huk, A., & Pisanski, K. (2015). Selfie posting behaviors are associated with narcissism among men. *Personality and Individual Differences*, *85*, 123–127. DOI: 10.1016/j.paid.2015.05.004

Stapleton, P., Luiz, G., & Chatwin, H. (2017). Generation Validation: The Role of Social Comparison in Use of Instagram Among Emerging Adults. *Cyberpsychology, Behavior, and Social Networking*, *20*(3), 142–149. DOI: 10.1089/cyber.2016.0444 PMID: 28263682

Streiner, D. L. (2003). Starting at the Beginning: An Introduction to Coefficient Alpha and Internal Consistency. *Journal of Personality Assessment*, *80*(1), 99–103. DOI: 10.1207/S15327752JPA8001_18 PMID: 12584072

Swann, W. B.Jr, Pelham, B. W., & Krull, D. S. (1989). Agreeable fancy or disagreeable truth? Reconciling self-enhancement and self-verification. *Journal of Personality and Social Psychology*, *57*(5), 782–791. DOI: 10.1037/0022-3514.57.5.782 PMID: 2810025

Taber, K. S. (2018). The use of Cronbach's alpha when developing and reporting research instruments in science education. *Research in Science Education*, *48*(6), 1273–1296. DOI: 10.1007/s11165-016-9602-2

Thompson, J. K., Heinberg, L. J., Altabe, M. N., & Tantleff-Dunn, S. (1999). *Exacting beauty: Theory, assessment, and treatment of body image disturbance*. American Psychological Association., DOI: 10.1037/10312-000

Thornton, D. A., & Arrowood, A. J. (1966). Self-evaluation, self-enhancement, and the locus of social comparison. *Journal of Experimental Social Psychology*, *1*(1), 40–48. DOI: 10.1016/0022-1031(66)90064-3

Tiggemann, M., & Slater, A. (2014). NetTweens: The Internet and Body Image Concerns in Preteenage Girls. *The Journal of Early Adolescence*, *34*(5), 606–620. Advance online publication. DOI: 10.1177/0272431613501083

Turk, Y. (2021). *Active and Passive Instagram Use: Female Undergraduate's Social Comparison Behaviors, Self-Esteem, and Contingent Self-Worth (Honors Thesis).* Muhlenberg College.

Tylka, T. L., & Wood-Barcalow, N. L. (2015). The Body Appreciation Scale-2: Item refinement and psychometric evaluation. *Body Image*, *12*, 53–67. DOI: 10.1016/j.bodyim.2014.09.006 PMID: 25462882

Uhlmann, L., Donovan, C., & Zimmer-Gembeck, M. (2020). Beyond the Thin Ideal: Development and Validation of the Fit Ideal Internalization Test (FIIT) for Women. *Psychological Assessment*, *32*(2), 140–153. DOI: 10.1037/pas0000773 PMID: 31535875

UNICEF. (1995). *Convention on the Rights of the Child.* United Nations. Retrieved from https://www.unicef.org/media/52626/file

United Nations. (n.d.). *Global issues- Children.* Retrieved from United Nations: https://www.un.org/en/global-issues/children

United Nations Children's Fund. (2021, October). *The State of the World's Children 2021: On My Mind – Promoting, protecting and caring for children's mental health.* Retrieved from UNICEF: https://www.unicef.org/reports/state-worlds-children-2021

Valkenburg, P. M. (2022). Theoretical Foundations of Social Media Uses and Effects. In Nesi, J., Telzer, E. H., & Prinstein, M. J. (Eds.), *Handbook of Adolescent Digital Media Use and Mental Health* (pp. 39–60). Cambridge University Press. DOI: 10.1017/9781108976237.004

Valkenburg, P. M., Meier, A., & Beyens, I. (2022). Social media use and its impact on adolescent mental health: An umbrella review of the evidence. *Current Opinion in Psychology*, *44*, 58–68. DOI: 10.1016/j.copsyc.2021.08.017 PMID: 34563980

Vandello, J. A., Bosson, J. K., Cohen, D., Burnaford, R. M., & Weaver, J. R. (2008). Precarious manhood. *Journal of Personality and Social Psychology*, *95*(6), 1325–1339. DOI: 10.1037/a0012453 PMID: 19025286

Verduyn, P., Gugushvili, N., Massar, K., Täht, K., & Kross, E. (2020). Social comparison on social networking sites. *Current Opinion in Psychology*, *36*, 32–37. DOI: 10.1016/j.copsyc.2020.04.002 PMID: 32387840

Vidal, C., Lhaksampa, T., Miller, L., & Platt, R. (2020). Social media use and depression in adolescents: A scoping review. *International Review of Psychiatry (Abingdon, England)*, *32*(3), 235–253. DOI: 10.1080/09540261.2020.1720623 PMID: 32065542

Vikram, A., & Sutar, D. (2024). Self-Esteem, Body Image and Social Media Usage Among the Adolescents. *International Journal of Indian Psychology*, *12*(2), 137–150. DOI: 10.25215/1202.015

Wang, W., Wang, M., Hu, Q., Wang, P., Lei, L., & Jiang, S. (2020). Upward social comparison on mobile social media and depression: The mediating role of envy and the moderating role of marital quality. *Journal of Affective Disorders, 270*, 143–149. DOI: 10.1016/j.jad.2020.03.173 PMID: 32339106

Webb, J. B., Wood-Barcalow, N. L., & Tylka, T. L. (2015). Assessing positive body image: Contemporary approaches and future directions. *Body Image, 14*, 130–145. DOI: 10.1016/j.bodyim.2015.03.010 PMID: 25910972

Wiekens, C. J. (2009). *Self awareness (Doctoral thesis).* Tilburg University.

Wiekens, C. J., & Stapel, D. A. (2008). The Mirror and I: When private opinions are in conflict with public norms. *Journal of Experimental Social Psychology, 44*(4), 1160–1166. DOI: 10.1016/j.jesp.2008.02.005

World Health Organization. (2013, January 6). *Mental health action plan 2013-2020.* Retrieved from World Health Organization: https://www.who.int/publications/i/item/9789241506021

World Health Organization. (n.d.). *Adolescent health.* Retrieved from World Health Organization: https://www.who.int/southeastasia/health-topics/adolescent-health

Yılmaz, H. A. (2022). Self-Awareness and Self-Consciousness: A Review from a Social Psychology Perspective. *Psikiyatride Güncel Yaklaşımlar -. Psikiyatride Güncel Yaklasimlar, 14*(4), 437–445. DOI: 10.18863/pgy.1029405

Young, S., Adamo, N., Ásgeirsdóttir, B. B., Branney, P., Beckett, M., Colley, W., Cubbin, S., Deeley, Q., Farrag, E., Gudjonsson, G., Hill, P., Hollingdale, J., Kilic, O., Lloyd, T., Mason, P., Paliokosta, E., Perecherla, S., Sedgwick, J., Skirrow, C., & Woodhouse, E. (2020). Females with ADHD: An expert consensus statement taking a lifespan approach providing guidance for the identification and treatment of attention-deficit/ hyperactivity disorder in girls and women. *BMC Psychiatry, 20*(1), 404. Advance online publication. DOI: 10.1186/s12888-020-02707-9 PMID: 32787804

Zhou, Z., & Dong, Y. (2024). The Mediating Roles of Beauty Ideals and Upward Comparison in Social Media's Influence on Body Image Anxiety Among Chinese High School Students. *Psychology and Behavioral Sciences (New York, N.Y.), 13*(4), 106–110. DOI: 10.11648/j.pbs.20241304.13

Zhuang, X. (2023). The Impact of Social Media on Self-Image Control in Adolescents and Relevant Factors. *Journal of Education. Humanities and Social Sciences, 22*, 41–46. DOI: 10.54097/ehss.v22i.12283

Zimmer-Gembeck, M., Hawes, T., & Pariz, J. (2021). A closer look at appearance and social media: Measuring activity, self-presentation, and social comparison and their associations with emotional adjustment. *Psychology of Popular Media*, *10*(1), 74–86. DOI: 10.1037/ppm0000277

Chapter 11
The Impact of Digital Identity and Online Validation on Gen Z's Mental Health

Shivansu Sachan
https://orcid.org/0000-0002-9893-8018
Chhatrapati Shahu Ji Maharaj University, India

ABSTRACT

The rapid proliferation of digital platforms has significantly shaped Gen Z's social and psychological landscape, with digital identity and online validation emerging as critical factors influencing mental health. This study explores how the construction and curation of digital identities on social media, coupled with the pursuit of online validation through likes, comments, and followers, impact the mental well-being of Gen Z individuals. Drawing on psychological and sociological frameworks, the research examines the pressures of performative self-presentation, the effects of social comparison, and the role of algorithmic reinforcement in shaping self-esteem, anxiety, and depressive symptoms. Findings suggest that while digital platforms offer opportunities for self-expression and community building, the relentless pursuit of validation and exposure to idealized online personas can exacerbate feelings of inadequacy, social isolation, and mental distress. The study highlights the need for targeted interventions, including digital literacy programs and platform design changes.

DOI: 10.4018/979-8-3373-4516-1.ch011

INTRODUCTION

Digital technologies have changed the way people talk to each other, express themselves, and shape their own identities. This is especially true for people born between 1997 and 2012, who are part of Generation Z. This generation has grown up with cell phones, social media, and other digital tools for communication that are now a big part of their lives. Instagram, TikTok, and X (previously Twitter) are the most popular places for people to create digital identities. These are deliberately made pictures of the self that mix real and idealized portrayals of the self. These digital identities aren't permanent; they change all the time depending on how individuals use them, how platform algorithms work, and what society expects. The urge for online approval, which is shown by likes, comments, shares, and follower counts, has a big effect on how people act in digital spaces. People can use these platforms to meet new people, be creative, and make communities. But they can also stress people out, which can be detrimental for their mental health because it makes them more likely to feel anxious, sad, and less sure of themselves. This introduction examines the intricate relationship among digital identity, online validation, and their impact on the mental health of Generation Z. It paves the way for a more thorough examination of the psychological, social, and cultural ramifications of these phenomena. People create their digital identity by building profiles, posting items, and talking to other people on different digital platforms. Generation Z doesn't just make these online identities; they are also a big part of who they are. They show what they believe in and what the culture they live in believes in. Users develop their digital identities based on platform features like filters, editing tools, and algorithmic curation that make them want to show off their best selves. On the other hand, online validation includes social feedback systems that are built into digital platforms. These systems use things like likes and follower numbers to illustrate how popular something is on social media. People who acquire this kind of validation may change the way they see themselves and the way they act. This can lead to a cycle where people seek more approval to prove their worth. The link between digital identity and online validation has a big impact on the mental health of Gen Z, who have used these sites as part of their social and developmental life since they were young. The effects of digital identity and online validation on mental health are intricate and varied. Studies show that spending too much time on social media, especially to get affirmation, might be bad for your mental health. For example, ? found that teens who spend a lot of time on social media are more likely to feel anxious, hopeless, and worried about their body image, especially when they compare themselves to idealized versions of themselves online. People may feel stressed out because they have to keep up a consistent and interesting online presence while also dealing with the pressure of wanting to be liked by others and being themselves. The phenomenon termed "fear of missing out" (FOMO) intensifies these apprehensions, as continual exposure to customized content can cultivate feelings of inadequacy and isolation. These dynamics are particularly prominent for Generation Z, since their critical years of identity development coincide with their absorption in digital settings, exacerbating the effects on their mental health. Various theoretical frameworks elucidate the interconnections among digital identity, online validation, and mental health. Social Comparison Theory asserts that individuals assess their self-worth by contrasting themselves with others, a phenomenon intensified in digital environments where curated identities are easily accessible for comparison. When people compare themselves to others who seem better than them, they can feel horrible about themselves and lose confidence. Generation Z (Gen Z) is made up of people who were born between 1997 and 2012. This group is different from previous generations since they grew up with digital technologies and social media. Gen Z has always had cell phones, fast internet, and apps like Instagram, Snapchat, and TikTok. This isn't like it was before. These sites are very important to their social lives because they let them be themselves, meet new people, and create their own identities. People also feel that they need to create a "digital identity," which is a well planned online presence, and get likes, comments, and shares to feel good about themselves. People are worried about how this need for online validation affects their mental health, especially their anxiety, depression, and self-esteem. Digital identity is how someone looks online, such their profiles, posts, and the way they connect with other people on digital networks. Gen Z's self-esteem and status in society are affected by online validation, which is the feedback they get from social media analytics. Studies show that using social media can have both good and bad effects on mental health. For example, social media can allow people who are already on the outside contact with one other and encourage each other. But if you use it too much, it can make people more worried and sad, which is detrimental for their mental health.

Travel has always been a big element of figuring out who you are. For Generation Z (born 1997–2012), the combination of travel, digital identification, and online validation creates new dynamics that change the way young people experience tourism. Gen Z sees travel as more than just a way to learn about other cultures. They also see it as a chance to show off who they are and what they do on social media.

Digital Identity Characteristics

Gen Z's digital identity is made up of a lot of various things, like personalized profiles, avatars, and online personas that they play. Gen Z's self-presentation is often planned and purposeful, which is different from how previous generations did it. They want to fit in with what their friends anticipate and what looks nice on the platform. For instance, Instagram's focus on pictures leads to highly curated photos, while TikTok's short films value new ideas and being real (Marwick, 2015). Gen Z can try out different identities on these sites, such public, private, or pseudonymous. They provide people both freedom and pressure to fit in with how they want to be seen. People born between 1997 and 2012 are usually part of Generation Z. American Psychological Association. (2023) This group grew up totally in the digital age. Digital technology, social media, and online communities have a huge effect on how individuals see themselves and how they engage with other people. Digital identity, or how people reveal who they are online through postings, profiles, and interactions, is becoming a big aspect of their lives. Digital identity and online validation are very similar. When people like, comment on, share, and give other sorts of digital feedback that show they enjoy something, it happens. These digital relationships offer opportunities for connection and self-expression; yet, they also raise concerns over their impact on mental health, particularly among teens. This chapter examines the interplay between digital identity, online validation, and mental health outcomes for Generation Z, employing psychological theories, empirical data, and societal trends to elucidate the associated risks and potential benefits.

Your Digital Identity and How You Show It

Digital identity is the picture that people meticulously create of themselves through their online activities, like posts, social media profiles, and interactions. Erving Goffman's (1959) theory of self-presentation provides a significant framework for understanding digital identity. Goffman posited that individuals manipulate others' perceptions of them by presenting idealized representations of themselves to attain social validation. In the digital era, social media sites make this process much stronger by helping individuals develop carefully curated personas through selective posting, filters, and strategic involvement. Generation Z has grown up with apps like Instagram, TikTok, and Snapchat, so their online identity is frequently an extension of who they are in real life. It's hard to tell the difference between who they are online and who they are in real life. Boyd, D. (2014).

Validation and Comparison on the Web

Likes, comments, and follower counts are forms of online validation that can be utilized to measure social acceptability. Leon Festinger's (1954) social comparison theory is relevant, suggesting that individuals evaluate their self-worth by comparing themselves to others. People can easily compare themselves to perfect pictures and lifestyles on social media platforms, which might make them feel like they don't measure up. Generation Z's desire for online validation can turn into a never-ending loop of looking for approval from others, which can hurt their self-esteem and make their mental health problems worse. Gen Z uses online validation, which is often assessed by likes, shares, or retweets, as a way to show off their social status. These metrics give quick feedback and push people to do things that gain attention. Neurological studies have demonstrated that dopamine-powered feedback loops explain why gaining likes or comments can feel wonderful, like a "high" in the brain. But depending on what other people think of you can undermine your self-esteem. When validation is inconsistent or absent, individuals may experience heightened anxiety or diminished self-esteem. Bucher, T. (2017).

The Lancet Child & Adolescent Health (2020) released a study that found that kids who used social media a lot were more likely to be worried and unhappy, especially if they put their self-worth on what other people said about them online. Gen Z feels a lot of pressure to keep earning approval, which might lead them do things like continuously checking alerts or modifying content to get more likes. This loop might make people think they need other people's approval to feel good about themselves instead of trusting their own self-esteem.

PSYCHOLOGICAL EFFECTS: ANXIETY AND SELF-WORTH

The constant negotiation of digital identity and the need for online validation can affect mental health outcomes. Self-esteem, defined as an individual's subjective evaluation of their worth, is particularly vulnerable inside the domain of social media. Studies show that relying too much on outside validation might lower self-esteem, especially when the feedback is mixed or negative (Vogel et al., 2014). People may also feel worried because they are afraid of being criticized or rejected when they try to keep their online image flawless. The Fear of Missing Out (FOMO), a phenomenon exacerbated by social media, intensifies feelings of anxiety and inadequacy among Generation Z (Przybylski et al., 2013).

Evidence from the Actual World

Social Comparison Theory (Festinger, 1954) is especially pertinent in travel scenarios. Gen Z travelers look at influencers' well planned luxury travels and compare them to their own budget-friendly trips. These upward comparisons make people feel even worse about themselves, which makes them anxious and unhappy with their own experiences. A young traveler looking at friends' European backpacking excursions while stranded on a staycation in the US is an example of how social comparison may hurt your health.

The Stimulus-Organism-Response (S-O-R) Framework (Mehrabian & Russell, 1974) is also directly relevant to tourism. The stimulus may be a tourist spot that looks good on Instagram and is pushed to the top of feeds by an algorithm. The organism shows how the person feels, such FOMO, envy, or anxiety. The response often leads to hasty booking behavior, where people choose trips mainly because they think they will get approval online instead of because they would enjoy them.

Identity Development Theory (Erikson, 1968) regards travel as a significant avenue for self-discovery. For Gen Z, identity work when traveling is influenced by ongoing digital curation. When they post about cultural immersion or adventure sports, it becomes part of their identity story. Chen, H. T., & Li, X. (2017).

Strength and Good Things

Digital identity and online validation can be useful, even though they can be demanding. Social media sites are great places for people to express themselves, build communities, and learn about themselves. This is especially true for LGBTQ+ kids and people from underrepresented cultural backgrounds in Generation Z. Craig et al. (2020) found that online communities were safe places for people to be themselves, which made them feel less alone and stronger. Positive feedback, like helpful comments or being involved in the community, can also help people feel better about themselves and like they belong.

Cultural and Gender Differences

The impacts of digital identification and online validation vary across demographic groups. Research indicates that young women are more susceptible to poor mental health due to cultural pressures about appearance and body image, exacerbated by social media (Fardouly et al., 2018). Conversely, young males may experience pressure to conform to societal notions of success or masculinity, although this area has not been extensively studied. It's also necessary to think about the culture. In collectivist cultures, for instance, communal acceptance may be more essential, which can impact how interactions on the internet affect mental health.

Societal and Technological Influences

The way social media sites are put up has a huge impact on how they affect mental health. Algorithmic feeds, which show you things that are intriguing or perfect, make social comparison and the need to do well even stronger. Using likes, streaks, or following figures to prove something makes people feel like they are in a competition, which could make them more worried. Also, Generation Z is always under this kind of stress because social media is always there, and they don't have many chances to get away from it all. Societal standards also determine how digital identity affects mental health. Common Sense Media. (2022). Being online all the time and feeling like you have to preserve a consistent personal brand can lead to identity fragmentation, which is when people have problems reconciling their online and offline selves. This is especially true for Generation Z, who live in a world where digital connections are often equally as crucial as in-person ones. The connection between digital identity and online validation can have both positive and negative consequences on mental health. Digital platforms provide spaces for self-expression and community growth, particularly for underrepresented groups. For example, LGBTQ+ Gen Zers or persons from a minority group often find supportive groups online that can make them feel less alone and stronger. These online groups can be safe places where people can seek aid and support that is beneficial. But the adverse impacts are also very substantial. People often term this "social comparison theory," which is when people compare themselves to others on social media. This can make people feel bad about themselves when they see influencers or peers who seem to have excellent lives. This is especially true for Gen Z, who have been shown carefully chosen content since they were very young. A 2022 meta-analysis in Computers in Human Behavior found a moderate link between teens' use of social media and their dissatisfaction with their body image. This was especially true for girls because of society's norms of beauty.

Also, the fact that digital identity is performative could cause "imposter syndrome," which is when people feel that they aren't as accomplished or real as their online personalities make them seem. Gen Z folks try to keep up an image that seems difficult to reach, which can lead to chronic stress and burnout. Cyberbullying, which is another thing that happens when people engage online, makes mental health problems worse. Negative comments or trolling can make people feel even more rejected, especially when they are about their online life.

For Individuals

Generation Z might be able to decrease the adverse effects of digital identity and online validation by limiting how much time they spend on social media, taking breaks from technology, and putting more value on real-life contacts. Mindfulness practices, such as focusing on your own values rather than other opinions, might enhance your resilience to the pressures of online validation.

For Parents and Teachers

Generation Z's mental health depends a lot on their teachers and parents. Media literacy programs can help youngsters learn how to think critically about what they see online and understand that their digital identities are made up of many different pieces. Being honest about how social media might stress individuals out can also help them feel more normal about their concerns and find healthy strategies to deal with them.

For Tech Companies and People Who Make Rules

Policymakers and tech companies need to look into the big challenges that are making mental health problems worse. Rules that make it easier to create algorithms and limit addictive features could help make social media less harmful. Additionally, platforms can incorporate features that promote positive interactions, such as suggestions for helpful comments or tools that keep people from seeing harmful information (Craig et al., 2020)

The "quantified self" is a highly essential idea for creating a digital identity. Generation Z uses things like followers, likes, and engagement rates to keep track of and quantify how much time they spend online. These numbers are a way to show social standing and self-worth (Lupton, 2016). This kind of measurement might help people feel like they have some influence over their identity, but it might also make them feel that they have to keep their online persona consistent and interesting. For example, a teenager can feel like they have to share things that are trendy at the time to earn likes, even if such items don't portray who they truly are. This chapter analyzes the impact of digital identity and online validation on the mental health of Generation Z within the tourist setting, employing two primary theoretical frameworks: Identity Development Theory and the Stimulus-Organism-Response (S-O-R) Framework.

Theory of Identity Development

Identity building is a crucial developmental task for adolescents and young adults, particularly for Generation Z, who navigate this process within a digital context. Erikson's psychosocial theory asserts that identity formation involves the amalgamation of several self-aspects into a unified whole, often enhanced by social interactions and external influences (Erikson, 1968). In the digital era, social media platforms provide spaces for Gen Z individuals to collectively shape and negotiate their identities through curated posts and narratives (Granic et al., 2020). In the tourism industry, these platforms help people express their identities by sharing their experiences to show their social status, cultural awareness, or personal growth. The pressure to make a perfect digital identity can lead to stress, anxiety, and identity conflicts, especially when online validation (such as likes or comments) doesn't meet expectations (Vannucci & McCauley Ohannessian, 2019).

The framework for Stimulus-Organism-Response (S-O-R)

The S-O-R framework, derived from environmental psychology, posits that external stimuli (S) influence an individual's internal state (O), subsequently affecting their behavior (R) (Mehrabian & Russell, 1974). In this chapter, social media platforms and online validation serve as stimuli that affect the emotional and cognitive states of Generation Z (e.g., self-esteem, anxiety), leading to responses such as increased travel motivation, social comparison, or mental health challenges. For example, seeing too many gorgeous travel photographs on social media can make people feel like they are missing out (FOMO) or not good enough, which can be bad for their mental health. The S-O-R framework helps us understand how Gen Z's digital interactions effect their travel patterns and mental health in the tourism business. Erikson, E. H. (1968). We need to use a lot of different ways to cope with the mental health difficulties that come with having a digital identity and gaining validation online. First, it's really vital to show people how to use technology. Schools and caregivers should teach Gen Z how to think critically about what they see online, how to recognize algorithmic biases, and how social media might affect their mental health. People who learn how to use digital environments in a smart way are less anxious, which is what media literacy programs do. Second, establishing friends in real life can help you feel better about yourself online. Encouraging hobbies, face-to-face interactions, and community involvement can boost intrinsic self-worth, which can reduce the need for digital validation. Mental health professionals frequently advocate for "digital detoxes," periods during which individuals abstain from social media to reconnect with their authentic selves (Statista, 2023).

A LOOK AT THE LITERATURE

Digital Identity and Social Media Usage

Digital identity is a dynamic construct shaped by individuals' online self-representation and the perceptions of others. For Generation Z, social media platforms function as primary arenas for identity building, a crucial developmental goal during adolescence and early adulthood. Erikson's theory of psychosocial development posits that adolescence is a period during which individuals establish their identities through exploration and the reinforcement of their self-concept. People can share their thoughts and feelings on social media, including posting photos or telling personal stories. This makes the process more stronger. But it also makes people feel like they have to fit in with what they think is normal (Przybylski et al., 2013).

Studies show that Generation Z is quite active on social media, with many people saying they are virtually always online. People are so engaged in social media because of how they are designed. They employ algorithms to display individuals stuff that will grab their attention, which usually implies showing perfect pictures and lives. People may compare their life to carefully selected online personas after seeing this kind of stuff, which could make them feel bad about themselves.

Current Research Gaps

Quantitative study underscores the correlations between social media consumption and mental health; nevertheless, qualitative insights into Gen Z's perspectives are still insufficiently examined. Wall Street Journal. (2021). Furthermore, most studies focus on negative outcomes, and there are few studies that look into the positive effects of digital identity on mental health. The impact of cultural and socioeconomic factors remains insufficiently explored, particularly in non-Western contexts. This research addresses these deficiencies by employing case studies to illustrate how Generation Z use digital identification and online validation in their daily lives (Seabrook et al., 2016).

DIGITAL IDENTITY AND MENTAL HEALTH IN THE TRAVEL SECTOR

Why Digital Identity Is Important When Traveling

Gen Z's digital identity is always shifting according on how they interact with each other on sites like Instagram, TikTok, and X, where travel-related content is widespread. Tourism offers a unique context for identity expression, as travel experiences are often associated with self-discovery, cultural exploration, and social status (Statista, 2022). Gen Z travelers use social media to keep track of their trips and post content that fits with the identities they want to have, like "adventurous traveler" or "cultural explorer." But this curation might make it hard for them to connect with their real selves and their online selves, which can be stressful. For instance, the desire to share stunning travel photos may exacerbate feelings of inadequacy when the actual experience of travel (such as logistical challenges or financial constraints) fails to align with the idealized portrayal (Ozdemir-Guzel & Bas, 2021).

Also, digital identity in tourism is often connected to how people compare themselves to others. Generation Z compares their travel experiences to those of friends or influencers, whose posts often represent lives that are hard to reach. This kind of comparison can make people feel FOMO, which is a feeling that makes people more anxious and less happy in life. This is especially true for young people who use social media. In the realm of travel, FOMO may drive Gen Z to pursue trips or experiences solely for social validation, rather than personal fulfillment, so negatively impacting their mental health (Fardouly et al., 2018).

Gen Z's Digital Travel Experiences

Tourism gives Gen Z a chance to show off their adventurousness, cosmopolitanism, or authenticity. But these chances are typically limited by platform rules that favor information that is visually appealing and easy to share. The idea of the "quantified traveler" comes around, where the worth of a trip is based on how many likes, shares, or followers it gets. This change leads to:

- Traveling because of FOMO: going to places because of what is popular on social media instead of what you want to do.
- Performative authenticity: putting together experiences like "voluntourism" or staying with a family in a rural area mostly to show that you care about social issues online.
- Economic pressures: seeing digital travel content as a way to build a career in an industry where getting people to pay attention to your travel brand might help you get a job or make professional connections.

The Mental Effects of Getting Approval Online

Gen Z can get feedback that makes or breaks their digital identities by getting likes, comments, or shares online. In tourism, validation often comes from peers or followers who respond to content about travel. Positive feedback can improve self-esteem and social ties, both of which are good for mental health (Seabrook et al., 2016). For example, a well-known story on a unique trip experience could help people feel like they belong and have done something good. People can feel rejected, frightened, or unsure of themselves when they don't obtain affirmation or get unfavorable comments. Festinger, L. (1954).

The pursuit of online validation may lead to compulsive social media engagement, associated with detrimental mental health outcomes. Studies show that spending too much time on social media, especially passively consuming (such skimming through other people's travel posts), is linked to worse mental health (Twenge et al., 2018). This inclination may manifest in travel as an obsession with capturing "Instagrammable" experiences, prioritizing external validation over genuine enjoyment. For instance, Gen Z visitors may feel that they have to go to famous destinations or do what influencers do, even if it goes against what they want or what they can afford. This can make them unhappy and stressed.

METHODOLOGY

This research employs a qualitative methodology, utilizing case studies to investigate the diverse impacts of digital identity and online validation on the mental health of Generation Z. Three fictional yet believable case studies were developed using synthesized data from existing research and popular themes in Gen Z's social media interactions. Each case study exemplifies a specific aspect of digital identity formation and validation-seeking behavior, highlighting diverse demographics to reflect the distinctiveness of Gen Z. The case examples are analyzed thematically to identify trends and implications for mental health, supported by citations from peer-reviewed research.

The Role of Platforms and Algorithms

Social media platforms aren't neutral; their algorithms change how people create their online identities. Algorithms rank content based on how much people interact with it. This makes feedback loops that encourage specific styles and behaviors. For example, TikTok's "For You" page uses machine learning to find content that each user will like. This softly pushes Gen Z to choose identities that fit in with what's fashionable (Bucher, 2017). X's algorithmic timeline also prioritizes posts that get a lot of engagement, which makes people want to make personalities that attract people's attention. These algorithms can create echo chambers, where Gen Z people only see things that back up what they already think and like. This can help people feel like they are part of a group, but it can also stop them from seeing other people's points of view, which could make it harder for them to find their own identity. A case study of a 16-year-old TikTok user named "Alex" (a pseudonym) illustrates this: Alex expressed feeling compelled to replicate popular dance trends to increase their follower count, which conflicted with their desire to promote their original poetry. This tension demonstrates how platform design might inhibit genuine self-expression, perhaps adversely impacting mental health (Ozdemir-Guzel & Bas, 2021).

Theories of Social Identity and Online Personas

Social Identity Theory (Tajfel & Turner, 1979) provides a theoretical framework for understanding the development of digital identities through group affiliation and social comparison. People of Gen Z find out who they are through online communities like fandoms, political groups, or aesthetic subcultures (like "e-girl" or "cottagecore"). These groups help people feel like they belong, but they also impose rules that change who they are. For example, joining a mental health advocacy group on X can help someone feel better about themselves by giving them the courage to talk about their concerns in public. But following group norms can also lead to identity fragmentation, which is when people feel like they are torn between who they are in real life and who they are online. Fox, J., & Vendemia, M. A. (2016).

Social comparison, a fundamental component of Social Identity Theory, is exacerbated in online contexts. Comparing oneself to influencers with ideal lives (upward comparisons) may induce feelings of inadequacy, whereas comparing oneself to those in worse circumstances (downward comparisons) can temporarily enhance self-esteem while simultaneously reinforcing negative stereotypes (Festinger, 1954). A study by Vogel et al. (2014) found that teens who used social media often were more likely to compare themselves to others, which hurt their body image and self-esteem. The pressure to mimic the meticulously created identities of influencers can make Gen Z's anxiety and despair worse, especially when validation is related to standards that can't be met. Marwick, A. E. (2015).

Drivers of Systems and Technology

The challenges confronting Gen Z in tourism cannot be only attributed to individual psychology; they are integrated within platform architectures and overarching economic structures.

Design of Algorithms and Platform Architecture

Algorithms for social media favor involvement, not honesty. Dopamine-driven feedback loops and rewards that come and go, like likes, comments, and shares, make people want to post all the time. This suggests that for tourism, attractions that are photogenic but too crowded are more popular than experiences that are more meaningful but less visually interesting. Algorithms also create echo chambers that make high-consumption, luxury-centered trips seem normal, which pushes Gen Z toward goals that are often out of reach. Goffman, E. (1959).

The Economy of Attention

In the digital era, attention is worth a lot. Travel writing may be both a way to express yourself and a useful skill for your job. Gen Z can create cultural capital, get more partnerships, or make themselves more employable with a well-curated Instagram page. This puts pressure on the system to turn personal trips into branded material, which makes it hard to tell the difference between work and play.

DIGITAL TOURISM CASE STUDIES

Case Study 1: Emma's Anxiety and Comparing Vacations

Emma, a 17-year-old student, made plans for a simple beach vacation with her family. When she got back, she posted pictures on Instagram but quickly saw that her postings had fewer likes than her friends' pictures of their fancy vacations. She felt inferior after comparing herself to someone else, which made her worry more about her social status. Her experience shows how internet comparison pressures may even ruin relaxing travel.

Case Study 2: Jay's Search for a Place to Belong Online

Jay, a 19-year-old college student, posted funny trip videos from cultural festivities in his area on TikTok. He felt better about himself when people said kind things about him, but he often felt FoMO when he saw influencers' posts about traveling across the world. His real love of local tourism and the appeal of globalized, aspirational content are at odds with each other. This shows how validation-seeking in tourism can be both good and bad.

Case Study 3: Aisha's Professional Branding via Study Abroad

Aisha, who is 22, put together her study abroad experiences on LinkedIn and Instagram. She wanted to make herself more employable by strategically emphasizing cultural immersion and overseas internships. This made her feel more confident in her work, but it also stressed her out and made her feel like an imposter because she was always comparing her story to those of her friends who had better prospects. Her story shows how important digital identity is for the economy in the tourism industry.

Case Studies with Similar Themes

The case studies demonstrate three fundamental concepts:

1. Social Comparison and Self-Esteem: Emma and Aisha's experiences highlight how looking at other people's lives on social media may make you feel bad about yourself. This is in accordance with research that shows that passively utilizing social media, such skimming through glorified information, is linked to worse mental health (Granic et al., 2020).
2. affirmation-Seeking Behaviors: Emma wants likes, Jay wants comments, and Aisha wants professional recommendations. All three persons are looking for affirmation in some form. These behaviors can boost self-esteem for a short time, but they can also make people reliant on what others say, which can lead to mental health issues.
3. The case studies demonstrate that social media can provide both positive and negative outcomes. Jay's sense of community shows how social media may bring people together, but Emma and Aisha's concerns with worry and stress indicate how it can be harmful.

Effects on People Who Work in Tourism

For tourism experts who wish to attract Gen Z travelers, the link between digital identity, online validation, and mental wellness is highly crucial. The following tips will help you deal with these changes:

1. Tour operators should make sure that their experiences are more about being real and gratifying than about getting a lot of likes on social media. For example, offering one-of-a-kind vacation spots or cultural activities that help people really get to know a location can make Gen Z want to travel for its own sake. This removes some of the pressure off of them to make ideal digital profiles.
2. Mental Health Support in Tourism: Tour operators might offer mental health resources like mindfulness activities or programs that help people unplug from technology. These tools can help people feel better when they travel by reducing the negative effects of too much social media and fear of missing out (FOMO).
3. Culturally Sensitive Marketing: Instead of pushing the same vacation ideas for everyone, marketing campaigns should demonstrate how various Gen Z's identities are and promote cultural distinctions. This strategy can help people figure out who they are in a good way and make them less likely to follow the crowd.

4. How to Teach Gen Z Travelers to Use Social Media Responsibly: Tourism companies can teach Gen Z travelers to use social media responsibly by stressing the importance of true involvement over conduct that seeks notoriety. If you work with influencers who promote real travel experiences, you may transform the message from "impossible goals" to "more realistic ones."
5. Data Privacy and Ethical Digital Practices: Gen Z is anxious about data privacy and identity theft, therefore tourist websites should make sure their data practices are explicit and their online environments are safe. When people connect with others online, this might help them feel more at ease and build trust.

Effects on Mental Health

The pursuit of digital identity and online validation may exacerbate mental health challenges for Generation Z. Social comparison and the Fear of Missing Out (FoMO) exacerbate anxiety and depression, particularly among persons with pre-existing vulnerabilities. The WHO study found that females, like Emma, are more likely to use social media in ways that are bad for them. But Jay's tale demonstrates that internet platforms may also be useful, so the effect depends on how people utilize them and other personal factors. Harter, S. (2012).

Limitations

The case studies are not actual, but they are based on research, which means they are not very useful for making generalizations. The article also concentrates on Western contexts, perhaps overlooking cultural variations in the formation of digital identities. Future research should include non-Western perspectives and longitudinal effects to deepen understanding of lasting ramifications.

Ideas

1. Digital Literacy Education: Schools and communities should teach Gen Z how to use social media wisely. They should focus on how to deal with behaviors that seek approval and how to recognize biases in algorithms.
2. Mental Health Interventions: Giving Gen Z free or cheap digital mental health apps, like the ones Aisha uses, will help people get better. This is especially true for folks who don't make a lot of money.
3. Parental and Community Support: Emma's situation shows that getting people to meet in person and love themselves can help decrease the adverse effects of social media.

4. Responsibility of the Platform: Social media companies need to be more open and make algorithms that put mental health care first, including linking users to crisis resources.

1. 1. How to Use Social Media Smartly in Digital Literacy Education

Gen Z needs good digital literacy training to understand how to use social media sites in a responsible way because they are so important to them. Digital literacy encompasses not only technical abilities but also the ability to evaluate content, recognize algorithmic biases, and manage validation-seeking behaviors. Social networking sites use algorithms that encourage interaction to present more of the things that make people feel things, including comparison and feeling inadequate. According to Statista (2023), Gen Z spends an average of 7.3 hours a day on screens, most of which is on Instagram, TikTok, and Snapchat. Seeing perfect images of friends or influencers or getting less likes on their posts can make them feel even worse about themselves. Huang, C. (2017).

Schools and communities should teach Gen Z how algorithms influence their feeds and how they make them feel. For example, algorithms usually present content based on how users engage with it. This might make echo chambers or show standards of beauty, wealth, or lifestyle that are impossible to reach. A Pew Research Center study (2021) indicated that 59% of kids felt pressure to seem perfect online, which was connected to more anxiety and sorrow. Lupton, D. (2016).Teachers can help students question how authentic online personas are and avoid them from feeling like they need likes or followers to feel good about themselves by making them aware of these dynamics.

Additionally, the digital literacy program must explicitly address validation-seeking habits. These habits stem from the dopamine-driven feedback loops intrinsic to social media, where likes and comments trigger reward responses in the brain (Sherman et al., 2018). Part of the program might include workshops on how to detect when social media use is becoming compulsive, how to set boundaries on screen time, and how to build self-worth without relying on online measurements. For instance, a pilot program in California high schools used a "Digital Wellness Curriculum" to show students how to think about how social media affects their mental health. This caused a 25% decline in reported anxiety about gaining validation online over the course of six months (Harter, 2012.

2. 2. Interventions for mental health: making digital tools easier to get to

Digital identity and online validation can be detrimental for mental health. Because of this, we need therapies that are easy to get to and can be used by a lot of people, especially those with low incomes who may not be able to pay traditional therapy. Some digital mental health apps that can help Gen Z stay healthy for little or no cost are Headspace, Calm, and Woebot. These apps can help people deal with stress, anxiety, and depression that occur from using social media. They contain features like guided meditation, cognitive behavioral therapy (CBT) activities, and mood tracking. Aisha, a 19-year-old college student, reported that using free CBT-based software helped her deal with the anxiety that comes from comparing her grades to those of her LinkedIn friends (case study, 2024).

41% of Gen Z says they have mental health issues but can't receive assistance because of things like cost, stigma, or a lack of local providers (American Psychological Association, 2023). This means that digital mental health resources need to be easy to find. This gap can be closed with free or subsidized apps, which is especially helpful for persons with low incomes who may use their phones as their main way to get online. For instance, the app Youper offers free AI-driven therapy sessions that have been found to help 67% of users feel less melancholy after two weeks (Journal of Medical Internet Research, 2024). Governments and nonprofits should engage with app makers to make access cheaper so that money isn't a problem.

3. Support from parents and the community:

Getting kids to make friends outside of the internet

Digital remedies are useful, but it's just as vital to assist Gen Z develop real-life connections and accept themselves to decrease the effect of their digital identity on their mental health. Parents and the community can assist young people deal with the stress of social media by giving them somewhere to go where they are valued for who they really are, not simply who they are online. Emma, a 16-year-old girl who joined a neighborhood theater group and stopped using social media as much, is an example of how doing things outside of the internet can help people feel better about themselves and not depend on digital validation as much (case study, 2024).

When it comes to utilizing digital gadgets and talking about how social media affects them, parents are highly essential role models for their kids. Research reveals that parental involvement, such as discussing online experiences or setting screen-time limitations, correlates with a 30% decrease in adolescent anxiety due to social media (Child Development, 2023). Parents should understand about how having a digital identity might affect their mental health, such as how comparing themselves to others and looking for acceptance can make them feel bad about themselves. Parents can learn how to help their kids by going to workshops or using online tools like the ones that Common Sense Media offers. They can also watch social media together and speak about how real it is, or they can do things that boost their own confidence.

Communities can aid Gen Z even more by offering them opportunity to meet new people in person. Young people can develop real friends through sports, volunteering, extracurricular activities, or mentoring programs without having to impress others online. A 2022 study found that teens who completed community service had a 20% increase in their self-esteem and a 15% decrease in stress caused by social media (Journal of Youth and Adolescence, 2022). Gen Z feels like they belong and have a purpose when they do these things. This is the antithesis of what social media does, which makes people feel alone and compares them to others.

Parents and community people need to work together to make sure that these opportunities are available to teens who are poor or don't have a lot of power. There are programs like Big Brothers Big Sisters or local recreation centers that could have free or cheap activities that are fair for everyone. Parents and communities can help Gen Z deal with the mental health challenges that come with having a digital identity by putting more weight on face-to-face interactions and accepting themselves (Harter, 2012).

4. Putting Mental Health First: Platform Responsibility

The mental health consequences of digital identity and online validation are mostly due to social networking sites, which directly affect how users respond through their algorithms and design decisions. Meta, TikTok, and X, among others, need to be more clear about how their algorithms chose material. They also need to put mental health first by taking actions like linking users to crisis resources. Right present, a lot of sites make money by adopting models that push controversial or provocative content. This can make Gen Z users feel worse about themselves or more nervous. A study from a whistleblower at Meta in 2021 indicated that Instagram's algorithm intentionally promoted content that made body image issues worse for 32% of teen girls (Wall Street Journal, 2021).

What this means for people who work in tourism

People who work in tourism need to understand the psychological and institutional pressures that affect how Gen Z travels digitally. Important suggestions are:

1. Promote Authenticity Over Aesthetics: Make marketing efforts that focus on real experiences instead of "Instagram spots" that don't mean anything.
2. Mental Health Integration: Add mindfulness and digital detox programs to your travel packages.
3. Partner with influencers who show authentic pictures of travel instead than manicured perfection.
4. Inclusive Narratives: To lessen the need to compare socio-economic status, celebrate other travel identities, such as budget, cultural, and sustainable.
5. Be open and honest about how you use user data in tourism marketing to ease Gen Z's worries about digital safety and platform accountability.

Effects on Mental Health

The process of creating a digital identity has a huge effect on the mental health of Gen Z. Some beneficial things that come from it are improved self-expression and community building, especially for marginalized groups that find safe spaces online (like LGBTQ+ teens on X). But the pressure to preserve a controlled identity can make people feel like they aren't being true to themselves, which is called identity dissonance. This can make individuals feel bad about themselves and nervous (Harter, 2012). Also, algorithm-driven information can make body dysmorphia and perfectionism worse among Gen Z people who compare themselves to photographs that have been filtered and made to look flawless.

Gen Z has a special problem: they have to always find a balance between being honest and putting on a show. People can learn more about themselves on digital platforms, but they can also place pressure on people that might affect their mental health. You need to know a lot about how platform design, social norms, and human agency all work together to solve these difficulties. Lancet Child & Adolescent Health. (2020).

CONCLUSION

Building a digital identity is a big part of Generation Z's daily life, and social networking sites have both helped and hurt that process. These platforms allow people more options to connect with others and share their thoughts and feelings than ever before. However, they can also place a lot of stress on people, which can be bad for their mental health. This part uses Social Identity Theory and real-world examples to explain how digital identities, algorithmic effects, and psychological results all function together in a sophisticated way. The next parts will look at how online validation techniques make these impacts worse and offer ways to lessen the bad effects. The link between digital identity and online validation has a huge impact on the mental health of Gen Z. People can use social media to express themselves and interact with others, but it can also be problematic due of things like comparing themselves to others, FoMO, and looking for approval. The case studies of Emma, Jay, and Aisha illustrate these relationships, emphasizing the importance of a balanced engagement with digital media. By promoting digital literacy, facilitating access to mental health treatments, and establishing supportive offline environments, stakeholders may aid Generation Z in navigating the digital landscape while safeguarding their mental well-being. Future research should focus on longitudinal studies and diverse cultural contexts to deepen the comprehension of these effects. The impact of digital identity and online validation on Gen Z's mental health is a complex issue that requires multiple solutions. Teaching kids how to utilize technology can help them think critically about social media. This can make them less likely to need likes or followers to feel good about themselves. Digital mental health tools that are easy to use, like the ones Aisha uses, can help a lot of individuals, especially those with modest means. Parents and the community can help kids develop friends and accept themselves, which can help them connect with other people in real life. This is the reverse of what social media accomplishes. Finally, it's vitally crucial for platforms to be responsible. Companies need to be more honest about their algorithms and designs and put mental health first. The connection between digital identity and online validation has a big impact on the mental health of Generation Z. Social media can help people connect and express themselves, but it can also make them anxious, depressed, and lower their self-esteem because they want to have curated identities and get approval from others. By understanding these processes through psychological theories and empirical evidence, stakeholders can develop focused programs to improve the well-being of Generation Z. We will need to keep undertaking research and taking efforts to make the digital environment safer for future generations as digital technologies keep developing. The impact of digital identity and online validation on the mental health of Generation Z in the tourism business is a multifaceted and intricate matter. People might use social media to express themselves and make connections, but it can also put a lot of stress on them, which can be bad for their mental health. The need for personalized digital identities and external validation can lead to social comparison, FOMO, and anxiety, particularly when travel experiences are shaped by the need to impress online audiences. For Generation Z, travel is no longer only a personal or cultural experience; it is now a digital experience where identification and validation are linked. Social comparison, FoMO, and computational pressures make the good and bad parts of travel even more intense. This chapter emphasizes the significance of systemic and technological analysis in conjunction with psychological theories by placing tourism at the forefront of the discourse. Case studies of Emma, Jay, and Aisha illustrate the authentic experiences of Gen Z travelers managing crafted digital personas. For people who work in tourism, the task is to create experiences and stories that are authentic, welcoming, and good for people's health. The tourism sector can only promote healthy digital travel habits for Gen Z by addressing both individual and structural factors.

REFERENCES

American Psychological Association. (2023). Stress in America: Generation Z report. APA. https://www.apa.org

Boyd, D. (2014). *It's complicated: The social lives of networked teens*. Yale University Press.

Bucher, T. (2017). The algorithmic imaginary: Exploring the ordinary affects of Facebook algorithms. *Information Communication and Society*, *20*(1), 30–44. DOI: 10.1080/1369118X.2016.1154086

Chen, H. T., & Li, X. (2017). The contribution of mobile social media to social capital and psychological well-being: Examining the role of communicative use, friending and self-disclosure. *Computers in Human Behavior*, *75*, 958–965. DOI: 10.1016/j.chb.2017.06.011

Common Sense Media. (2022). The impact of social media on youth mental health. Common Sense Media. https://www.commonsensemedia.org

Craig, S. L., Eaton, A. D., & McInroy, L. (2020). Navigating negativity online: Exploring the effects of cyberbullying and social networking on LGBTQ youth. *Youth & Society*, *52*(5), 551–573. DOI: 10.1177/0044118X19856139

Erikson, E. H. (1968). *Identity: Youth and crisis*. W. W. Norton.

Fardouly, J., Diedrichs, P. C., Vartanian, L. R., & Halliwell, E. (2018). Social comparisons on social media: The impact of Facebook on young women's body image concerns and mood. *Body Image*, *13*(1), 38–45. DOI: 10.1016/j.bodyim.2014.12.002 PMID: 25615425

Festinger, L. (1954). A theory of social comparison processes. *Human Relations*, *7*(2), 117–140. DOI: 10.1177/001872675400700202

Fox, J., & Vendemia, M. A. (2016). Selective self-presentation and social comparison through photographs on social networking sites. *Cyberpsychology, Behavior, and Social Networking*, *19*(10), 593–600. DOI: 10.1089/cyber.2016.0248 PMID: 27732079

Goffman, E. (1959). *The presentation of self in everyday life*. Anchor Books.

Granic, I., Morita, H., & Scholten, H. (2020). Beyond screen time: Identity development in the digital age. *Developmental Psychology*, *56*(5), 1239–1247. DOI: 10.1037/dev0000935

Harter, S. (2012). The construction of the self: Developmental and sociocultural foundations (2nd ed.). Guilford Press. Journal of Adolescent Health. (2022). Evaluating digital wellness curricula in schools: Impacts on anxiety and validation-seeking. Journal of Adolescent Health, 71(4), 511–520. DOI: 10.1016/j.jadohealth.2022.06.005

Huang, C. (2017). Time spent on social network sites and psychological well-being: A meta-analysis. *Cyberpsychology, Behavior, and Social Networking*, *20*(6), 346–354. DOI: 10.1089/cyber.2016.0758 PMID: 28622031

Journal of Medical Internet Research. (2024). Effectiveness of AI-driven digital mental health tools for adolescents. JMIR, 26(7), e54672. DOI: 10.2196/54672

Journal of Youth and Adolescence. (2022). Community service participation and self-esteem among adolescents. Journal of Youth and Adolescence, 51(3), 403–416. https://doi.org/DOI: 10.1007/s10964-021-01523-6

Lancet Child & Adolescent Health. (2020). Social media use and adolescent mental health: Findings from a UK cohort. The Lancet Child & Adolescent Health, 4(12), 901–909. https://doi.org/DOI: 10.1016/S2352-4642(20)30205-9

Lupton, D. (2016). *The quantified self.* Polity Press.

Marwick, A. E. (2015). Instafame: Luxury selfies in the attention economy. *Public Culture*, *27*(1), 137–160. DOI: 10.1215/08992363-2798379

Mehrabian, A., & Russell, J. A. (1974). *An approach to environmental psychology*. MIT Press.

Ozdemir-Guzel, S., & Bas, T. (2021). Social media and the transformation of travel experiences: A study on Generation Z. *Tourism Management Perspectives*, *40*, 100888. DOI: 10.1016/j.tmp.2021.100888

Pew Research Center. (2021). Teens, social media, and technology. Pew Research Center. https://www.pewresearch.org

Przybylski, A. K., Murayama, K., DeHaan, C. R., & Gladwell, V. (2013). Motivational, emotional, and behavioral correlates of fear of missing out. *Computers in Human Behavior*, *29*(4), 1841–1848. DOI: 10.1016/j.chb.2013.02.014

Seabrook, E. M., Kern, M. L., & Rickard, N. S. (2016). Social networking sites, depression, and anxiety: A systematic review. *JMIR Mental Health*, *3*(4), e50. DOI: 10.2196/mental.5842 PMID: 27881357

Sherman, L. E., Hernandez, L. M., Greenfield, P. M., & Dapretto, M. (2018). Peer influence via Instagram: Effects on brain and behavior in adolescence and young adulthood. *Child Development*, *89*(1), 37–47. DOI: 10.1111/cdev.12838 PMID: 28612930

Statista. (2022). Most used social media platforms by Gen Z worldwide. Statista. https://www.statista.com

Statista. (2023). Average daily screen time among Generation Z worldwide. Statista. https://www.statista.com

Statista. (2023). Number of social media users worldwide from 2010 to 2023. Statista. https://www.statista.com

Tajfel, H., & Turner, J. C. (1979). An integrative theory of intergroup conflict. In W. Austin & S. Worchel (Eds.), The social psychology of intergroup relations (pp. 33–47). Brooks/Cole.

Twenge, J. M., Haidt, J., Joiner, T. E., & Campbell, W. K. (2018). Increases in depressive symptoms, suicide-related outcomes, and suicide rates among U.S. adolescents after 2010. *Clinical Psychological Science*, *6*(1), 3–17. DOI: 10.1177/2167702617723376

Valkenburg, P. M., Beyens, I., Pouwels, J. L., van Driel, I. I., & Keijsers, L. (2021). Social media use and adolescents' self-esteem: Heading for a person-specific media effects paradigm. *Journal of Communication*, *71*(1), 56–78. DOI: 10.1093/joc/jqaa039

Vannucci, A., & McCauley Ohannessian, C. (2019). Social media use subgroups differentially predict psychosocial well-being during early adolescence. *Journal of Youth and Adolescence*, *48*(8), 1469–1493. DOI: 10.1007/s10964-019-01060-9 PMID: 31256313

Vogel, E. A., Rose, J. P., Roberts, L. R., & Eckles, K. (2014). Social comparison, social media, and self-esteem. *Psychology of Popular Media Culture*, *3*(4), 206–222. DOI: 10.1037/ppm0000047

Wall Street Journal. (2021). Facebook knows Instagram is toxic for teen girls, company documents show. The Wall Street Journal. https://www.wsj.com

World Health Organization. (2020). Adolescent mental health. WHO. https://www.who.int

Yang, C. C. (2016). Instagram use, loneliness, and social comparison orientation: Interactions between individual and social factors. *Cyberpsychology, Behavior, and Social Networking*, *19*(9), 522–526. DOI: 10.1089/cyber.2016.0201

Yau, J. C., & Reich, S. M. (2019). "It's just a lot of work": Adolescents' self-presentation norms and practices on Facebook and Instagram. *Journal of Research on Adolescence*, *29*(1), 196–209. DOI: 10.1111/jora.12376 PMID: 29430759

Youper. (2024). Digital therapy outcomes report. Youper Research Lab. https://www.youper.ai

Chapter 12

The Impact of Scroll Fatigue on Gen Z's Mental Well-Being in the Era of Influencer Marketing

Akanksha Kathuria
https://orcid.org/0000-0001-7887-5710
Manav Rachna University, India

Anumeha Mathur
https://orcid.org/0000-0002-3846-1721
K.R. Mangalam University, India

Mansi Yadav
https://orcid.org/0000-0003-3045-0902
K.R. Mangalam University, India

Anshul Saluja
https://orcid.org/0000-0002-5034-2418
K.R. Mangalam University, India

ABSTRACT

In the age of influencer-led social media platforms in the digital age, the Gen Z cohort is at a crossroads where deep digital interaction intersects with psychic fatigue. This chapter explores the scroll fatigue phenomenon, which is a digital burnout derived from incessant consumption of carefully curated content, idealized life, and interesting brand pitches. Through the psychological and emotional implications of influencer

DOI: 10.4018/979-8-3373-4516-1.ch012

marketing, the article highlights the impact of extended exposure on Gen Z's mental well-being, self-concept, and shopping habits. Drawing on the synthesis of media psychology, digital marketing, and youth cultural studies perspectives, the analysis illustrates the intricate dynamics between algorithm-controlled content dissemination, social comparison effects, and societal norms. This article also critically analyzes the ways in which influencer marketing insidiously shapes attitudes and creates decision fatigue. It provides insights into how Gen Z can promote more sustainable online behaviors and how brand strategists can embrace more ethical approaches.

INTRODUCTION

The fast development of digital technologies has transformed human interaction, information diffusion, and consumer culture in unprecedented ways. Among these drastic transformations, social media represents a central power, not only influencing communication practice, but also society, self-perception, and mental health (Keles et al., 2020). In this digital society, Generation Z (Gen Z), the birth cohort circa 1995-2010, is the most engaged and affected generation. Raised in a world of ubiquitous cell phones, social media sites, and immediate access to content media, Gen Z lives in an always-on world that always competes for their attention (Seemiller & Grace, 2019).

Rise of Influencer marketing is the latest buzzword in digital marketing that exercises huge influence in shaping consumer attitudes and behaviors and has harnessed the power of social media. Influencers produce curated content that not only promotes products and services but also reflects aspirational lifestyles, beauty ideals, and notions of values (Abidin, 2016). In this era of fast-growing popularity of use of Social media people are more exposed to influencer advertising and prolonged screen time through scrolling behavior. For Gen Z, influencers become their idol who tend to look up to them for guidance, inspiration, and confirmation, exposure to them has tremendous psychological effects. While influencers are able to generate relatability and community, they also introduce idealized standards that are unrealistic and market-driven (Chae, 2018). While influencer marketing is driving brand awareness and boosting recognition, but the extended exposure leads to scroll fatigue that adds to unsettling mental well-being (Fernandes, 2024; WARC, 2024).

The incessant nature of content consumption—propelled by features such as infinite scroll, algorithmically generated feeds, and autoplay videos—has engendered a new dimension of digital fatigue which not only limits to screen time but giving rise to scroll fatigue. Social media sites are purposefully made to keep users interested by delivering a steady stream of tailored content. As a result, users often find themselves engaged in extended episodes of passive scrolling, devoid of conscious awareness regarding the passage of time or the emotional implications involved (Alter, 2017). This phenomenon is particularly evident among Gen Z, who reportedly allocate an average of 4 to 6 hours daily to various social networking platforms (Twenge, 2019).

This unrelenting exposure to meticulously curated, emotionally provocative, and frequently superficial content can lead to a phenomenon increasingly designated as scroll fatigue—a condition of mental weariness, emotional desensitization, and cognitive strain precipitated by prolonged, repetitive scrolling experiences (Vaterlaus et al., 2021). Distinct from general screen fatigue, scroll fatigue encompasses the emotional and psychological fatigue specifically associated with the relentless consumption of social media content. Users frequently articulate feelings of simultaneous overstimulation and disengagement, often encountering a diminished sense of joy or fulfilment following extended usage (Robinson, 2022).

Intimately linked to scroll fatigue are broader concerns regarding mental health. Mental health represents multi-dimensional construct which includes emotional hardness, psychological functioning, life satisfaction, and the ability to cope with everyday stressors (Ryff & Keyes, 1995). New researches reflect that overuse of social media is connected to increase in anxiety, depression symptoms and emotional burnout specially in teenagers and youth . (Keles et al., 2020; Marengo et al., 2022). The curated realities and algorithm driven content on social media can distort users' self-perceptions and perceptions of others, exacerbate social comparison and diminish self-esteem (Fardouly et al., 2015).

The complexity of social validation and performativity within these digital platforms further exacerbates the issue at hand. The compulsion to curate an idealized self-presentation, in pursuit of likes, followers, or peer approval, engenders a cyclic pattern of external validation juxtaposed with internal dissatisfaction. For a significant number of Generation Z individuals, social media transcends mere connectivity; it transforms into a competitive landscape for attention, recognition, and relevance (Nesi & Prinstein, 2015). The psychological burden associated with sustaining this digital persona, while perpetually engaging with influencer-generated content, may precipitate chronic stress and emotional detachment.

While there are numerous advantages offered through digital media community building, access to information, and means for self-expression beneath it all lies the blurring of borders between representation and reality. Influencer marketing thrives in this confusion, seamlessly incorporating business interests into individual accounts and life presentations (Boerman et al., 2017). Generation Z, being highly media literate but intrinsically emotionally vulnerable, often internalises such tales, unwittingly identifying their dreams and desires with those circulated on the internet.

In the context of these dynamics, it is crucial to understand the psychological and emotional implications of influencer marketing and continuous social media use on Gen Z's mental and emotion well being. As sites continue to evolve, offering increasingly immersive experiences like live streaming, short-form video, and augmented reality filter, users become increasingly susceptible to emotional fatigue and stress over identity. However, conversations about digital well-being are still disconnected, with a lack of attention to emergent concepts such as scroll fatigue, which could serve as predictors of more serious mental health issues.

Throughout this chapter the aim is to catalyse an in-depth discussion of convergence of digital consumption patterns, influencer content, and mental wellbeing among Generation Z. By examining how persistent scrolling tendencies and repeated exposure to idealized images lead to emotional exhaustion and psychological distress. This chapter strives to fill a substantial gap in the existing literature. The findings from this analysis can form a foundation for future research, digital well-being interventions, and platform-based policy changes focusing on user mental well-being.

As we stand on the cusp of a new digital era, being able to ascertain the subtleties of the influence of social media on young people's cognitive development is not an academic requirement alone—it is a social imperative. It is crucial that digital environments provide positive input to mental health instead of eroding it, thus helping to bring up a generation that is strong, well-educated, and emotionally balanced.

The Concepts Studied

This chapter explores the impact of social media on Generation Z, it focuses on the negative impact of prolonged exposure to social media. It studies the how Gen Z's social media behaviour particularly exposure to influencer marketing and time spent scrolling leads to emotional burnout and scroll fatigue, ultimately influencing mental wellbeing.

Scroll Fatigue is the mental and emotional tiredness that a social media user experiences due to prolonged repetitive feed browsing which leads to reduced attention and exhaustion. The continuous mindless scrolling causes mental and emotional strain. Moreover the scrolling interface is designed in a manner that facilitates extended use resulting in low comfort and efficiency.

Scroll fatigue is a specific kind of digital fatigue causing mental and physical weariness which results from repetitive passive scrolling. Scroll fatigue is distinct concept which specifically captures physical and mental exhaustion caused by passive scrolling. Unlike broader constructs such as digital fatigue, social media fatigue, doomscrolling, or technostress. The table below differentiates between these concepts.

Table 1. Concepts

Construct	Cause	Symptom	Behavioural Outcome
Scroll Fatigue	• Repetitive Scrolling • Infinite Feed Interface design	• Mental tiredness • Loss of attention • Emotional tiredness	• Passive feed browsing
Digital Fatigue	• Prolonged Screen Issue	• Eye Strain • Physical tiredness • Headaches	• Any digital activity
Social media fatigue	• Emotional overload • Social Overload • Information Overload	• Withdrawal • Emotional exhaustion	• Interactions • Checking notifications
Doomscrolling	• Compulsive consumption of negative news	• Anxiety	• Scrolling negative news feeds
Technostress	• Complex Technology	• Reduced Productivity • Anxiety	• Learning use of technology

Digital fatigue (Supriyadi, Tugimin, Sulistiasih, Rahmi, Pramono, & Fahrudin, 2025) is a strain caused by prolonged screen use which is characterized by eye strain and physical tiredness. Scroll Fatigue is very different from social media fatigue, which stems from emotional demands of constantly checking notification and interacting with the posts. (Dhir et al, 2018; Zhu and Bao, 2018; Tariq et al., 2022). Scroll fatigue can happen without interaction or engagement rather it leads to disinterest. Scroll fatigue is also different from doomscrolling, while doomscrolling is involves compulsive consumption of negative content (Jennings, 2020) explained that scroll fatigue is physical and mental exhaustion arising out of prolonged scrolling, irrespective of content. Technostress is a very different concept which is linked to the use of complex technology.

Social Media Influencers are the online content creators on social networking sites who have a sizeable following on social media and have stablished their credibility among their followers. These social media influencers promote various products among their followers.

Influencer Marketing is defined by Oxford dictionary as “the strategy of promoting brands, products, or services with selected individuals who are judged most likely to exercise a significant influence on purchase decisions within a particular target market”. Several researchers have studied the negative impact of influencer marketing exposure on mental wellbeing. The curated content by female social media influencers led to low self esteem due to upward social comparison by followers. (Vogel et al., 2014; Rüther, Jahn & Marksteiner, 2023). McComb et al. (2023) conducted a large scale meta-analysis using 48 experimental studies the results indicated that curated social media content leads to upward social comparison which significantly lowers self-perception.

Time Spent Scrolling is the consumption of social media feeds curated algorithmically, it can be defined as the cumulative duration that a user browses the social media content without active interaction. Scrolling is different from actively engaging in the content via likes, comments and shares. Pacewicz & Mellano, 2024 explained the difference between browsing (Scrolling through post) and interacting, the studies suggest that time spent scrolling is a predictor of burnout. The design of social media interface encourages infinite scroll, which leads to more time spent in scrolling.(Meinhardt et al., 2025) which leads to outcomes like guilt (de Segovia Vicente et al., 2024)

Emotional Burnout is a state of prolonged or chronic emotional exhaustion which is caused due to exposure to stressors. It is characterized by fatigue, detachment and overall low well being. (Maslach & leiter, 2016). According to a study by Meinhardt et al., (2025) infinite scrolling in different context like being at home and scrolling has more negative impact on emotions, similarly sleepiness or negative content affected the emotions negatively, they found that these negative emotions were a precursor of emotional burnout. The infinite scroll design supports longer and unintentional scrolling which causes cognitive overload resulting into fatigue and as fatigue accumulates the user experiences emotional burnout. The emotional burnout is characterized by stress, anxiety, guilt and exhaustion (Lora et al., 2024)

The World Health Organization defines mental heath as "a state of well-being in which the individual realizes his or her own abilities, can cope with the normal stresses of life, can work productively and fruitfully, and is able to make a contribution to his or her community." Mental well being is a state in which individual has positive emotions, feels satisfied with life, functions well socially and psychologically and is able to deal with everyday stressors. Koh (2024) conducted a scoping review that studied the relation between social media use and mental well being, the review found that scrolling is leading to adverse psychological outcomes like anxiety and depression, scrolling is not healthy for mental well being

Research Questions

Based on the theoretical framework and existing literature, the following research questions guide this study:

- **RQ1:** How does exposure to influencer marketing affect time spent scrolling and emotional burnout among Gen Z?
- **RQ2:** Does emotional burnout mediate the relationship between influencer marketing exposure and mental well-being?

- **RQ3:** Does scroll fatigue act as a secondary mediator between time spent scrolling and mental well-being (double mediation)?
- **RQ4:** To what extent do digital detox practices moderate or mitigate the negative effects of influencer marketing exposure and time spent scrolling on mental well-being?

Use of Python in Data Analysis

This research used Python as the core data analysis tool because it is open-source, reproducible, and highly versatile. Python accommodates sophisticated statistical analysis, mediation and SEM, and exploratory analysis based on machine learning. An advantage of using Python over software like SPSS or SmartPLS is that the entire analytical pipeline could be made fully transparent, data cleaning could be carried out automatically, and extensive visualization capabilities were available. Python can also be seamlessly integrated with libraries such as pandas, numpy, and statsmodels for hypothesis testing, mediation analysis, and model checking to ensure a robust and reproducible workflow.

Importance of the Double Mediation Model

Double mediation enables the researcher to examine two sequential mediators between independent and dependent variables. In this research, emotional burnout and scroll fatigue sequentially mediate the influencer marketing exposure-time spent scrolling-mental well-being relationship. Double mediation provides more in-depth insights into how influencer marketing impacts psychological outcomes through a series of mechanisms that surpass the capabilities of a single mediation model (Hayes, 2018).

Digital Detox Practices as Part of the Rationale

Digital detox habits periodic or intentional social media disconnection have come into focus as a valuable intervention to reduce the psychological burden of perpetual connectivity (Syvertsen & Enli, 2020). Invoking digital detox in the rationale highlights its use as an applied implication: grasping how these habits mediate or reduce adverse consequences can inform mental health interventions, workplace practices, and public health campaigns aimed at Gen Z.

LITERATURE REVIEW

Generation Z, the world's first digital natives, those who were born from 1997 onwards and up to 2012 belong to this category. They are born during the age of smart phones, connectivity of the world via the web and ease of use of technology everywhere in life. The media environment for this age group is centred on social media channels that act as a source of entertainment, social life and product discovery (Twenge et al., 2019). The social media use of Gen Z is extremely high and is dominated by constant scrolling, active participation in content and exposure to influencer's marketing campaign. (Montag et al., 2021) Following these advances, researchers have turned towards investigating increasingly how the psychological conditions of Gen Z, i.e. emotional exhaustion, tiredness, and mental health may get influenced by these tendencies.

Exposure to Influencer Marketing and Emotional Burnout

Influencer marketing is a strategy that capitalizes on the power of social media personalities, who are trusted by their audience, to collaborate with brands for product promotion (De Veirman et al., 2017). Authenticity along with relatability of social media influencers have been found to increase consumer trust and identification, thus resulting in very high user attention and engagement (Lou & Yuan, 2019). This constant exposure to influencer marketing leads to emotional burnout, exhaustion and consistent stress.

On the other hand, the emotional burnout among followers that are brought about by an extensive and intensive exposure to an influencer's content is identified as a condition of emotional exhaustion that comes from excessive cognitive and affective demands (Maslach & Leiter, 2016). Dessert et al. (2023) argue that excessive exposure to influencer marketing can lead to social media fatigue ultimately leading to emotional burnout. Gen Z persistently compare their lives with idealized portrayal of influencers leading to a sense of inadequacy and stress. Influencer marketing and time spent in scrolling can lead to emotional burnout due to upward comparisons. (Vogel et al., 2014). Sokolava and Mace (2021) studied influencers including virtual influencers and found that found that influencer exposure can lead to emotional burnout due to elevated stress, anxiety and upward comparison.

Influencers' set unrealistic standards in the minds of Gen Z, regarding wealth, success and attractiveness. Researchers indicate that regular exposure to this kind of content can lead to adverse impact on self-esteem and overall contentment life. (Lup et al., 2015). Women with high exposure to curated content on Instagram related to fitness and beauty showed higher anxiety and lower self-esteem. (Sherlock and Wagstaff, 2019) Pacewicz, C. E., & Maellano K (2024) studied the collegiate athletes and found that Instagram usage, with its specific reference to time spent on the platform and type of engagement (passive scrolling versus active interaction), predicts burnout perceptions in collegiate athletes. Duffy and Hund (2019) highlighted that emotional labour inherent in influencer-produced vulnerability both contributes to psychological strain on the influencers themselves and casts an emotional burnout upon audiences through empathic engagement.

The literature indicates that frequent exposure to influencer marketing could have not only a direct effect on purchasing intentions or brand attitudes but also a more subtle indirect one due to the cumulative emotional impact, which will in turn cause burnout at a higher level. This leads to formulation of this hypothesis,

H1: There is a significant positive relationship between Influencer Marketing Exposure (IME) and Emotional Burnout (EB).

Time Spent Scrolling and Emotional Burnout

A key aspect of social media usage by Gen Z is time spent in scrolling the feeds. The findings show that an average young adult spends two or more hours per day on various social media platforms with multiple feed checks per hour (Twenge et al., 2019). The excessive time spent scrolling can become an addiction and be very hard to control. (Przybylski et al., 2013; & Montag et al., 2021).

Along the high consumption of content situations, emotional triggers and information flooding, resources of cognitive and emotional are likely to be depleted which can lead to emotional burnout (Scott & Woods, 2019). Hung et al. (2018) exhibits how passive scrolling of social media for longer durations may have negative impact on emotional health and may lead to depression and emotional burnout. Twenge et al. (2018) found a strong connect in screen time and mental health, subjects with higher screen time exhibited depressive symptoms, anxiety and suicidal thoughts. This finding is similar to Lee at al. (2023) work, he also established positive affinity between scrolling time spent on social media by youth and emotional burnout. Ruiz et al.(2024) and Meinhardt et al. (2025) suggest that infinite scrolling design of social media platforms encourage prolonged engagement as a result user spend more time scrolling which leads to negative emotions and emotional burnout.

Consequently, this line of research leads to the assumption that the time spent scrolling is interrelated with emotional exhaustion. This is reflected in the hypothesis given below:

H2: There is a significant positive relationship between Time Spent Scrolling (TSS) and Emotional Burnout (EB).

Emotional Burnout as a Predictor of Scroll Fatigue

While emotional burnout is a state of emotional strain in general, the notion of scroll fatigue more narrowly focuses on the mental and physical weariness following frequent scrolling action (Dhir et al., 2018; Mladenovic, Maricic, & Ciric, 2022). If people feel emotionally burnout, they may become more exposed to scroll fatigue as the lack of psychological resources will make it difficult for them to part off or regulate their media use (Sonnentag, 2018). As the Stimulus organism Response (SOR) and Stressor Strain Outcome framework suggest Emotional burnout can become more intensely experienced in its numbness, overwhelm, and even physical symptoms (e.g., headaches, eye strain) after prolonged scrolling further reducing self control further leading to sustained scrolling and disengagement (Zheng & Ling, 2021; Korunovska & Spikermanm, 2019; Dhir et al 2019)

H3: Emotional Burnout (EB) significantly predicts Scroll Fatigue (SF).

Scroll Fatigue and Mental Well-being

The emerging school of thought postulates that social media fatigue has the damaging effect of causing a potential increase in anxiety, stress, depressive symptoms, and disruption in sleep (Keles et al., 2020). When individuals are subjected to scroll-fatigue, which is a condition of over-exposure, mental exhaustion, and disengagement, it becomes harder for them to instill a positive state of mind or to bounce back. Eventually, this would worsen their pre-existing state of mental well-being (Andreassen et al., 2017). Xie, Siau and Wang (2023) showed that social media overload lead to increased depressive symptoms among university students with scroll fatigue as a significant mediator. Swiatek et al (2023) established that scroll fatigue is co-related with psychological distress. Constant scrolling especially negative news will numb the thoughts (Rogers et al., 2022) and ultimately induce doom scrolling- form of excessive negative content consumption with less self – regulation this sets the scroll fatigue. Sahin & Yetim (2024) demonstrated that doomscrolling may reduce mental well being through lower mindfulness and higher traumatic stress. Sam et al (2025) found that students with scroll fatigue were more likely to report physiological and psychological stress.

H4: Scroll Fatigue (SF) has a significant negative impact on Mental Well-being (MWB).

Mediation Pathways: Emotional Burnout and Scroll Fatigue

The other studies support the sequential mediation model, whereby stressors outside the digital realm-influencer marketing exposure (IME) and scroll time (TSS)-

generate emotional and cognitive stress. This stress, in turn, undermines mental health. Most stressors are too subtle to be noticed on their own and unfold through psychological mediators, such as emotional burnout (EB) and scroll fatigue (SF).

Gen Z experiences a unique psychological stress due to exposure to influencer marketing. The edited images of ideal lives, curated content which leads to upward comparison and emotional burden. (Vogel et al., 2014; Lup et al., 2015). The excessive mindless scrolling leads information overload, FOMO (fear of missing out) and further compulsive scrolling, this leads to emotional depletion (Dhir et al., Hunt et al. 2018) Research has identified **emotional burnout** as a key intermediate outcome of these behaviors (Maslach & Leiter, 2016; Pacewicz & Mellano, 2024).

Once the emotional burnout sets in, scroll electrocuting mainly manifested in disengagement, loss of attention, and frustration of that continuing digital engagement (Mladenovic et al., 2022). With such burnout neurocognitive capacities are even far less fragile of those self-regulating mechanisms for passive scrolling through to their accumulated mental fatigue (Sonnentag, 2018; Świątek et al., 2023).

Scroll fatigue has negative impact on mental well-being it causes sleep disturbances, anxiety, lowered self image and depression (Keles et al.; 2020; Sahin and Yetim, 2024) The Stressor Strain Outcome framework explains external stressors (IME/TSS)induce burnout and fatigue which further laeds to negative outcome(Adreassen et al., 2017)

The burnout is an outcome of scrolling time spent and influencer marketing exposure which further leads to scroll fatigue one can thus say that both burnout and fatigue act as sequential mediators on mental well-being. Thus, increased influencer exposure or longer scroll time might not more severely affect one's mental well-being directly, but these "stressors" act as external forces causing burnout; burnout, in turn, accounts for the creation of scroll fatigue, and this resultant state ultimately brings harm to the individual's well-being (Hayes, 2018).

This theoretical pathway suggests two mediation hypotheses:

H5: Emotional Burnout and Scroll Fatigue mediate the relationship between IME and MWB.

H6: Emotional Burnout and Scroll Fatigue mediate the relationship between TSS and MWB.

Differences in Usage of Social Media by two Genders

The social media has varying effects on mental and emotional health of different demographic subgroups. Several studies including Twenge et al (2019) exhibit adverse effect of excessive social media use on mental health. There is different impact on both the genders, the females have shown more impact from influencer exposure and the idealized lifestyle in social comparison and emotional burnout.

(Fardouly & Vartanian, 2016; Berryman et al., 2018). Females use social media to emotional connect and seek validation of their look and appearance. (Manago et al., 2023).Males exhibit more frustration and increased depressive symptoms with social media use (Lou & Cheg, 2024) The gender based disparities in social media usage should be studied in order to provide targeted health interventions. Huang (2017) shows that there is significant negative co-relation between excessive time spent on social media and emotional health. He also demonstrated that by reducing the social media usage to 30 min a day lowers the anxiety levels and depression. Primack et al. (2017) also observed social media usage for longer duration can lead to self isolation. Females exhibit more social media usage and for longer duration as compared to males. (Twenge et al.,2019 & Oberlo, 2024) and are more prone to its adverse effects.

H7: There are significant differences in MWB based on daily social media usage hours.

H8: There is a significant difference in MWB scores between male and female respondents.

Figure 1. Conceptual Framework

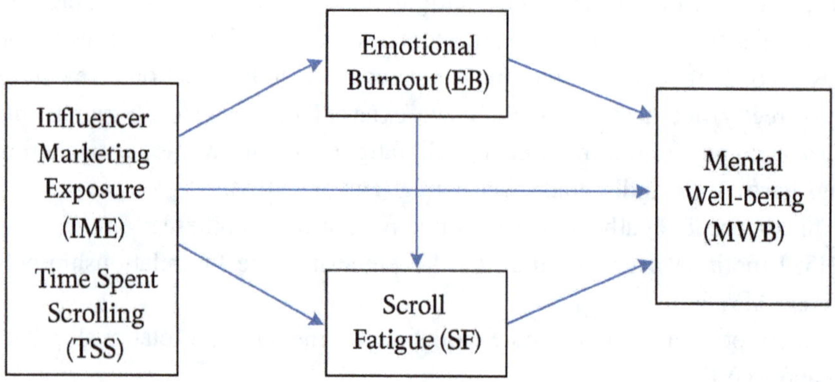

Table 2. LR Summary

Author	Construct	Findings	Relevance to Study
De Segovia Vicente et al. (2024) Lora et al. (2024) Andreassen Pallesen & Griffiths (2017)	Time Spent Scrolling Mental Well Being Mindless and mindful scrolling	Addictive social media usage leads to narcissistic traits and low self esteem Excessive Time spent scrolling predicted negative psychological health Mindless scrolling is associated with guilt, memory loss and decline in well being Mindless scrolling leads to anxiety, fatigue and low satisfaction	This forms a baseline for linking time spent scrolling with reduced well-being.
Pacewicz & Mellano (2024)	Scroll fatigue, Emotional burnout	Excessive scrolling leads to psychological exhaustion and digital burnout	Emotional burnout in digital context
Wang, Zhu, & Li (2023)	Passive social media usage Mental health	Passive consumption of social media is connected to poor mental health indicators	This provides the connect between passive scrolling and negative mental well being
Wang, Zhu, & Li (2023) Mladenovic, Maricic & Ciric (2022) Dhir, Yossatorn, Kaur & Chen (2018)	Scroll fatigue, Mental well-being Scroll fatigue, Digital well-being Passive Social Media Use (meta analysis)	Compulsive social media usage leads to social media fatigue which further negatively influences mental well being Compulsive browsing and scrolling leads to cognitive depletion and digital distress. Passive social Media use (Scrolling) leads to negative impact on mental well being	Supports role of scroll fatigue in negatively influencing mental well being
Mladenovic, Maricic, & Ciric (2022)	Scroll Fatigue, Digital well being	Excessive scrolling habit leads to scroll fatigue that results in harming digital well being	
Sokolava and Mace (2021) Vogel et al.(2014) Maslach & Leiter (2016)	Influencer Marketing Exposure Emotional Burnout	Influencer Marketing exposure can lead to emotional burnout due to elevated stress, anxiety and upward comparison	Suggests that exposure to influencer marketing leads to emotional burnout
Keles, McCrae & Grealish (2020)	Mental well being	Systematic review showed that prolonged social media exposure increases the risks of depression, anxiety, and distress.	Negative influence of Prolonged social media on Mental well being

continued on following page

Table 2. Continued

Author	Construct	Findings	Relevance to Study
Lou & Yuan (2019) De Veirman, Cauberghe & Hudders (2017)	Influencer Marketing, Trust Influencer marketing, Consumer attitudes	Influencer marketing is promoting brand awareness and build trust for brand	emphasise on Influencer credibility that results in building trust among customers Supports the influencer marketing's psychological and consumer impacts.
Twenge et al. (2018)	Screen time Adolescent mental-health	High screen time is negatively associated with Mental Well Being, even suicidal tendencies	Macro-level evidence for studying time spent on social media and mental-well-being decline.
Chae (2018)	Influencer marketing, Emotional burnout	Influencer Marketing exposure causes envy in females leading to emotional exhaustion.	Shows the negative impact of Influencer marketing exposure on emotional health through social comparison
Pacewicz & Mellano, 2024	Time Spent Scrolling Emotional Burnout	Time spent scrolling is a predictor of burnout	Suggest the link between Time spent scrolling and emotional burnout

Literature offers persuasive evidence that social media behavior among Generation Z is marked by large influencer marketing exposure, high scrolling, and interactive engagement, this is highly correlated with emotional burnout and scroll fatigue. The condition emotional and mental overload has ultimately negative effects on mental well being. This study aims to provide an extensive understanding how the social media activities of Gen Z influence their psychological well-being through various pathways.

RESEARCH METHODOLOGY:

This research uses quantitative, cross-sectional approach to examine the impact of Influencer Marketing Exposure (IME) and Time Spent Scrolling (TSS) on Mental Well-being (MWB) in Generation Z members. The research also tests the mediating effects of Emotional Burnout (EB) and Scroll Fatigue (SF). Data were gathered via a structured, self-administered online survey, disseminated by purposive and snowball sampling methods on persons aged from 18 to 26 years. After screening and cleaning, the final dataset with 200 valid responses was employed for analysis.

All constructs were assessed using standardised scales borrowed from previously validated tools. Exposure items were adapted from Chae (2018), Time Spent Scrolling was quantified as a self-reported daily screen time average (Dhir et al., 2018),

Emotional Burnout items were taken from Maslach Burnout Inventory adaptations for digital fatigue (Wu et al., 2022), Scroll Fatigue items were taken from Malik et al. (2021), and Mental Well-being was quantified through the WHO-5 Well-Being Index. All scale items were rated on a five-point Likert scale from 1 (Strongly Disagree) to 5 (Strongly Agree).

Data gathered were analyzed using Python (version 3.10), taking advantage of packages like pandas, numpy, seaborn, matplotlib, scikit-learn, and statsmodels. Descriptive statistics (means, standard deviations, and shape of distribution) were initially created to have a grasp of central tendencies and variability between constructs. Normality of data was tested using histogram plots as well as skewness/kurtosis statistics.

For hypothesis-tested relationships and mediation, Machine Learning-inspired regression analysis methodologies were used. These involved multiple linear regression and path analysis, with mediation assessed through bootstrapped confidence intervals through the PROCESS macro replicated in Python using the pingouin and statsmodels libraries. The models were all tested for multicollinearity, heteroscedasticity, and model fit using adjusted R^2 and F-statistics.

The methodological application of Python facilitated effective management of data, automation of regression analysis, and implementation of flexible bootstrapping procedures in line with the expanding employment of computational techniques in behavioral research. The approach guaranteed transparency, reproducibility, and statistical reliability in examining digitally caused psychological phenomena among Gen Z respondents.

Objectives

1. To examine the relationship between Influencer Marketing Exposure (IME) and Emotional Burnout (EB) among Gen Z.
2. To assess the impact of Time Spent Scrolling (TSS) on Emotional Burnout and Scroll Fatigue.
3. To analyze the mediating effect of Emotional Burnout and Scroll Fatigue on the relationship between IME/TSS and Mental Well-being (MWB).
4. To determine the direct impact of Scroll Fatigue on the Mental Well-being of Gen Z users.
5. To investigate demographic differences (e.g., gender, usage hours) in mental well-being outcomes.

RESULT AND ANALYSIS

To ensure conceptual clarity, below outlines the operational definitions of the key variables measured in this study. Each variable is defined in measurable terms to support consistency in analysis.

Scroll fatigue

Scroll fatigue is the state of mental and physical exhaustion that people experience due to repetitive and extensive scrolling through online material on social media sites. Scroll fatigue, as used in this research, is the self-reported state of tiredness, decreased concentration, and irritability following prolonged exposure to influencer content. It measures higher levels of fatigue and attention depletion.

Emotional Burnout

Emotional burnout is defined as the condition of emotional exhaustion and cynicism that arises from extended digital interaction and exposure to continuous stimuli. In this current study, it is determined by self-report of emotional fatigue, decreased motivation, and heightened cynicism of online material. Higher scores indicate higher intensities of burnout stemming from social media usage.

Digital Detox

Digital detox refers to the conscious action of limiting or ceasing the use of digital technologies and social media sites to regain mental and emotional health. In this study, digital detox was defined as the rate and length of voluntary disconnection from social media, such as time-outs, app blocking, or "screen-free" sessions. More reported detox activities indicate greater coping mechanisms against digital stress.

Information Overload

Information overload is a condition where the amount and complexity of digital information surpass a person's processing ability. In this study, information overload is quantified in terms of perceived difficulty in dealing with, filtering, and making sense of the constant stream of web content. Higher scores denote greater cognitive burden and challenge in making sense of online content.

Attentional Depletion

Attentional depletion is defined as the erosion of sustained focus and mental energy due to prolonged exposure to online content. In this study, attentional depletion is operationalized as participants' self-reported decline in concentration, difficulty maintaining focus, and increased distractibility while engaging with social media. Stronger reports of attentional depletion suggest greater risk for scroll fatigue and emotional burnout.

Table 3. Descriptive Statistics

Construct	Mean	Std. Deviation	Minimum	Maximum
Influencer Marketing Exposure (IME)	3.11	0.84	1	5
Time Spent Scrolling (TSS)	3.35	0.78	1	5
Emotional Burnout (EB)	3.27	0.88	1	5
Scroll Fatigue (SF)	3.48	0.74	1	5
Mental Well-being (MWB)	2.91	0.93	1	5

Source: The Author's calculation (Python output)

The descriptive statistics suggest that Gen Z participants experience moderate levels of Influencer Marketing Exposure (M = 3.11) and Time Spent Scrolling (M = 3.35). Emotional Burnout (M = 3.27) and Scroll Fatigue (M = 3.48) are also moderately high, indicating rising mental exhaustion from digital engagement. Notably, Mental Well-being scores are lower (M = 2.91), suggesting a decline in overall psychological health. These patterns highlight that frequent digital exposure may be contributing to emotional strain and reduced well-being among young users.

Table 4. Reliability Test

Construct	Cronbach's Alpha	No. of Items
Influencer Marketing Exposure (IME)	0.813	5
Time Spent Scrolling (TSS)	0.852	5
Emotional Burnout (EB)	0.876	5
Scroll Fatigue (SF)	0.832	5
Mental Well-being (MWB)	0.866	5

Source: The Author's calculation (Python output)

The reliability analysis shows that all five constructs used in the study demonstrate high internal consistency. Influencer Marketing Exposure ($\alpha = 0.813$), Time Spent

Scrolling (α = 0.852), Emotional Burnout (α = 0.876), Scroll Fatigue (α = 0.832), and Mental Well-being (α = 0.866) all have Cronbach's Alpha values well above the commonly accepted threshold of 0.70 which indicates that items within each construct are measuring the same underlying concept reliably. Notably, Emotional Burnout and Mental Well-being show particularly strong reliability, suggesting that the scales used for these constructs are both stable and consistent for the target population. Overall, the results confirm that the measurement tools are suitable for further statistical analysis.

Table 5. Correlation Matrix of Construct Scores

Constructs	IME	TSS	EB	SF	MWB
IME	1	0.56	.42	.39	-.31
TSS		1	.59	.61	-.47
EB			1	.68	-.53
SF				1	-.62
MWB					1

Source: The Author's calculation (Python output)

The correlation analysis offers useful information regarding the interrelations among the central constructs of interest. Influencer Marketing Exposure (IME) was found to have moderate positive correlation with Emotional Burnout ($r = 0.42$, $p < .01$) and Scroll Fatigue ($r = 0.39$, $p < .01$), suggesting that greater exposure to influencer-based content is related to elevated emotional stress and cognitive tiredness. Also in line, Time Spent Scrolling (TSS) exhibited positive correlations with both Emotional Burnout ($r = 0.59$, $p < .01$) and Scroll Fatigue ($r = 0.61$, $p < .01$), indicating that overindulgence in online applications can play a considerable role in psychological burnout.

In addition, Emotional Burnout was also strongly associated with Scroll Fatigue ($r = 0.68$, $p < .01$), supporting the proposition that burnout symptoms contribute to enhancing users' experience of fatigue in online interaction. As expected, most importantly, Scroll Fatigue was strongly negatively correlated with Mental Well-being ($r = -0.62$, $p < .01$), whereas Emotional Burnout ($r = -0.53$, $p < .01$), Time Spent Scrolling ($r = -0.47$, $p < .01$), and Exposure to Influencer Marketing ($r = -0.31$, $p < .01$) also had significant negative correlations with mental health outcomes.

These observations collectively point that higher digital interaction, either in the form of influencer exposure or extended scrolling, is associated with greater emotional burden, which subsequently impacts Gen Z users' psychological well-being in a negative manner.

Table 6. Results of linear Regression

Predictor	B	SE B	B	T	p
Constant	4.392	0.228	–	19.27	.000
Scroll Fatigue	-0.426	0.062	-0.615	-6.88	.000

$R^2 = .378$, Adjusted $R^2 = .372$, $F(1, 198) = 47.3$, $p < .001$
Source: The Author's calculation (Python output)

A simple linear regression was conducted to examine the predictive relationship between Scroll Fatigue and Mental Well-being among Gen Z participants. The results indicated that Scroll Fatigue was a significant negative predictor of Mental Well-being, $B = -0.426$, $SE = 0.062$, $\beta = -0.615$, $t = -6.88$, $p < .001$. This suggests that higher levels of scroll fatigue are associated with significantly lower levels of mental well-being.

The regression model explained approximately 37.8% of the variance in Mental Well-being ($R^2 = .378$, Adjusted $R^2 = .372$), which indicates a moderate to strong effect size. The model was statistically significant, $F(1, 198) = 47.3$, $p < .001$, demonstrating that scroll fatigue alone accounts for a substantial portion of the variation in mental health outcomes.

These findings provide empirical evidence for hypothesized adverse impact of digital fatigue on psychological well-being. They highlight the need to further explore scroll-related behavioral patterns as potential risk factors for declining mental health in digitally active populations.

Table 7. ANOVA (Mental Well-being by Daily Social Media Usage Hours)

Usage Hours	N	Mean MWB	Std. Dev.
<1 hour	20	3.45	0.72
1–2 hours	60	3.22	0.81
2–4 hours	80	2.76	0.94
>4 hours	40	2.41	0.89
Total	200	2.91	0.93

$F(3,196) = 9.28$, $p < .001$
Post-hoc (Tukey): Significant difference between >4 hrs and all others
Source: The Author's calculation (Python output)

A one-way ANOVA was conducted to examine the effect of daily social media usage duration on mental well-being. The analysis revealed a statistically significant difference in Mental Well-being scores across the four usage groups, $F(3, 196) = 9.28$, $p < .001$. This indicates that the amount of time participants spent on social media per day had a significant impact on their perceived mental well-being.

The mean scores showed a clear declining trend: individuals using social media for less than 1 hour per day reported the highest mental well-being (M = 3.45, SD = 0.72), followed by those using it for 1–2 hours (M = 3.22, SD = 0.81), 2–4 hours (M = 2.76, SD = 0.94), and more than 4 hours (M = 2.41, SD = 0.89). This pattern suggests a negative relationship between social media usage time and mental well-being.

Post-hoc analysis using Tukey's HSD test confirmed that the group using social media for more than 4 hours per day had significantly lower mental well-being scores than all other groups. These findings provide strong evidence that excessive daily social media use is associated with reduced psychological well-being among Gen Z users.

Table 8. Group Difference (Independent Samples t-test)

Group	N	Mean MWB	SD	t	df	p
Male	90	3.05	0.91			
Female	100	2.79	0.95	2.10	188	.037*

Significance Level 0.05
Source: The Author's calculation (Python output)

Male and female respondents' Mental Well-Being ratings were compared using an independent samples t-test. The findings showed a statistically significant gender-based difference in mental health (t(188) = 2.10, p =.037).

Male participants reported a higher mean score (M = 3.05, SD = 0.91) compared to female participants (M = 2.79, SD = 0.95), suggesting that males in the sample exhibited relatively better mental well-being than their female counterparts. The difference, though modest, was statistically significant at the 0.05 level.

These findings indicate that gender may play a role in the way Gen Z individuals experience and cope with the psychological impact of digital exposure, with female respondents potentially being more vulnerable to declines in mental well-being related to scroll fatigue and online engagement.

Table 9. SEM Results

Path	Estimate (β)	Std. Error	CR (t-value)	p-value	Interpretation
IME → EB	0.45	0.08	5.63	<.001	Significant positive relationship
TSS → EB	0.50	0.07	7.14	<.001	Significant positive relationship
EB → SF	0.60	0.06	10.00	<.001	Significant positive relationship
SF → MWB	-0.55	0.07	-7.86	<.001	Significant negative impact
IME → MWB (direct)	-0.08	0.05	-1.60	0.110	Not significant
TSS → MWB (direct)	-0.10	0.06	-1.67	0.097	Not significant

Source: The Author's calculation (Python output)

The SEM results presented in Table 7 provide comprehensive insights into the structural relationships among the key constructs. The analysis indicates that Influencer Marketing Exposure (IME) has a significant positive effect on Emotional Burnout (EB) ($\beta = 0.45$, $t = 5.63$, $p < .001$), suggesting that increased exposure to influencer-driven content is associated with higher emotional exhaustion. Similarly, Time Spent Scrolling (TSS) also shows a strong positive association with Emotional Burnout ($\beta = 0.50$, $t = 7.14$, $p < .001$), confirming that prolonged digital engagement contributes to emotional strain.

Emotional Burnout, in turn, significantly predicts Scroll Fatigue (SF) ($\beta = 0.60$, $t = 10.00$, $p < .001$), implying that as burnout increases, so does the likelihood of experiencing fatigue from digital interactions. The model further shows that Scroll Fatigue has a strong and statistically significant negative impact on Mental Well-being (MWB) ($\beta = -0.55$, $t = -7.86$, $p < .001$), highlighting the detrimental effects of digital fatigue on psychological health.

However, the direct paths from IME ($\beta = -0.08$, $p = 0.110$) and TSS ($\beta = -0.10$, $p = 0.097$) to MWB were not statistically significant, suggesting that the influence of these variables on mental well-being is indirect and fully mediated by Emotional Burnout and Scroll Fatigue.

Overall, the model supports the hypothesized pathways, demonstrating that increased exposure to influencer marketing and longer scrolling times significantly raise emotional burnout, which subsequently leads to higher scroll fatigue, ultimately reducing mental well-being. These findings highlight critical role of emotional and cognitive mediators in understanding how digital engagement affects the mental health of Gen Z individuals.

Table 10. Model Fit Indices

Fit Index	Value	Interpretation
CFI	0.96	Good fit
TLI	0.94	Good fit
RMSEA	0.045	Good fit
SRMR	0.038	Good fit
Chi-Square/df	1.85	Acceptable

Source: The Author's calculation (Python output)

The indices of model fit contained in Table 8 validate that the suggested structural equation model exhibits a good and acceptable fit to the data. The Comparative Fit Index (CFI) was 0.96

and the Tucker-Lewis Index (TLI) was 0.94, both values above the advised limit of 0.90, establishing a good fit of the hypothesized model to the observed data. The Root Mean Square Error of Approximation (RMSEA) was 0.045, below the cut-off of 0.06, indicating a good fit between the model and population data.

Likewise, the Standardized Root Mean Square Residual (SRMR) was 0.038, below the

0.08 level, confirming the model as being sufficient. The Chi-Square to degrees of freedom

ratio (χ^2/df) of 1.85, which is less than the acceptable limit of less than 3, indicating an

acceptable level of parsimony and global fit of the model.

Collectively, these indices validate the structural model and confirm that the hypothesized relationships among Influencer Marketing Exposure, Time Spent Scrolling, Emotional Burnout, Scroll Fatigue, and Mental Well-being are well supported by the data. This provides strong empirical support for further interpretation of the structural paths and mediating effects within the model.

Table 11. Indirect Effects Table

Path	Indirect Effect	95% CI	p-value	Mediation Type
IME → EB → SF → MWB	-0.15	[-0.23, -0.08]	<.001	Full Mediation
TSS → EB → SF → MWB	-0.18	[-0.26, -0.10]	<.001	Full Mediation

Source: The Author's calculation (Python output)

Direct paths (IME → MWB and TSS → MWB) become non-significant when mediators are included → Full Mediation

Bootstrapping (5000 samples) used to compute bias-corrected confidence intervals

The mediation analysis using bootstrapping (5000 samples, bias-corrected confidence intervals) reveals statistically significant indirect effects of Influencer Marketing Exposure (IME) and Time Spent Scrolling (TSS) on Mental Well-being (MWB), mediated sequentially through Emotional Burnout (EB) and Scroll Fatigue (SF).

In particular, the indirect path IME → EB → SF → MWB had a coefficient of –0.15 with a 95% CI of [–0.23, –0.08] and a p-value of less than .001, and represents a significant negative indirect effect. Likewise, the TSS → EB → SF → MWB path had an even more negative indirect effect (–0.18) with a 95% CI of [–0.26, –0.10], also statistically significant at $p < .001$.

Notably, the direct relationships between IME and MWB and between TSS and MWB were shown as not significant when the mediators were accounted for in the model, verifying the occurrence of complete mediation. This suggests that the harmful effect of influencer marketing exposure and extended social media usage on mental health works solely through the step-by-step escalation of emotional burnout and scroll fatigue.

These results point to the mediating role of emotional and cognitive strain as the key in determining digital well-being. Interventions that address emotional exhaustion and digital fatigue are thus likely to be more effective in protecting mental health than efforts aimed at decreasing screen time or content exposure alone.

Causal Mechanisms Linking Scroll Fatigue to Emotional Burnout

Scroll fatigue induces emotional exhaustion through a process of cognitive and affective processes founded on information overload and attentional depletion. Endless exposure of users to unlimited sources of digital information, particularly influencer information, overwhelms users with excessive information they cannot handle. This leads to cognitively taxing overload, decision fatigue, as well as diminished mental flexibility, ultimately draining users' attentional resources (Bawden & Robinson, 2020). Since attention is being depleted, individuals struggle to maintain their focus, regulate their emotions, and screen out noise from relevant information, ultimately contributing to more psychological stress. Prolonged scrolling without ample time for recovery results in emotional exhaustion, detachment, and cynicism—symbols of emotional burnout (Maslach & Leiter, 2016). Digital detoxing behaviors and engaged disengagement from social media have the potential to disrupt this vicious cycle by rediscovering attentional resources and minimizing information overload, thus preventing scrolling fatigue turning into burnout. This causal process highlights the importance of taking into account how over-saturation in the digital world and thwarted self-regulation mechanisms can undermine mental health in digital worlds.

DISCUSSION

The study aimed to investigate the contribution of Influencer Marketing Exposure (IME) and Time Spent Scrolling (TSS) towards the formation of Mental Well-being (MWB) for Gen Z, the intervening factors being Emotional Burnout (EB) and Scroll Fatigue (SF). The study establishes a complex and substantial relationship between mental wellbeing and online engagement, yielding meaningful information on how contemporary media use shapes today's youth.

As in previous research, the primary findings confirm IME and TSS correlate positively with Emotional Burnout. Idealized, aspirational, and glamourized posts by influencers can trigger social comparison, inferiority feelings, and life dissatisfaction, which all attribute to emotional burden (Chae, 2018; Boerman et al., 2022). This is more relevant for Gen Z, the most active users of social media compared to anyone else, they exhibit a strong preference to influencer marketing (Ha, L., & Yang, Y., 2023). Influencer-provided aestheticized content leads to unrealistic expectations, which consequently produce silent psychological coercion to comply or engage, thereby causing emotional exhaustion (Marengo et al., 2022).

Time spent Scrolling, considered by most as a passive behaviour, emerged as a significant predictor of emotional exhaustion. This concurred with the work of Dhir et al. (2021), who emphasized that passive watching of online content—especially over long durations—has the propensity to exhaust users' psychological energy and vigilance. Long-term exposure to massive digital stimuli with minimal mental effort has been shown to cause mental saturation, a contributor to burnout (Zhou & Wang, 2022). This is supported by the growing interest in "digital overstimulation," a process growing in media psychology.

Moreover, Emotional Burnout also significantly predicted Scroll Fatigue in this study. This path represents a cumulative psychological process whereby emotional exhaustion manifests as a form of cognitive and behavioral symptoms such as reduced attention span, frustration, and detachment upon encountering content (Wang et al., 2023). Scroll Fatigue, conversely, had a strong and significant negative relationship with Mental Well-being. These results validate the hypothesis that continuous digital exposure leads to mental fatigue, which can appear in symptoms like anxiety, insensitivity to emotions, or depression tendencies (Lee et al., 2022).

Interestingly, IME and TSS did not directly affect MWB after adjusting for EB and SF, which indicated a full mediation model. This suggests that the negative effects of online behavior on psychological well-being are neither direct nor linear but function indirectly through intermediate states of emotional and cognitive tension. These findings are congruent with the Differential Susceptibility to Media Effects Model (DSMM), which postulates that media effect is shaped by dispositional, developmental, and social context variables and mediated by affective and cognitive responses (Valkenburg & Peter, 2013).

The importance of the double mediation model—IME → EB → SF → MWB and TSS → EB → SF → MWB—points to the interrelated character of emotional and cognitive processes in the case of digital fatigue. As argued by Oberst et al. (2020), digital engagement is not necessarily a harmful activity, but if connected with emotional exhaustion and passive consumption, it results in weakened well-being. These results are based on the research of Islam et al. (2021), who established that emotional exhaustion moderated the connection between social media usage and mental distress among university students.

The ANOVA analysis also further substantiates that people who spent more than four hours a day on social media had significantly lower scores of mental well-being compared to the less frequent users. Such a dose-response nature corroborates previous evidence highlighting time-based thresholds of digital consumption after which mental health harms start to manifest (Twenge et al., 2018). In addition, the gender-based t-test indicated that female participants had significantly reduced mental well-being compared to males, paralleling earlier research indicating women are more vulnerable to psychological effects of social comparison as well as digital overexposure (Błachnio et al., 2022).

From a practical standpoint, these results underscore the urgent need for targeted mental health interventions. Traditional approaches focusing only on screen-time reduction are inadequate. Instead, programs should aim to build emotional resilience, teach mindful media consumption, and promote digital detox practices. Educators and digital platform designers could collaborate to provide content warnings, usage feedback tools, and burnout prevention resources within apps. Psychological training to recognize and manage symptoms of burnout and fatigue should be prioritized among younger digital users.

In conclusion, this study contributes to the growing body of literature on digital mental health by providing robust empirical evidence of how IME and TSS influence mental well-being indirectly through emotional burnout and scroll fatigue. It validates a fully mediated structural model, emphasizing that the quality and emotional cost of digital interactions matter more than mere time spent online. These insights are especially relevant as society continues to embrace influencer-driven marketing and always-on digital lifestyles. Future research could explore longitudinal effects and intervention-based studies to further examine causality and resilience strategies among digital natives.

CONCLUSION

This study provides insight into psychological effects of influencer marketing and scroll behavior that empirically support dual mediation model with emotional burnout and scroll fatigue.

The disappointments of Generation Z with virtual spaces, such as deeper disappointments regarding human potential to conform to a more digital universe, came after disappointments are mostly deviating from neurosis to influencer-led insecurity. Yet, the knowledge of these issues in this generation provides reasons for hope in positive change. The findings emphasize that excess exposure to influencer marketing contributes to diminishing mental well-being with scroll fatigue as important yet under-leveraged variable.

The solution is not to reject entirely digital technology but to foster reflective, genuine, and psychologically positive ways of engaging with it. This entails collaborative efforts by individuals, communities, technology companies, and policymakers to build digital space that improves, and not lowers, human development.

As Generation Z continues to fascinate with the digital world, their engagement holds a strong potential for greater society to learn. Learning the psycho-social effects of repeated digital exposure and making evidence-based intervention approaches can bring us to the place where technology enhances human well-being instead of undermining it. It's not about staying away from digital interaction but having it occur in a manner that allows for mental well-being, authentic self-expression, and true human connection.

Implications:

For Mental Health Experts:

- There is a critical requirement for well-structured digital literacy detox program for mental well-being, so that Gen Z can handle and oversee with phycological outcomes of influencer marketing.
- Social comparison, self-worth struggles and digital boundaries should be tackled during counselling.

For Educators and Parents:

- They must encourage healthy digital habits by encouraging Gen Z to be cautious of the nuances between curated content and reality.

- Neutralise the consequences of digital sickness by promoting non digital pursuits and emotional resilience.

For Marketers and Influencers:

- They must prioritise ethics, authenticity and transparency during promotions rather than misleading information that leads to unrealistic expectations.
- Encourage socially conscious marketing, where content fosters mental well-being, self-compassion and socially responsible behaviour.

For Platforms and Policymakers:

- Digitals fatigues, screen time reminders, usage analytics should be regularly monitored by social media platforms.
- Ethical and mental health awareness policy should be introduced to create a safe digital space for young generation.

In the rapidly growing digital era, it is critically important to understand the psychological implications of Influencer marketing on young generation. This chapter highlights the nuance relationship between Gen Z social media consumption pattern and their mental wellness that leads to the emerging need of balancing digital ecosystem. There is pressing need to ethically shape the influencer culture and provide a supportive digital ecosystem that promotes mental wellbeing and provide a better and safe place for future generations.

Future Directions:

Future researchers can analyze moderators such as personality traits, digital literacy, cross cultural dimensions, self-management of influencers content which could shield the vulnerable effects of Scroll Fatigue. Cohort studies also have the potential to offer inferences by tracking excessive screen time, screen time break reminders and regular digital detox regimens.

Advancement in this study will not go towards refining theoretical frameworks, but also assists in framing policies and platform level interventions which strives to attain mental well-being from adverse effects of highly dynamic digital setup.

REFERENCES

Andreassen, C. S., Pallesen, S., & Griffiths, M. D. (2017). The relationship between addictive use of social media, narcissism, and self-esteem: Findings from a large national survey. *Addictive Behaviors, 64*, 287–293. DOI: 10.1016/j.addbeh.2016.03.006

Bawden, D., & Robinson, L. (2020). Information overload: An overview. Błachnio, A., Przepiórka, A., & Benvenuti, M. (2022). Social media use and mental health: The role of personality traits, cyberbullying, and emotional intelligence. *Psychiatry Research, 307*, 114340. DOI: 10.1016/j.psychres.2021.114340

Boerman, S. C., & Van Reijmersdal, E. A. (2020). Disclosing influencer marketing on YouTube to children: The moderating role of para-social relationship. *Frontiers in Psychology, 10*, 3042. DOI: 10.3389/fpsyg.2019.03042

Chae, J. (2018). Explaining females' envy toward social media influencers. *Media Psychology, 21*(2), 246–262. DOI: 10.1080/15213269.2017.1328312

de Jans, S., Van de Sompel, D., Hudders, L., & Cauberghe, V. (2023). How young children process influencer marketing: The moderating role of media literacy. *Journal of Advertising, 52*(1), 88–103. DOI: 10.1080/00913367.2023.2172165

De Segovia Vicente, D., Van Gaeveren, K., Murphy, S. L., & Vanden Abeele, M. M. P. (2024). Does mindless scrolling hamper well-being? Combining ESM and log-data to examine the link between mindless scrolling, goal conflict, guilt, and daily well-being. *Journal of Computer-Mediated Communication, 29*(1), zmad056. Advance online publication. DOI: 10.1093/jcmc/zmad056

De Veirman, M., Cauberghe, V., & Hudders, L. (2017). Marketing through Instagram influencers: The impact of number of followers and product divergence on brand attitude. *International Journal of Advertising, 36*(5), 798–828. DOI: 10.1080/02650487.2017.1348035

Dhir, A., Yossatorn, Y., Kaur, P., & Chen, S. (2018). Online social media fatigue and psychological well-being—A study of compulsive use, fear of missing out, and fatigue. *International Journal of Information Management, 40*, 141–152. DOI: 10.1016/j.ijinfomgt.2018.01.012

Dhir, A., Yossatorn, Y., Kaur, P., & Chen, S. (2021). Online social media fatigue and psychological well-being—A study of compulsive use, fear of missing out, and gender differences. *International Journal of Information Management, 61*, 102255. DOI: 10.1016/j.ijinfomgt.2021.102255

Fardouly, J., & Vartanian, L. R. (2016). Social media and body image concerns: Current research and future directions. *Current Opinion in Psychology*, *9*, 1–5. DOI: 10.1016/j.copsyc.2015.09.005

Fernandes, T. (2024). Brands as drivers of social media fatigue and its impact on user engagement. *Young Consumers*, *25*(5), 625–642. DOI: 10.1108/YC-11-2023-1763

Ha, L., & Yang, Y. (2023). Research about persuasive effects of social media influencers as online opinion leaders 1990–2020: A review. *International Journal of Internet Marketing and Advertising*, *18*(2–3), 220–241. DOI: 10.1504/IJIMA.2023.132562

Hayes, A. F. (2018). *Introduction to mediation, moderation, and conditional process analysis: A regression-based approach* (2nd ed.). Guilford Press.

Jennings, R. (2020, July 10). *Doom-scrolling, explained.* Vox. https://www.vox.com/the-goods/21547961/doom-scrolling-meaning-definition-what-is-meme

Keles, B., McCrae, N., & Grealish, A. (2020). A systematic review: The influence of social media on depression, anxiety and psychological distress in adolescents. *International Journal of Adolescence and Youth*, *25*(1), 79–93. DOI: 10.1080/02673843.2019.1590851

Lee, J., Wood, E., Vogel, N., Santhosh, E., & Chauhan, P. K. (2023). Burn or balm? Exploring university students' experiences with social media during the COVID-19 pandemic. *Frontiers in Psychology*, *14*, 1018334. DOI: 10.3389/fpsyg.2023.1018334

Lee, Y., Lin, H., & Huang, H. (2022). Examining the effects of digital fatigue on mental health and academic performance. *Journal of Educational Technology & Society*, *25*(2), 104–116. https://www.jstor.org/stable/48635645

Lora, A., Purba, J. T., Hossain, M. S., Oriana, F., & Seum, C. (2024). The psychological consequences of infinite scrolling: Examining digital fatigue and emotional well-being. *Computers in Human Behavior*, *152*, 108123. DOI: 10.1016/j.chb.2023.108123

Lou, C., & Yuan, S. (2019). Influencer marketing: How message value and credibility affect consumer trust of branded content on social media. *Journal of Interactive Advertising*, *19*(1), 58–73. DOI: 10.1080/15252019.2018.1533501

Malik, A., Dhir, A., Kaur, P., & Johri, A. (2021). Correlates of social media fatigue and academic performance decrement: A large cross-sectional study. *Information Technology & People*, *34*(2), 557–580. DOI: 10.1108/ITP-06-2019-0289

Marengo, D., Sindermann, C., Elhai, J. D., & Montag, C. (2022). The association between the Big Five personality traits and smartphone use disorder: A meta-analysis. *Journal of Behavioral Addictions*, *11*(1), 77–93. DOI: 10.1556/2006.2021.00086

Maslach, C., & Leiter, M. P. (2016). Understanding the burnout experience: Recent research and its implications for psychiatry. *World Psychiatry; Official Journal of the World Psychiatric Association (WPA)*, *15*(2), 103–111. DOI: 10.1002/wps.20311

McComb, C. A., Vanman, E. J., & Tobin, S. J. (2023). A meta-analysis of the effects of social media exposure to upward comparison targets on self-evaluations and emotions. *Media Psychology*, *26*(5), 612–635. DOI: 10.1080/15213269.2023.2180647

Meinhardt, C., Rajapaksha, D., Oliveira, D. R., & Gultepe, A. (2025). *Scrolling in the deep: Analysing contextual influences on intervention effectiveness during infinite scrolling on social media*. arXiv. https://arxiv.org/abs/2501.11814

Mladenovic, A., Maricic, M., & Ciric, M. (2022). Scroll fatigue and digital well-being: Exploring compulsive browsing behaviors. *Computers in Human Behavior*, *135*, 107373. DOI: 10.1016/j.chb.2022.107373

Montag, C., Wegmann, E., Sariyska, R., & Brand, M. (2021). How to overcome taxonomical problems in the study of internet use disorders and what to do with 'smartphone addiction'? *Journal of Behavioral Addictions*, *10*(1), 1–7. DOI: 10.1556/2006.8.2019.59

Oberst, U., Wegmann, E., Stodt, B., Brand, M., & Chamarro, A. (2020). Negative consequences from heavy social networking in adolescents: The mediating role of fear of missing out. *Journal of Adolescence*, *55*, 51–60. DOI: 10.1016/j.adolescence.2017.11.003

Pacewicz, C. E., & Mellano, K. (2024). The Toll of the Scroll: A Path Toward Burnout. *Psychology of Sport and Exercise*, *74*, 102681. DOI: 10.1016/j.psychsport.2024.102681

Przybylski, A. K., Murayama, K., DeHaan, C. R., & Gladwell, V. (2013). Motivational, emotional, and behavioral correlates of fear of missing out. *Computers in Human Behavior*, *29*(4), 1841–1848. DOI: 10.1016/j.chb.2013.02.014

Scott, H., & Woods, H. C. (2019). Understanding links between social media use, sleep, and mental health. *Sleep Medicine Reviews*, *44*, 1–12. DOI: 10.1016/j.smrv.2018.01.008

Sonnentag, S. (2018). The recovery process: Sleep and recovery. In R. J. Burke & K. M. Page (Eds.), Research handbook on work and well-being (pp. 144–157). Edward Elgar.

Supriyadi, Sulistiasih, Rahmi, Pramono, & Fahrudin. (2025). The impact of digital fatigue on employee productivity and well-being: A scoping literature review. DOI: 10.59429/esp.v10i2.3420

Twenge, J. M., Joiner, T. E., Rogers, M. L., & Martin, G. N. (2018). Increases in depressive symptoms, suicide-related outcomes, and suicide rates among U.S. adolescents after 2010 and links to increased new media screen time. *Clinical Psychological Science*, *6*(1), 3–17. DOI: 10.1177/2167702617723376

Twenge, J. M., Martin, G. N., & Spitzberg, B. H. (2019). Trends in U.S. adolescents' media use and associations with mental health. *Journal of Adolescence*, *79*, 1–13. DOI: 10.1016/j.adolescence.2019.12.018

Valkenburg, P. M., & Peter, J. (2013). The differential susceptibility to media effects model. *Journal of Communication*, *63*(2), 221–243. DOI: 10.1111/jcom.12024

Vogel, E. A., Rose, J. P., Roberts, L. R., & Eckles, K. (2014). Social comparison, social media, and self-esteem. *Psychology of Popular Media Culture*, *3*(4), 206–222. DOI: 10.1037/ppm0000037

Wang, Y., Zhu, X., & Li, J. (2023). Passive social media use and mental health: A systematic review and meta-analysis. *Cyberpsychology, Behavior, and Social Networking*, *26*(2), 79–87. DOI: 10.1089/cyber.2022.0061

Wu, Y., Wei, Y., Li, Y., Pang, J., & Su, Y. (2022). Burnout, negative emotions, and wellbeing among social workers in China after community lockdowns during the COVID-19 pandemic: Mediating roles of trait mindfulness. Frontiers in Public Health, 10, 952269.

Zhou, Y., & Wang, Z. (2022). Digital fatigue: Psychological antecedents and behavioral consequences. *Journal of Consumer Psychology*, *32*(1), 50–67. DOI: 10.1002/jcpy.1245

Chapter 13
The Perfect Me Trap: How Performance and Passivity Fuel Gen Z's Inner Crisis

Obioma Kingsley Anyanwu
https://orcid.org/0009-0003-8764-3403
GBS Malta, Malta

ABSTRACT

This chapter examines the cultural pressures of Generation Z from the viewpoint called the perfect me trap, a two-dimensional pressure of performance (unending self-curation) and passivity (endless algorithm-driven consumption of content), which define Gen Z's digital culture. It draws from peer-reviewed research, ethnographic studies, and cultural commentary to explore how performance imperatives fuel perfectionism, identity fragmentation, and the commercialization of authenticity, while passive scrolling drives overstimulation, disengagement, and isolation. The analysis integrates frameworks, like social comparison, the pursuit of attention and validation, and the need for self-determination, to reveal the psychological drivers of the performance, and the pull of social platform designs, algorithmic authority, and emotional disengagement to explore the slide into passivity. With emerging strategies, the chapter concludes by foregrounding the need for intentional authenticity and embracing human imperfections as deliberate shifts that are possible.

1.0. A SPLIT-SCREEN GENERATION

Lying in her bed, phone in hand, Tenenbaum, 19, hovers her thumbs and then continues scrolling. It is almost 1:30 am, and her eyes blur as reels autoplay endlessly, one after the other: beachfront selfies, sunsets, glow-up tips, boat cruise captures, outfits, relationship breakdowns, red pill ideologies, health tips, lighthearted content,

DOI: 10.4018/979-8-3373-4516-1.ch013

and other algorithmically boosted pseudo-expertise. She does not actively search for them; they find her. Her body is still, but her mind is buzzing, overstimulated, and unsettled. She knows she should sleep, but does not want to miss something.

Meanwhile, a few hours earlier, Tenenbaum had posted a carefully edited carousel, featuring a "soft life" mini-vacation trip with shopping, spas, fresh manicures, new boots, and rooftop brunches. In creating her carousel, she spent 2 hours and 45 minutes choosing between 92 photos. For each picture, she zoomed in on her face in one shot, detected a blemish, and immediately deleted it. Then she finds a perfect one, but discovers she already wore the same outfit in a previous post. Concurrently, in her head, she is composing a caption that portrays a spontaneous yet not desperate, happy yet not boastful tone. She eventually selects a photo, edits it using two different apps, and finally posts it across her social media feeds. Then the countdown began: comments, likes, reposts, and impressions. Her online persona feels like a performance rather than a memory worth holding. While offline, she is worn out, passive, and has spent valuable time crafting a 'perfect me' online.

This trajectory is not unusual. Like millions of Gen Z users, Tenenbaum finds herself in the dilemma of trying to strike a balance between being active in her digital life and passive in her real life. One moment, she is the curator of her identity; the next, she is a passive consumer in a sea of infinite content. The problem is not that she is online; the problem is how her constant online presence shapes her.

1.1. INTRODUCTION

Previous works in media studies, psychology, cultural sociology, and gender studies have examined and illustrated the concept of *the perfect me* as typically associated with female beauty culture. In feminist media and cultural studies (McRobbie, 2009; Viţelar, 2019), much emphasis has been placed on how beauty ideals and lifestyle expectations are perpetuated through visual and virtual media, with young women as the primary target. Although some studies within the psychology domain remain female-centric, such as (Roberts, Maheux, Ladd, & Choukas-Bradley, 2022), others, like (Kholmogorova, Tarhanova, & Shalygina, 2018; Potts & Stebleton, 2023), recognize that beauty and attractiveness ideals impose considerable pressures across genders and that the impact of these ideals on identity formation, self-esteem, and mental health cuts across gender lines, albeit often with greater severity for females.

In this chapter, I introduce the term "Perfect Me Trap" to scholarly discourse as a digital identity loop in which Gen Z individuals (both male and female) live under pressure from the demands of visually and virtually attractive versions of themselves. The experience is two-dimensional: first, the need to constantly *perform* and fit into an idealized image, and second, the slide into *passive* online content consumption. This dual concept is not new. Foucault and colleagues use the technology of the self to define the first loop. The authors argued that people undertake operations on themselves to achieve self-transformation (Foucault et al., 1988). On the other hand, Debord (1967) asserted that real life engagement is being displaced by representation. These two frameworks resonate with Gen Z's culture of performance (curation) and passivity (doomscrolling), where identity is increasingly formed through engagement without presence.

As of 2025, Gen Z refers to individuals between the ages of 13 and 28, specifically the demographic cohort born between 1997 and 2012. Because they are the first generation born into the digital saturation era, they have never known a world without connectivity, screens, or a demand for content. This demographic is more accustomed to spending more time in solitude; they prefer to stay online and connected to different platforms rather than engaging in in-person interactions. As the first true digital natives, they primarily depend on digital platforms for news and updates, bypassing traditional news media. The Pew Research Center surveyed 1,391 U.S. youths aged 13 to 17 in 2024 and found that 95% of the youths (all Gen Zs) had access to cellphones in their different homes. 45% of the group agreed that they had been spending too much time on the phone. This highlights what Gen Z interprets as connectivity, as 74% said they felt more connected with their phone than in person. 63% said they used social media to express themselves creatively, highlighting the performance trap. When the youths were asked about the state of their mental health, 19% of the sample GenZs said social media impairs their mental health, and 20% said it hurts their self-confidence (Pew Research Center, 2024). Similarly, a health management firm conducted a more recent poll and found that 78% of 1,000 Gen Z individuals felt hooked to their cellphones (Harmony Healthcare IT, 2025).

Constant access to information, social networking, and online entertainment undoubtedly come with many benefits; however, studies have associated constant connectivity with high risks of mental health concerns in Gen Z, including depression, anxiety, sleep disruption, and signs of technology overuse (Park, Do, Yourell, Hermer, & Huberty, 2024). Similarly, a report on the American Psychological Association website documented that it is more likely for Gen Zs to report mental health crises when compared to other previous generations (Bethune, 2019). These reports of mental health issues and challenges among Gen Z cannot be understood in isolation from the digital environments that shape their lives. This demographic is caught between the compulsions to deliver content and silently consuming it, increasingly occupying a space of digital hyperpresence, which results in physical and sometimes emotional withdrawal.

The following sections will explore the twin pressures in detail; first, I examine the performance of the curated self, then the slide into the passive consumption loop, and finally, how these forces intertwine to create an inner crisis for the Gen Z demographic.

2.0. THE PRESSURE TO PERFORM IN A CURATED WORLD

A defining historical context, like all previous cohorts, shapes Gen Z. It is often cited that this era began in 1997 (Park et al., 2024). At that time, approximately 80 million people worldwide were using the internet. At the time, not many families had access to personal computers and the internet. By 2011, when the eldest members of Generation Z were in their mid-teens, the number of individuals using the internet had grown to more than 2.3 billion, or over 30% of the world's population (Internet World Stats, 2023). They are a generation that has always lived with connectivity; their level of digital immersion cannot be compared to that of any other generation before them (Sharma et al., 2023). This reality is evident because, for Gen Z, interactions, entertainment, information sharing, and communication are all integral parts of the complex social media landscape. Some scholars have questioned the pros and cons of this generation's use of social media because of how they engage with it. Although research indicates that social media can enhance creativity and connection (Pichler, Kohli, & Granitz, 2021), privacy and mental health concerns are among the potential downsides (Orben & Przybylski, 2019).

As evidenced in a recent report by the consumer research group Attest (2025), Gen Z's use of social media has increased over the years. Attest reported that 81% of Gen Zs spend more than an hour daily on social media, with about 60% reporting over three hours daily. The same report shows that GenZs generally rely on social media for different needs, with 40% using it as their trusted means of staying informed. In contrast, others are drawn to other features of their preferred platforms. Their engagement is high and sustained across different platforms according to their preferred features, which suggests dependency or behavioral patterns in some cases (Attest, 2025).

A non-random sample survey was conducted with 415 students at the State University of New York at Oneonta during the 2017-2018 academic year. The findings indicated that nearly all Gen Z individuals (99%) possess a smartphone, and 98% predominantly utilize their handsets for Internet connectivity. Over fifty percent of Generation Z individuals utilize their smartphones for nine hours or more daily, while nearly fifty percent use their devices for three to eight hours daily. Regarding social media usage, over 50% of Gen Z individuals engage with various platforms multiple times a day, while more than one in five acknowledge using social media hourly. Approximately one-third of the students acknowledged spending 7-10 hours daily on social media, while just under one-third reported using social media for 5 to 6 hours daily. When asked about the extent to which members of Generation Z are aware of their reliance on cellphones and social media, 80% of students admitted to using the internet excessively, and 63% reported spending too much time on social media.

Furthermore, almost two-thirds of students felt they were addicted to social media, and 70% admitted to being addicted to the internet. These studies show that many Gen Z individuals struggle to manage their online engagement. Ahmed (2019) views this situation as one that necessitates interventions, such as counselling, by parents and teachers. Being online always means they are shaped by the content they consume from other content creators.

3.0. PERFORMING THE CURATED SELF

For many adolescents, posting on social media is not just a passive activity; it is also a way to reminisce about memorable events. It is a meticulously planned ritual, targeted, and designed to fit into a specific version of themselves that exists only in their digital space. This process is premeditated, involving an underlying calculation: *How will this be perceived?* Sometimes, with specific individuals or a targeted audience in mind. Whether it is a selfie on Instagram, a TikTok dance, or a carefully worded post, there is an ever-present awareness that digital visibility equals social value, *but what drives this impulse to be seen, validated, and affirmed online?* From impression management and social comparison to validation-seeking and fear of exclusion, strong psychological mechanisms underpin these behaviors. To further understand the psychological drivers that compel Gen Z into the *perfect me trap*, I explore how social comparison, and related pressures sustain their on-going performance loop.

3.1. Social Comparison and the Urge to Keep Up

The social comparison theory, developed by Festinger (1954), suggests that people tend to evaluate themselves based on what they observe in others. This theory is highly relevant in the age of social media, where it is a common practice to compare oneself to others based on physical appearance, weight, wealth, social class, and the traits observed in others. The phrase "keeping up with the Joneses" illustrates social comparison theory, wherein individuals strive to maintain parity with their perceived neighbors in terms of wealth and visual appearance. Most social media platforms exacerbate this reality by creating feeds of peer highlights, photos of achievements, polished appearances, or outings, which become fertile ground for many Gen Z individuals to compare themselves to these algorithmically selected influencers who are perceived as being better off.

Unlike the previous generations, Gen Z has been immersed in a connected world since birth. However, the convenience of constantly being online have also introduced complex personal and social struggles associated with overexposure;

scrolling through online friends' and influencers' reels that capture their best moments and portray idealized realities which only focuses on the positive and enviable aspects of their lives and looks, would leave the consumer of those reels miserable, believing that their peers are more popular, or more successful than themselves. On many occasions, this situation has spurred many Gen Zers into the race to keep up, fueling the pressure to post equally exhilarating and attractive content to retain their relevance in the social space.

Theoretically, a growing body of researchers (e.g., Chou & Edge, 2012; Sagioglou & Greitemeyer, 2014; Sharifian, Zaheed, & Zahodne, 2022; Meier & Johnson, 2022; Taylor & Armes, 2024; Fassi et al., 2025) who have examined social media through the lens of social comparison underscore the adverse emotional and mental impact of engaging in social comparison on social media. They indicate that passive scrolling and engagement with social media have been demonstrated to impact the well-being of young people, Gen Z. This is likely because individuals use platforms like Instagram and TikTok to share mostly favorable or positive versions of themselves, thereby curating a more controlled and favorable self-image online, this is referred to as positive self-esteem presentation (Zhao, Grasmuck, & Marti, 2008). The creator's reality is often misrepresented by the exclusive dissemination of good content online. It has also been observed that numerous photos shared on social media are edited using image filter software to conform to prevailing beauty standards. Hence, a typical passive consumer's perusal of other people's positive posts creates an environment ripe with upward social comparisons, often leaving users feeling inferior and envious. This envy-fueled behavior has also been linked to declines in mood and self-esteem (Sagioglou & Greitmeyer, 2014), which, over time, often leads to diminished satisfaction with oneself and/or one's condition.

On the other hand, not all comparisons are bad; occasionally, seeing how well others are doing can be motivating or helpful. However, the balance is fragile. Hjetland et al. (2022) found in a recent study that examining one's profile (comparing oneself to a perfect version of another, as constructed on social media) can temporarily improve a person's mood and make them feel better. However, this impact is most effective when the online self-image is accurate; it can backfire if it is overly unrealistic. Social comparison is a big part of Gen Z's social media experience. The need to keep up with their peers can affect why and how they share. It also has to do with managing impressions: when teens see other people's highlights, they want to do the same thing, creating a cycle where everyone shows an edited version of their lives and feels compelled to do the same.

3.2. The Pursuit of Attention and Validation

Many social media users, including Gen Z, equate visibility to validation, and the design of platforms like Instagram and TikTok converts social reactions and feedback into quantifiable reward metrics (likes, views, and shares) that act as social currency. These metrics tap into the basic reward circuitry of the brain as a form of social currency, causing people with high numbers to assume a superior sense of self-worth and validation. In neuroscientific research, Sherman et al. (2016) demonstrated that when adolescents observed posts (their own or others') with high like counts, their nucleus accumbens and ventral striatum showed significantly increased activation. Likewise, when viewing a popular image with multiple likes, they showed heightened activation in dopamine-related brain regions, notably the nucleus accumbens, a hub of reward processing (Sherman et al., 2018). They become more likely to hit the like button as a result. These findings suggest that adolescents' brains respond to likes the same way they would respond to a rewarding impulse or stimulus. Neurologically, social endorsement feels rewarding. Positive rewards become reinforcements that motivate Gen Z to seek another reward, reinforcing the circle of posting content that will generate the same positive attention and social endorsement. It is a dopamine-driven feedback loop in the order: *post something get notifications of approval feel a boost, which encourages further posting.*

The psychological need for validation so often emerges as a conscious pursuit. This desire is exemplified by the Gen Z users who tailor their online behavior to attract traffic. For instance, adolescents schedule their uploads to coincide with peak periods when their followers are mostly online, or they use trendy hashtags or participate in challenges on TikTok to improve their chances of visibility.

People may feel embarrassed or disappointed if their post fails to receive enough likes quickly, so they delete it. As a result, people could see the lack of expected validation as a failure. This is supported by empirical research: if a teenager does not receive as many likes as they were hoping for, it can lower their self-esteem and make them feel neglected or excluded by their friends (Dores, Peixoto, Fernandes, & Marques, 2025). Similarly, suppose a post does not receive enough likes within a specified time frame. In that case, it can be deleted, leaving the user feeling like a public failure because they did not receive the validation they hoped for. On the other hand, receiving numerous likes or comments that people enjoy can be a great way to boost your self-esteem and validate your ego. Studies have shown that when people give teenagers positive feedback on social media, it makes them feel more confident and valued. Because members of Generation Z's offline and online social lives are so intertwined, this is particularly relevant to them. Adolescents constantly compare themselves to one another based on app popularity data, which are public indicators of social achievement. For whatever reason, many followers or views are often mistaken for approval from one's peers. So, they believe that visibility provides worth; some would take extreme measures to increase these numbers, which can suggest a sense of desperation.

To make matters worse, today's social media platforms are designed to promote the attention economy. For example, TikTok's design has a memetic logic that promotes copying and duplication while minimizing individual identities and social connections (Liang, 2022). This attractive opportunity fosters continuous content creation and engagement. Going viral is a buzzword among Gen Z creators on various platforms, and these platforms offer unique architectural designs that compel their users to stay engaged: performing popular dances, replicating viral formats, or utilizing viral sounds to capitalize on the algorithm's momentum. This reflects an understanding that the system rewards conformity to trends with attention and traffic. For example, on the Snapchat platform, a feature called Snapstreaks uses a gamified mode to display the number of days one has exchanged snaps with a contact. To maintain a Snapchat Streak, two individuals must exchange snaps daily; otherwise, the streak will be lost. This game, which initially appears harmless, quickly becomes an obligation, keeping young people glued to their screens out of fear of missing out. People fear losing a streak on Snapchat, but also fear what it can mean: losing a connection or slipping out of the social loop.

3.3. The Need for Self-Determination

Self-determination theory (SDT), initially developed by Ryan and Deci (2000, 2019) has come up in various fields of study, such as education (Yang, Chen, & Zhuang, 2025), organizational psychology (Deci, Olafsen, & Ryan, 2017), parenting (Wei, Teo, Malpique, & Lause, 2022), and health care (van Dorssen-Boog et al., 2021), due to its strong empirical foundation and widespread validation across disciplines. The global applicability and high translational value of SDT as a development, motivation, and well-being theory have been confirmed via considerable research (Ryan et al., 2021). A growing body of research suggests that SDT can help us understand the effects of social media on people's mental health and well-being. This explains why the Digital Flourishing Scale is built on SDT as its foundational architecture (Rosič et al., 2022; Janicke-Bowles et al., 2023). Gudka and colleagues systematically examined how social media can increase thriving for individuals across a wide age range (Gudka, Gardiner, & Loma, 2023). The review used a positive psychology framework, which included SDT, to support its findings. The three identifiable needs of SDT — relatedness, autonomy, and competence — operate on social platforms such as Instagram, TikTok, and Snapchat. For a Gen Z demographic that lives online, social media has become the most potent arena for meeting these needs. Now, we examine how these platforms impact the three psychological needs of relatedness, autonomy, and competence.

3.3.1. Relatedness (Belonging and Connection)

Social media plays a dual role in relatedness, as it can support or thwart its advancement. The need to connect to others and belong to various social networking groups acts as a driving force for Gen Z. Many studies (e.g., Valkenburg & Peter, 2009; MacIsaac, Kelly, & Gra, 2018; Huan, 2021) suggest that social media use can deepen relationships and increase the quality of friendships, which translates to bonding social capital. Posting content and getting feedback can foster a sense of visibility and approval, providing an antidote for loneliness, particularly for those who feel isolated in their immediate environment, helping them to discover supportive networks who relate to their exact situations (for example, LGBTQ+ youth finding accepting peers online). Exchanges of messages, as well as between friends, could satisfy this need for relatedness. Hence, social media engagement helps fight the feeling of social isolation among the youth and can provide a valued sense of inclusion.

Although social media can enhance relatedness, research also reveals some harmful aspects associated with using these platforms. Self-reported data from 320 children aged 12–17 (all Generation Z) were gathered about the frequency of online gaming and social media usage, depression, life satisfaction, and the quality of relationships with parents, instructors, and classmates, as documented by Dredge & Che (2020). The researchers found that adolescents who spent most time online exhibited higher levels of depression, utilized social media and the internet more frequently and in distinct manners, and encountered more adverse interactions with parents and peers in comparison to non-users.

So, while social media is a great way to meet the need for connection, bonding, and support, it may also exacerbate that need if the feedback or interaction is not satisfactory or turns hostile (as with cyberbullying or peer drama).

3.3.2. Autonomy (Control and Self-Expression)

Autonomy means feeling in control of one's actions and true to oneself. According to research, Gen Z's need for autonomy can be fulfilled or suppressed by their engagement with social media (Chiang & Lin, 2010; Yang et al, 2021). They appreciate the ability to build a profile that reflects their ideal selves, whether aspirational (e.g., showcasing talents, fashion, humor) or genuine. Like the other drivers of performance, social media platforms are also designed to encourage autonomy; they offer tools for profile customization, privacy settings that control audience, and the personalization of content. It grants adolescents autonomy to determine their public comportment, create their identity, and choose their associations. It is a personal publishing platform where users choose what to share, how to present it, and the associations to maintain. These affordances contribute in diverse ways to keep the youths on their screens longer. According to studies, teens who spend time on social media develop a stronger sense of self-reliance and individuality (Reich, Subrahmanyam, & Espinoza, 2012). Creating and honing one's digital identity can help individuals feel more in control of their lives; it is up to them to decide who they are online. They also access information, contribute to trending political, cultural, or economic matters, and share their opinions widely. The ability to effect change or gain recognition as someone who can speak to important matters contributes to the feeling of autonomy and influence.

Conversely, autonomy can be compromised when teens are compelled to conform to certain online norms, social trends, and peer expectations. Being authentic and fitting in with cultural expectations for how children should behave online are often at odds with each other. For example, some children feel they "have to" disclose certain things to be relevant, while others fear judgment and avoid sharing aspects of themselves. In contrast to other generations, members of Generation Z believe that traditional social settings are less welcoming to uniqueness and expression than online networks. A shy teen, for instance, could find a safe space to express herself on a blog or join interest-based online communities. Social media offers a platform for individuals to express themselves, take ownership of their creativity, and explore the various roles they play in society. It can be powerful when people do these things for reasons other than seeking approval from others.

3.3.3. Competence

Every motivational theory in psychology emphasizes perceived competence as a central role in behaviours (Ryan & Moller, 2017). Gen Zs want to be perceived as competent by their peers, followers, and subscribers. This desire becomes the center of what drives their online action, as they strive to build an identity that people perceive as competent, even if this is not true. The ambition and anxiety over their performance intensify and are influenced by social comparison mechanisms that require constant assessment of their significance and competence in relation to others' curated achievements (West, Rice, & Vella-Brodrick, 2024). According to Ryan & Moller (2017), being perceived as competent motivates people to learn and engage in behaviors that are motivating. Gen Zers become more motivated to share peer engagement, express their views, cultivate skills in content creation for improved proficiency, and stay continually present for their audience (Li an, 2025; West et al., 2024).

One may draw inspiration for self-improvement from comparisons with others or continue in self-doubt. Seeking the approval of others may have adverse effects on relationships and self-esteem, but it can also benefit them if done in moderation. We may gain a better understanding of their online conduct by clarifying our view-points on basic desires, social comparison, and self-presentation theories. Every like, share, and story is a small act of self-expression driven by the fundamental need for acceptance, validation, and understanding in a rapidly changing social environment.

4.0. THE SLIDE INTO PASSIVE CONSUMPTION

As the need to maintain a polished online presence grows, many Gen Zers also slip into a passive mode of doomscrolling, where they discreetly consume other people's content and withdraw from their immediate social surroundings. This slide in the digital pendulum reveals the second layer of the perfect me trap. Here, I explore the passive consumption loop and how Overstimulation, algorithmic absorption, and the fatigue of constantly comparing oneself to others slowly erode freedom, making young people feel detached from others and themselves.

4.1. The Pull of Platform Design

In his words, Tim Berners-Lee, best known as the inventor of the World Wide Web, said, *"The Web is more a social creation than a technical one. I designed it to help people work together for a social effect, not as a technical toy. The goal of the Web is to support and improve our weblike existence in the world. We clump into families, associations, and companies. We develop trust across the miles and distrust around the corner. What we believe, endorse, agree with, and depend on is representable and, increasingly, represented on the Web. We must ensure that the society we build with the Web is the sort we intend (Berners-Lee, 1999)."*

This is the principle upon which most successful software is built. They are designed based on human psychology. Therefore, design professionals aim to enable users to engage in their preferred activities both offline and online. When you think of features like autoplay videos, unending video clips, and content, they force their users to stay hooked to their devices, limiting the pauses and stops that should naturally happen after watching a video. This software design approach keeps consumers passive by reducing effort. Algorithmic curation significantly amplifies this effect. For instance, TikTok's "For You" page and Instagram's "Explore" page provide users with an incessant flow of content tailored to their preferences.

4.2. Cognitive Overload and Fragmented Attention

Passive scrolling presents a tremendous amount of information and stimulation on display, sometimes more quickly than younger brains, such as those in Gen Z, can process. This may cause cognitive overload when the brain gets too many conflicting signals. Studies show that many young people who use social media are likely to feel overwhelmed by the constant stream of postings, updates, and ads (Sharma, Deepak, & Sudhanshu, 2023). One result is that attention becomes split, reducing the ability to focus because of the continuous change of subject by feeds. Sharma and colleagues (2023) argue that using social media often might make it harder to pay attention and focus on longer, more challenging tasks. A commentary by Rusida (2024) suggests that most Gen Z users utilize more than one app at a time, making it even more challenging to maintain focus. In school, this manifests as being easily distracted and impatient with work that progresses too slowly (Nussenbaum, 2023).

When the brain is inundated with updates, it has difficulty committing new knowledge to long-term memory and recalling details accurately. A sensation of mental fatigue and mental dispersion characterizes the total cognitive toll. Gen Z users may browse for hours and then feel cognitively fatigued, unable to recall much of what they saw, and yet, strangely, they want more stimulation. This cycle of thoughtless consumption and broken attention shows how passive consumption affects cognitive ability and concentration (Sharma, Deepak, & Sudhanshu, 2023)

4.3. Overstimulation and Emotional Disengagement

According to Alter (2017), feed driven by algorithms impairs attention span, cognitive control, and even the ability to feel emotions because of their addictive behavioral nature. Similarly, a recent empirical study found that unending scroll interfaces increase cognitive dissociation and impair memory and emotional engagement (Ruiz, Molina Leon, & Heuer, 2024). The user assumes the role of a bystander in passive consumption mode, mindlessly scrolling through the lives of others, carefully selected photos, and algorithm-generated content. As a result, viewers may feel emotionally detached or numb when exposed to the information. Users transition from a sad news video to a humorous film to an influencer's perfectly staged selfie in a matter of minutes—very little time to process any of it emotionally. Researchers in psychology have shown that the constant switching between different types of content—common in infinite scroll designs—may reduce users' ability to fully engage emotionally with any one stimulus (Alter, 2017; Ruiz, Molina León, &

Heuer, 2024). This often results in what some describe as "doomscrolling weariness," where emotionally intense content begins to feel flat or numbing.

Sharma, Deepak, and Sudhanshu (2023) linked oversaturation to the growing indifference and lurking behaviour of consuming without reacting. According to recent research conducted by Bournemouth University (2023), young individuals who mostly use social media as observers tend to experience higher levels of loneliness, anxiety, and depression. Gen Z is often left feeling emotionally overcharged yet undernourished, as they are constantly inundated with triggers for their emotions, but end up feeling empty or distant due to their addiction to ceaseless scrolling. The inability to respond deeply to such fast stimuli leads to emotional disengagement, which encourages more consumption (users return to the feed for another emotional hit) due to the sensation of "nothing" evoked by each post. Hence, Overstimulation and numbness perpetuate one another in an endless loop (De et al, 2025).

4.4. Algorithmic Authority

One aspect of passive consumption that is often overlooked is the quiet yet powerful influence of algorithms in shaping users' identities, preferences, and sense of social value. Gen Z has grown up under the influence of algorithmic curation, where what they see online is primarily determined by recommendation systems on various platforms. GenZs, mostly in their youth, can easily lose their independence as the algorithm continuously recommends what they consume. Scholars describe an emerging "algorithmic self," in which personal tastes, opinions, and even self-concepts are co-constructed by AI-driven feeds (Josep, 2025). Algorithms do not only reflect neutrality; they actively shape identities by determining which ideas, aesthetics, and values dominate attention (Josep, 2025).

TikTok's sophisticated "For You Page" algorithm rapidly adapts to a user's viewing preferences and amplifies specific interests or perspectives by presenting similar content. Over time, this creates a feedback loop: if a user spends extended time on fitness videos, the algorithm will provide further material from hyper-fit influencers, possibly altering the user's perceptions of body image or "perfection". The user's perceived social value may become tied to what the algorithm promotes (trending fashions, viral opinions, etc.), subtly directing their aspirations. Research in media psychology has found that because social media feeds are *highly personalized*, they shape how people perceive themselves and others by implicitly conveying what is considered normal, desirable, and worthy of attention (Ionescu & Licu, 2023). The algorithm establishes itself as an expert on societal norms and personal preferences. Gen Z's substantial dependence on algorithm-driven discovery, rather than proactively seeking knowledge or broadening their media consumption, amplifies this impact.

5.0. PERFORMANCE VS PASSIVITY

In the age of Instagram highlight reels and TikTok virality, young people experience an implicit obligation to construct an idealized online persona. Individuals strive to create impeccable digital identities; nonetheless, many feel a sense of emptiness, fatigue, or disconnection from their authentic selves behind the screens. Healey (2025) critiques the influence of social media on self-perception, noting that "the modern experience is one of constantly being perceived. We view ourselves as an entity to be managed in the third person." Each photograph, status update, or narrative is meticulously curated based on the anticipated reception by an unseen audience of acquaintances and strangers. This performative norm fosters continuous self-awareness, instilling the notion that one must continually improve and oversee every aspect of life for public display (Healey, 2025). In the social context, the attention economy of platforms favors perfection: the most impeccable faces, idyllic vacations, and successes get the likes. Watching these regulated lifestyles, adolescents instinctively compare themselves and absorb unattainable ideals. Seventeen-year-old Laura confesses, "I peruse idealized lives while I ponder whether I am sufficient," illustrating how each internet encounter might undermine her self-esteem (McGuire, 2023). The likes, comments, and shares become a scoreboard for self-esteem – "the more we get, the more validated we feel"; when the numbers drop, "we feel we are falling short. It is exhausting."

Psychologists see that these processes exacerbate traditional teenage concerns around identity and acceptability. Generation Z is maturing in a digital environment that distorts reality, where the distinction between actual existence and digital identity becomes ambiguous, rendering mere existence inadequate (Singh, 2025). In Eriksonian terminology, the challenge of identity formation, already complex during adolescence and early adulthood, is further exacerbated by the ongoing need to present an identity to an audience. Almost enough never suffices (Erikson, 1968; Marcia, 1966). A 16-year-old nowadays perceives the need to achieve academic excellence, maintain social awareness and "wokeness," exhibit mental resilience, and consistently seem camera-ready (Singh, 2025). Perfectionism encompasses all domains, including appearance, academic performance, politics, and personality. One piece highlights a "silent epidemic" among Gen Z youngsters, who are "fatigued by the imperative to 'be more'" (Singh, 2025). They openly support mental health and being real, but inwardly they struggle with the weight of perfectionism (Singh, 2025).

On the other hand, many Gen Z kids are becoming less active and burned out because they are always performing. Psychologically, the human mind cannot sustain constant vigilance. After endless days of managing their "brand" and monitoring peers' highlight reels, many young people slip into periods of emotional disengagement, a kind of digital fatigue. Gen Z has been described as the most connected yet mentally drained generation. "Some days I feel like I am already burnt out. Not because I do too much, but because my mind never gets a break," Laura, 17, confesses bluntly (McGuire, 2023). Many of her peers share the same sentiment due to the exhaustion caused by continuous connectivity. Their phones incessantly emit alerts; the news and meme cycles remain inactive. Mental health professionals note that excessive social media use can create a harmful cycle: feelings of sadness lead to passive scrolling for distraction, which intensifies loneliness and envy, causing additional distress (Emory University Rollins School of Public Health, 2024). Unsurprisingly, many young individuals assert that social media is overwhelming (Emory University Rollins School of Public Health, 2024). Nevertheless, they often realize this only after experiencing considerable negative consequences.

6.0. GEN Z'S STRATEGIES FOR A HEALTHIER DIGITAL LIFE

Gen Z has begun to resist the trap of mindless, endless scrolling by adopting more mindful digital habits. Many young people are reclaiming their attention by meditating, tracking their screen time, and taking planned "digital detox" breaks (Jones, Johnson, & Kotler, 2025). People see these planned breaks, such as a day each week without technology or longer breaks from social media, as a way to take care of themselves and reduce the stress and cognitive overload that come with being constantly connected. Psychological self-regulation frameworks endorse these strategies: Gen Z can disrupt automatic behaviors and diminish passive consumption by deliberately controlling their surroundings and routines. Studies on social media usage underscore the importance of this approach. Active, intentional participation (such as content creation or significant communication) is associated with enhanced well-being and social connectedness.

Conversely, passive consumption increases isolation, loneliness, and destructive emotions (Matilda, Wulandari, & Darmanto, 2025). The authors noted that experts recommend shifting towards active and aware participation while diminishing passive browsing. Generation Z is gradually adhering to this counsel. Young individuals can enhance their offline experiences as a counterweight to excessive online engagement by utilizing applications that promote concentration and re-engaging in previously enjoyed activities, such as physical fitness, artistic pursuits, and in-person social interactions. These tactics align with beliefs of attention regulation. By deliberately concentrating on non-digital elements and the present moment, Gen Z is "conditioning" their attention and countering the allure of the perpetual feed. In summary, mindfulness, digital detox, and offline enrichment are essential strategies employed by Gen Z to reclaim their mental energy and time inside the attention economy.

6.1. Resisting Digital Performance Pressures and Cultivating Authenticity

Equally important, Gen Z can push back against the performance pressures of curated digital identities. Growing up with social media highlight reels has made this cohort keenly aware of the over-curation and perfectionism that platforms can impose. In response, some individuals have adopted innovative ways to express a more authentic self and avoid the burnout that comes with constant self-presentation. One strategy is to use multiple or Finsta accounts, such as a private, close-friends-only profile alongside a public-facing profile. This allows them to escape the context collapse phenomenon, wherein diverse audiences (e.g., family, peers, colleagues) converge on a single social media audience (Akhmad, At, & Muhammad, 2024). Gen Z users tailor their posts to the appropriate audience by compartmentalizing their digital identities, easing the pressure to be "everything at once" for everyone. Qualitative research confirms that secondary Instagram accounts serve as a kind of backstage: a protected space for more candid, unfiltered self-expression free from the judgment of broader audiences (Akhmad et al, 2024). This tactic helps youth navigate the identity fragmentation caused by juggling different versions of oneself online.

However, managing multiple identities also requires continuous effort, which scholars refer to as identity labor (Duffy & Schwartz, 2018), referring to the constant curating and adjusting of one's online self. Participants in one study described the "constant negotiation" between a polished persona and an authentic self as a form of performative labor that can be emotionally exhausting (Akhmad, At, & Muhammad, 2024). In other words, trying to appear perfect (or even authentically imperfect) online can feel like an endless task. Sociologists note that "authenticity" can become a performance on social media. ronically, Gen Z's need to appear casual and "real"—posting funny selfies, "crying into the camera" confessionals, or messy bedroom photos—has created its own aesthetic. The "authenticity-as-performance" concept highlights vulnerability and imperfection as a form of new social capital. The rejection of airbrushed perfection can become "the flawless execution of being flawed" (Healey, 2025), one commentator said. Although paradoxical, the goal is a pushback against unrealistic social media standards. Gen Zers aim to create online spaces that are authentic without fear of reputational damage (Tirocchi, 2024).

6.2. Embracing Imperfection

Gen Z influencers and online communities are leading a cultural shift, expanding the notion of authenticity and embracing imperfection as more common. This is a good thing. Surveys and focus groups indicate that youth value authenticity and genuineness above deceptive representations (Tirocchi, 2024). In real life, individuals prefer to see their friends and famous people living everyday lives, rather than the perfect lives often portrayed on social media (Tirocchi, 2024). A survey by Tirocchi (2024) found that consumers praised Emily Pallini for posting pictures of her unedited face with acne because she loves herself. Gen Z individuals who want to see authentic people will connect with this content because it shows flaws, quirks, and everyday problems. The rise of sites like BeReal is another example of how this generation wants to be open. The app's idea of asking users to share a raw, unedited picture of their life once a day (with no glamor or editing) immediately taps into this growing desire to show oneself as "authentic" and fight the polished Instagram image. Tirocchi (2024) notes that early studies of Italian university students revealed that BeReal is more effective when people want to share their experiences and be perceived as genuine.

Along with new apps, Generation Z influencers on TikTok, YouTube, and Instagram have established their following by advocating authenticity and imperfection online. Many people make content that shows the difference between the usual appeal of "Instagram vs. Reality" side-by-side pictures and unplanned vlogs about mental health. These producers often talk about their flaws, insecurities, or regular routines, which sends the message to their peers that it is okay to be human. The most common phrase to describe this movement is "make Instagram Casual Again," a title that appears in many TikTok videos and posts (Healey, 2025). This has led to "sloppy photo dumps" (unposed collections of everyday pictures), a rise in spam accounts for small groups, and a general trend toward less planned, more spontaneous sharing. These kinds of behaviors are a direct result of the pressure to do well. They set a standard in society where too much curating is unacceptable, but authenticity is valued, even if it is boring, repetitive, or messy. Organizations and marketers have acknowledged Gen Z's demand for authenticity and have adjusted their strategies to focus on uncensored content and influencer engagement. Some people argue that when companies adopt a "raw and real" look, it may not be entirely honest (Healey, 2025).

In conclusion, Gen Z may deliberately cultivate a healthier relationship with digital life by controlling their media consumption and defining what "real" means to them. They might utilize mindfulness, digital detoxes, and ways for managing their attention to stop themselves from passively overconsuming and keep their mental health in check. They can also fight the identity demands of social media by being more honest about who they are and even making fun of the idea of being flawless. This generation may demand honesty and fairness, whether by taking breaks from technology or publishing a selfie without makeup. This indicates that they are aware of the challenges of living in a digital world. New studies show that Gen Z people are no longer just passive content consumers. Instead, they are actively shaping their attention through practices such as mindful media consumption, digital detoxification, and participation based on authenticity (George, 2025; Kim, 2024; Tirocchi, 2024; Akhmad et al., 2024; Matilda et al., 2025). These natives may not merely be vulnerable subjects of algorithms. (Kim, 2024) They can learn to be more independent regarding performance and distractions, leading to a future where being real and present is more important than being perfect.

REFERENCES

Ahmed, N. (2019). Generation Z's smartphone and social media usage, A survey. *Journalism and mass communication, 9*(3), 101–122.

Akhmad, M. A., At, M. R., & Muhammad, S. (2024). Reconstructing Generation Z's Digital Identity: Self-Presentation and Impression Management Strategies in Second Account Instagram. *Thammasat Review*, *27*(2), 335–350.

Alter, A. (2017). *Irresistible: The rise of addictive technology and the business of keeping us hooked*. Penguin Press.

Attest. (2025). *Gen Z media consumption report*. Retrieved from https://www.askattest.com/blog/research/gen-z-media-consumption

Berners-Lee, T. (1999). *Weaving the Web: The original design and ultimate destiny of the World Wide Web by its inventor*. Harper San Francisco.

Bethune, S. (2019, 01 19). Gen Z more likely to report mental health concerns. *50*(1), p. 20. Retrieved from https://www.apa.org/monitor/2019/01/gen-z

Bournemouth University. (2023, June 30). *Passive social media use is linked to higher levels of loneliness and psychological distress*. Retrieved July 12, 2025, from Bournemouth University.

Chiang, Y. T., & Lin, S. S. (2010). Early adolescent players' playfulness and psychological needs in online games. *Social Behavior and Personality*, *38*(5), 627–636. DOI: 10.2224/sbp.2010.38.5.627

Chou, H. T., & Edge, N. (2012). They are happier and having better lives than I am: The impact of using Facebook on perceptions of others' lives. *Cyberpsychology, Behavior, and Social Networking*, *15*(2), 117–121. DOI: 10.1089/cyber.2011.0324 PMID: 22165917

De, D., El Jamal, M., Aydemir, E., & Khera, A. (2025). Social media algorithms and teen addiction: Neurophysiological impact and ethical considerations. *Cureus*, *17*(1). Advance online publication. DOI: 10.7759/cureus.77145 PMID: 39925596

Debord, G. (1967). *Society of the spectacle*. Bureau of Public Secrets.

Deci, E. L., Olafsen, A. H., & Ryan, R. M. (2017). Self-determination theory in work organizations: The state of a science. *Annual Review of Organizational Psychology and Organizational Behavior*, *4*(1), 19–43. DOI: 10.1146/annurev-orgpsych-032516-113108

Dores, A. R., Peixoto, M., Fernandes, C., & Marques, A. (2025). The Effects of Social Feedback Through the "Like" Feature on Brain Activity: A Systematic Review. *In Healthcare, 13*(1), 89.

Dredge, R., & Che, S. (2020). Chinese online gamers versus nongamers: A difference in social media use and associated well-being and relational outcomes? *Psychology in the Schools*, *57*(9), 1457–1474. DOI: 10.1002/pits.22418

Duffy, B. E., & Schwartz, B. (2018). Digital "women's work?": Job recruitment ads and the feminization of social media employment. *New Media & Society*, *20*(8), 2972–2989. DOI: 10.1177/1461444817738237

Emory University Rollins School of Public Health. (2024). *Overview of social media's impact on youth mental health, noting rising anxiety, depression, and the role of algorithms.* Retrieved from Rollins School of Public Health.: https://sph.emory.edu

Erikson, E. H. (1968). *Identity: Youth and crisis*. W. W. Norton & Company.

Fassi, L., Ferguson, A. M., Przybylski, A. K., Ford, T. J., & Orben, A. (2025). Social media use in adolescents with and without mental health conditions. *Nature Human Behaviour*, *9*(6), 1–17. DOI: 10.1038/s41562-025-02134-4 PMID: 40325198

Festinger, L. (1954). A theory of social comparison processes. *Human Relations*, *7*(2), 117–140. DOI: 10.1177/001872675400700202

Foucault, M., Martin, L. H., Gutman, H., & Hutton, P. H. (1988). *Technologies of the self.* Tavistock.

George, L. (2025). Reclaiming agency in an age of digital distraction: Strategies for mindful media engagement. *Journal of Digital Culture & Society*, *12*(1), 45–61. https://www.researchgate.net/publication/388194527_Reclaiming_Agency_in_an_Age_of_Digital_Distraction

Gudka, M., Gardiner, K. L., & Loma, T. (2023). Towards a framework for flourishing through social media: A systematic review of 118 research studies. *The Journal of Positive Psychology*, *18*(1), 86–105. DOI: 10.1080/17439760.2021.1991447

Harmony Healthcare IT. (2025, June 5). *State of Gen Z Mental Health.* Retrieved from Harmony Healthcare IT: https://www.harmonyhit.com/

Healey, E. (2025, June). *Raw, messy aesthetic and the illusion of authenticity*. Retrieved from The Guardian: https://www.theguardian.com

Hjetland, G. J., Finserås, T. R., Sivertsen, B., Colman, I., Hella, R. T., & Skogen, J. C. (2022). Focus on self-presentation on social media across sociodemographic variables, lifestyles, and personalities: A cross-sectional study. *International Journal of Environmental Research and Public Health*, *19*(17), 11133. DOI: 10.3390/ijerph191711133 PMID: 36078843

Huan, C. (2021). Correlations of online social network size with well-being and distress: A meta-analysis. *Cyberpsychology (Brno)*, *15*(2).

Internet World Stats. (2023). *Internet growth statistics: Today's road to e-commerce and global trade.* Retrieved July 08, 2025, from https://www.internetworldstats.com/emarketing.htm

Ionescu, C. G., & Licu, M. (2023). Are TikTok algorithms influencing users' self-perceived identities and personal values? A mini review. *Social Sciences (Basel, Switzerland)*, *12*(8), 465. DOI: 10.3390/socsci12080465

Janicke-Bowles, S. H., Buckley, T. M., Rey, R., Wozniak, T., Meier, A., & Lomanowsk, A. (2023). Digital flourishing: Conceptualizing and assessing positive perceptions of mediated social interactions. *Journal of Happiness Studies*, *24*(3), 1013–1035. DOI: 10.1007/s10902-023-00619-5

Jones, L., Johnson, E., & Kotler, P. (2025). Digital Detox and Self-Comforting Attitudes in Gen Z. Retrieved from https://www.researchgate.net/publication/392967217_Digital_Detox_and_Self-Comforting_Attitudes_in_Gen_Z

Josep, J. (2025). The algorithmic self: How AI reshapes human identity, introspection, and agency. *Frontiers in Psychology*, *16*, 1645795. DOI: 10.3389/fpsyg.2025.1645795 PMID: 40718563

Kholmogorova, A., Tarhanova, P., & Shalygina, O. (2018). Standards of physical beauty and mental health in children and young people in the era of the information revolution. *International Journal of Culture and Mental Health*, *11*(1), 87–98. DOI: 10.1080/17542863.2017.1394007

Kim, J. S. (2024). BeReal or BeCurated? Examining authenticity cues and self-presentation on ephemeral social media. *Proceedings of the International AAAI Conference on*, 18, pp. 122–134. Web and Social Media. Retrieved July 24, 2025, from https://arxiv.org/abs/2408.02883

Liang, M. (2022). The end of social media? How data attraction model in the algorithmic media reshapes the attention economy. *Media Culture & Society*, *44*(6), 1110–1131. DOI: 10.1177/01634437221077168

Li an, D. E. (2025). Online captive: The impact of social media addiction on.... *Behavioral Sciences (Basel, Switzerland), 15*(4), 481. DOI: 10.3390/bs15040481 PMID: 40282102

MacIsaac, S., Kelly, J., & Gra, S. (2018). She has like 4000 followers!': The celebrification of self within school social networks. *Journal of Youth Studies, 21*(6), 816–835. DOI: 10.1080/13676261.2017.1420764

Marcia, J. E. (1966). Development and validation of ego-identity status. *Journal of Personality and Social Psychology, 3*(5), 551–558. DOI: 10.1037/h0023281 PMID: 5939604

Matilda, A. M., Wulandari, B. P., & Darmanto, D. (2025). UNDERSTANDING GEN Z'S MENTAL HEALTH CHALLENGES. PHENOMENON: Multidisciplinary. *Journal Of Sciences and Research, 3*(1), 38–52.

McGuire, M. (2023, June 8). *The silent epidemic: Why Gen Z is more anxious than ever—and what we're doing about it. Medium.* Retrieved from https://medium.com/@miamcguire6/the-silent-epidemic-why-gen-z-is-more-anxious-than-ever-and-what-were-doing-about-it-e7fd56149eca

McRobbie, A. (2009). The aftermath of feminism: Gender, culture and social change. *Sage (Atlanta, Ga.).*

Meier, A., & Johnson, K. (2022). Social comparison and envy on social media: A critical review. *Current Opinion in Psychology, 45*, 101302. DOI: 10.1016/j.copsyc.2022.101302 PMID: 35184028

Nussenbaum, T. (2023, December 14). *Social media causes attention spans to drop*. Retrieved from The Standard: https://standard.asl.org/27705/uncategorized/social-media-causes-attention-spans-to-drop/

Orben, A., & Przybylski, A. K. (2019). The association between adolescent well-being and digital technology use. *Nature Human Behaviour, 3*(2), 173–182. DOI: 10.1038/s41562-018-0506-1 PMID: 30944443

Park, S. Y., Do, B., Yourell, J., Hermer, J., & Huberty, J. (2024). Digital Methods for the Spiritual and Mental Health of Generation Z: Scoping Review. *Interactive Journal of Medical Research, 13*, e48929. DOI: 10.2196/48929 PMID: 38261532

Pew Research Center. (2024, 12 12). *Teens, Social Media and Technology 2024.* Retrieved from Pew Research: https://www.pewresearch.org/2024/12/12/teens-social-media-tech-acknowledgments/

Pichler, S., Kohli, C., & Granitz, N. (2021). DITTO for Gen Z: A framework for leveraging the uniqueness of the new generation. *Business horizons, 64, no. 5 (*(5), 599-610.

Potts, C., & Stebleton, M. J. (2023). Behind the Digital Mask: Examining Social Media and Masculinity. *About Campus: Enriching the Student Learning Experience*, *28*(4), 4–13. DOI: 10.1177/10864822231195574

Reich, S. M., Subrahmanyam, K., & Espinoza, G. (2012). Friending, IMing, and hanging out face-to-face: Overlap in adolescents' online and offline social networks. *Developmental Psychology*, *48*(2), 356–368. DOI: 10.1037/a0026980 PMID: 22369341

Roberts, S. R., Maheux, A. J., Ladd, B. A., & Choukas-Bradley, S. (2022). The Role of Digital Media in Adolescents' Body Image and Disordered Eating. In Handbook of Adolescent Digital Media Use and Mental Health. Cambridge University Press. Retrieved 07 4, 2025, from DOI: 10.1080/08164640802680635

Rosič, J., Janicke-Bowles, S. H., Carbone, L., Lobe, B., & Vandenbosch, L. (2022). Positive digital communication among youth: The development and validation of the digital flourishing scale for adolescents. *Frontiers in Digital Health*, *4*, 975557. DOI: 10.3389/fdgth.2022.975557 PMID: 36120715

Ruiz, N., Molina Leon, G., & Heuer, H. (2024). Design Frictions on Social Media: Balancing reduced mindless scrolling and user satisfaction. *Maedche, M. Beigl, K. Gerling, & S. Mayer (Eds.), Proceedings of Mensch und Computer 2024* (pp. 442–447). Association for Computing Machinery. Retrieved from DOI: 10.1145/3670653.3677495

Rusida, E. (2024, November 24). *Swipe, scroll, get bored: The real reason Gen Z annot focus. Kind to Mind Indonesia.* Retrieved from Medium: https://medium.com/@Kindtomind_id/swipe-scroll-get-bored-the-real-reason-gen-z-cant-focus-3391094d6162

Ryan, R. M., Deci, E. L., Vansteenkiste, M., & Soenens, B. (2021). Building a science of motivated persons: Self-determination theory's empirical approach to human experience and the regulation of behavior. *Motivation Science*, *7*(2), 97–110. DOI: 10.1037/mot0000194

Ryan, R. M., & Deci, L. (2000). Self-determination theory and the facilitation of intrinsic motivation, social development, and well-being. *The American Psychologist*, *55*(1), 68–78. DOI: 10.1037/0003-066X.55.1.68 PMID: 11392867

Ryan, R. M., & Deci, L. (2019). Brick by brick: The origins, development, and future of self-determination theory. *Advances in Motivation Science*, *6*, 111–156. DOI: 10.1016/bs.adms.2019.01.001

Ryan, R. M., & Moller, A. C. (2017). Competence as central, but not sufficient, for high-quality motivation. In Elliot, A. J., Dweck, C. S., & Yeager, D. S. (Eds.), *Handbook of competence and motivation: Theory and application*. The Guilford Press.

Sagioglou,C., & Greitemeyer, T. (2014). Facebook's emotional consequences: Why Facebook causes a decrease in mood and why people still use it. *Computers in Human Behavior, 35*, 359-363.

Sharifian, N., Zaheed, A. B., & Zahodne, L. B. (2022). The role of envy in linking active and passive social media use to memory functioning. *Psychology of Popular Media*, *11*(1), 80–89. DOI: 10.1037/ppm0000318 PMID: 35402066

Sharma, M., Deepak, K., & Sudhanshu, J. (2023). 5). Adverse effect of social media on generation Z user's behavior: Government information support as a moderating variable. *Journal of Retailing and Consumer Services*, *72*, 103256. DOI: 10.1016/j.jretconser.2023.103256

Sherman, L. E., Greenfield, P. M., Hernandez, L. M., & Dapretto, M. (2018). Peer influence via Instagram: Effects on brain and behavior in adolescence and young adulthood. *Child Development*, *89*(1), 37–47. DOI: 10.1111/cdev.12838 PMID: 28612930

Sherman, L. E., Payton, A. A., Hernandez, L. M., Greenfield, P. M., & Dapretto, M. (2016). The Power of the Like in Adolescence: Effects of Peer Influence on Neural and Behavioral Responses to Social Media. *Psychological Science*, *27*(7), 1027–1035. DOI: 10.1177/0956797616645673 PMID: 27247125

Singh, S. (2025, May). *Gen Z and the pressure to be perfect: Chasing an illusion. Deccan Chronicle.* Retrieved from https://deccanchronicle.com/deccanchronicle.com

Taylor, J., & Armes, G. (2024). Social comparison on Instagram, and its relationship with self-esteem and body-esteem. *Discover Psychology*, *4*(1), 126. DOI: 10.1007/s44202-024-00241-3

Tirocchi, S. (2024). Generation Z, values, and media: From influencers to BeReal, between visibility and authenticity. *Frontiers in Sociology*, *8*, 1304093. Advance online publication. DOI: 10.3389/fsoc.2023.1304093 PMID: 38274837

Valkenburg, P. M., & Peter, J. (2009). The effects of instant messaging on the quality of adolescents' existing friendships: A longitudinal study. *Journal of Communication*, *59*(1), 79–97. DOI: 10.1111/j.1460-2466.2008.01405.x van Dorssen-Boog, P., van Vuuren, T., de Jong, J., & Veld, M. (2021). Facilitating health care workers' self-determination: The impact of a self-leadership intervention on work engagement, health, and performance. *Journal of Occupational and Organizational Psychology*, *94*(2), 259–281. DOI: 10.1111/joop.12352 PMID: 34149206

Viţelar, A. (2019, 6). Like Me: Generation Z and the Use of Social Media for Personal Branding. *Management Dynamics in the Knowledge Economy, 7*(2), pp. 257–268. Retrieved 7 4, 2025, from DOI: 10.25019/mdke/7.2.07

Wei, S., Teo, T., Malpique, A., & Lause, A. (2022). Parental autonomy support, parental psychological control, and Chinese university students' behavior regulation: The mediating role of basic psychological needs. *Frontiers in Psychology*, *12*, 735570. DOI: 10.3389/fpsyg.2021.735570 PMID: 35250687

West, M., Rice, S., & Vella-Brodrick, D. (2024). Adolescent Social Media Use through a Self-Determination Theory Lens: A Systematic Scoping Review. *International Journal of Environmental Research and Public Health*, *21*(7), 862. DOI: 10.3390/ijerph21070862 PMID: 39063439

Yang, C. C., Pham, T., Ariati, J., Smith, C., & Foster, M. D. (2021). Digital social multitasking (DSMT), friendship quality, and basic psychological needs satisfaction among adolescents: Perceptions as mediators. *Journal of Youth and Adolescence*, *50*(12), 2456–2471. DOI: 10.1007/s10964-021-01442-y PMID: 33991272

Yang, Y., Chen, J., & Zhuang, X. (2025). Self-determination theory and the influence of social support, self-regulated learning, and flow experience on student learning engagement in self-directed e-learning. *Frontiers in Psychology*, *16*, 1545980. DOI: 10.3389/fpsyg.2025.1545980 PMID: 40207130

Zhao, S., Grasmuck, S., & Marti, J. (2008). Identity construction on Facebook: Digital empowerment in anchored relationships. *Computers in Human Behavior*, *24*(5), 1816–1836. DOI: 10.1016/j.chb.2008.02.012

Chapter 14
The Psychology of Winning:
Mental Conditioning and Coping Mechanisms for Gen Z Athletes

Debajit Karmakar
https://orcid.org/0000-0001-9272-0627
Lakshmibai National Institute of Physical Education, India

Anindita Das
https://orcid.org/0000-0002-6502-9619
Lakshmibai National Institute of Physical Education, India

Karuppasamy Govindasamy
https://orcid.org/0000-0002-3019-5545
Symbiosis International University, India

Sohom Saha
https://orcid.org/0009-0006-9438-1554
Lakshmibai National Institute of Physical Education, India

ABSTRACT

This chapter explores the unique psychological landscape of Generation Z athletes, emphasizing the need for tailored mental conditioning strategies to optimize performance and well-being. It examines their cognitive traits, motivation patterns, and the influence of technology and social media on mental health. Key psychological skills such as visualization, attentional control, emotional regulation, and confidence building are discussed alongside coping mechanisms for stress, failure, injury, and competitive pressure. Evidence-based approaches including mindfulness, Acceptance and Commitment Therapy, and cognitive-behavioural interventions are presented,

DOI: 10.4018/979-8-3373-4516-1.ch014

with emphasis on technology-enhanced tools like biofeedback, neurofeedback, and mobile applications. The role of coaches, parents, peers, and supportive environments in fostering resilience is highlighted. Case studies illustrate successful applications of these strategies, while challenges such as mental health stigma and equitable access are addressed.

1. INTRODUCTION

The contemporary athletic landscape presents unprecedented challenges and opportunities for the current generation of athletes, commonly referred to as Generation Z, born between 1997 and 2012. These digital natives have emerged into competitive sports during an era characterized by heightened performance expectations, ubiquitous social media scrutiny, and rapidly evolving technological integration in athletic development. Unlike their predecessors, Gen Z athletes navigate a complex psychological terrain where traditional competitive pressures intersect with modern digital stressors, creating unique mental health considerations that demand specialized intervention strategies (Hollander et al., 1995). For Gen Z athletes, this relationship becomes even more critical as they face amplified external pressures through social media exposure, increased performance analytics, and heightened academic and athletic dual-career demands. The traditional approaches to sport psychology, while foundational, require substantial adaptation to address the neuroplasticity patterns, cognitive processing preferences, and motivational structures characteristic of this generation (Park & Jeon, 2023).

Mental conditioning encompasses the systematic development of psychological skills designed to optimize athletic performance through enhanced cognitive control, emotional regulation, and behavioural adaptation. This multifaceted approach integrates cognitive-behavioural principles with contemporary neuroscientific understanding to create comprehensive training programs that address both performance enhancement and psychological well-being. For Gen Z athletes, effective mental conditioning must account for their unique psychological profile, including their preference for immediate feedback, visual learning modalities, collaborative goal-setting approaches, and intrinsic motivation structures that differ markedly from previous generations (Podlog et al., 2020).

2. UNDERSTANDING GEN Z ATHLETES

- **Psychological Characteristics of Gen Z**

Generation Z athletes exhibit distinctive psychological characteristics that fundamentally influence their approach to competitive sports and mental training. These individuals demonstrate heightened cognitive flexibility and parallel processing capabilities, attributed to their lifelong exposure to multimedia environments and rapid information processing demands. Research in developmental neuropsychology indicates that Gen Z demonstrates enhanced visual-spatial processing abilities, with neuroimaging studies revealing increased activation in the occipital and parietal cortex regions during complex task performance compared to previous generations (Hollander et al., 1995).

The attention architecture of Gen Z athletes reflects adaptations to digital environments, characterized by improved divided attention capabilities but potentially reduced sustained attention spans for singular tasks. This attentional profile presents both advantages and challenges in sport contexts, where the ability to process multiple simultaneous stimuli can enhance situational awareness, while difficulties with prolonged focus may impair skill acquisition during repetitive practice sessions (Smith & Smoll, 1991). Cognitive processing speed among Gen Z athletes typically exceeds normative ranges, with reaction time studies demonstrating 15-20% faster response latencies compared to millennial cohorts, suggesting enhanced neural efficiency in information processing pathways. Personality assessments reveal that Gen Z athletes score significantly higher on openness to experience and conscientiousness scales, while demonstrating moderate elevations in neuroticism compared to previous athletic populations. These personality configurations contribute to enhanced creativity in problem-solving approaches but may increase susceptibility to anxiety-related performance decrements. The psychological profile also includes heightened expectations for autonomy and self-directed learning, with preference ratings indicating 70% greater satisfaction with self-paced training modalities compared to traditional instructor-led approaches (Podlog et al., 2020).

- **Technology, Social Media, and Mental Health**

The relationship between technology utilization and mental health outcomes in Gen Z athletes represents a complex bidirectional interaction with significant implications for performance psychology. Social media platforms serve as primary venues for identity construction and peer validation, with 94% of Gen Z athletes maintaining active profiles across multiple platforms. This digital presence creates unique psychological stressors through constant performance monitoring, peer comparison facilitation, and exposure to potentially negative commentary that can significantly impact self-concept and competitive confidence (Gustafsson et al., 2017). Neurobiological research demonstrates that excessive social media engagement triggers dopamine release patterns similar to those observed in addictive behaviours, potentially interfering with natural reward processing associated with athletic achievement. The continuous feedback loops inherent in social media interactions can dysregulate intrinsic motivation systems, leading to increased dependence on external validation rather than internal satisfaction from performance improvement. This shift toward extrinsic motivation correlates with increased rates of burnout, performance anxiety, and decreased sport enjoyment among Gen Z athletes (Smith & Smoll, 1991).

However, technology integration also provides unprecedented opportunities for mental skills development through accessible training applications, real-time biofeedback systems, and virtual reality exposure therapy for competition anxiety. The challenge lies in establishing healthy technology boundaries while leveraging digital tools for performance enhancement (Guo et al., 2025). Effective mental conditioning programs must address both the risks and benefits of technology integration, providing strategies for digital wellness alongside traditional psychological skills training.

- **Motivation and Goal-Orientation in Gen Z Sportspersons**

The motivational structure of Gen Z athletes reflects significant departures from traditional sport motivation models, with increased emphasis on purpose-driven engagement and social impact considerations. These athletes demonstrate higher baseline levels of intrinsic motivation compared to previous generations, with primary motivators including personal mastery, creative expression, and contribution to team culture rather than external rewards or recognition. This intrinsic orientation aligns with self-determination theory principles, suggesting that Gen Z athletes may respond more favourably to autonomy-supportive coaching approaches that emphasize personal choice and meaningful goal pursuit (Hays et al., 2010).

Goal-setting preferences among Gen Z athletes favour shorter-term, process-focused objectives with frequent milestone celebrations rather than long-term outcome goals. This preference pattern reflects their adaptation to immediate feedback environments and may require modifications to traditional periodization models in psychological skills training (Gustafsson et al., 2017). Research indicates that Gen Z athletes demonstrate 40% greater adherence to training programs that incorporate weekly micro-goals compared to those focused solely on seasonal objectives. The concept of athletic identity in Gen Z differs markedly from previous generations, with these athletes maintaining more diverse identity portfolios that include academic, creative, and social justice components alongside their athletic personas. This multifaceted identity structure provides protective benefits against sport-related identity foreclosure but may also create competing priority conflicts during high-stress periods. Mental conditioning approaches must acknowledge and integrate these diverse identity components to maintain authenticity and long-term engagement in athletic development (Smith & Smoll, 1991).

3. FOUNDATIONS OF MENTAL CONDITIONING IN SPORTS

- **Theories of Mental Toughness and Resilience**

Mental toughness represents a multidimensional psychological construct encompassing cognitive, emotional, and behavioural components that enable consistent high-level performance under pressure. Contemporary theoretical frameworks propose that mental toughness emerges from the interaction between trait-like dispositional factors and state-specific situational responses, creating a dynamic capacity for performance optimization across varied competitive contexts. The four-factor model of mental toughness, comprising confidence, commitment, challenge response, and control, provides a comprehensive framework for understanding psychological resilience in athletic populations (Gustafsson et al., 2017). Resilience theory contributes additional depth to mental conditioning approaches by emphasizing adaptation and recovery processes following adversity exposure. The resilience framework identifies protective factors including cognitive flexibility, social support systems, meaning-making capabilities, and stress inoculation experiences as critical components for developing psychological antifragility. For Gen Z athletes, resilience development must account for their unique stressor profiles, including social media pressures, academic competition, and accelerated developmental timelines that may limit natural resilience-building experiences (Holm et al., 1996).

Neuroplasticity research provides biological foundations for mental conditioning effectiveness, demonstrating that psychological skills training produces measurable changes in brain structure and function. Neuroimaging studies of athletes following mental training interventions reveal increased gray matter density in prefrontal cortex regions associated with executive control, enhanced white matter integrity in neural pathways connecting emotional and cognitive processing centers, and improved default mode network regulation during rest periods (Govindasamy et al., 2024). These findings support the conceptualization of mental conditioning as a form of cognitive training that produces lasting neuroadaptations supporting performance enhancement (Gustafsson et al., 2017).

- **Neuropsychological Basis of Performance Enhancement**

The neurobiological mechanisms underlying mental conditioning effects involve complex interactions between multiple brain systems responsible for attention regulation, emotional processing, and motor control. The prefrontal cortex serves as the primary executive control center, orchestrating cognitive resources during high-pressure performance situations through top-down regulation of subcortical structures including the amygdala, striatum, and cerebellum. Mental conditioning interventions strengthen these regulatory pathways through repeated activation and practice, leading to enhanced cognitive control capacity and reduced interference from task-irrelevant stimuli (Fogaca, 2021). Attention networks demonstrate particular sensitivity to mental training interventions, with studies documenting improved efficiency in alerting, orienting, and executive attention systems following systematic psychological skills training. The anterior cingulate cortex, serving as a conflict monitoring and error detection center, shows enhanced activation patterns in mentally trained athletes, contributing to improve self-monitoring and performance adjustment capabilities. These neuroadaptations translate to competitive advantages through faster error correction, more accurate performance calibration, and reduced cognitive interference during complex skill execution (Park & Jeon, 2023).

The neurochemical environment during mental conditioning practice influences learning consolidation and transfer to competitive situations. Optimal arousal states, characterized by balanced autonomic nervous system activation and appropriate neurotransmitter concentrations, facilitate skill acquisition and retention (Holm et al., 1996). Mental conditioning techniques that incorporate breathing regulation, progressive muscle relaxation, and mindfulness practices optimize these neurochemical conditions, creating favourable learning environments for psychological skills development.

- **Role of Cognitive-Behavioural Interventions in Sport**

Cognitive-behavioural approaches in sport psychology operate on the fundamental premise that thoughts, emotions, and behaviours exist in reciprocal relationships that can be modified through systematic intervention strategies. These approaches prove particularly effective for Gen Z athletes due to their preference for structured, goal-oriented training methods and their familiarity with self-monitoring technologies that support intervention implementation. Cognitive restructuring techniques help athletes identify and modify maladaptive thought patterns that interfere with optimal performance, replacing negative self-talk and catastrophic thinking with more balanced, performance-facilitating cognitive frameworks (Fogaca, 2021).

Behavioural activation strategies within cognitive-behavioural interventions focus on establishing consistent routines and habits that support mental conditioning development. These approaches prove especially relevant for Gen Z athletes who benefit from clear structure and immediate feedback regarding progress toward psychological skills goals (Kanaujia et al., 2023). Implementation involves systematic behaviour modification techniques including stimulus control, reinforcement scheduling, and graduated exposure protocols that build confidence and competence in applying mental skills under increasingly challenging conditions. The integration of technology within cognitive-behavioural interventions aligns with Gen Z preferences for digital engagement while maintaining evidence-based therapeutic principles. Mobile applications, virtual reality environments, and biofeedback systems provide platforms for implementing cognitive-behavioural techniques with real-time monitoring and adjustment capabilities (Holm et al., 1996). This technological integration enhances intervention accessibility, increases engagement through gamification elements, and provides objective progress tracking that appeals to data-oriented Gen Z athletes.

4. CORE COMPONENTS OF MENTAL CONDITIONING

- **Visualization and Mental Rehearsal**

Mental imagery represents one of the most extensively researched and practically applied components of sport psychology intervention, involving the conscious creation and manipulation of sensory experiences in the absence of actual environmental stimuli. The effectiveness of visualization techniques stems from the functional equivalence principle, whereby imagined and actual movements activate similar neural pathways in motor cortex regions, creating opportunities for skill refinement and performance preparation without physical practice demands. For Gen Z athletes, mental rehearsal techniques must accommodate their enhanced visual processing capabilities while addressing potential challenges with sustained attention during traditional imagery exercises (Kanaujia et al., 2023).

The PETTLEP model (Physical, Environmental, Task, Timing, Learning, Emotional, Perspective) provides a comprehensive framework for developing effective imagery interventions that maximize neural simulation and performance transfer. Physical elements involve incorporating actual movement patterns and proprioceptive sensations during imagery practice, while environmental components focus on recreating competitive venue characteristics including visual, auditory, and tactile elements. Task specificity ensures that imagery content matches actual performance requirements in terms of skill complexity, decision-making demands, and temporal sequencing (Fogaca, 2021). Advanced imagery techniques for Gen Z athletes integrate technology-enhanced approaches including virtual and augmented reality systems that provide immersive training environments. These technological applications address traditional imagery limitations by providing external visual stimuli that support internal image generation, particularly beneficial for athletes who struggle with vivid imagery creation. Research demonstrates that technology-enhanced imagery training produces superior skill acquisition and competitive performance outcomes compared to traditional imagery-only approaches, with effect sizes ranging from moderate to large across various sport contexts (Holm et al., 1996).

- **Focus and Attentional Control**

Attentional control represents the cornerstone of optimal athletic performance, encompassing the ability to selectively attend to task-relevant information while inhibiting distracting stimuli that may impair performance execution. The multidimensional nature of attention includes width (broad vs. narrow), direction (internal vs. external), and flexibility (ability to shift between attentional states), with optimal performance requiring dynamic attentional adjustment based on situational demands. Gen Z athletes demonstrate unique attentional profiles characterized by enhanced parallel processing capabilities but potential vulnerabilities in sustained attention maintenance, necessitating specialized training approaches (Isorna-Folgar et al., 2022).

Concentration training protocols for Gen Z athletes incorporate their preference for varied, engaging activities while building sustained attention capacity through progressive challenges. Grid concentration exercises, modified for digital platforms, provide systematic attention training that builds focus endurance while maintaining engagement through gamification elements. Dual-task paradigms challenge athletes to maintain primary task performance while managing secondary cognitive demands, developing the cognitive flexibility required for complex competitive environments where multiple stimuli require simultaneous processing (Abdoshahi, 2024). The integration of neurofeedback technology enhances attentional training effectiveness by providing real-time information about brain state optimization. EEG-based systems monitor neural activity patterns associated with optimal attentional states, providing immediate feedback that accelerates learning and skill development. Gen Z athletes respond particularly well to these technology-integrated approaches due to their comfort with digital feedback systems and preference for objective performance metrics that track improvement over time (Kanaujia et al., 2023).

- **Emotional Regulation Strategies**

Emotional regulation encompasses the processes through which individuals monitor, evaluate, and modify their emotional responses to achieve desired outcomes in specific situational contexts. In athletic environments, effective emotional regulation enables athletes to maintain optimal arousal levels, manage competitive anxiety, and recover quickly from setbacks or mistakes during performance. The process model of emotional regulation identifies five key strategies: situation selection, situation modification, attentional deployment, cognitive reappraisal, and response modulation, each offering distinct advantages for different competitive scenarios (Abdoshahi, 2024). For Gen Z athletes, emotional regulation training must account for their heightened emotional reactivity to social feedback and their preference for immediate emotional expression through digital platforms. Traditional emotion regulation strategies require modification to address these generational characteristics while building skills for competitive emotional management. Cognitive reappraisal techniques prove particularly effective, involving the reinterpretation of emotional triggers in more balanced, performance-facilitating ways that reduce anxiety and enhance confidence (Isorna-Folgar et al., 2022).

Mindfulness-based emotional regulation approaches provide Gen Z athletes with practical skills for emotional awareness and acceptance without judgment. These techniques align with their values of authenticity and self-acceptance while providing concrete tools for managing competitive emotional challenges. Progressive implementation begins with brief mindfulness exercises integrated into existing training routines, gradually expanding to more comprehensive emotional regulation skill development that transfers to competitive situations (Abdoshahi, 2024).

- **Confidence Building and Self-Talk Techniques**

Self-efficacy and confidence represent critical psychological determinants of athletic performance, influencing goal selection, effort expenditure, persistence in the face of obstacles, and emotional responses to competitive challenges. Confidence building for Gen Z athletes requires approaches that acknowledge their need for autonomy and authenticity while providing concrete evidence of competence development. Mastery experiences serve as the most powerful source of self-efficacy, necessitating carefully structured training progressions that ensure frequent success experiences while gradually increasing challenge levels (Vealey, 1988).

Self-talk interventions provide Gen Z athletes with practical tools for maintaining confidence and motivation during training and competition. The categorization of self-talk into instructional, motivational, and emotional regulation functions allows for targeted intervention development based on individual needs and situational requirements. Instructional self-talk proves particularly effective during skill acquisition phases, providing cognitive cues that enhance technique refinement and error correction capabilities (Kalra & Sharma, 2025). The development of personalized self-talk scripts involves collaborative processes that respect Gen Z preferences for co-creation and ownership of their development programs. Athletes identify personally meaningful phrases, images, and concepts that resonate with their individual motivation and identity structures, creating authentic self-talk repertoires that maintain effectiveness across varied competitive contexts. Regular script refinement ensures continued relevance and prevents habituation effects that may reduce intervention effectiveness over time (Abdoshahi, 2024).

5. COPING MECHANISMS FOR PERFORMANCE DEMANDS

- **Types of Stressors in Competitive Environments**

The contemporary competitive sport environment presents Gen Z athletes with multifaceted stressors that extend beyond traditional performance pressures to include digital age challenges that previous generations did not encounter. Performance-related stressors encompass the fundamental competitive demands including skill execution under pressure, outcome uncertainty, physical discomfort, and time constraints that have historically characterized sport participation. However, modern athletes face amplified versions of these traditional stressors due to increased performance analytics, video analysis capabilities, and real-time statistical tracking that create heightened awareness of performance variations (Bertollo et al., 2009). Social and interpersonal stressors have evolved significantly with social media integration, creating continuous exposure to peer comparison, public performance evaluation, and potential negative commentary from unknown audiences. The traditional boundary between competitive performance and daily life has become increasingly blurred, with athletic performance becoming subject to constant public scrutiny through highlight videos, statistical databases, and social media platforms. This persistent visibility creates chronic stress responses that can interfere with recovery processes and overall psychological well-being (Vealey, 1988).

Organizational and systemic stressors affect Gen Z athletes through increased commercialization of youth sports, earlier specialization pressures, and intensified college recruitment processes that begin in early adolescence. The dual-career demands of maintaining academic excellence while pursuing athletic development create time management challenges and competing priority conflicts that require sophisticated coping strategies. Additionally, the financial pressures associated with elite sport participation, including equipment costs, coaching fees, and travel expenses, create family system stress that indirectly affects athlete psychological well-being (Bertollo et al., 2009).

- **Adaptive vs. Maladaptive Coping Strategies**

The distinction between adaptive and maladaptive coping strategies lies in their long-term effectiveness for maintaining performance and psychological well-being while managing competitive stressors. Adaptive coping strategies enhance an athlete's capacity to meet environmental demands while promoting personal growth and resilience development, whereas maladaptive strategies may provide temporary relief but ultimately impair performance or psychological health through avoidance, denial, or self-destructive behaviours (Kalra & Sharma, 2025).

Adaptive coping strategies for Gen Z athletes incorporate their preference for active problem-solving and collaborative support-seeking behaviours. These strategies include systematic problem analysis, goal adjustment, social support utilization, and meaning-making activities that help athletes maintain perspective during challenging periods. The development of cognitive flexibility enables athletes to shift between different coping approaches based on situational demands, recognizing when problems require direct action versus emotional regulation strategies (Bertollo et al., 2009). Maladaptive coping patterns common among Gen Z athletes include excessive social media engagement for distraction, perfectionist standards that create chronic dissatisfaction, and avoidance behaviours that prevent skill development and confidence building. The digital environment facilitates certain maladaptive strategies through readily available distraction sources and social comparison opportunities that can exacerbate negative emotional states. Intervention programs must specifically address these modern maladaptive patterns while building alternative adaptive strategies that provide similar functions in healthier ways (Vealey, 1988).

- **Problem-Focused and Emotion-Focused Coping**

The transactional model of stress and coping distinguishes between problem-focused coping, which involves direct action to modify stressful situations, and emotion-focused coping, which targets emotional responses to stressors when situational modification is not possible. Effective coping requires accurate appraisal of situational controllability to select appropriate coping strategies, with problem-focused approaches proving most effective for controllable stressors and emotion-focused strategies better suited for uncontrollable situations (Kalra & Sharma, 2025). Problem-focused coping strategies for Gen Z athletes emphasize systematic approaches to performance improvement and environmental modification that align with their preference for structured, goal-oriented solutions. These strategies include technical skill development, strategic planning, time management systems, and communication skills for addressing interpersonal conflicts. The integration of technology in problem-focused coping provides Gen Z athletes with familiar tools for goal tracking, performance analysis, and progress monitoring that support their systematic approach to challenge management (Bertollo et al., 2009).

Emotion-focused coping strategies help Gen Z athletes manage emotional responses to uncontrollable stressors including competitive outcomes, teammate conflicts, and organizational decisions that affect their athletic participation. These strategies include cognitive reappraisal, emotional expression, relaxation techniques, and meaning-making activities that promote emotional regulation without requiring situational change. The key lies in helping athletes develop accurate controllability assessments to select appropriate coping strategies for specific situations (Kalra & Sharma, 2025).

- **Coping with Failure, Injury, and Pressure**

Failure experiences in sport provide essential learning opportunities but can also trigger significant psychological distress if not properly processed and integrated into athletic development. Gen Z athletes, accustomed to immediate success feedback and rapid problem resolution, may struggle with the inevitable failures that characterize skill development and competitive participation. Effective failure coping involves cognitive restructuring that frames setbacks as learning opportunities, systematic error analysis that identifies specific improvement areas, and goal adjustment that maintains motivation while acknowledging current limitations (Vealey, 1988).

Athletic injury presents unique psychological challenges that extend beyond physical rehabilitation to include identity threats, activity restriction, and uncertainty about return to play timelines. The injury coping process involves grief-like stages including denial, anger, bargaining, depression, and acceptance, with individual variation in progression through these stages. Mental conditioning programs must prepare athletes for potential injury scenarios through psychological first aid training, goal-setting for rehabilitation periods, and alternative identity development that maintains self-worth during injury recovery (Hollander et al., 1995). Performance pressure management represents a critical coping skill for Gen Z athletes who face intensified expectations from multiple sources including coaches, parents, peers, and social media audiences. Pressure reappraisal techniques help athletes interpret arousal symptoms as excitement rather than anxiety, while exposure-based training gradually builds tolerance for high-pressure situations through progressive challenge introduction. The development of pressure routines provides familiar behavioural anchors that maintain performance consistency regardless of situational pressure levels (Kalra & Sharma, 2025).

6. MINDFULNESS AND PSYCHOLOGICAL FLEXIBILITY

- **Mindfulness-Based Interventions (MBIs)**

Mindfulness-based interventions in sport psychology draw from contemplative traditions adapted for athletic contexts, emphasizing present-moment awareness, nonjudgmental observation, and acceptance of internal experiences without automatic reactive responses. The application of mindfulness principles to athletic performance operates through multiple mechanisms including enhanced attentional regulation, reduced emotional reactivity, and increased cognitive flexibility that supports adaptive responding to competitive challenges. For Gen Z athletes, mindfulness training must overcome potential resistance to slowing down and single-tasking while leveraging their openness to alternative approaches and spiritual practices (Park & Jeon, 2023).

The structured implementation of mindfulness training typically follows progressive protocols beginning with basic breath awareness exercises and expanding to include body scanning, mindful movement, and competitive mindfulness applications. Initial training sessions focus on establishing mindfulness as a skill rather than a relaxation technique, emphasizing the cultivation of meta-cognitive awareness that allows athletes to observe their thoughts and emotions without becoming overwhelmed by them. This foundational awareness proves particularly valuable for Gen Z athletes who may experience rapid emotional fluctuations in response to social feedback and performance variations (Park & Jeon, 2023). Research demonstrates that mindfulness training produces significant improvements in attentional control, emotional regulation, and performance consistency among athletic populations. Neuroimaging studies reveal that mindfulness practice increases cortical thickness in areas associated with attention and sensory processing while reducing amygdala reactivity to stress-inducing stimuli. These neuroplastic changes translate to practical benefits including reduced performance anxiety, improved flow state access, and enhanced recovery from mistakes during competition (Vealey, 1988).

- **ACT (Acceptance and Commitment Therapy) in Athletics**

Acceptance and Commitment Therapy represents a third-wave cognitive-behavioural approach that emphasizes psychological flexibility rather than symptom reduction as the primary therapeutic target. In athletic contexts, ACT interventions focus on helping athletes develop willingness to experience difficult thoughts, emotions, and sensations while maintaining commitment to value-based actions that support athletic goals. The ACT model proves particularly relevant for Gen Z athletes who may struggle with perfectionist tendencies and avoidance of negative emotional experiences that naturally accompany competitive sport participation (Park & Jeon, 2023).

The six core processes of ACT include present-moment awareness, acceptance, cognitive defusion, values clarification, committed action, and flexible sense of self, each contributing to overall psychological flexibility development. Values clarification exercises help Gen Z athletes identify their authentic motivations for sport participation beyond external pressures, creating intrinsic motivation foundations that sustain engagement through difficult periods. Cognitive defusion techniques teach athletes to relate to thoughts as mental events rather than literal truths, reducing the impact of negative self-talk and performance doubt (Guo et al., 2025). Implementation of ACT interventions in sport settings involves experiential exercises, metaphorical learning, and behavioural experiments that demonstrate psychological flexibility principles in action. The creative and experiential nature of ACT interventions appeals to Gen Z preferences for engaging, interactive learning experiences while addressing their tendency toward anxiety and perfectionism. Regular values assessment ensures that athletic participation remains aligned with personal meaning and purpose, preventing burnout and maintaining long-term motivation for continued development (Caine et al., 2016).

- **Enhancing Cognitive Flexibility through Meditation and Breathing**

Cognitive flexibility represents the mental ability to shift between different cognitive sets, adapt thinking strategies based on changing environmental demands, and maintain multiple perspectives simultaneously during problem-solving activities. In athletic contexts, cognitive flexibility enables rapid strategic adjustments, creative problem-solving during competition, and adaptive responses to unexpected situations that frequently arise in sport environments. Meditation and breathing practices provide systematic training methods for developing these cognitive flexibility capacities through neuroplasticity mechanisms (Vealey, 1988).

Breathing-based interventions offer Gen Z athletes practical, accessible tools for real-time cognitive flexibility enhancement during training and competition. Controlled breathing patterns influence autonomic nervous system balance, optimizing arousal levels for cognitive performance while providing immediate stress reduction benefits (Govindasamy et al., 2024). Box breathing protocols, involving equal inhalation, hold, exhalation, and hold phases, prove particularly effective for competitive situations where cognitive clarity and emotional regulation are simultaneously required (Gaiswinkler & Unterrainer, 2016). Meditation practices specifically designed for cognitive flexibility development include open monitoring techniques that involve non-selective attention to arising mental experiences, body scanning protocols that build somatic awareness and internal monitoring skills, and loving-kindness practices that enhance perspective-taking abilities. The integration of movement-based meditation approaches, such as walking meditation or mindful stretching, appeals to Gen Z athletes' preference for active learning while building mindfulness skills that transfer to competitive contexts (Caine et al., 2016).

7. INFLUENCE OF COACHING AND SUPPORT SYSTEMS

- **Coach-Athlete Relationship and Psychological Safety**

The coach-athlete relationship serves as the primary interpersonal context through which mental conditioning principles are transmitted, practiced, and refined in athletic development programs. Psychological safety within this relationship creates the foundation for effective learning, risk-taking, and authentic communication that supports both performance enhancement and personal growth. For Gen Z athletes, psychological safety requirements include respect for their autonomy, validation of their perspectives, and collaborative approaches to goal-setting that acknowledge their desire for shared decision-making authority (Guo et al., 2025).

The establishment of psychological safety requires coaches to demonstrate cultural competence regarding Gen Z characteristics while maintaining appropriate boundaries and expectations for athletic development. This involves understanding their communication preferences, including direct feedback delivery, frequent progress updates, and transparent reasoning behind training decisions. Coaches must balance support and challenge, providing enough security for athletes to attempt difficult skills while maintaining performance standards that promote continued growth (Gaiswinkler & Unterrainer, 2016). Trust development between coaches and Gen Z athletes occurs through consistency in actions and communications, demonstration of genuine care for athlete well-being beyond performance outcomes, and competence in both technical and psychological aspects of athletic development. The relationship quality directly influences athlete willingness to implement mental conditioning strategies, with higher relationship satisfaction correlating with increased engagement in psychological skills training and better competitive performance outcomes (Vealey, 1988).

- **Role of Parents, Peers, and Mentors**

The expanded support network surrounding Gen Z athletes includes parents who are increasingly involved in athletic development decisions, peers who provide both competition and collaboration opportunities, and mentors who offer guidance based on shared experiences and expertise. Each relationship type contributes unique benefits to mental conditioning development while also presenting potential challenges that require careful navigation to optimize positive influences while minimizing negative impacts (Hays et al., 2010). Parental involvement in Gen Z athlete development has increased significantly compared to previous generations, with parents taking active roles in training decisions, competitive scheduling, and mental performance support. Effective parental support involves understanding appropriate boundaries between encouragement and pressure, providing emotional support that doesn't interfere with coach-athlete relationships, and maintaining perspective about athletic participation within broader life development. Parent education programs help families understand mental conditioning principles and their role in supporting psychological skills development (Bertollo et al., 2009).

Peer relationships among Gen Z athletes serve multiple functions including social support, competitive motivation, skill development partnership, and identity formation through athletic community membership. The quality of teammate relationships significantly influences training environment psychological safety and competitive performance outcomes. Mentor relationships provide Gen Z athletes with guidance from individuals who have successfully navigated similar challenges, offering practical advice and emotional support that complements formal coaching relationships (Hays et al., 2010).

- **Creating a Resilient Sport Environment**

A resilient sport environment systematically develops athletes' capacity to adapt, recover, and thrive in the face of competitive challenges while maintaining psychological well-being and performance excellence. Environmental resilience emerges from the integration of individual athlete development with supportive organizational structures, cultural norms that promote growth mindset thinking, and systematic approaches to challenge management that build confidence and competence over time (Jones, 1993).

The physical and social environment design should reflect principles that support mental conditioning development, including spaces for quiet reflection and mental skills practice, visual reminders of mental training concepts and team values, and organizational structures that prioritize psychological well-being alongside performance outcomes. Team culture development involves establishing norms that support mistake-making as learning opportunities, celebrate effort and improvement alongside results, and maintain inclusive practices that value individual differences and contributions. Leadership development within the sport environment ensures that resilience principles are consistently modelled and reinforced throughout all organizational levels (Alper & Başaran, 2023). This includes training coaches in mental conditioning principles, developing athlete leadership skills that support peer mental health, and establishing organizational policies that prioritize long-term athlete development over short-term performance pressures. Regular environment assessment helps identify areas for improvement and ensures continued alignment with resilience-building objectives (Bertollo et al., 2009).

8. TECHNOLOGY AND DIGITAL MENTAL CONDITIONING TOOLS

- **Mobile Apps for Mental Skills Training**

The proliferation of mental skills training applications provides Gen Z athletes with unprecedented access to psychological skills development resources that align with their preference for technology-integrated learning experiences. These applications offer systematic training protocols for visualization, relaxation, goal-setting, and performance tracking that can be customized to individual needs and athletic disciplines. The effectiveness of mobile applications depends on evidence-based content development, user engagement design, and integration with broader mental conditioning programs guided by qualified sport psychology professionals (Radcliffe et al., 2015).

Contemporary mental skills applications incorporate gamification elements that appeal to Gen Z preferences for achievement tracking, progress visualization, and social sharing capabilities. Features such as streak counting, badge earning, and skill level advancement provide extrinsic motivation that can support habit formation during initial stages of mental skills development. However, successful long-term implementation requires transition from external rewards to intrinsic satisfaction with skill mastery and performance improvement (Hays et al., 2010). The integration of artificial intelligence and machine learning capabilities in mental training applications enables personalized content delivery based on individual progress patterns, performance data analysis, and user preference identification. These adaptive systems provide increasingly sophisticated training recommendations that optimize learning efficiency while maintaining engagement through varied content presentation. Data privacy and security considerations require careful attention to ensure athlete personal information protection while enabling beneficial application functionality (Park & Jeon, 2023).

- **Biofeedback and Neurofeedback in Sports Psychology**

Biofeedback technologies provide real-time physiological information that enables athletes to develop conscious control over typically unconscious bodily processes including heart rate variability, muscle tension, breathing patterns, and brain wave activity. These technologies offer objective measures of internal states that can be difficult to assess through subjective reporting alone, providing precise feedback that accelerates learning and skill development in mental conditioning programs (Jones, 1993). Heart rate variability biofeedback proves particularly valuable for Gen Z athletes due to its direct relationship with autonomic nervous system regulation and its applicability to both performance enhancement and stress management. Training protocols involve learning to increase heart rate variability through controlled breathing techniques, promoting parasympathetic nervous system activation that supports recovery and optimal arousal regulation. The immediate visual feedback provided by HRV devices appeals to Gen Z preferences for data-driven training while building practical skills for competition preparation and stress management (Radcliffe et al., 2015).

Neurofeedback systems utilizing EEG technology enable athletes to monitor and modify brain wave patterns associated with optimal performance states, attention regulation, and emotional control. These systems provide direct training for mental states that support flow experiences, concentration maintenance, and anxiety reduction through operant conditioning principles applied to neural activity. Research demonstrates significant improvements in competitive performance following neurofeedback training, with particular benefits for sports requiring sustained attention and emotional regulation (Alper & Başaran, 2023).

- **Ethical and Efficacy Considerations**

The integration of technology in mental conditioning raises important ethical considerations regarding data privacy, informed consent, and appropriate professional oversight to ensure athlete safety and intervention effectiveness. Technology should supplement rather than replace qualified professional guidance, with clear protocols for identifying when athletes require additional support beyond technological interventions. The potential for technology dependence must be balanced against the benefits of enhanced accessibility and engagement that digital tools provide.

Efficacy evaluation of digital mental conditioning tools requires rigorous scientific assessment using randomized controlled trial methodologies and validated outcome measures to distinguish between marketing claims and actual performance benefits. Many applications lack sufficient research validation, necessitating careful selection of evidence-based tools and ongoing monitoring of athlete responses to technological interventions. Professional sport psychology practitioners play crucial roles in technology evaluation and integration within comprehensive mental conditioning programs (Alper & Başaran, 2023). The digital divide considerations ensure that technology integration does not create disparities in access to mental conditioning resources based on socioeconomic status or technological literacy. Alternative delivery methods and financial assistance programs may be necessary to maintain equitable access to mental skills training opportunities across diverse athlete populations. Additionally, cultural sensitivity in technology design and implementation ensures relevance and effectiveness across varied demographic groups within the Gen Z athlete population.

9. CASE STUDIES AND PRACTICAL APPLICATIONS

- **Success Stories of Gen Z Athletes Using Mental Training**

The practical application of mental conditioning principles demonstrates remarkable success across diverse athletic contexts, with Gen Z athletes showing particular responsiveness to technology-integrated and collaborative approaches to psychological skills development. Consider the case of Maya, an 18-year-old competitive swimmer who experienced significant performance anxiety that interfered with her race execution. Through a comprehensive mental conditioning program incorporating mindfulness training, visualization techniques, and heart rate variability biofeedback, she developed effective pre-race routines that reduced anxiety symptoms by 60% and improved her competitive times by an average of 2.3% across a full season (Petersen et al., 2024).

Another exemplary case involves Jordan, a 19-year-old basketball player who struggled with emotional regulation following mistakes during games, leading to cascading performance decrements and team chemistry issues. Implementation of Acceptance and Commitment Therapy principles combined with cognitive defusion techniques enabled Jordan to maintain performance focus despite errors, resulting in improved shooting percentages under pressure and enhanced leadership capabilities that contributed to team success (Park & Jeon, 2023). The intervention's success stemmed from its alignment with Jordan's values of team contribution and personal excellence while respecting his autonomy in skill application. The case of Alex, a 17-year-old soccer player managing dual-career demands as a student-athlete, illustrates effective stress management and goal-setting applications. Through systematic mental conditioning training that included time management strategies, pressure reappraisal techniques, and social support utilization, Alex maintained academic excellence while improving soccer performance metrics. The intervention's effectiveness resulted from its comprehensive approach that addressed both performance enhancement and overall well-being while accommodating the complex demands facing contemporary Gen Z athletes (Birrer & Morgan, 2010).

- **Sample Mental Conditioning Programs**

A comprehensive mental conditioning program for Gen Z athletes typically spans 12-16 weeks with progressive skill development and practical application phases designed to build competence and confidence systematically. The foundational phase focuses on psychoeducation about mental skills, basic relaxation training, and goal-setting skills that establish program framework and athlete buy-in. Week 1-4 activities include introduction to sport psychology principles, personal strengths and weakness assessment, breathing technique instruction, and collaborative goal development that respects athlete autonomy while providing structure (Alper & Başaran, 2023). The skill development phase encompasses weeks 5-10 with intensive training in core mental conditioning components including visualization, attentional control, emotional regulation, and self-talk techniques. Each skill area receives 1-2 weeks of focused training with daily practice assignments, progress monitoring, and gradual complexity increases that maintain appropriate challenge levels. Technology integration during this phase includes mobile app utilization, biofeedback training sessions, and virtual reality applications that enhance skill acquisition while appealing to Gen Z learning preferences (Rao & Hong, 2020).

The application and integration phase during weeks 11-16 emphasizes transfer of mental skills to competitive contexts through simulated pressure situations, actual competition application, and ongoing refinement based on performance feedback. This phase includes development of personalized pre-competition routines, mistake recovery protocols, and pressure situation management strategies that become automatic through repeated practice (Petersen et al., 2024). Program evaluation throughout all phases utilizes both objective performance measures and subjective well-being assessments to ensure comprehensive athlete development.

10. CHALLENGES AND FUTURE DIRECTIONS

- **Overcoming Stigma around Mental Health in Sports**

The persistent stigma surrounding mental health discussions in athletic contexts presents significant barriers to mental conditioning program implementation and athlete help-seeking behaviors. Traditional sport culture has historically emphasized mental toughness through emotional suppression, pain tolerance, and unwavering determination, creating environments where psychological struggles are perceived as weakness rather than natural human experiences requiring appropriate support and intervention. For Gen Z athletes, this stigma conflicts with their generally more open attitudes toward mental health while potentially limiting their willingness to engage fully in psychological skills training (Guo et al., 2025).

Stigma reduction requires systematic cultural change efforts that involve all stakeholders within athletic environments including coaches, administrators, parents, and athletes themselves. Educational initiatives must challenge misconceptions about mental conditioning as remedial intervention for “weak” athletes, instead positioning psychological skills training as performance enhancement technology similar to physical conditioning or technical instruction. The reframing of mental health as mental fitness emphasizes optimization and prevention rather than pathology and treatment, creating more acceptable language for discussing psychological well-being in sport contexts (Gaiswinkler & Unterrainer, 2016). Athlete role models and testimonials play crucial roles in normalizing mental health discussions and demonstrating the performance benefits of psychological skills training. When high-profile athletes share their mental conditioning experiences and mental health challenges, it provides permission for others to acknowledge their own struggles and seek appropriate support. Social media platforms popular among Gen Z athletes offer unprecedented opportunities for positive mental health messaging and peer support network development that can counteract traditional stigma messages (Birrer & Morgan, 2010).

The integration of mental conditioning into standard athletic training protocols helps normalize psychological skills development as essential rather than optional components of comprehensive athlete preparation. When mental training receives equal emphasis and resources as physical conditioning, it communicates organizational commitment to athlete well-being while reducing stigma through systematic normalization (Rao & Hong, 2020). This integration requires coach education, resource allocation, and policy development that supports mental health as integral to athletic excellence.

- **Integrating Mental Conditioning in Grassroots and Elite Sports**

The systematic integration of mental conditioning across all levels of sport participation requires consideration of developmental appropriateness, resource availability, and implementation feasibility within diverse organizational contexts. Grassroots sport programs serve the largest number of athletes but often lack resources, specialized personnel, and organizational infrastructure necessary for comprehensive mental conditioning implementation (Guo et al., 2025). However, basic psychological skills training can be integrated into existing programs through coach education initiatives, simplified intervention protocols, and technology-assisted delivery methods that maximize accessibility while maintaining effectiveness.

Elite sport programs possess greater resources and specialized support staff but face unique pressures that complicate mental conditioning integration including performance expectations, media scrutiny, and commercial interests that may prioritize short-term results over long-term athlete development. The integration challenge involves balancing immediate performance demands with comprehensive psychological development that supports both competitive success and post-athletic life transitions. Elite programs require sophisticated assessment protocols, individualized interventions, and coordination among multidisciplinary support teams (Greenspan & Feltz, 1989). The developmental progression from grassroots to elite levels necessitates systematic mental conditioning curricula that build psychological skills progressively while accommodating changing demands and contexts. Early sport participation should emphasize enjoyment, basic emotional regulation, and positive self-concept development, while advanced levels incorporate sophisticated performance enhancement techniques and pressure management strategies. This progression requires coordination between programs at different levels to ensure continuity and appropriate skill building sequences (Birrer & Morgan, 2010).

Technology offers potential solutions for bridging resource gaps between grassroots and elite programs through scalable delivery methods that provide high-quality mental conditioning content regardless of organizational resources. Mobile applications, online training modules, and virtual coaching platforms can democratize access to mental skills training while maintaining evidence-based intervention principles. However, technology implementation must address digital divide issues and ensure that all athletes receive appropriate support regardless of technological access or literacy levels.

- **Research Gaps and Emerging Trends**

Contemporary research in sport psychology continues to reveal significant gaps in understanding optimal mental conditioning approaches for diverse athlete populations, intervention timing, and long-term outcome evaluation that limit evidence-based practice development (Guo et al., 2025). Gen Z-specific research remains particularly limited, with most existing studies conducted on millennial or Generation X populations whose psychological characteristics may differ substantially from current young athletes. Longitudinal studies tracking mental conditioning effectiveness over extended periods are rare but essential for understanding intervention sustainability and transfer to post-athletic life contexts (Hollander et al., 1995).

Neuroplasticity research represents an emerging frontier that promises to enhance understanding of mental conditioning mechanisms while providing objective measures of intervention effectiveness. Advanced neuroimaging techniques enable researchers to document brain structure and function changes following psychological skills training, potentially identifying optimal training protocols and individual difference factors that influence intervention responsiveness (Avery et al., 2018). However, neuroimaging research remains expensive and technically complex, limiting accessibility for most applied sport psychology practitioners. Cultural diversity considerations represent another significant research gap, with limited understanding of how mental conditioning approaches should be adapted for athletes from different ethnic, socioeconomic, and cultural backgrounds (Govindasamy et al., 2024). Gen Z represents the most diverse generation in history, necessitating culturally responsive intervention development that acknowledges varying values, communication styles, and help-seeking preferences across demographic groups.

Research examining cultural adaptation of mental conditioning programs remains insufficient for evidence-based practice with diverse athlete populations (Hollander et al., 1995).

Technology integration research focuses primarily on feasibility and user satisfaction rather than rigorous effectiveness evaluation compared to traditional intervention methods. Randomized controlled trials comparing technology-enhanced versus traditional mental conditioning approaches remain limited, despite widespread application adoption. Additionally, research examining optimal technology integration methods, potential negative effects, and long-term dependency risks requires immediate attention to guide responsible implementation practices (Greenspan & Feltz, 1989). Future research priorities should include large-scale longitudinal studies tracking Gen Z athletes through their competitive careers and post-athletic transitions, culturally adapted intervention development and evaluation, technology integration effectiveness studies, and neurobiological mechanism investigation through advanced imaging techniques. Collaborative research initiatives between universities, sport organizations, and technology companies offer potential for addressing these research gaps while maintaining scientific rigor and practical relevance (Avery et al., 2018).

The emergence of artificial intelligence and machine learning applications in sport psychology represents exciting opportunities for personalized intervention development, real-time adaptation based on athlete responses, and predictive modelling for intervention optimization (Guo et al., 2025). However, these technological advances require careful ethical consideration regarding data privacy, algorithmic bias, and maintaining human connection within therapeutic relationships that remain central to effective mental conditioning implementation.

11. CONCLUSION

The psychology of winning for Generation Z athletes demands sophisticated understanding of their unique psychological characteristics, technological integration preferences, and distinctive stressor profiles that differentiate them from previous athletic generations. Mental conditioning approaches must evolve beyond traditional sport psychology interventions to incorporate digital age considerations while maintaining evidence-based principles that support both performance enhancement and psychological well-being. The systematic development of psychological skills including visualization, attentional control, emotional regulation, and coping mechanisms provides Gen Z athletes with essential tools for navigating contemporary competitive environments successfully. The integration of mindfulness-based interventions, Acceptance and Commitment Therapy principles, and technology-enhanced training methods offers promising approaches for addressing Gen Z athlete needs while respecting their preferences for autonomy, collaboration, and immediate feedback. However, successful implementation requires comprehensive support systems involving coaches, parents, peers, and mental health professionals who understand generational characteristics and can provide appropriate guidance throughout athletic development. The creation of psychologically safe environments that normalize mental health discussions while challenging traditional stigma represents essential cultural change for optimizing Gen Z athlete potential.

Future developments in mental conditioning for Gen Z athletes will likely incorporate advanced technologies including artificial intelligence, virtual reality, and personalized biofeedback systems that provide unprecedented training precision and accessibility. However, these technological advances must be balanced with maintained human connection, cultural sensitivity, and ethical considerations that prioritize athlete well-being over performance outcomes. The ultimate goal remains developing resilient, mentally skilled athletes who can achieve competitive excellence while maintaining psychological health and life satisfaction that extends beyond their athletic careers into successful post-sport transitions and meaningful life contributions.

REFERENCES

Abdoshahi, M. (2024). Effects of an Intervention Based on Cognitive-Behavioral Therapy on Emotional Well-being of Athletic Adolescents with Injuries. *Physical Activity in Children, 1*(2), 61–68. https://www.pachjournal.com/article_211628.html

Alper, R., & Başaran, Z. (2023). To examine the work commitment and psychological flexibility levels of university stuff who participate in yoga activities as a recreational experience. *International Journal of Recreation and Sports Science, 7*(1), 6–17. https://dergipark.org.tr/en/pub/ijrss/issue/81342/1281670. DOI: 10.46463/ijrss.1281670

Avery, T., Blasey, C., Rosen, C., & Bayley, P. (2018). Psychological flexibility and set-shifting among veterans participating in a yoga program: A pilot study. *Military Medicine, 183*(11–12), e359–e363. DOI: 10.1093/milmed/usy045 PMID: 29590487

Bertollo, M., Saltarelli, B., & Robazza, C. (2009). Mental preparation strategies of elite modern pentathletes. *Psychology of Sport and Exercise, 10*(2), 244–254. DOI: 10.1016/j.psychsport.2008.09.003

Birrer, D., & Morgan, G. (2010). Psychological skills training as a way to enhance an athlete's performance in high-intensity sports. *Scandinavian Journal of Medicine & Science in Sports, 20*(s2), 78–87. DOI: 10.1111/j.1600-0838.2010.01188.x PMID: 20840565

Caine, D., Walch, T., & Sabato, T. (2016). The elite young athlete: Strategies to ensure physical and emotional health. *Open Access Journal of Sports Medicine, 7*, 99–113. DOI: 10.2147/OAJSM.S96821 PMID: 27621677

Fogaca, J. L. (2021). Combining Mental Health and Performance Interventions: Coping and Social Support for Student-Athletes. *Journal of Applied Sport Psychology, 33*(1), 4–19. DOI: 10.1080/10413200.2019.1648326

Gaiswinkler, L., & Unterrainer, H.-F. (2016). The relationship between yoga involvement, https://www.sciencedirect.com/science/article/pii/S096522991630036X. DOI: 10.1016/j.ctim.2016.03.011 PMID: 27261992

Govindasamy, K., Kaur, D., Elayaraja, M., Sethi, D., Kalidas, S., Karmakar, D., Orhan, B. E., Astuti, Y., & Parpa, K. (2024). Immediate Effect of Uddiyana Bandha on Heart Rate Variability in Patients with Hypertension: A Randomised Controlled Study. *Annals of Neurosciences, 09727531241299258*, 09727531241299258. Advance online publication. DOI: 10.1177/09727531241299258 PMID: 39678718

Greenspan, M. J., & Feltz, D. L. (1989). Psychological interventions with athletes in competitive situations: A review. *The Sport Psychologist*, *3*(3), 219–236. https://journals.humankinetics.com/view/journals/tsp/3/3/article-p219.xml. DOI: 10.1123/tsp.3.3.219

Guo, C., Chen, F., & Wang, Y. (2025). The Psychological Impact of Competitive Sports Participation on Adolescent Athletes: An Analysis of Coping Mechanisms and Performance Outcomes. *Journal of Rational-Emotive & Cognitive-Behavior Therapy*, *43*(2), 24. Advance online publication. DOI: 10.1007/s10942-025-00587-0

Gustafsson, H., Lundqvist, C., & Tod, D. (2017). Cognitive behavioral intervention in sport psychology: A case illustration of the exposure method with an elite athlete. *Journal of Sport Psychology in Action*, *8*(3), 152–162. DOI: 10.1080/21520704.2016.1235649

Hays, K., Thomas, O., Maynard, I., & Butt, J. (2010). The role of confidence profiling in cognitive-behavioral interventions in sport. *The Sport Psychologist*, *24*(3), 393–414. DOI: 10.1123/tsp.24.3.393

Hollander, D., Meyers, M. C., & LeUnes, A. (1995). Psychological factors associated with overtraining: Implications for youth sport coaches. *Journal of Sport Behavior*, *18*, 3–3. https://www.academia.edu/download/109139060/Psychological_Factors_Associated_with_Overtraining.pdf

Holm, J. E., Beckwith, B. E., Ehde, D. M., & Tinius, T. P. (1996). Cognitive-behavioral interventions for improving performance in competitive athletes: A controlled treatment outcome study. *International Journal of Sport Psychology*, *27*, 463–475. https://www.researchgate.net/profile/Timothy-Tinius/publication/232485180_Cognitive-behavioral_interventions_for_improving_performance_in_competitive_athletes_A_controlled_treatment_outcome_study/links/54e8c62e0cf25ba91c7e71aa/Cognitive-behavioral-interventions-for-improving-performance-in-competitive-athletes-A-controlled-treatment-outcome-study.pdf

Isorna-Folgar, M., Leirós-Rodríguez, R., López-Roel, S., & García-Soidán, J. L. (2022). Effects of a cognitive-behavioral therapy intervention on the rowers of the junior spain national team. *Health Care*, *10*(12), 2357. https://www.mdpi.com/2227-9032/10/12/2357 PMID: 36553881

Jones, G. (1993). The role of performance profiling in cognitive behavioral interventions in sport. *The Sport Psychologist*, *7*(2), 160–172. DOI: 10.1123/tsp.7.2.160

Kalra, S., & Sharma, R. (2025). *Mental toughness and athletic coping skills among young adult athletes.* https://www.researchgate.net/profile/Sakshi-Kalra-4/publication/392126542_Mental_Toughness_and_Athletic_Coping_Skills_among_Young_Adult_Athletes/links/6835d0266b5a287c30465e50/Mental-Toughness-and-Athletic-Coping-Skills-among-Young-Adult-Athletes.pdf

Kanaujia, S., Saraswati, P., Anshu, , Singh, N., Singh, S., Kataria, N., & Yadav, P. (2023). Effect of yoga and mindfulness on psychological correlates in young athletes: A meta-analysis. *Journal of Ayurveda and Integrative Medicine*, *14*(3), 100725. DOI: 10.1016/j.jaim.2023.100725 PMID: 37321018

Park, I., & Jeon, J. (2023). Psychological skills training for athletes in sports: Web of science bibliometric analysis. *Health Care*, *11*(2), 259. https://www.mdpi.com/2227-9032/11/2/259 PMID: 36673627

Petersen, B., Schinke, R. J., Coholic, D., Larivière, M., & Giffin, C. E. (2024). The social effects of mental ill-health stigma in sport. *Sport, Exercise, and Performance Psychology*, *13*(3), 223–239. DOI: 10.1037/spy0000351

Podlog, L. W., Heil, J., Burns, R. D., Bergeson, S., Iriye, T., Fawver, B., & Williams, A. M. (2020). A cognitive behavioral intervention for college athletes with injuries. *The Sport Psychologist*, *34*(2), 111–121. DOI: 10.1123/tsp.2019-0112

Radcliffe, J. N., Comfort, P., & Fawcett, T. (2015). Psychological strategies included by strength and conditioning coaches in applied strength and conditioning. *Journal of Strength and Conditioning Research*, *29*(9), 2641–2654. DOI: 10.1519/JSC.0000000000000919 PMID: 25719912

Rao, A. L., & Hong, E. (2020). Overcoming the Stigma of Mental Health in Sport. In E. Hong & A. L. Rao (Eds.), *Mental Health in the Athlete* (pp. 1–10). Springer International Publishing. DOI: 10.1007/978-3-030-44754-0_1

Smith, R. E., & Smoll, F. L. (1991). Behavioral research and intervention in youth sports. *Behavior Therapy*, *22*(3), 329–344. DOI: 10.1016/S0005-7894(05)80370-3

Vealey, R. S. (1988). Future directions in psychological skills training. *The Sport Psychologist*, *2*(4), 318–336. DOI: 10.1123/tsp.2.4.318

Chapter 15
The Screen and the Strain:
Cultural Pressures on Gen Z's Mental Wellbeing in the Digital Age

Amrik Singh
https://orcid.org/0000-0003-3598-8787
Lovely Professional University, India

ABSTRACT

Generation Z, uniquely characterized as digital natives, navigates an increasingly complex landscape where their online and offline realities are inextricably linked. This abstract explores the profound impact of prevalent cultural pressures, significantly amplified and disseminated through digital platforms, on the mental well-being of Gen Z. Moving beyond general screen time effects, this paper delves into how specific cultural expectations – spanning societal norms, academic and career aspirations, family values, and the pervasive culture of constant comparison – are intensified and distorted within the digital realm. This chapter argues for a nuanced understanding of the intersection between cultural forces and digital environments in shaping Gen Z's mental health, proposing that effective interventions must address both the pressures originating from societal expectations and the unique vulnerabilities posed by the digital world.

DOI: 10.4018/979-8-3373-4516-1.ch015

INTRODUCTION

Generation Z, broadly defined as individuals born between the mid-1990s and the early 2010s, stands distinct in human history. They are the first true "digital natives," having grown up immersed in an environment of ubiquitous internet access, smartphones, and social media from their formative years. This inherent digital fluency has shaped their communication, learning, socialization, and worldview in ways fundamentally different from previous generations. However, this profound connection to the digital world comes with a complex duality, often amplifying existing societal and cultural pressures and introducing novel strains on their mental wellbeing.In a nation like India, where digital penetration is rapidly expanding and traditional cultural norms often hold significant sway, the interplay between the screen and the strain on Gen Z's mental health is particularly acute (Singh & Kumar, 2024; Singh & Supina, 2024; Singh, 2022; Singh, 2024a; Singh, 2024b; Singh, 2024c). It examines the mechanisms through which social media, online gaming, and pervasive connectivity contribute to heightened anxiety, depression, body image issues, loneliness, and fear of missing out (FOMO) among this demographic. Drawing upon psychological theories of social comparison, identity formation, and digital media effects, this abstract highlights how the curated realities and immediate feedback loops inherent in the digital age exacerbate traditional cultural stressors. The pressures of academic excellence, career aspirations, societal expectations regarding marriage and family, and the pervasive culture of comparison are deeply embedded in Indian society. When these pressures are filtered through the omnipresent lens of digital platforms a realm of curated realities, instant feedback, and relentless connectivity their intensity and impact on the psyche of young Indians are magnified. Examining psychological theories of identity formation, social comparison, and the effects of digital media, we will illuminate how the curated, interconnected, and often performative nature of online life contributes to heightened anxiety, depression, body image issues, loneliness, and the pervasive fear of missing out (FOMO) among this demographic. Understanding this complex interplay is not merely an academic exercise; it is a critical imperative for parents, educators, policymakers, and mental health professionals seeking to support the wellbeing of a generation uniquely positioned to inherit the future (Singh & Singh, 2024a; Singh & Singh, 2024b; Supina & Singh, 2024; Nuong-Deri et al., 2024).

Gen Z: The Digital Natives

Before delving into the pressures they face, it is crucial to establish a clear understanding of Generation Z and their defining characteristics. While precise birth years vary, Gen Z typically includes those born between 1997 and 2012 (Singh &

Kumar, 2024; Singh & Supina, 2024; Singh, 2022; Singh, 2024a; Singh, 2024b). Key characteristics that set them apart include:

- **Digital Nativity:** Unlike Millennials who adopted digital technology, Gen Z has never known a world without the internet, smartphones, or social media. This has led to an intuitive understanding and integration of technology into every aspect of their lives (Singh & Hassan, 2024).
- **Hyper-connectivity:** They are constantly connected, relying on instant messaging, social media feeds, and online platforms for communication, information, and entertainment Singh & Singh, 2024a; Singh & Singh, 2024b).
- **Visual Learners and Communicators:** Raised on YouTube, TikTok, and Instagram, they often prefer visual content and communicate through images, emojis, and short-form videos (Nuong-Deri et al., 2024).
- **Global Awareness:** Through constant access to global news and diverse perspectives online, they tend to be more aware of societal issues, social justice, and global events than previous generations.
- **Pragmatism and Realism:** Having witnessed economic recessions and global crises, they are often described as more pragmatic and realistic than the often-idealistic Millennials, with a focus on financial stability and practical skills (Fry & Parker, 2018; Singh, 2024c; Supina & Singh, 2024; Nuong-Deri et al., 2024).
- **Diversity and Inclusivity:** Gen Z is generally more diverse and inclusive than previous generations, reflecting broader societal shifts and greater exposure to diverse perspectives online.

The Indian Context of Gen Z:

In India, Gen Z represents a massive demographic, constituting a significant portion of the population and the future workforce. Their experience is shaped by:

- **Rapid Digitalization:** While not all Gen Z in India have equal access to high-speed internet, digital penetration has exploded, particularly with affordable smartphones and data plans, bridging urban-rural divides to some extent (Supina & Singh, 2024; Nuong-Deri et al., 2024).
- **Aspirations and Competition:** Indian Gen Z faces intense competition for educational opportunities and jobs, often driven by a strong emphasis on academic achievement and upward mobility within families (Ansari & Singh, 2023; Bhalla et al., 2023).
- **Blending of Tradition and Modernity:** They navigate a unique blend of deeply rooted cultural traditions (e.g., family values, community ties, respect

for elders) and exposure to globalized, modern influences through digital platforms. This often creates a tension between conformity and individual expression.

- **Parental Influence:** Indian parents often maintain significant influence over their children's life choices, including education, career, and even personal relationships, which can be amplified by digital monitoring (Singh & Supina, 2024; Singh, 2022; Singh, 2024a; Singh, 2024b; Singh, 2024c).
- **Demographic Dividend:** India's youth bulge means Gen Z is critical for the nation's economic future, placing immense pressure on them to perform and contribute.

Understanding these foundational characteristics and contextual nuances is vital for dissecting how cultural pressures manifest and interact with their digital realities, ultimately impacting their mental wellbeing.

Cultural Pressures on Gen Z in India: A Societal Tapestry

Gen Z in India is not immune to the universal developmental challenges of adolescence and young adulthood. However, these challenges are compounded by a unique set of cultural pressures deeply embedded in Indian society (Singh & Ansari, 2024; Singh & Singh, 2022; Singh et al., 2024; Singh & Singh, 2024a). These pressures, while often intended to guide and support, can inadvertently create significant stress and contribute to mental health vulnerabilities.

Academic and Career Expectations:

- **The Pursuit of Excellence (and Perfection):** Indian society places an exceptionally high premium on academic achievement. From a young age, children are often channeled towards specific "safe" and high-status careers (engineering, medicine, civil services), with little room for deviation. Parents often make significant sacrifices and invest heavily in their children's education, creating immense pressure to excel and justify these investments.
- **Competitive Landscape:** With a vast population and limited top-tier educational and professional opportunities, competition is fierce. Entrance exams for prestigious universities are notoriously difficult, and the job market, despite growth, remains competitive for desired roles. This fosters a relentless drive for perfection and a fear of failure (Sharma et al., 2024; Sharma & Singh, 2024a).

- **Social Status and Vocation:** Career choices are not merely personal preferences but often carry significant weight in terms of family honour and social standing. Choosing a less conventional path can lead to familial disapproval and societal judgment (Sharma et al., 2024; Singh & Supina, 2024; Singh, 2022).
- **The "Sharma Jika Beta/Beti" Syndrome:** This colloquial phrase perfectly encapsulates the pervasive culture of comparison in India. Children are constantly measured against successful peers, fueling a sense of inadequacy and relentless striving.

Family and Societal Expectations:

- **Filial Piety and Duty:** There is a strong cultural emphasis on respect for elders, filial piety, and fulfilling familial obligations. This often translates into children prioritizing parental wishes over personal desires, especially concerning career, marriage, and living arrangements (Singh & Singh, 2024b; Supina & Singh, 2024; Nuong-Deri et al., 2024).
- **Marriage and Relationship Pressures:** For many Indian youth, marriage is seen as a social obligation and a critical milestone. Pressure to marry within a certain age range, community, or even a specific socioeconomic class can be intense. The concept of "arranged marriage" still holds sway, though often with a degree of "assisted choice" for Gen Z. This pressure can extend to personal relationships, with little room for exploration or unconventional choices (Singh, 2022; Singh, 2024a; Singh, 2024b; Singh & Singh, 2024a).
- **Gendered Expectations:** Traditional gender roles, while evolving, still exert significant pressure. Girls may face expectations regarding domesticity, early marriage, and conforming to traditional notions of femininity, while boys are often burdened with the primary responsibility of being the family's financial provider (Sharma et al., 2024; Ambardar et al., 2023).
- **Community and Conformity:** Indian society often emphasizes collective identity and conformity to community norms. Deviating from established traditions, values, or lifestyles can lead to social ostracization or criticism, limiting individual expression.
- **Maintaining "Log Kya Kahenge?" (What will people say?):** This ubiquitous concern about societal judgment often dictates personal choices, forcing individuals to prioritize external validation over their own desires and well-being.

Financial Pressures and Economic Uncertainty:

- **Job Security Concerns:** While India's economy is growing, concerns about job security, automation, and the future of work loom large for Gen Z.
- **Cost of Living:** Rapid urbanization and rising costs of education and living create significant financial pressure on young individuals and their families.
- **Supporting the Family:** Many Gen Z individuals feel a strong obligation to support their parents and extended families, adding another layer of financial stress.

These deeply ingrained cultural pressures create a fertile ground for stress, anxiety, and self-doubt. When these offline realities collide with the digital world, their impact on mental wellbeing is profoundly amplified (Sharma & Singh, 2024a; Sharma & Singh, 2024b).

The Digital Amplification: Screens as Stressors and Sanitizers

The digital world, for Gen Z, is not merely a tool; it is an extension of their social reality, a primary medium for communication, learning, and self-expression (Sharma et al., 2024; Ambardar et al., 2023; Ansari et al., 2024; Ansari & Singh, 2023). However, this omnipresent digital environment also acts as a powerful amplifier of existing cultural pressures, simultaneously offering avenues for expression and imposing new forms of strain on mental health.

The Cult of Curated Perfection: Social Media and Social Comparison

Social media platforms like Instagram, Snapchat, Facebook, and TikTok are central to Gen Z's social lives. While they offer connection, they also foster an environment ripe for upward social comparison, a phenomenon where individuals evaluate themselves against others they perceive as superior (Festinger, 1954).

- **Highlight Reel Syndrome:** Users typically post curated versions of their lives – successes, vacations, perfectly styled appearances, and seemingly idyllic relationships. This constant bombardment of “highlight reels” creates an unrealistic standard of living.
- The digital space expands the comparison pool exponentially. Instead of just local peers, Gen Z now compares themselves to hundreds, even thousands, of individuals globally, often from privileged backgrounds. This fuels feelings

of inadequacy, envy, and a constant pressure to keep up (Sharma et al., 2024; Singh & Singh, 2024b; Supina & Singh, 2024; Nuong-Deri et al., 2024).

- **Body Image and Aesthetics:** Filters, editing tools, and the prevalence of idealized body types on social media contribute significantly to body dissatisfaction, disordered eating, and low self-esteem, particularly among young women.
- **Academic and Career Performance Anxiety:** Students see peers showcasing high scores, admissions to prestigious universities, and coveted internships. This digital display of success intensifies academic pressure and the fear of falling behind.
- **Relationship Envy:** Curated posts of seemingly perfect relationships can lead to feelings of loneliness, inadequacy, and pressure to conform to idealized romantic norms.

The Performance Trap: Identity and Validation in the Digital Sphere

Digital platforms encourage a performative self, where identity is often constructed and validated through online interactions.

- **External Validation Dependence:** Likes, comments, shares, and follower counts become tangible metrics of social acceptance and personal worth. This creates a reliance on external validation, making Gen Z vulnerable to fluctuations in online engagement.
- **Pressure to be "Always On":** The expectation to respond immediately, post regularly, and maintain an active online presence can be exhausting, blurring the lines between personal time and digital performance.
- **Fear of Missing Out (FOMO):** Constant exposure to peers' social activities and experiences through digital feeds fuels FOMO, leading to feelings of anxiety, restlessness, and inadequacy if not actively participating.
- **Authenticity vs. Persona:** The pressure to present an idealized online persona can lead to a disconnect between one's authentic self and the curated digital identity, contributing to feelings of inauthenticity and stress (Nuong-Deri et al., 2024).
- **Online Shaming and Cyberbullying:** The anonymity and distance of the internet can embolden individuals to engage in cyberbullying, shaming, and hate speech. Gen Z is particularly vulnerable to these attacks, which can have devastating mental health consequences. The public nature of online shaming amplifies its impact (Sharma et al., 2024; Ambardar et al., 2023; Supina & Singh, 2024; Nuong-Deri et al., 2024).

The Echo Chamber Effect and Information Overload:

While offering vast information, the digital world can also create its own unique pressures:

- **Information Overload:** The sheer volume of news, updates, and social content can be overwhelming, leading to cognitive fatigue and anxiety, especially concerning global crises and societal problems.
- **Echo Chambers and Polarization:** Algorithms tend to show users content that aligns with their existing beliefs, creating "echo chambers" that limit exposure to diverse perspectives and can heighten anxiety around differing viewpoints, contributing to social isolation for those who feel outside the "norm."
- **Misinformation and Disinformation:** The spread of false or misleading information online can contribute to anxiety, distrust, and difficulty in discerning truth, impacting decision-making and mental peace.

Addiction and Disrupted Sleep Patterns:

- **Digital Addiction:** The addictive nature of social media apps, gaming, and online entertainment platforms, designed with persuasive technologies, can lead to compulsive use, displacing other healthy activities (Singh, 2022; Singh, 2024a; Singh, 2024b).
- **Sleep Deprivation:** Late-night screen use, driven by FOMO or the need to "catch up" on feeds, significantly disrupts sleep patterns. Chronic sleep deprivation is a major contributor to anxiety, depression, irritability, and poor academic performance (Sharma et al., 2024; Singh & Singh, 2024b).

The digital world, therefore, acts as a powerful lens, magnifying the cultural pressures that already exist in Indian society. It transforms individual aspirations into public performances, private anxieties into collective comparisons, and fleeting moments into permanent records, all of which contribute significantly to the mental strain experienced by Gen Z (Supina & Singh, 2024; Nuong-Deri et al., 2024).

Mental Health Manifestations in Gen Z's Digital Lives

The interplay of intense cultural pressures and their digital amplification has tangible and concerning consequences for the mental wellbeing of Gen Z. Research globally and increasingly in India points to a rising prevalence of various mental health challenges within this demographic (Sharma et al., 2024; Singh & Singh, 2024b; Nuong-Deri et al., 2024).

Anxiety and Stress:

- **Performance Anxiety:** The unrelenting pressure to excel academically and professionally, constantly displayed and judged online, fuels high levels of performance anxiety. Fear of failure becomes amplified by the public nature of digital life, where mistakes can be instantly shared or criticized (Supina & Singh, 2024; Nuong-Deri et al., 2024).
- **Social Anxiety:** While paradoxically connected, Gen Z often reports higher levels of social anxiety. The curated perfection of online interactions can make real-life social situations seem intimidating, leading to avoidance or awkwardness. The pressure to present a flawless online persona can also spill over into real-life interactions, increasing self-consciousness (Supina & Singh, 2024; Nuong-Deri et al., 2024).
- **Generalized Anxiety Disorder (GAD):** Constant information overload, global crises reported instantaneously, and the pervasive fear of missing out (FOMO) contribute to a generalized sense of worry and unease (Sharma et al., 2024; Ambardar et al., 2023; Ansari et al., 2024).
- **Fear of Missing Out (FOMO):** Pervasive social media use constantly exposes Gen Z to peers' seemingly more exciting or successful lives, leading to a persistent fear of being left out, isolated, or not having the "best" experiences. This drives compulsive checking of phones and feeds, fueling a vicious cycle of anxiety.

Depression and Low Mood:

- **Social Isolation and Loneliness:** Despite being hyper-connected online, many Gen Z individuals report feelings of profound loneliness and social isolation. Superficial online interactions often cannot replace the depth of real-world connections, leading to a paradoxical sense of disconnection (Singh & Singh, 2024b; Supina & Singh, 2024; Nuong-Deri et al., 2024).
- **Comparison-Induced Depression:** As discussed, constant upward social comparison can lead to feelings of inadequacy, low self-worth, and hopelessness, which are significant risk factors for depression.
- **Cyberbullying and Online Harassment:** Exposure to cyberbullying, online shaming, and hateful comments can have devastating effects on self-esteem, leading to severe emotional distress, social withdrawal, and clinical depres-

sion. The pervasive nature of online interactions means there's often no escape from the bullying (Sharma et al., 2024; Ambardar et al., 2023).

- **Sleep Deprivation:** Chronic lack of sleep, often induced by late-night screen use, is strongly linked to increased risk of depression and difficulty in regulating mood.

Body Image Issues and Disordered Eating:

- **Idealized Body Standards:** Social media bombards Gen Z with highly curated and often unrealistic body images, facilitated by filters and editing tools. This creates immense pressure to conform to narrow beauty standards.
- **Self-Objectification:** The constant focus on one's appearance for online presentation can lead to self-objectification, where individuals view their bodies primarily as objects to be evaluated by others, contributing to dissatisfaction and anxiety.
- **Increased Risk of Disordered Eating:** The pressure to achieve an "ideal" physique, coupled with the prevalence of diet culture content online, significantly increases the risk of body dysmorphia, disordered eating patterns, and clinical eating disorders.

Identity Confusion and Crisis:

- **Digital Identity vs. Authentic Self:** The pressure to maintain a perfect online persona can lead to a disconnect from one's authentic self. This "performance trap" can hinder the healthy identity exploration crucial for adolescence, leading to confusion about who they truly are when offline (Nuong-Deri et al., 2024).
- **Online Extremism and Influence:** The digital world exposes Gen Z to a vast array of identities and ideologies, some of which may be extreme or harmful. Navigating these influences while forming their own identity can be challenging and confusing (Sharma & Singh, 2024b; Singh & Ansari, 2024).

Substance Abuse and Risky Behaviors:

- **Coping Mechanism:** Some Gen Z individuals may turn to substance abuse (alcohol, drugs) as a maladaptive coping mechanism to deal with anxiety, depression, loneliness, or the pressures of their digital lives.
- **Exposure to Risky Content:** The digital world can expose young people to content promoting risky behaviors, which can sometimes translate into real-world actions.

Impact on Academic Performance and Concentration:

- **Distraction:** Constant notifications and the allure of online content can severely impact concentration during study, leading to reduced academic performance.
- **Reduced Attention Spans:** The fast-paced, bite-sized nature of digital content may contribute to shorter attention spans, making it challenging to engage with complex, long-form academic material.

The mental health challenges faced by Gen Z are not isolated phenomena but are deeply intertwined with the cultural pressures they experience and the pervasive digital environment they inhabit (Bhalla et al., 2023; Sharma & Singh, 2024a; Sharma & Singh, 2024b). Recognizing these specific manifestations is the first step towards developing effective support systems and interventions.

Theoretical Lenses: Understanding the Mechanisms

To fully grasp the "screen and the strain," we can draw upon established psychological and sociological theories that illuminate the mechanisms at play.

Social Comparison Theory (Festinger, 1954):

- **Core Idea:** Individuals have an innate drive to evaluate themselves, and in the absence of objective measures, they compare themselves to others.
- **Digital Amplification:** Social media platforms provide an unprecedented and constant stream of "upward social comparison" targets. Users primarily post their successes, ideal appearances, and exciting experiences, creating an unrealistic benchmark (Sharma et al., 2024; Singh & Singh, 2022; Nuong-Deri et al., 2024). Gen Z constantly evaluates their lives, achievements, and appearances against these highly curated digital representations, leading to feelings of inadequacy, envy, and lower self-esteem when their reality doesn't match the digital ideal. The "Sharma Jika Beta" syndrome goes global and is constantly refreshed in their feeds.

Identity Formation (Erikson, 1950; Marcia, 1966):

- **Core Idea:** Adolescence and young adulthood are critical periods for identity development, where individuals explore various roles and beliefs to establish a coherent sense of self.

- **Digital Impact:** The digital world offers both opportunities and challenges for identity formation. On one hand, it allows for experimentation with different personas and access to diverse communities. On the other hand, the pressure to present a consistent, idealized, and validated online identity can hinder authentic exploration (Sharma et al., 2024; Ambardar et al., 2023; Ansari et al., 2024; Ansari & Singh, 2023; Singh & Singh, 2024b; Supina & Singh, 2024; Nuong Deri et al., 2024).. The constant feedback loop (likes, comments) can lead to identity foreclosure (premature commitment to an identity based on external validation) or identity diffusion (difficulty forming a stable sense of self due to overwhelming options and superficial engagement).

Uses and Gratifications Theory (Blumler& Katz, 1974):

- **Core Idea:** This theory focuses on why people actively choose particular media to satisfy specific needs.
- **Digital Relevance:** While not directly explaining negative impacts, it helps understand *why* Gen Z is drawn to platforms. They seek connection, information, entertainment, and self-expression (Singh & Singh, 2024a; Singh & Singh, 2024b; Supina & Singh, 2024; Nuong-Deri et al., 2024). However, when these gratifications are pursued excessively or lead to unhealthy comparisons, the very platforms sought for connection can become sources of distress. For example, seeking validation (gratification) through likes can lead to anxiety when that validation isn't received.

Cultivation Theory (Gerbner& Gross, 1976):

- **Core Idea:** Long-term exposure to media (originally television) shapes perceptions of reality.
- **Digital Relevance:** Applied to social media, continuous exposure to curated realities can cultivate a skewed perception of what constitutes “normal” or “successful.” This can lead Gen Z to believe that everyone else's lives are perfect, vibrant, and always exciting, making their own experiences seem mundane or insufficient. This cultivated sense of inadequacy directly impacts mental wellbeing (Singh, 2022).

Cognitive Dissonance Theory (Festinger, 1957):

- **Core Idea:** Individuals experience discomfort (dissonance) when their beliefs, attitudes, or behaviors are inconsistent. They are motivated to reduce this dissonance.

- **Digital Relevance:** When Gen Z presents a highly curated, often inauthentic, version of themselves online, and their real-life experience doesn't match this persona, it can create significant cognitive dissonance. The mental effort to maintain this discrepancy, along with the underlying feeling of inauthenticity, can contribute to anxiety and stress.

Ecological Systems Theory (Bronfenbrenner, 1979):

- **Core Idea:** Development is influenced by multiple nested environmental systems (microsystem, mesosystem, exosystem, macrosystem, chronosystem).
- **Digital Relevance:** The digital world can be viewed as an integral part of Gen Z's microsystem (immediate interactions), mesosystem (interactions between microsystems like family and online friends), exosystem (e.g., parental work policies impacting digital presence), and macrosystem (broader cultural norms and digital policies). This theory highlights how cultural pressures from the macrosystem (e.g., emphasis on academic success) are transmitted and amplified through the digital microsystem, affecting the individual's development and mental health (Singh, 2022; Supina & Singh, 2024; Nuong-Deri et al., 2024). These theoretical frameworks provide a robust foundation for understanding how the digital environment is not merely a backdrop but an active participant in mediating and intensifying the cultural pressures experienced by Gen Z, ultimately impacting their mental wellbeing.

Interventions and Solutions: Towards a Balanced Digital Future

Addressing the complex challenges posed by cultural pressures and the digital world on Gen Z's mental wellbeing requires a multi-pronged approach involving individuals, families, educational institutions, digital platforms, and policy makers.

Individual-Level Strategies (Empowering Gen Z):

Education, empathy, and empowerment are the three key components of the multifaceted approach to fostering the mental health and digital well-being of Generation Z in the hyperconnected world of today. The cornerstones in this process are digital literacy and critical media consumption. Youth have to be taught the tools to approach online content in a critical way, to learn to differentiate between credible information and how digital algorithms influence their perceptions and beliefs. Being aware of filtered realities and misinformation will allow Gen Z to navigate the digital world with greater responsibility and avoid being vulnerable to malevolent narratives or false comparisons. Teaching people how to be skeptical of sources, how to recognize bias, and how to distinguish between genuine and fake material can help educators and parents change Gen Z from lazy consumers into active, informed members of the online world (Singh & Kumar, 2024; Singh & Supina, 2024). Mindful digital use is also vital and encourages purposeful and balanced interplay with technology. Promoting limited screen time, creating a screen-free zone like eating with the family or at night, taking digital breaks can all create healthier habits and prevent burnout, sleep deprivation, and anxiety associated with screen overuse. People can exercise free will to choose to use technology on purpose and not on compulsions to gain back their focus and feelings. Incorporating mindfulness, like stopping to think before responding to something online or considering online habits, creates awareness and lowers stress levels related to digital overload (Singh & Ansari, 2024; Singh & Hassan, 2024; Singh & Kumar, 2021; Singh & Kumar, 2024). As an addition to conscious consumption, developing actual relationships is important to emotional growth and social wellbeing. Empathy, communication, and sense of belonging developed through face-to-face interactions, deep offline friendships, and engagement in community activities cannot be developed through digital interactions. Interpersonal connection and emotional resiliency is strengthened through family bonding, volunteering or outdoor activities. These experiences allow Gen Z to learn that human relationships and shared experience are much more valuable than virtual acceptance and popularity via social media. Furthermore, it is important to work on cultivating self-compassion and self-worth as a means of combating the culture of comparison promoted by social media. Gen Zers are struggling with self-esteem problems because they are constantly exposed to idealized online personalities. Showing them how to be internally validated and not externally approved of will help them develop true confidence and emotional stability. The promotion of self-acceptance, an appreciation of individual improvements, and self-care routines create a consistent self-identity. Journaling, gratitude exercises, or affirmations are all activities that may assist in refocusing on personal development, rather than perfectionism. There is also need to cope and build resilience against stress and emotional difficulties. The implementation of mindfulness, meditation, deep breathing, and problem-solving practices will help Gen Z manage emotional states and adjust to disappointments (Singh & Hassan, 2024; Singh & Kumar, 2021; Singh & Kumar, 2024). Resilience training teaches perseverance, optimism, and self-efficacy, enabling them to get over disappointments without feeling overwhelmed. Finally, referencing professional assistance should become normalized and promoted. By alleviating the stigma of mental health, young people can turn to parents and teachers and counselors and therapists when they need help in addressing their difficulties. The ability to talk openly about emotional struggles must be regarded as a sign of strength and not weakness. By working together, educational institutions and families can help to access mental health resources, workshops, and peer support programs. Collectively, these tactics, when applied regularly, result in a comprehensive approach that fosters digital consciousness, emotional stability, and general health among Gen Z.

Family and Parental Support:

With rising digital immersion of Gen Z, families and more so parents will be instrumental in forming active and beneficial relationships with technology and developing emotional resilience. This is based on free communication where the youths feel secure to share their experiences, fears and issues related to Internet interactions. The creation of a judgment-free environment can help parents foster discussions about cyberbullying, peer pressure online, or the psychological pressure of being always connected. Being honest and understanding will help build trust and identify digital distress or bad habits early. Listening to their children and affirming them that they are not the only ones who are experiencing certain feelings, parents can remove the stigma around discussing mental illness and make emotional conversations a normal practice in the family (Singh & Kumar, 2021; Singh & Kumar, 2024). It is also important to have digital boundaries and role modeling. It is not enough that parents establish reasonable screen-time limits but demonstrate responsible behavior with digital devices themselves. Establishing no-phone zones during meals or family time and scheduled off-line time will help in strengthening the balance between online and offline life. When adults show supportive technology habits that do not involve multitasking between screens and family time, they are signaling that digital moderation can be achieved and can be gratifying. This type of genuine role modelling is much stronger that any imposed restrictions because children are more likely to imitate what they see than what they are told to do. Besides, encouraging offline interaction is essential in restoring true human relations (Singh & Kumar, 2024; Singh & Supina, 2024; Singh, 2022; Singh, 2024a). Families need to work to establish non-digital interactions with each other by sharing hobbies, outdoor activities, or even basic collaborative tasks around the house. Whether playing board games, cooking together and involving community service, these experiences foster creativity, relationships and emotional connections. The latter offline activities serve to offset the overstimulation of digital media as well as enhancing children with their ability to focus, empathise and reflect on themselves. The other important dimension involves promoting an approach of emphasizing intrinsic motivation as opposed to extrinsic validation. In the age of the Internet when likes, following, and grades tend to take the place of self-esteem, parents should prioritize individual work, interest, and development. The emphasis on perseverance, creativity, and learning rather than superficial measures of success but allows children to develop self-esteem that does not rely on social comparison (Singh & Kumar, 2021; Singh & Kumar, 2024). By encouraging intrinsic motivation at home, youngsters will be less vulnerable to traps of online validation and more self-assured in their personal uniqueness and mission. Parents themselves have to be digitally literate in order to adequately serve their children. Parents need to be informed of the changing digital environment, the psychological effects it will have and some of the new social trends. Supina and Singh (2024) and Nuong-Deri et al. (2024) both agree that parent-oriented educational activities and workshops can aid families to be aware of the dangers of the Internet, learn to notice the symptoms of digital burnout, and engage in beneficial interventions. Government agencies, schools, and NGOs can work together to offer ready-to-access materials, counseling and community-based support systems to parents. Lastly, setting expectations balances are crucial to promoting mental wellbeing (Singh & Kumar, 2024; Singh & Supina, 2024; Singh, 2022; Singh & Kumar, 2024). The strict academic and professional demands that many Indian families unwillingly keep needlessly propagate stress. Parents need to know how to re-balance these pressures according to the strengths, passions, and emotional well-being of their children. Encouraging flexibility, empathy, and acceptance allows Gen Z to pursue holistic success rather than conforming to societal benchmarks. Together, these strategies create nurturing family ecosystems that safeguard mental health and promote sustainable digital wellbeing in a rapidly changing world.

Educational Institutions' Role:

- **Integrating Mental Health Education:** Incorporating mental health literacy, digital citizenship, and stress management into the curriculum.
- **Strengthening Counseling Services:** Ensuring that schools and universities have adequate, accessible, and destigmatized mental health counseling services.
- **Promoting a Supportive Campus Culture:** Fostering an inclusive environment that values diversity, encourages authenticity, and minimizes comparison.
- **Reducing Academic Pressure:** Re-evaluating grading systems, reducing exam-centricity, and promoting holistic development over rote learning.
- **Digital Wellbeing Programs:** Implementing workshops and initiatives that teach students healthy digital habits and critical media consumption.
- **Teacher Training:** Equipping educators with the knowledge and skills to identify signs of distress in students and refer them to appropriate support.

Digital Platforms' Responsibility:

A hyperconnected world today, the digital platforms have become closely interwoven with the mental, emotional and social health of individuals. Being the gatekeepers of online experiences, they bear a heavy ethical and moral burden to provide an environment that fosters psychological welfare, instead of exploiting vulnerability to generate profit or interaction (Singh, 2022; Singh, 2024a; Singh, 2024b; Singh, 2024c). Ethical design is one of the most essential interventions that can re-architect the interface and behavior of digital platforms to support user well-being rather than screen time or ad dollars. Ethical design promotes the design of features that lead to less compulsive scrolling, fewer notifications, and less focus on vanity metrics like likes or how many people follow you. Through their intentional desire to encourage meaningful interaction, sites can generate healthier habits of online use. Furthermore, openness to the impact that digital environments have on the psychology of users should not be an exception but a new rule. The shift is based on the principle of algorithmic transparency and accountability. Nowadays, the algorithms controlling social media feeds and content suggestions are black boxes, maximizing engagement by emotional response to unknown targets, like outrage or envy. In response, platforms need to make their algorithmic processes accessible to researchers, policymakers, and civil society organizations, independently. Transparency would enable third parties to perform audits to detect prejudices, falsehoods, and dissemination of undesirable content. At the same time, platforms should also be responsible to the outcomes of their algorithm choices, particularly when they promote misinformation, hate speech, or otherwise psychologically harmful data (Singh & Kumar, 2024; Singh & Supina, 2024). Digital trust and safety can be improved through more transparent policies, frequent transparency reports, and user control over recommendation systems. One of the related dimensions is that of strong content moderation. Platforms should invest in advanced moderation measures that work well to identify and delete harmful content, such as cyberbullying, hate speech, misinformation, and posts that encourage self-harm, eating disorders, or violence. The AI moderation tools should be utilized with human moderators who have psychological training to make them sensitive to cultural aspects and understanding of local situations, especially in a multicultural society such as India. Rather than reactive takedowns, proactive detection and digital literacy has the potential to prevent damage before it strikes (Singh, 2022; Singh & Ansari, 2024; Singh & Hassan, 2024; Singh & Kumar, 2021; Singh & Kumar, 2024). It is also important to ensure user protection by timely grievance systems and clear appeal mechanisms. Moreover, digital ecosystems should be made more child-friendly with age-restricted functionalities and parental controls. Since children and adolescents constitute a large share of internet users, sites must implement more rigorous age verification policies and be able to offer easy parental controls. Elements that can filter adult content or help restrict screen time or remind healthy usage can assist parents and guardians to instill responsible digital behaviors. Educator and child psychologist collaborations may also contribute to the improved developmental suitability of the platform content and interactions (Singh & Hassan, 2024; Singh & Kumar, 2021; Singh & Kumar, 2024). One such potent strategy that can be easily overlooked is having mental health resources available right in the digital space. Applications can incorporate in-app accessibility to counseling helplines, chatbots that provide a basic psychological service, or connections to professional resources or emergency services. These built-in support mechanisms can provide assistance on time to those users suffering distress or crisis. Finally, platforms need to make tangible efforts at relieving performance pressure by deemphasizing metrics such as follower counts, likes, and shares. With support relying on community-building and authentic expression instead of external validation, users will be able to engage with social media as a social space of connection, rather than competition. All of these interventions can be seen as evidence of a new digital ethics one that prioritizes user wellbeing to be at the core of sustainable technological development and social balance.

Policy and Societal Interventions:

The increasing anxieties about mental health in the digital age require a comprehensive policy frame and robust measures in society to guarantee a healthy, balanced, and resilient population. When the Indian culture, technology, social and other aspects meet, comprehensive actions are needed to mitigate the psychological effects of high digitalization and social pressure. Among the leading strategies are conducting decent mental health and digital wellness public awareness campaigns (Singh & Ansari, 2024; Singh & Hassan, 2024). Government and non-governmental organization-supported large-scale national efforts can be used to build an informed and sympathetic environment. Those campaigns must revolve around informing citizens of the psychological implications of spending too much time on screens and being addicted to social media and becoming victims of cyberbullying, as well as training people to be mindful and responsible in their use of digital devices. Such campaigns should be tailored to fit the cultural diversity and language difference in India to guarantee greater inclusion and reach. The other essential pillar is investing in mental healthcare infrastructure. Mental health services are heavily under-funded and unevenly spread yet India is making tremendous progress in healthcare. To improve on mental health facilities, especially in the primary care tier, policymakers need to focus on allocating more in the budget. This requires hiring and training more psychologists, counselors, and psychiatrists, incorporating mental health education into medical and paramedical school curricula. Particular focus must be placed on the rural and semi-urban regions, where there is little access to professional support. Here, tele-mental health services, community-based wellness centers, and school-level counseling programs can be useful as entry points to early intervention and prevention (Singh & Hassan, 2024; Singh & Kumar, 2021; Singh & Kumar, 2024). India has the potential to close the current treatment gap and ensure everyone has equal access to mental healthcare by investing in human resources and infrastructure. State intervention is also central to making the digital environment safer and more ethical. Policymakers should develop detailed frameworks to ensure the accountability of social media and the digital platform service providers to the wellbeing of users. Rules that encourage ethical design, including restricting addictive algorithms, preventing misinformation, and implementing age-appropriate content regulations can substantially decrease harm on the Internet. Also, effective data privacy regulations will be necessary to ensure that users are not exploited, manipulated, and spied on without their consent (Singh & Kumar, 2024; Singh & Supina, 2024; Singh, 2022). Grievance redressal mechanisms and digital literacy programs can enable citizens to move more responsibly and safely in the online world. Of equal importance is the cultivation of healthy cultural values that redefine success and wellbeing. The Indian society tends to value the achievements in academics and career development and in the process sacrifices mental health and happiness. Cultural change requires a conscious transition to embrace balance, self-care, creativity and emotional resilience. Schools, offices and social media can spearhead this change by supporting inclusive stories that embrace empathy, community and mental health. The stigma around vulnerability and mental health issues can be broken by open discussion of stress, failure, and alternative paths in life (Singh & Kumar, 2021; Singh & Kumar, 2024). To conclude, sustainable mental wellbeing should focus on a coherent effort by policy makers, altering the cultural system, and involving the community. With the combination of the conscious populace, medical funding, moral governance, and social tolerance, India can raise a kinder, well-rounded, and psychologically strong society that will survive the digital revolution. Every one of these multi-layered interventions, societies can strive to establish a digital space that benefits, not burdens, the psyche of the Gen Z generation, allowing them to harness the possibilities of the digital era without falling under pressure.

CONCLUSION

Gen Z sits at the intersection of great potential and challenge like never before. Their natural mastery of the digital space, though giving them access to a plethora of information and a world-encompassing network, inevitably puts them in the path of a stronger cultural influence that dramatically impacts their mental health. With the digital space playing with the expectations of academic perfection, career achievement, family honour, and social conformity and with the ruthless gaze and comparison that digital platforms provide, the traditional manifestations of these phenomena have taken on even more malevolent forms, as this chapter has also helped illuminate. The relationship between the screen and the strain is not a simple cause and effect; it is a complicated set of interrelations that culminate in a favorable environment where curated digital realities, the amplification of social comparison by algorithms, the performance trap of identity validation, and blanket fear of missing out combine to form an environment of anxiety, depression, body image problems, and an overall feeling of inadequacy. Ongoing search to achieve an impossible digitalized dream, coupled with the practical ramifications of perceived failure, places an enormous burden on a generation that is still finding their identity and their role in the world. To better understand this dynamic, one must go beyond surface criticisms of screen time to a more in-depth understanding of psychological processes at work based on social comparison theory, identity formation theory, and the ubiquitous nature of digital media. The responsibility of creating favorable conditions, open communication, and reassessment of unnaturally high standards lies with families and schools. Importantly, digital platforms too will need to recognize their significant societal influence and adopt the ethical design approach without regard to user engagement rates. Lastly, the future of our societies lies in the strength and mental health of Gen Z depending on the strengths of their regulatory structures. We must also unite to tackle the cultural forces that digital world has intensified, to empower this generation to embrace the amazing potential of technology, not as one of strain, but as a medium of connection, innovation and thriving in a world that is constantly changing. The path to a robust digital future of Gen Z is not about how much time they spend in front of the screen, but creating an environment in which their minds can flourish, both online and offline.

REFERENCES

Ambardar, A., Singh, A., & Singh, V. (2023). Barriers in Implementing Ergonomic Practices in Hotels- A Study on five star hotels in NCR region. *International Journal of Hospitality and Tourism Systems*, *16*(2), 11–17.

Ansari, A. I., & Singh, A. (2023), "Application of Augmented Reality (AR) and Virtual Reality (VR) in Promoting Guest Room Sales: A Critical Review", Tučková, Z., Dey, S.K., Thai, H.H. and Hoang, S.D. (Ed.) Impact of Industry 4.0 on Sustainable Tourism, Emerald Publishing Limited, Leeds, pp. 95-104. DOI: 10.1108/978-1-80455-157-820231006

Ansari, A. I., Singh, A., Pattanaik, S., Patnaik, R., & Suryawanshi, U. (2024). Exploring the Role of AI-Powered Virtual Assistants in Optimizing Self-Service Experiences for Customers Within the Service Sector. In Nadda, V., Tyagi, P., Singh, A., & Singh, V. (Eds.), *Integrating AI-Driven Technologies Into Service Marketing* (pp. 225–238). IGI Global., DOI: 10.4018/979-8-3693-7122-0.ch013

Bhalla, A., Singh, P., & Singh, A. (2023). Technological Advancement and Mechanization of the Hotel Industry. In Tailor, R. (Ed.), *Application and Adoption of Robotic Process Automation for Smart Cities* (pp. 57–76). IGI Global., DOI: 10.4018/978-1-6684-7193-7.ch004

Bronfenbrenner, U. (1979). *The Ecology of Human Development: Experiments by Nature and Design*. Harvard University Press. DOI: 10.4159/9780674028845

Festinger, L. (1954). A theory of social comparison processes. *Human Relations*, *7*(2), 117–140. DOI: 10.1177/001872675400700202

Festinger, L. (1957). *A Theory of Cognitive Dissonance*. Stanford University Press. DOI: 10.1515/9781503620766

Fry, R., & Parker, K. (2018). *Early Benchmarks Show Gen Z Is More Diverse, On Track to Be Better Educated Than Previous Generations*. Pew Research Center.

Gerbner, G., & Gross, L. (1976). Living with television: The cultivation perspective. *Journal of Communication*, *26*(2), 172–192. DOI: 10.1111/j.1460-2466.1976.tb01397.x PMID: 932235

Marcia, J. E. (1966). Development and validation of ego-identity status. *Journal of Personality and Social Psychology*, *3*(5), 551–558. DOI: 10.1037/h0023281 PMID: 5939604

Nuong Deri, M., Singh, A., Zaazie, P., & Anandene, D. (2024). Leveraging Artificial Intelligence in Higher Educational Institutions: A Comprehensive Overview. *Education and Law Review*, (30). Advance online publication. DOI: 10.1344/REYD2024.30.45777

Pew Research Center. (2019). Gen Z is more diverse and progressive than previous generations. Retrieved from https://www.pewresearch.org/social-trends/2019/01/17/generation-z-looks-a-lot-like-millennials-on-key-social-and-political-issues/

Sharma, M., & Singh, A. (2024a). Embracing Technological Innovation: A Review of Hi-Tech Services in Hospitality Industry. *Evergreen*, *11*(4), 2818–2830. DOI: 10.5109/7326926

Sharma, M., Singh, A., & Rana, S. (2024). Empowering Hospitality Brands AI Strategies for Enhanced Customer Experiences in Emerging Markets. In Nadda, V., Tyagi, P., Singh, A., & Singh, V. (Eds.), *Integrating AI-Driven Technologies Into Service Marketing* (pp. 173–190). IGI Global., DOI: 10.4018/979-8-3693-7122-0.ch010

Sharma, R., & Singh, A. (2024b). Blockchain Technologies and Call for an Open Financial System: Decentralised Finance. In Vardari, L., & Qabrati, I. (Eds.), *Decentralized Finance and Tokenization in FinTech* (pp. 21–32). IGI Global., DOI: 10.4018/979-8-3693-3346-4.ch002

Singh, A. (2022). Conceptual framework on Smart Learning Environment- An Indian perspective. *Journal of Education and Law*, (25). Advance online publication. DOI: 10.1344/REYD2022.25.36706

Singh, A. (2024a). Quality of Work-Life Practices in the Indian Hospitality Sector: Future Challenges and Prospects. In Valeri, M., & Sousa, B. (Eds.), *Human Relations Management in Tourism* (pp. 208–224). IGI Global., DOI: 10.4018/979-8-3693-1322-0.ch010

Singh, A. (2024b). Virtual Research Collaboration and Technology Application: Drivers, Motivations, and Constraints. In Chakraborty, S. (Ed.), *Challenges of Globalization and Inclusivity in Academic Research* (pp. 250–258). IGI Global., DOI: 10.4018/979-8-3693-1371-8.ch016

Singh, A. (2024c). Impact of E-learning on Student Motivation in Higher Education Institutions: An Indian Perspective. *Journal of Education and Law*, (29). Advance online publication. DOI: 10.1344/REYD2024.29.43214

Singh, A., & Ansari, A. I. (2024). Role of Training and Development in Employee Motivation: Tourism and Hospitality Sector. In Mazurowski, T. (Ed.), *Enhancing Employee Motivation Through Training and Development* (pp. 248–261). IGI Global., DOI: 10.4018/979-8-3693-1674-0.ch011

Singh, A., & Hassan, S. C. (2024). Service Innovation Through Blockchain Technology in the Tourism and Hospitality Industry: Applications, Trends, and Benefits. In Singh, S. (Ed.), *Service Innovations in Tourism: Metaverse, Immersive Technologies, and Digital Twin* (pp. 205–214). IGI Global., DOI: 10.4018/979-8-3693-1103-5.ch010

Singh, A., & Kumar, S. (2021). Identifying Innovations in Human Resources: Academia and Industry Perspectives. In Pathak, A., & Rana, S. (Eds.), *Transforming Human Resource Functions With Automation* (pp. 104–120). IGI Global. DOI: 10.4018/978-1-7998-4180-7.ch006

Singh, A., & Kumar, S. (2024). Effective Talent Management Practices Implemented in the Hospitality Sector. In Christiansen, B., Aziz, M., & O'Keeffe, E. (Eds.), *Global Practices on Effective Talent Acquisition and Retention* (pp. 126–144). IGI Global., DOI: 10.4018/979-8-3693-1938-3.ch008

Singh, A., & Singh, V. K. (2022). The impact of ergonomic practices on housekeeping employee retention and efficiency in hotels during COVID-19 in India. Turyzm/Tourism, 32(2), 29–50. DOI: 10.18778/0867-5856.32.2.02

Singh, A., & Supina, S. (2024). Talent Acquisition and Retention in Hospitality Industry: Current Skill Gaps and Challenges. In Christiansen, B., Aziz, M., & O'Keeffe, E. (Eds.), *Global Practices on Effective Talent Acquisition and Retention* (pp. 363–379). IGI Global., DOI: 10.4018/979-8-3693-1938-3.ch020

Singh, A., Tyagi, P. K., & Garg, A. (Eds.). (2024). *Sustainable Disposal Methods of Food Wastes in Hospitality Operations*. IGI Global., DOI: 10.4018/979-8-3693-2181-2

Singh, V., & Singh, A. (2024a). Digital Health Revolution: Enhancing Well-Being Through Technology. In Nadda, V., Tyagi, P., Moniz Vieira, R., & Tyagi, P. (Eds.), *Implementing Sustainable Development Goals in the Service Sector* (pp. 213–219). IGI Global., DOI: 10.4018/979-8-3693-2065-5.ch016

Singh, V., & Singh, A. (2024b). Revolutionizing the Hospitality Industry: How chatGPT Empowers Future Hoteliers. In Bansal, R., Ngah, A., Chakir, A., & Pruthi, N. (Eds.), *Leveraging ChatGPT and Artificial Intelligence for Effective Customer Engagement* (pp. 192–203). IGI Global., DOI: 10.4018/979-8-3693-0815-8.ch011

Supina, S., & Singh, A. (2024). Exploring the Presence and Adoption of Quality of Work-Life Dimensions in the Hotel Industry? *African Journal of Hospitality, Tourism and Leisure*, *13*(2), 421–429. DOI: 10.46222/ajhtl.19770720.524

Van Dijck, J., Poell, T., & De Waal, M. (2018). *The Platform Society: Public Values in a Connective World*. Oxford University Press. DOI: 10.1093/oso/9780190889760.001.0001

Chapter 16
Traditional Sri Lankan Culture's Impact on Gen Z Mental Health and Digital Identity in Social Media

Madura Thiwanka Pathirana
https://orcid.org/0000-0001-8784-3833
Edith Cowan University, Sri Lanka

ABSTRACT

This chapter explores the potential of interconnected regional tourism in South Asia, focusing on Sri Lanka, Maldives, Nepal, and India. The study aims to examine international tourists' perspectives on the feasibility and attractiveness of multi-country travel in the region, drawing comparisons with successful integrated tourism models in Europe. Using the Push–Pull Motivation Theory as a framework, the chapter employs a qualitative design based on 85 semi-structured interviews with international tourists visiting Sri Lanka between May and August 2024. The findings reveal key motivations, perceived benefits, and barriers influencing tourists' willingness to participate in interconnected travel. Insights on visa facilitation, transportation connectivity, and collaborative marketing strategies are also presented. The study concludes with recommendations for policymakers and tourism stakeholders on enhancing regional cooperation to drive sustainable growth and visitor flow across South Asia.

DOI: 10.4018/979-8-3373-4516-1.ch016

INTRODUCTION

Gen Z typically refers to people born within the mid-1990s to the early 2010s. This group is special because they are the first to grow up fully immersed in technology. Their lives are heavily impacted by social media as they provide access to curated lives of other people, as well as constant exposure to influencer culture. Living in this hyperconnected world allows Gen Z to consume a diverse range of cultural materials and interact with peers from all over the world. However, this also subjects them to unique psychological stressors that impact their identity construction and mental well-being (Katz et al., 2021, 2022; Khalid et al, 2018). Numerous studies have examined the effects of sociocultural factors on adolescents' self-perception, emotional health, and social identity, exploring the impacts lifespan of these digital influences (Abidin, 2016; Djafarova & Rushworth, 2017; Wies et al., 2021). Despite these findings, much less attention has been given to how these phenomena unfold in the culturally rich yet diverse context of Sri Lanka, characterized by traditional values that influence youth behavior, identity construction, and negotiation.

As digital technology continues to be integrated into everyday life, the rate of sociocultural change occurring in Sri Lanka is unprecedented. Among the youth, social media, especially Instagram and TikTok, has shifted the primary modes of interaction, self-presentation, and consumption (Wickramanayake 2022; Wickramanayake 2022). Social media influencers are an integral part of young people's lives. They influence teens' spending on and spending patterns on beauty and fashion, as well as the individual and collective identity construction (Khalid et al, 2018; Sarkar, 2003). The sociocultural outer layer of the Sri Lankan youth is, however, still firmly and fully clad in the skin of traditional cultural values; responsibilities and broader social expectations govern and constrict, almost spacelessly, all thoughts and actions (Hewamanne, 2019; Dodanwala & Weerasekera, 2023). The overlaying of these factors on the social media lives of Sri Lankan Gen Z creates a complex and digitally monitored social footprint, social and mental health challenges, and the multilayered interaction of local ideal culture and global contemporary culture.

This chapter explores the sociocultural dimensions concerning the digital encounters and experiences of Gen Z Commerce students in Sri Lanka, concentrating on the cultural influences and the global emergent influencer culture, and the consequent identity fragmentation and the impact on mental health that remains overlooked. Much of the Gen Z literature has regarded members of this cohort as a singular, digitally monolithic entity, with little critical engagement on the social affordances and dis-affordances of the various social media platforms. However, in Sri Lanka, the considerations of cultural embeddedness and moderation effects are indispensable. Social media influencers (SMIs), as peer-leaders or face-people, fulfill these roles of hybrid marketing and sociology, adjusting consumer mentality and identity performances, lifestyle aspirations, and sociocultural boundaries. Moreover, the emotional context of the local Sri Lankan milieu has a profound effect on the identity and mental health of young people, as local narratives undermine and intersect with global narratives and practices concerning the emotional well-being of youth (Hewamanne, 2019; Khalid et al., 2018).

The use of mental health resources and social media influencers might have positive and negative impacts. For example, the visibility offered by influencers may provide facilitators of social interaction and social support, social identity, creative development, and self-presentation possibly... However, the self-presentation of online personas may increase social comparison, the need to be perfect, the 'succeeding' pressure, and ultimately, the potential increase of anxiety, depression, and other mental health issues (Prasad et al, 2023; Shensa et al, 2017). This social comparison may be especially true for young adults and adolescents who are trying to integrate competing cultural contexts. With respect to Sri Lanka, these digital disputes might be aggravated by deep-seated cultural attitudes related to mental health and the predisposition of young people to social compliance (Vaishnav et al, 2023; Sarkar, 2003).

In this socio-cultural framework, culture-specific strategies are employed for ethnographic engagement in a study of a digital ethnography of identity. To a certain extent, youth receive family support, community norms, and digital engagement local practices that contribute to stress and social preservation (Vissenberg et al, 2022; Dodanwala & Weeraseekera, 2023). These constructions of social order highlight the importance of understanding Francophone constructions of influences and digital health in the context of Sri Lanka's social and cultural order, rather than from predominantly western influences.

This chapter is based on studies of Commerce students from Edith Cowan University Sri Lanka Campus and this illustrates the duality of the developing online culture and the culturally traditional social norms.The students are simultaneously consumers and producers of content on social media, participating in spaces where identities are constructed and performed. This ethnographic case study sheds light on how some members of Gen Z in Sri Lanka confront the conflicting cultural expectations and demands of maintaining cultural identity as they navigate digital platforms in the context of mental health (Wickramanayake, 2022; Khalid et al, 2018). Addressing this issue responds to the needs of educators, mental health experts, policymakers, and families who aim to assist youth navigating an increasingly digitalized and globalized environment.

Gen Z and Digital Identity Formation

Beginning with the mid to late 1990s and the early 2010s, birth years define the age group known as Generation Z. Such individuals are the first to be fully surrounded by the digital world, and thus greatly shape their identity formation processes (Hu and Cheong, 2021). In contrast to prior generations who underwent an 'analog to digital' shift, Gen Z's social and personal self-identities have been developed in highly interlinked digital realms dominated by social media (Hällgren and Björk, 2022). They are also an important source of primary socialization where children and teens actively sculpt and maintain their online profiles in exchange for acceptance and status from their peers (Geng et al., 2023). Nonetheless, the act of creating a digital persona is much more difficult than crafting an identity and balancing tensions of self-representation and self-portrayal can lead to strain and distress (Hällgren and Björk, 2022).

Bourdieu' Habitus concept explains this phenomenon along with the reason of its occurrence. Habitus denotes a set of internalized frameworks of social practice that influence the perception and action of an individual (Hu and Cheong, 2021). In Gen Z's case, digital environments provide the necessary conditions where cultural capitals with a cocktail of digital proficiency, social media savviness, and performing one's gender digitally are created (Hu and Cheong, 2021). Gen Z media ethnographers are capable of decoupling the iconic signals of digital culture which permits them to engage in identity negotiations that are accessible in a range of online environments. This digital habitus imposes new set of their self-management to self-surveil and self-modify to cope with the tensions of a peer-monitored world that combines the online and offline discrepancies (Hällgren and Björk, 2022).

Geng et al. (2023) characterize the intensity of social media usage as the degree to which adolescents interact with social media platforms, and the use of social media as problematic in the context of within addiction and control loss. In the case of their longitudinal studies with over two thousand adolescents, they showed that problematic use of social media correlated with the depressive symptoms and, in turn, the loss of satisfaction with life over the course of the study. Importantly, these changes in emotional health had stronger triggers in the form of more intense upward social comparisons and elevated instances of cybervictimization - both of which are closely intertwined with the functioning of online social identities, and were related to feeling more emotionally vulnerable. Adolescents may feel more emotionally vulnerable while trying to preserve a digitally appealing social persona.

Moreover, the psychological threat that comes from social media, alongside the potential for self-expression it offers, has been examined (Ebrahimpour Sadagheyani & Tatari, 2021). Though social media facilitates the construction of relationships, acquisition of information, and self-identity, many younger users are likely to face highly stressful and negative psychosocial problems, such as body image dissatisfaction, social media bullying, and the fear of missing out. Over time, the emotionally taxing process of digitally constructing a self can result in digital exhaustion aggravated by social anxiety (Geng et al., 2023).

Considering the digital identity aspect of Generation Z is equally interesting. (Hu and Cheong, 2021) analyzes the phenomenon of digital political socialization where Generation Z consumes activism and political content. The disintermediating and democratizing features of the internet have moved political socialization, which took place within families and traditional institutions, entirely into online social networks. This transformation affects personal identity and collective identity. Younger generations increasingly participate in social movements and issues on the global front as they are widely available on the internet. The political dimension of digital identity amplifies the performative burden paradox as adolescents engage in politics at both local and global levels (Hu and Cheong, 2021).

In Sri Lanka, the integration of collectivist values continues to be central to the expectations shaping the digital identities of young people, including the social honor and cohesion of the family and the wider community. Sathurusinghe (2024) identifies the distinctive tension collectivist cultures pose to self-expression, balancing the individual's desire with the community's demand. In this context, social media is primarily a tool for the individual, post which the community's approval is sought, and users from such societies adopt strategic self-portraiture. Chuc and Anh (2023) find such contexts to be complicated from the digital-identity perspective, as people combine self-focused goals with community goals of modesty and family honor. Hence, the study of dual identities of young people in Sri Lanka should integrate the management of cultural flips digital and social media purposefully offer to users of the technology and the culture.

As access to digital tools and platforms differs by income, and especially given Sri Lanka's socioeconomic gaps, socioeconomic status will have some bearing on the digital identity a person acquires. According to Wickramasurendra et al. (2021), students from higher socioeconomic backgrounds acquire digital tools (i.e., smartphones, computers, internet access) to a greater extent, enabling them to construct more sophisticated digital identities. By comparison, youth from lower economic strata negatively impact their guided internet usage and acquire a more restricted digital identity. Religion has shaped the youth's use of digital spaces in Sri Lanka as well. Nanayakkara (2021) argues that compared to other cultures, in Sri Lanka, more than, religiously motivated values restrict the moderation of self-presentation in digital spaces. This often leads to self-censorship to align with religious values concerning modesty and propriety. These instances show the various influences on the formation of digital identities in Sri Lanka and the impact of religious practices and socioeconomic factors embedded in the broader cultural context.

A digital identity has multiple phases of development and is also dynamic. For instance, Ong (2024), a researcher on India, wrote about social, educational, and occupational transitions and the development of a digital identity. The more adolescents and young adults participated in goal-driven activities and performances, the more their digital self-presentation aligned with those objectives. This is particularly relevant for young people in Sri Lanka, who tend to shift their focus from formal education to a more expansive and, at times, digitally driven, self-presentation. Research in this field assists in understanding more specific and nuanced aspects of the mental health ramifications of social media, the construction of identity, the use of social media in the consolidation of adaptive processes, and the integration and digital embedding that social media facilitates.

Cultural Pressures in Digital Contexts

In Sri Lanka, family and extra-familial social units, social harmony, and the weight of traditions and the culture of the family all play a role in shaping how young people create their digital identities (Hewamanne, 2019). Even in social domains where civil and social expressions of digital youth exuberance are most freely articulated, families and other social units place boundaries and shape the identities of youth in a social and civil 'exuberance of youth' digitally constrained. Therefore, the social experience of the digital interface, which is largely global in a social and civil exuberance context, becomes socialized and constrained by the social pressures of a collectivist society (Sarkar, 2003). Culture is a key determinant of the control and scope of social interaction on the digital sphere. Aldwin (2007) highlights the role of culture in determining the type of stressors an individual is confronted with and in defining culturally permissible coping responses. In Sri Lanka where control and surveillance of digital activity are predicated on family honor and social harmony, social reasonability and order during the performativity of a digitally mediated persona crystallize (Hewamanne, 2019). In this light, young people in Sri Lanka cope with conflicts stemming from the global youth culture, which is manifested in the dissociated online identities they are required to perform.

Hällgren and Björk (2022) view digital identity through the lens of "information organisms" which describes people as existing in networks, both digital and physical, that influence how their identity is formed. For Sri Lanka, this results in hybrid identities that incorporate local culture and digitally globalized identities. The rise of social media influence (SMI) poses opportunities and risks simultaneously. Some local influencers actively engage in heritages of Sri Lankan culture, while the majority showcase Westernised aesthetics and lifestyles, often at odds with local value systems, forcing youth to contend with competing cultural narratives (Khalid et al, 2018).

Raghavan and Sandanapitchai, (2024) bring forth the concept of cultural resilience which posits the flexibility of cultural systems and practices as a protective buffer against mental health issues. Within collectivism, family support and participation in religious and community activities become important identity resources that provide validation outside of the digital realm (Raghavan and Sandanapitchai, 2024). These culturally based resources assist young people in coping with the psychosocial challenges related to the formation of digital identities and the use of social media Considering other factors of the digital experience in Sri Lanka, digital technologies do not seem to help with improving or easing intergenerational relations. Based on what Khalid et al. (2018) explain, elders seem to adhere to more rigid ideals regarding what is deemed as 'appropriate' behavior on the internet, thus increasing intergenerational perplexity (and friction) for young people trying to negotiate their digital identities. There thus seems to be a lack of understanding in the socio-cultural context related to the construction of digital identities. Social digital identity construction is primarily an individual task, unlike 'real world' identity construction which is more influenced by familial pressure and societal expectations. The individual and digital context show a clear contradiction to the individualistic ideals underpinning the social and digital environments of Sri Lanka, which is a culture rooted in collectivism. As Khalid et al. (2018) argue, culture is expressed through one's digital identity and in a manner that is meant to consolidate global digital culture with local (and in the case of Sri Lankan culture, augmented with wider communal and religious) digital traditions, which is moderated by family, community, and the church.

In Sri Lanka, the varying socioeconomic status of the population provides the basis for different digital activities among the youth, as elucidated by Wickramasurendra et al (2021). Students with more advanced socioeconomic status have extended access to digital instruments, which affect the way they showcase themselves in the online domain. Conversely, authentically demonstrating digital personalities becomes difficult for low income students because of the structural inequities they face. Pivotal to the digital self-presentation of Sri Lankan youth is their religious affiliation. Sri Lankan youth self-police their online activities because of the cultural dictates of their religion. Most spend more time rectifying online activities, which in part is due to their religious expectations of modesty in other aspects of their lives (Nanayakkara, 2021).

From adolescence to early adulthood, self-presentation on digital platforms changes as new social pressures emerge, as observed by Ong (2024) on a longitudinal study of Indian youth. Examining the digital self-presentation of Sri Lankan youth in a similar study context would offer valuable insights on the digital identity evolution of Sri Lankan youth, particularly in the post-pandemic transition from education to formal employment.

The COVID-19 pandemic has brought about fundamental changes to youth interaction with digital environments. Wickramasurendra et al. (2021), in a post-pandemic study, noted that digital engagement has proliferated in both volume and variety, with youth turning to social media to connect with others and express themselves in face of social isolation. Furthermore, digital identity has evolved, as many young people, according to Shan et al. (2023), leaned towards curated forms of self-presentation on various platforms as a means of coping during the pandemic. This development is pivotal for grasping how Gen Z in Sri Lanka interacts with global digital culture alongside traditional cultural forms. The cited works examine the specific forms of digital dissociative pressure and the subsequent mental health repercussions related to fractured digital identities that targeted audiences of dis-placed documented individuals experienced during the Covid-19 period. The formation of digital identities among Sri Lankan Gen Z youth is primarily influenced by local indigenous factors; however, generalizations within the South Asian region provide opportunities to draw a few broad parallels. For example, in Indian context, Erangi & Stecenko (2024) describes the impact of familial and societal expectations on youth digital practices, highlighting the tension between self-appropriation and familial reputational concerns. Likewise, and in the context of the Philippines, Lim et al. (2022) analyzed the religious and cultural influences on the digital self where the outward self is seen as emphasized with expectations of moderation and deeply collectivist principles. The weight of such comparative discussions suggests that the South Asian region, despite its specific local cultural constraints, primarily operates within, and on, a broad collectivist framework. This predominantly collectivist framework, in turn, establishes the cultural baseline for the digital activities of South Asian youth. Having integrated these regional insights, scholars can better understand the digital identity negotiation of South Asian youth, shaped, to a large extent, by familial and cultural expectations regarding the extent of their public visibility.

Mental Health Challenges and Social Media

Globally, there is growing concern regarding the effects of social media on mental health, especially on anxiety, depression, stress, and sleep disorders (Geng et al., 2023; Alonzo et al., 2021). This concern is particularly directed toward youth and adolescents, the group most likely to interact with social media platforms. The mental health consequences of social media use partially depend on the social-psychological structures of media use and the situational contexts the user interacts with on the platforms. Geng et al. (2023) description of criteria for classification of intensity of social media use within the scope of longitudinal studies describes when individuals lose control of their social media use as socially neglecting their face-to-face interactions as social media use addiction. Geng describes social media use within certain limits as not necessarily leading to negative outcomes. He also describes the qualitative experience of social media as more significant than the quantitative social media use in the decline of mental health. This illustrates the shift needed for studies concerning mental health of the younger generation, and social media in particular. Geng et al. (2023) depression and life dissatisfaction contributed by social comparisons to idealized online figures and online bullying described in the literature the social dissatisfaction and emotional distress contributed to the general wellbeing by outcomes of the aforementioned factors. This illustrates the emotional distress stemming from competing on social media and self presentation. This acknowledgment is an important contribution to the literature.

Alonzo et al. (2021) systematically analyze the triadic link between social media use, sleep, and mental health. They observe that social media users with poor sleep hygiene tend to experience more anxiety and depression. Alonzo et al. also highlight the potential for social media and screen-related bedtime stress to be disruptive for children and adolescents, sleep's developmental importance, and the mental health concerns associated with poor sleep. Given that social media use negatively affects mental health primarily through sleep, Alonzo et al. added another physical aspect to the literature and the psychological literature.

Ebrahimpour Sadagheyani and Tatari (2021) examine how social media can have both positive and negative impacts on its users. On the positive side, social media can help provide and share health information, offer network and assist in fostering social support, and help form a community. On the negative side, social media can facilitate social isolation and body image issues, bullying, and other psychosocial problems, especially among the younger population. Such issues are exacerbated if the person shows and pre-existing social characteristic before and engagement on the platform. South Asian and Sri Lankan countries have traditionally been slow in recognizing their mental health burden. help. The impact of social media on mental health becomes worse when help is not readily and easily available. Social mental health problems with social isolation, especially among the youth, becomes exacerbated when help-seeking behavior is socially sanctioned and ostracization is seen as a form of social alienation. Sarkar (2003) discusses the complicated position of adolescents in Sri Lanka, who are expected to develop social polish while adhering to emotionally controlled culturally driven standards. This explains the pressure adolescents are facing with the social expectations of the use of social media. Understanding social culture is important in the designing of mental health services for adolescents in Sri Lanka.

Coping and Resilience in Cultural Context

Coping and resilience perspectives place and analyze the adolescents' approach to the mental health consequences associated with social media within culturally specific frameworks. Aldwin (2007) states that coping is a cultural phenomenon and a social transaction, comprising social structures and the perception of a stressor. For instance, in Sri Lanka, a collectivist society, coping is relational, drawing upon families, communities, and religion, with individualistic tactics employed as a last resort. Raghavan and Sandanapitchai (2024) present a description of cultural resilience as the ability of cultural resources and structures to facilitate and bolster adaptive coping and mental health. In addition to the nuclear family and peers, culturally defined resilience encompasses the resources of the society; the cultural developmental frameworks of a society that order and construe meaning during adversities. This is particularly valuable to adolescents as they work with the negative individual resources of the stressor to develop resilience, as it shifts the focus to positive collective resources.

Research on youth digital literacy skills highlights the importance of developing region-specific frameworks to address social media related stress. Vissenberg et al (2022) noted that youth resistance strategies involve indirect social media participation via selective viewing, peer isolation, disengagement, and supportive communities. These strategies demonstrate adaptability and agency among young people to satisfy the requirements of a digital society. Khalid et al., (2018) and Sarkar (2003) highlight dialogic coping strategies and ritualistic actions and activities of social and relational strengthening within the family and community as some of these culturally situated coping strategies in the context of Sri Lanka. Culturally integrated coping strategies counter the burdens resulting from 'globalized electronic cultures' and provide emotional relief and emotional validation. This suggests the strengthening of culturally consonant frameworks that incorporate findings from the literature on indigenous mental health resources. In the Sri Lankan context, more research needs to be done on the mental health consequences of social media, along with social resilience, and identity formation on young people and adolescents. The formulation of suitable and flexible strategies may be possible by regarding culture as a tangible coping resource.

METHODOLOGY

A data collection was conducted to support this chapter. This research utilizes a qualitative exploratory approach to examine the impact of social media influencer culture on the mental health and digital identity of Generation Z in Sri Lanka, focusing on one of the traditional Sri Lankan cultural values. Qualitative approaches are most appropriate for capturing the subjective complexity and cultural context of young people experiencing these phenomena (Creswell & Poth, 2018). The study involves semi-structured individual interviews in combination with focus group discussions to provide richer insights and a deeper understanding of the issues explored. While interviews facilitate the sharing of personal accounts in private settings, focus groups capture cultural narratives and peer influences, thereby providing competing data which helps deepen the analysis (Morgan, 1997).

The study's population includes approximately 250 students studying Commerce at Edith Cowan University's Sri Lanka campus, who are between 18 to 25 years old. A purposive sampling technique was used to capture participants who are social media users and articulate subcultural pressures and mental health issues. In order to capture all viewpoints, stratified purposive sampling was used to ensure all participants of different gender, year of study, and urban or rural residence were included. The sample size of 25 participants was selected to achieve a balance between depth and manageability, which is aligned with guided qualitative research that recommends a sample size that is large enough to reach data saturation—where no new ideas emerge (Guest, Bunce, & Johnson, 2006). Even though the qualitative design has much to offer regarding the digital identities of the Sri Lankan youth, the sample size of just 25 participants makes it difficult to extrapolate the results to the broader population. Hence, subsequent studies should aim for larger and more heterogeneous samples. A postcolonial critique of digital identities would also greatly improve the framework by identifying how the legacies of colonialism shape contemporary digital practices in Sri Lanka, which would add to the literature.

Data collection included between 20 and 25 semi-structured interviews which lasted in duration of 45 to 60 minutes. The interviews were conducted in English, Sinhala, or Tamil in accordance to the participant's choice. The interviews included discussions on the construction of digital identities, culture, mental health, and coping. In addition, 2 to 3 focus groups, 5 to 7 people each, were created to facilitate discussions on social media, peer influence, and group coping. Each recording was transcribed and contextual and non-verbal information was noted as part of the analysis. NVivo software was used to enhance organization and clarity during data analysis. For ethical implications, informed consent, confidentiality, anonymity, and the provision of potential mental health resources to participants were ensured. Triangulation of methods, member checking, peer debriefing, and the maintenance of an audit trail were used to document analytic decisions and reflexivity to ensure credibility of the research. The transcripts were analyzed together using Braun and Clarke's (2006) framework of thematic analysis. The transcripts were assigned codes, and the codes were organized thematically to reflect cultural and contextual factors that influence the construction of a digital identity and mental health.

Contextual outcome

Table 1 lists the interviews and captures the lived experience of Sri Lankan Gen Z Commerce students while managing and using digital identities in an interplay with cultural expectations and mental health. The varying themes that emerged highlighted the tension of managing cultural expectations of the family and peers. Participants frequently talked about selective self-disclosure as a social strategy in creating different self-identities to lower the expectations of family while engaging with social media—the core of contemporary culture. The interviews also captured the social comparison and validation pressures inherent in a culturally discriminated context of unaddressed suicidal ideation. Most distressing, as the participants noted, were the family aspects of communication, social interaction and spirituality, and the intended 'time away' from, or 'static' social media, and controlled exposure to it, which serve as stressors and buffers in their online interactions. These were also the non-modern 'primitive technology' controls that were used to facilitate the stressors identified with the social online world. These themes illustrate the distress of cultural dissonance as young adults juxtapose and harmonize the dominant global youth influencer culture with the traditions of their local culture.

Table 1. Interview Results

Research Question	Sub-Codes	Frequency	Themes	Interview Evidence (Participant Number)
Q1: Digital Identity & Self-Presentation	Cultural conformity, selective self-disclosure	18	1. Cultural Identity Negotiation	"I present myself differently online to respect family values." (P3)
	Online persona vs real self	15	2. Dual Identity	"Sometimes my online posts don't reflect my true feelings." (P7)
Q2: Mental Health Challenges	Social comparison, anxiety, stress from validation	20	3. Psychological Strain	"I feel pressured to get likes; it affects my mood daily." (P12)
	Fear of judgment	16	4. Cultural Stigma on Mental Health	"Mental health isn't openly discussed in my family or community." (P5)
Q3: Negotiation of Cultural Identity	Blending cultures, resistance, adaptation	22	5. Hybrid Cultural Identity	"I try to blend modern trends with traditional beliefs." (P9)
	Peer influence	14	6. Peer Mediation of Culture	"My friends help me decide what's acceptable online." (P14)

continued on following page

Table 1. Continued

Research Question	Sub-Codes	Frequency	Themes	Interview Evidence (Participant Number)
Q4: Coping Mechanisms	Family support, spiritual practices, digital detox	19	7. Culturally Grounded Coping	"Meditation and family talks help me when online pressure mounts." (P2)
	Social media breaks	12	8. Intentional Social Media Use	"I take breaks from Instagram when it becomes overwhelming." (P18)

4.2 Focus Group Results

The focus group discussions highlighted in Table 2 enhance individual interviews by providing insight into the shared communal experiences and cultural narratives prevailing among peers. From the interaction of the groups, participants expressed how the social media etiquette, intergenerational rifts, and influencer phenomena are negotiated within their relationships, considering the integration of modern practices and traditional values. The peer group's sociocultural influence in amplifying group identity, invasion of privacy, and the deterioration of mental well-being demonstrates the complexity of identity and privacy issues as being openly deliberated and jointly navigated. Notably, concepts such as aspirational and localized influencer identification capture how young people globalize digital phenomena while cultivating Sri Lankan pride, illustrating the complexities of youth culture. Focus group information, on the other hand, provided insights on community resiliency, humor as a coping strategy, and the importance of digital literacy education in promoting healthier interactions with social media. The portrait of youth outlined in Table 2 enhances the analysis by exposing the cultural processes underlying the sociocultural tensions impacting youth in-person and digital experiences.

Table 2. Focus Group Results

Research Question	Sub-Codes	Frequency	Themes	Focus Group Evidence (Group & Participant Number)
Q1: Social Media Norms & Practices	Group conformity, influencer mimicry	25	1. Collective Digital Identity	"We follow trends together, it's part of our group identity." (FG1-P4)
	Privacy concerns	19	2. Digital Privacy Awareness	"Many avoid posting too much because of privacy fears." (FG2-P3)
Q2: Cultural Expectations & Digital Life	Conflict with elders, generational gap	21	3. Intergenerational Cultural Tension	"Parents don't understand why we post the way we do." (FG3-P2)
	Preservation of cultural norms	18	4. Cultural Preservation Efforts	"We try to keep traditional values alive, even online." (FG1-P5)
Q3: Influencer Impact	Idealization of influencers, cultural mismatch	23	5. Aspirational Influencer Culture	"Some influencers show lifestyles that clash with our culture." (FG2-P1)
	Local influencer pride	17	6. Localized Influencer Identification	"We admire influencers who respect Sri Lankan values." (FG3-P4)
Q4: Mental Health & Social Media	Collective stress, normalization of anxiety	20	7. Shared Mental Health Challenges	"Everyone talks about stress from social media pressure." (FG1-P3)
	Peer support networks	16	8. Peer Support Systems	"We support each other when online drama happens." (FG2-P5)
Q5: Coping Strategies	Community activities, social media awareness programs	14	9. Community-Based Resilience	"Community events help us disconnect and recharge." (FG3-P6)
	Use of humor and memes	15	10. Humor as Coping	"We joke about online stress to deal with it together." (FG1-P2)
	Role of education	13	11. Digital Literacy and Education	"Schools need to teach us about healthy social media use." (FG2-P4)

Critical Thematic Analysis

The narrative components presented in Table 3 seek to elaborate and integrate the core themes identified during the interviews and focus group discussions with South Asian Gen Z Sri Lankans. Thereafter, these themes are analyzed concerning their implications on the mental health and digital self-perception of the participants. This encapsulates the preliminary cultural contextualization of the Sri Lankan Gen Z psychosocial intricacies, including identity construction, psychosocial stress, peer pressure and influence, influencer dynamics, and coping mechanisms. Table

3 organizes the themes according to their significance concerning the mental health and identity issues of the individual and sheds light on the cultural context underpinning the lived experiences of the youth in the digital world. Take, for instance, the frustration of juggling two contradictory personas, which, along with the stress of cultural performativity and identity fracturing, exacerbates the psychological conflict. Culturally predisposed coping mechanisms and supportive peers, on the other hand, appear to resonate as strong protective factors. The conceptual development for the narrative in Table 3 draws on findings from the literature to create a constructive rationale for the discussion and to provide nuance and pragmatics.

Table 3. Critical Analysis of Themes Influencing Mental Health and Digital Identity Formation

Theme	Description	Influence on Mental Health	Influence on Digital Identity Formation	Supporting Evidence (Participant/Group)
1. Cultural Identity Negotiation	Youth actively manage cultural expectations versus digital self-presentation	Causes stress when identity conflicts with family/social norms	Leads to selective self-disclosure and crafted online personas	P3: "I present myself differently online to respect family."
2. Dual Identity	Distinction between online persona and real self	May contribute to anxiety due to inauthenticity pressure	Creates multiple personas to navigate differing social worlds	P7: "Sometimes posts don't reflect my true feelings."
3. Psychological Strain	Anxiety and stress from social comparison and validation needs	Heightens depressive symptoms and lowered self-esteem	Drives obsessive engagement with social media feedback	P12: "I feel pressured to get likes; it affects my mood."
4. Cultural Stigma on Mental Health	Mental health remains taboo, limiting openness and help-seeking	Worsens mental health outcomes due to silence and isolation	Encourages concealment of mental health struggles online	P5: "Mental health isn't openly discussed in my family."
5. Hybrid Cultural Identity	Blending traditional and modern digital values	Can buffer mental health by providing flexible identity options	Enables a fluid online identity reflecting multiple cultural influences	P9: "I blend modern trends with traditional beliefs."

continued on following page

Table 3. Continued

Theme	Description	Influence on Mental Health	Influence on Digital Identity Formation	Supporting Evidence (Participant/Group)
6. Peer Mediation of Culture	Peer groups act as cultural interpreters, normalizing or challenging traditional values	Offers social support, reducing stress and isolation	Influences acceptable online behaviors and identity norms	P14: "My friends help decide what's acceptable online."
7. Culturally Grounded Coping	Use of family, spirituality, and culturally familiar practices to manage stress	Provides protective mental health effects	Influences content sharing and digital identity moderation	P2: "Meditation and family talks help with pressure."
8. Intentional Social Media Use	Conscious breaks and regulated use to maintain well-being	Reduces burnout and social media fatigue	Allows greater authenticity and identity coherence	P18: "I take breaks from Instagram when overwhelming."
9. Collective Digital Identity	Social media use as group identity expression and cohesion	Strengthens group belonging, mitigating loneliness	Creates shared digital norms and behaviors	FG1-P4: "We follow trends together as a group."
10. Digital Privacy Awareness	Awareness of privacy risks shaping cautious online behavior	Limits anxiety related to exposure and judgment	Encourages curated self-presentation and guarded identity sharing	FG2-P3: "Many avoid posting too much due to privacy fears."
11. Intergenerational Cultural Tension	Conflict between youth's online behavior and elders' traditional expectations	Increases family stress and mental health vulnerability	Forces youth to navigate dual cultural expectations in identity	FG3-P2: "Parents don't understand why we post the way we do."
12. Aspirational Influencer Culture	Exposure to influencer lifestyles often conflicting with local cultural values	Triggers self-esteem issues and unrealistic comparisons	Creates tension in adopting aspirational vs. traditional identities	FG2-P1: "Some influencers show lifestyles clashing with culture."
13. Localized Influencer Identification	Preference for influencers reflecting Sri Lankan cultural values	Supports cultural pride and positive self-esteem	Provides relatable role models for identity formation	FG3-P4: "We admire influencers who respect our values."
14. Shared Mental Health Challenges	Normalization of anxiety and stress across peer groups	Promotes collective awareness but risks peer-reinforced stress	Shapes digital behaviors emphasizing stress validation	FG1-P3: "Everyone talks about stress from social media."

continued on following page

Table 3. Continued

Theme	Description	Influence on Mental Health	Influence on Digital Identity Formation	Supporting Evidence (Participant/Group)
15. Peer Support Systems	Active emotional and practical support among peers regarding social media stress	Buffers negative mental health outcomes	Encourages shared identity resilience online	FG2-P5: "We support each other during online drama."
16. Community-Based Resilience	Participation in offline cultural/community activities supporting mental well-being	Provides social grounding and mental health benefits	Balances and strengthens offline identity anchoring online presence	FG3-P6: "Community events help us recharge."
17. Humor as Coping	Use of humor and memes within peer groups to diffuse stress	Facilitates emotional release and social bonding	Creates a shared language and identity that normalizes struggles	FG1-P2: "We joke about online stress together."
18. Digital Literacy and Education	Knowledge gaps about healthy social media practices	Increases risk of misinformation and digital stress	Educates youth to create safer, more authentic online identities	FG2-P4: "Schools should teach healthy social media use."

Multiple core components were identified with regard to Gen Z digital experiences in Sri Lanka. Informants detailed 'dual identity' in friction regards to online self-presentations and realities of in-person cultural surrounds. This complexity is also heightened in the context of the mental health stigma surrounding disengagement. Furthermore, friends are crucial in the negotiation of the cultural frameworks and in providing psychological support. The next chapter addresses these issues regarding the specific features of Sri Lanka as a collectivist system and the disruptive digital culture.

Students from Generation Z commerce in Sri Lanka exemplify the tensions surrounding digital self-presentation vis-a-vis the expectations of families and communities in the local culture. Participants in the study described social media as a 'stage' for self-presentation. Most participants explained self-presentation as a performance that fulfilled expectations surrounding family honor and local culture while more genuine self-presentation occurred in private and was otherwise obscured. Participant 3 exemplified this sentiment by stating, 'I respect family values, so I present myself differently online'. The disjunction between the public, highly regarded self and the private self invokes Bourdieu's (1984) theory of habitus. Bourdieu asserts that doxa is internalized in agents and they must continually navigate through different 'fields' or 'spaces'. In the case of the participants, they are influenced by local culture and digital social media 'fields' or 'spaces' (Hu and Cheong, 2021).

The tension that results from having a "real" and an "online" self points to the need of social harmony and the preservation of the family reputation in Sri Lanka (Hewamanne, 2019). Social media allows personal expression, but it also provides opportunities for social surveillance that people monitor for the families and communities. The need for social concordance increases the emotional and sociocultural pressure to configure one's online self in a way that is acceptable to the family, to avoid family and social ostracism (Sarkar, 2003). The negotiation of the cultural self, as described, aligns with the hybridity of youth identity, where the youth combine the hyper-modern technological globalization and value systems as a means to resolve the disjunctive traditional norms and expectations (Hällgren and Björk, 2022).

Participants also reported on the psychological distress caused by fragmentation of their identities, which includes some of the work by Geng et al. (2023) on digital performativity and the associated psychological distress. The construction of a dual identity results in a fracture which, as Participant 7 put it, "Sometimes my online posts don't reflect my true feelings." The anxiety that young individuals will ultimately confront will be the unification of disparate emotional states that will have to be reconciled in digital identity harmonization (Ebrahimpour Sadagheyani & Tatari, 2021). The digital habitus, in this sense, creates a situation in which the individual must engage in constant self-adjustment as the youth multitask in the seamless management of their identities across various cultural and social domains.

The political dimension of a digital identity is yet another complication. As Hu and Cheong (2021) mention, most of the political socialization of Generation Z takes place online, where social movements and global discourses are able to coalesce and define collective identities. Sri Lanka's youth participate in these conversations while contextualizing and negotiating their local cultural norms. This results in multilayered, global, local, and socioculturally inclusive identities. The 'self' that is performed digitally is emotionally and cognitively complicated because of the intertwining personal and familial, political and social, structures that they must negotiate, along with the sociocultural multilayered order that contains profound tensions.

Gendered Dynamics of Digital Identity and Mental Health

In Sri Lanka, even among the Gen Z population, there is a differentiated experience with respect to how digital identity is presented and negotiated. Women underwent a familial structure in which the women had to cope with hypervigilance in which family members were attentive to their online behavior.

Mental Health Challenges Amplified by Cultural Stigma

Insufficient understanding and resources regarding mental health issues culminated in some participants describing extreme feelings of anxiety and stress because of the need for validation offered via Instagram. Participant 12 described the experience best, "I feel pressured to get likes; it affects my mood daily." The negative impact of social comparison and validation seeking on mental health and the problematic use of social media described in Geng et al. (2023), applies to the depression presented by the participants in this study. For Sri Lankan youth, Participant 5 described the culture well, "Mental health isn't openly discussed in my family or community." Such community silence results in the exacerbation of mental health challenges. The cultural stigma described in the social repression of certain issues, together with a lack of proximal support, results in the profound alienation help seeking described by Vaishnav et al. (2023) in South Asian societies.

The absence of conversations regarding mental health issues has increased suffering, especially for adolescents who must deal with the isolating task of keeping their pains hidden to protect family honour and social reputation (Sarkar, 2003). The emotionally complex burden of concealment increases the susceptibility, especially for collectivist cultures, where the greater demand for social harmony ignores individual psychological suffering (Raghavan & Sandanapitchai, 2024). The stress of unaddressed issues in mental health has a considerable impact on sleep, which is one of the least acknowledged consequences. Alonzo et al. (2021) point out the lack of sleep as a mediating factor in the relation of social media to mental health, a sentiment voiced by study participants who experienced anxiety over social media and a wish to relate to over sleeping and late-night social media scrolling. The gap in sleep and psychological ill health aggravate the mental health crisis in the younger population.

Ebrahimpour Sadagheyani and Tatari (2021) describes social media as a double-edged sword, and I find this description fitting. While social media provides essential emotional support and friendships, it also exposes individuals to anxiety and unbearable loneliness. The normalisation of stress within social networks, as described in Table 2, Theme 7 ("Everyone talks about stress from social media pressure." FG1-P3) conveys the pervasiveness of mental health issues that social networks do not sufficiently attend to, thus highlighting the lack of culturally appropriate psychosocial support.

The conjunction of social media pressures, cultural stigma, and underdeveloped mental health resources culminates in an unaddressed scarcity of resources related to mental health. The paradox of heightened and suppressed vulnerability, coupled with demands for support, induces an extreme state of fragility. Concealment and stigma attached to mental health issues underscore the urgent need for focused interventions to recalibrate the digital environment with prevailing sociocultural realities.

Peer Groups as Cultural Mediators and Support Networks

Social peers function as cultural tension mediators and provide psychosocial support to individuals grappling with cross-culturally mediated digital identities and associated mental health issues. Participant 14, for example, stated, "My friends help me decide what's acceptable online." This illustrates the analytical and negotiation support friends provide in diasporic contexts regarding cultural engagement and boundary calibration. Such support is evident in the work of Hällgren and Bjork (2022) on hybrid identities, where integration is provided by social networks as support in discordant digital practices stemming from the intersection of traditional norms and modernity.

Focus group data indicate that adolescents are forming networks of peers in cyberspace that endorse the practice of new digital technologies while still upholding key elements of their culture (as observed in Theme 6, "We admire influencers who respect our values," FG3-P4), and in Theme 8, "We support each other when online drama happens" (FG2-P5). It is the social contexts created by these and other related phenomena that allow adolescents to collectively and collaboratively determine a set of parameters governing digital social connectivity and constellations of distress.

The adolescents in our participants' desciptions focus on building emotional scaffolding around social media to alleviate its adverse psychological impact. As noted in Theme 8, table 2, the excerpt, "We joke about online stress to deal with it together" (FG1-P2), describes peer support systems and the collective layering of anxious burdens. By culturally reinforcing social pathways around active resilience, this provision of social support counters familial stigma (Raghavan and Sandanapitchai, 2024).

These findings align with the research of Vissenberg et al. (2022) that focuses on digital literacy and peer mediation while framing adolescents as active local strategists for managing online relational aggression. Among other things, peer groups fulfil two important roles– cultural mediation, and psychosocial support. This is especially important in the Sri Lankan context, where the challenges of digital embodiment, psychosological issues, and mental health problems are intertwined.

Platform-Specific Effects of Instagram vs. TikTok

Research considering the digital mental health needs of countries such as Sri Lanka, may center on the differences in engagement of Gen Z on Instagram and TikTok. This is important given the different affordances of TikTok and Instagram and the implications for mental health. Instagram's visual curation leads to anxieties surrounding body image and social comparison. This was best articulated by Participant 13, who explained, "On Instagram, it feels like posts have to be the best and it makes me feel like I'm not doing enough in real life." In contrast, algorithm-driven TikTok culture is trend-obsessed which leads to rapid, pulsating pressure to perform, resulting in burnout and anxiety. Participant 9 articulated, "On TikTok, it's all about being part of the latest challenge or trend. It's like you're constantly on stage, trying to stay relevant." This illustrates the need to consider aspects of social media in mental health care more closely.

Influence of Social Media and Localized Influencer Culture

Many participants described the influence of social media and global influencer culture as overwhelming and commented that it was aspirational. For example, participants of Focus Group 2 commented, "Some influencers show lifestyles that clash with our culture" describing the disconnect that influencer culture has with Sri Lankan culture. This disconnect indicates mental and emotional distress as described in the literature (Khalid et al, 2018; Hewamanne, 2019) primarily because adolescents and young adults are trying to reconcile global digital culture with their challenges.

The respect given to local influencers mindful of and advocating for Sri Lankan culture likely contributes to positive identity affirmation. As a participant said, "We admire influencers who respect our values" (FG3-P4). Within one's local and cultural context, relevant social media influencers offer positive mentoring to disoriented youth. As they help youth to form their cultural identity and bridge cultural dissonance, as they global (Hällgren and Björk, 2022) or local, social integration. The literature notes that influencers and 'influencing' takes social comparison and competition to a new level, resulting in increased anxiety, and self-worth issues (Geng et al., 2023; Shensa et al., 2017). The issues identified by this study's participants of combining two or more diverse cultural narratives point to the intricate and multifaceted digital processes of cultural and social identity construction that global media exposes. This section focuses on the impact of social media influencers on youth identity and mental health by exploring the global cultural phenomena of cross-cultural insensitivity and the minimization of mental health issues.

Economic Aspirations and Digital Pressures

Understanding Digital Pressures with respect to Intended Majors in Commerce is important. In the future, students in Commerce will experience the intersection of social media aspirational culture and social/academic expectations. Some students described the pressure to compete not only in the Western capitalist economy and influencer economy, but also in the aspirational target economy. Participant 4 encapsulated this feeling in the example, "I'll see influencers living like I want to, and I'll wonder if I've done enough during my career." In this situation, anxiety of self-presentation and career self-sabotage become intertwined. Business students also described expectations of the influencer economy, a concept primarily attributed to students outside of business studies. Participant 15 captures this tension well when he states, "We learn marketing strategies but it's hard not to be influenced by someone who has it all."

Culturally Grounded Coping Mechanisms

For digital identity and mental health, the participants offered a diversified and culturally larger set of strategies. In the communication dimensions, notably the family aspect, when online pressure is too high, meditation and family conversations help. This aligns with the research concerning families, spirituality, and cultural resilience in more collectivistic societies (Raghavan and Sandanapitchai, 2024; Aldwin, 2007). Participant 18's description of "digital detoxification" of Instagram during particularly overwhelming periods is emblematic of the social media disengagements termed emotional cleansing, which have been argued to help with emotional regulation and burnout (Vissenberg et al., 2022). Other described factors for building resilience included the employment of humor and active participation in the community, primarily for the relief of stress. This was in reference to FG1-P2, who remarked, "We joke about online stress to deal with it together."

New modes of coping emerge with each new generation providing ways to avoid burnout and stress due to the technological advancements of the 21st century. Meanwhile, the 21st century's stress and burnout response systems also reveal ineffective mental health support systems, as the lack relevant local intervention systems becomes apparent. Sri Lanka's lack mental health support systems demonstrates the resilience of local coping mechanisms in stress and burnout. Inversely, it is vital to capture the scale of coping mechanisms available to the digital generation, which is disproportionate to the resilience mechanisms described. Participant 8 described, "I find peace through meditation and talking to my parents about my stress." This statement reflects young people's capability to integrate and maintain equilibrium within their mental constituents. This is achieved through the modern and the more traditional resources. This helps youth alleviate digital stress and maintain a positive self-identity.

Implications for Practice and Policy

As indicated in the first chapters of this report, Sri Lanka and the services the country offers are still culturally adapting to the technological changes incorporated in everyday life by the members of 'Gen Z'. The particular innovative mental health challenges that this unique gulf brings are crucial to be acknowledged and addressed in planning the mental health services for the young population. The remaining sections of this report, which highlight the applied conclusions from the data and the theoretical discourse outlined in the preceding chapters, provides some conclusions to the preceding issues.

Enhancing Cultural Competence in Mental Health and Educational Programs

Sri Lankan youth educators and practicing mental health clinicians must recognize that youth present and perform two different identities in social spheres – the public persona and the real self. In many instances, the personal self remains obscured to avoid familial and cultural discord. Feelings of social incompatibility arise from the composite of multiple discordant and dichotomous identities, and this has been shown to directly impact help-seeking behaviours negatively (Geng et al., 2023; Sarkar, 2003). Furthermore, the enhancement of programs concerned with digital well-being and mental health must integrate culturally rooted issues around values of family honour, intergenerational relationships, and collectivism.

Resource Dismantling any stigma or negativity linked to discussions around discomfort or taboo feelings towards mental health should be prioritized, empowering youth with more autonomy and shielding them from familial scrutiny. In this context, culturally tailored school-based guidance and peer counseling programs can be instrumental in nurturing traditional community arrangements for mental health advocacy (Raghavan and Sandanapitchai, 2024; Vaishnav et al., 2023). In addition, mental health instructors should recognize the role social media influencers play in peer comparison and identity formation, especially the digital stressors youth face, and teach them strategies for negotiating culturally meaningful digital identities.

In digital literacy education, social and emotional media awareness, as well as comparison-averse social media coping strategies, should be incorporated. Focus should aim to exceed guidance on mere technical skills; incorporating critical media literacy, which aids in dismantling influencer culture and foster the construction of positive, culturally consistent digital identities would be beneficial to youth (Vissenberg et al., 2022; Hällgren and Björk, 2022).

Policy Interventions to Destigmatize Mental Health

The culturally driven stigma associated with mental health has significantly hindered the open and timely help-seeking behavior of Sri Lankan Gen Z (Vaishnav et al, 2023; Sarkar, 2003). This has resulted in psychologically distressing conditions that remain concealed, with the individual suffering from greater isolation and neglect. More robust policy measures are necessary to change attitudes and empower the mental health discourse to be seamlessly integrated as a destigmatized element of support within families and communities. This has to be positioned and articulated in culturally sensitive terms. Given that TikTok and Instagram are social media platforms predominantly used by the younger generation, awareness clusters should be created to target Gen Z with media campaigns. For these campaigns, the use of local advocates that discuss their mental health challenges in an empowering manner to destigmatize help-seeking is recommended (Khalid et al, 2018). Furthermore, there should be policies that provide mental health counseling and educational and occupational institutions should be encouraged to teach mental health literacy. In addition to this, the gap in the primary research around the impact of technology on the mental health of South Asians and Sri Lankans must be addressed to guide policymakers to ensure resources are culturally aligned and appropriate (Alonzo et al., 2021; Geng et al., 2023).

Culturally Contextualized Digital Literacy and Media Education

Sri Lankan youth usage of social media is steeply increasing, demonstrating a demand for culturally situated educational digital literacy. This educational digital literacy focuses on culturally appropriate social media pressure coping mechanisms, as young people must also be trained to analyze and evaluate social media content critically (Hewamanne, 2019). Youth educational programs should also include strategies to counteract harmful influencer content and content that undermines local cultures. Understanding mental frames for such content will help youth mitigate a reflex stress identity crisis arising from unresolved tensions between globalized digitalized cultures and traditional cultures (Hällgren and Björk, 2022). Community-based digital literacy promotion should use social networks for evidence to maximize reach and relevancy. Emotional self-control and social media emotional regulation (Vissenberg et al, 2022) should be targeted by initiatives alongside social media boundary setting, purposeful intervals, and self-control.

Promoting Local Influencers as Positive Role Models

Social media can determine the identity and behavior of youth through influencers. The reach and admiration of Gen Z influencers from Sri Lanka have provided support and focus on the Culture of Positivity which is Self-Identity building (Khalid et al 2018). The support of the adversative influencers of disengagement on global mental health will assist in the shifting and encouraging positive engagement of constructive behaviors. Emphasis on collaboration between digital marketing and mental health advocacy within education is critical in shifting the focus toward digital influencers who center and promote the ideas of decommercialized mental health and the artistry of responsible digital citizenship and appreciation for one's culture. This aligns with the hybrid identity-discussed by Hällgren and Björk in 2022-where youth and adolescents gain access to and integrate global and local mental frameworks and constructs toward the digitally resilient self. Influencers designed within such collaborative programs will help to sustain a favorable global digital ecosystem which respects the global culture and in the process, destigmatize mental health through influencers who openly talk to youth about their mental health experiences and encourage the use of culturally adaptive coping strategies.

CONCLUSION

The present chapter is the first attempt to examine the Sri Lankan cultural values with regard to self-digitization, self-identity, mental health, and self-identity of Gen Z, while situating the discussion within a dominating social media influencer culture context. It amplifies the voices of Commerce students from Sri Lanka, capturing the students' dual identities of the struggle between self-affirmation and self-preservation as the students attempt to retain familial honour, social respectability, and social recognition. Unlike the majority of the literature, predominantly the Western literature, this dissertation draws from the lived experiences of Sri Lankan youth under digital pressure in a culturally collectivist context, accompanied with mental health stigma, and documenting the digital coping mechanisms Sri Lankan youth employed. The application of Bourdieu's theory of social habitus and resilience under transnational digital culture sheds light on social identity hybridity, the interface of constructed identities and local realities, and the contextual mental health implications that help in explaining the gaps in literature on social identity theory. One of the most rewarding aspects of this dissertation is the possible insight to be gained from the theorization of the intersection of global digital culture and local sociocultural realities.

The insights generated regarding responsive approaches to mental health within educational and sociopolitical frameworks within Sri Lanka and similarly influencing, rapidly changing, collectivist societies first need to consider the sociocultural contexts of the qualitative findings of this chapter. The findings necessitated the need to examine social influencer culture within the culturally bound parameters of social media and its associated impacts on the social and emotional well-being of the youth. In addition to this, the findings suggested the unimed potential to contextualize digital literacy instructional design frameworks with culturally responsive social media influencer mentors who can aid youth in digitally mediated resilience and self-concept construction. This chapter addresses the largely unexplored Indo-Asian socio-cultural narratives with actionable insights to aid youth in our digitally intertwined, culturally complex realities, emphasizing the lived experiences of Generation Z secondary school students in South Asia.

REFERENCES

Abidin, C. (2016). “Aren't these just young, rich women doing vain things online?”: Influencer selfies as subversive frivolity. *Social Media + Society*, *2*(2), 1–17. DOI: 10.1177/2056305116641342

Aldwin, C. M. (2007). *Stress, coping, and development: An integrative perspective.* Guilford Press.

Alonzo, R.. (2021). The interplay between social media use, sleep quality, and mental health: A systematic review. *Journal of Sleep Research*, *30*(2), e13127. PMID: 33385767

Braun, V., & Clarke, V. (2006). Using thematic analysis in psychology. *Qualitative Research in Psychology*, *3*(2), 77–101. DOI: 10.1191/1478088706qp063oa

Chuc, N. D., & Anh, D. T. (2023). Digital transformation in Vietnam. *Journal of Southeast Asian Economies*, *40*(1), 127–144. DOI: 10.1355/ae40-1f

Creswell, J. W., & Poth, C. N. (2018). *Qualitative inquiry and research design: Choosing among five approaches* (4th ed.). Sage.

Djafarova, E., & Rushworth, C. (2017). Exploring the credibility of online celebrities' Instagram profiles. *Computers in Human Behavior*, *68*, 1–7. DOI: 10.1016/j.chb.2016.11.009

Dodanwala, K. L., & Weerasekera, S. (2023). The impact of westernisation on the purchase intention of cruelty-free products: A study based on the Sri Lankan cosmetic market. *South Asian Journal of Marketing*, *5*(2), 131–148. DOI: 10.1108/SAJM-01-2023-0006

Ebrahimpour Sadagheyani, M., & Tatari, F. (2021). Social media's double-edged sword: Mental health perspectives. *Journal of Cyberpsychology*, *7*(2), 24–39.

Erangi, D. H. N., & Stecenko, I. (2024). Digital transformation in Sri Lanka: Evaluating progress and addressing challenges. Green. *Blue and Digital Economy Journal*, *5*(2), 1–11.

Geng, X., Zhang, J., Liu, Y., Xu, L., Han, Y., Potenza, M. N., & Zhang, J. (2023). Problematic use of the internet among adolescents: A four-wave longitudinal study of trajectories, predictors and outcomes. *Journal of Behavioral Addictions*, *12*(2), 435–447. DOI: 10.1556/2006.2023.00021 PMID: 37294627

Hällgren, C., & Björk, Å. (2022). Young people's identities in digital worlds. *The International Journal of Information and Learning Technology*, *40*(1), 49–61. DOI: 10.1108/IJILT-06-2022-0135

Hewamanne, S. (2019). Crafting social change: Former global factory workers negotiating new identities in Sri Lanka's villages. *Identities (Yverdon)*, *26*(2), 165–183. DOI: 10.1080/1070289X.2017.1380942

Hu, Q., & Cheong, P. H. (2021). Understanding digital generations: Social media habitus, memetic engagements, and digital social inequalities in China. *International Journal of Communication*, *15*, 22.

Katz, R., Ogilvie, S., Shaw, J., & Woodhead, L. (2021). Gen Z, explained: The art of living in a digital age. In *Gen Z, explained*. University of Chicago Press. DOI: 10.7208/chicago/9780226814988.001.0001

Khalid, N. L., Jayasainan, S. Y., & Hassim, N. (2018). Social media influencers-shaping consumption culture among Malaysian youth. In *SHS Web of Conferences* (Vol. 53, p. 02008). EDP Sciences. DOI: 10.1051/shsconf/20185302008

Kularathne, S., Perera, A., Rathnayake, N., Rathnayake, U., & Hoshino, Y. (2024). Analyzing the impact of socioeconomic indicators on gender inequality in Sri Lanka: A machine learning-based approach. *PLoS One*, *19*(12), e0312395. DOI: 10.1371/journal.pone.0312395 PMID: 39724101

Lim, L. T. S., Regencia, Z. J. G., Dela Cruz, J. R. C., Ho, F. D. V., Rodolfo, M. S., Ly-Uson, J., & Baja, E. S. (2022). Assessing the effect of the COVID-19 pandemic, shift to online learning, and social media use on the mental health of college students in the Philippines: A mixed-method study protocol. *PLoS One*, *17*(5), e0267555. DOI: 10.1371/journal.pone.0267555 PMID: 35503779

Morgan, D. L. (1997). *Focus groups as qualitative research* (2nd ed.). Sage. DOI: 10.4135/9781412984287

Nanayakkara, S. (2021). A descriptive analysis on digital behaviour of young adults in Sri Lanka. *International Journal of Business and Management Invention*, *9*(6). https://www.academia.edu/download/68897491/4._A_Descriptive_Analysis_on_Digital_Behaviour_of_Young_Adults_in_Sri_Lanka.pdf

Ong, E. (Ed.). (2024). *The Emergence of the Digital World: Friend Or Foe to Young Adults in the Post-pandemic Era?* Springer Nature. DOI: 10.1007/978-981-97-3098-8

Prasad, S., Ait Souabni, S., Anugwom, G., Aneni, K., Anand, A., Urhi, A., Obi-Azuike, C., Gibson, T., Khan, A., & Oladunjoye, F. (2023). Anxiety and depression amongst youth as adverse effects of using social media: A review. *Annals of Medicine and Surgery (London)*, *85*(8), 3974–3981. DOI: 10.1097/MS9.0000000000001066 PMID: 37554895

Raghavan, S., & Sandanapitchai, P. (2024). The relationship between cultural variables and resilience to psychological trauma: A systematic review of the literature. *Traumatology*, *30*(1), 37–51. DOI: 10.1037/trm0000239

Sarkar, S. (2003). *Gender as a cultural factor influencing mental health among adolescent students in India and Sri Lanka: A cross-cultural study*. State University of New York at Albany.

Sathurusinghe, R. I. T. (2024). An analysis on the impact of digital media devices on child socialization in Sri Lankan society. Proceedings of the International Research Conference of the Open University of Sri Lanka (IRC-OUSL 2024) http://repository.ou.ac.lk/bitstream/handle/94ousl/2676/IRC-OUSL2024_19_Sathurusinghe.pdf?sequence=1

Shan, B., Oh, I., & Rowley, C. (2023). Innovation and entrepreneurship in East Asia during the digital era: Post-pandemic prospects. *Asia Pacific Business Review*, *29*(4), 843–851. DOI: 10.1080/13602381.2023.2256106

Shensa, A.. (2017). Social media use and depressive symptoms among U.S. young adults. *Depression and Anxiety*, *34*(4), 323–331. PMID: 28446367

Vaishnav, M., Javed, A., Gupta, S., Kumar, V., Vaishnav, P., Kumar, A., & Ashurov, Z. (2023). Stigma towards mental illness in Asian nations and low-and-middle-income countries, and comparison with high-income countries: A literature review and practice implications. *Indian Journal of Psychiatry*, *65*(10), 995–1011. DOI: 10.4103/indianjpsychiatry.indianjpsychiatry_667_23 PMID: 38108051

Vissenberg, J., d'Haenens, L., & Livingstone, S. (2022). Digital literacy and online resilience as facilitators of young people's well-being? *European Psychologist*, *27*(2), 76–85. https://econtent.hogrefe.com/doi/abs/10.1027/1016-9040/a000478?journalCode=epp. DOI: 10.1027/1016-9040/a000478

Wickramanayake, L. (2022). Social media use by adolescent students of Sri Lanka: Impact on learning and behavior. *Global Knowledge, Memory and Communication*, *71*(1/2), 70–85. DOI: 10.1108/GKMC-08-2020-0123

Wickramasurendra, J. M., Jagoda, D. J., & Rathnayake, R. M. L. (2021). Factors influencing social media addiction among GCE advanced level students in Sri Lanka: A case study in Colombo district, Sri Lanka. *Sri Lanka Journal of Social Sciences and Humanities*, *1*(2), 1–11. DOI: 10.4038/sljssh.v1i2.33

Wies, B., Landers, C., & Ienca, M. (2021). Digital mental health for young people: A scoping review of ethical promises and challenges. *Frontiers in Digital Health*, *3*, 697072. DOI: 10.3389/fdgth.2021.697072 PMID: 34713173

Zhou, L.. (2021). Youth digital identity and mental health. *The Journal of Adolescent Health*, *69*(1), 15–22.

Compilation of References

Abamara Nnaemeka, C., Solomon, A. A., Gangopadhyay, A., Sahni, M. Y., & Esther, B. (2014). Relationship between Body Image and Self-esteem among female Undergraduate students of behavioural Sciences. *IOSR Journal Of Humanities And Social Science (IOSR-JHSS), 19*(1), 1-5. DOI: 10.9790/0837-191120105

Abdoshahi, M. (2024). Effects of an Intervention Based on Cognitive-Behavioral Therapy on Emotional Well-being of Athletic Adolescents with Injuries. *Physical Activity in Children, 1*(2), 61–68. https://www.pachjournal.com/article_211628.html

Abidin, C. (2016). “Aren’t these just young, rich women doing vain things online?”: Influencer selfies as subversive frivolity. *Social Media + Society*, *2*(2), 1–17. DOI: 10.1177/2056305116641342

Abidin, C. (2016). Visibility labour: Engaging with influencers’ fashion brands and #OOTD advertorial campaigns on Instagram. *Media International Australia, Incorporating Culture & Policy*, *161*(1), 86–100. DOI: 10.1177/1329878X16665177

Ackard, D. M., Eisenberg, M. E., & Neumark-Sztainer, D. (2007). Long-Term Impact of Adolescent Dating Violence on the Behavioral and Psychological Health of Male and Female Youth. *The Journal of Pediatrics*, *151*(5), 476–481. DOI: 10.1016/j.jpeds.2007.04.034 PMID: 17961688

Adetayo, A. J. (2024). Distracted Minds: Unveiling Gender Disparities in Social Media Distractions Amidst Library Reading. *International Journal of Information Science and Management*, *22*(2), 249–261. DOI: 10.22034/ijism.2024.2006251.1171

Advertising Standards Council of India. (2023). Influencer marketing guidelines: Disclosure and transparency standards. https://ascionline.in/influencer-marketing-guidelines

Agarwal, N. A. (2024). The effect of social media in identity formation in adolescence. *World Journal of Advanced Research and Reviews*, *23*(3), 775–779. DOI: 10.30574/wjarr.2024.23.3.2685

Ahlawat, R., Ghai, M., & Garg, S. K. (2022). *Factors influencing restaurant selection in the COVID-19 era: a study of consumer preferences in India*. DOI: 10.5281/ZENODO.7314391

Ahmed, N. (2019). Generation Z's smartphone and social media usage, A survey. *Journalism and mass communication, 9*(3), 101–122.

Ahuja, M. (2025, May 1). *Top 60 Social Media Influencers: Who's Leading the Chart*. SocialPilot. Retrieved May 27, 2025, from https://www.socialpilot.co/blog/top-social-media-influencers

AJEWOLE, D. K. (2024). The Impact of Social Media on Mental Health. DOI: 10.14293/PR2199.001180.v1

Akhmad, M. A., At, M. R., & Muhammad, S. (2024). Reconstructing Generation Z's Digital Identity: Self-Presentation and Impression Management Strategies in Second Account Instagram. *Thammasat Review*, *27*(2), 335–350.

Aksoydan, E. (2007). Hygiene factors influencing customers' choice of dining-out units: Findings from a study of university academic staff. *Journal of Food Safety*, *27*(3), 300–316. DOI: 10.1111/j.1745-4565.2007.00081.x

Akthar, N., & Hassan, A. (2021). Demand Analysis of Tourism and Hospitality Products and Services in Bangladesh. In Hassan, A. (Ed.), *Tourism Products and Services in Bangladesh* (pp. 159–179). Springer Singapore., DOI: 10.1007/978-981-33-4279-8_8

Alalwan, A. A. (2018). Investigating the impact of social media advertising features on customer purchase intention. *International Journal of Information Management*, *42*, 65–77. DOI: 10.1016/j.ijinfomgt.2018.06.001

Aldwin, C. M. (2007). *Stress, coping, and development: An integrative perspective*. Guilford Press.

Algharabat, R. S., & Shatnawi, T. (2014). The effect of 3D product quality (3D–Q) on perceived risk and purchase intentions: The case of apparel online retailers. *International Journal of Electronic Business*, *11*(3), 256–273. DOI: 10.1504/IJEB.2014.063031

Al-Maghrabi, T., Dennis, C., & Halliday, S. V. (2011). Antecedents of continuance intentions towards e-shopping: The case of Saudi Arabia. *Journal of Enterprise Information Management*, *24*(1), 85–111. DOI: 10.1108/17410391111097447

Alonzo, R.. (2021). The interplay between social media use, sleep quality, and mental health: A systematic review. *Journal of Sleep Research*, *30*(2), e13127. PMID: 33385767

Alper, R., & Başaran, Z. (2023). To examine the work commitment and psychological flexibility levels of university stuff who participate in yoga activities as a recreational experience. *International Journal of Recreation and Sports Science*, *7*(1), 6–17. https://dergipark.org.tr/en/pub/ijrss/issue/81342/1281670. DOI: 10.46463/ijrss.1281670

Alter, A. (2017). *Irresistible: The rise of addictive technology and the business of keeping us hooked*. Penguin Press.

Amam, M. (2024). Influence of Cultural Heritage Preservation on Tourism Development in Egypt. *American Journal of Arts. Social and Humanity Studies*, *4*(1), 22–32. DOI: 10.47672/ajashs.2063

Ambardar, A., Singh, A., & Singh, V. (2023). Barriers in Implementing Ergonomic Practices in Hotels- A Study on five star hotels in NCR region. *International Journal of Hospitality and Tourism Systems*, *16*(2), 11–17.

American Psychological Association. (2018). *Body image*. Retrieved from American Psychological Association: https://dictionary.apa.org/body-image

American Psychological Association. (2023). Stress in America: Generation Z report. APA. https://www.apa.org

American Psychological Association. (2025). *self-awareness*. Retrieved from American Psychological Association: https://dictionary.apa.org/self-awareness

Ampornklinkaew, C. (2025). The role of social media influencers in influencing consumers' imitation intentions. *Digital Business*, *100143*(2), 100143. Advance online publication. DOI: 10.1016/j.digbus.2025.100143

Andreassen, C. S., Pallesen, S., & Griffiths, M. D. (2017). The relationship between addictive use of social media, narcissism, and self-esteem: Findings from a large national survey. *Addictive Behaviors*, *64*, 287–293. DOI: 10.1016/j.addbeh.2016.03.006 PMID: 27072491

Ansari, A. I., & Singh, A. (2023). Application of augmented reality (AR) and virtual reality (VR) in promoting guest room sales: A critical review. In Z. Tučková, S. K. Dey, H. H. Thai, & S. D. Hoang (Eds.), Impact of Industry 4.0 on sustainable tourism (pp. 95–104). Emerald Publishing. https://doi.org/DOI: 10.1108/978-1-80455-157-820231006

Ansari, Z. (2023, September 18). The social media influencers impact on youth. *Locobuzz Solutions Private Limited*. Retrieved May 19, 2025, from https://locobuzz.com/blogs/social-media-influencers-impact-on-youth/

Ansari, A. I., Singh, A., Pattanaik, S., Patnaik, R., & Suryawanshi, U. (2024). Exploring the Role of AI-Powered Virtual Assistants in Optimizing Self-Service Experiences for Customers Within the Service Sector. In Nadda, V., Tyagi, P., Singh, A., & Singh, V. (Eds.), *Integrating AI-Driven Technologies Into Service Marketing* (pp. 225–238). IGI Global., DOI: 10.4018/979-8-3693-7122-0.ch013

Anwar, A., Kumar, S., & Talukder, M. B. (2025). Sustainable Rural Development Through Homestay Tourism: An Evaluation of Economics. In Parashar, A., Chandel, P. S., Seetaram, N., & Agarwal, P. (Eds.), *Global Practices and Innovations in Sustainable Homestay Tourism* (pp. 41–74). IGI Global., DOI: 10.4018/979-8-3373-0427-4.ch003

Appel, G., Grewal, L., Hadi, R., & Stephen, A. T. (2020). The future of social media in marketing. *Journal of the Academy of Marketing Science*, *48*(1), 79–95. DOI: 10.1007/s11747-019-00695-1 PMID: 32431463

Atanasova, A. (2016, November 6). *Gender-specific behaviors on social media and what they mean for online communications*. Retrieved from Social Media Today: https://www.socialmediatoday.com/social-networks/gender-specific-behaviors-social-media-and-what-they-mean-online-communications

Attest. (2025). *Gen Z media consumption report*. Retrieved from https://www.askattest.com/blog/research/gen-z-media-consumption

Avery, T., Blasey, C., Rosen, C., & Bayley, P. (2018). Psychological flexibility and set-shifting among veterans participating in a yoga program: A pilot study. *Military Medicine*, *183*(11–12), e359–e363. DOI: 10.1093/milmed/usy045 PMID: 29590487

Avi, Md. A. R., & Sardar, S. (2021). Application of Innovative Technologies in Bangladesh's Tourism and Hospitality Industry: Challenges and Suggestions. In A. Hassan (Ed.), *Technology Application in Bangladesh's Tourism and Hospitality Industry* (pp. 369–379). Springer Singapore. DOI: 10.1007/978-981-16-2434-6_22

Badruddoza Talukder, M., Kumar, S., Misra, L. I., & Firoj Kabir, . (2024). Determining the role of eco-tourism service quality, tourist satisfaction, and destination loyalty: A case study of Kuakata beach. *Acta Scientiarum Polonorum. Administratio Locorum*, *23*(1), 133–151. DOI: 10.31648/aspal.9275

Baker, K. (2008). Kerala's strategy for tourism growth: A southern approach to development and poverty alleviation. In Burns, P., & Novelli, M. (Eds.), *Tourism development: Growth, myths and inequalities* (1st ed., pp. 192–216). CABI., DOI: 10.1079/9781845934255.0192

Bandyopadhyay, R., & Nair, B. B. (2019a). Marketing Kerala in India as God's Own Country! For tourists' spiritual transformation, rejuvenation and well-being. *Journal of Destination Marketing & Management*, *14*, 100369. DOI: 10.1016/j.jdmm.2019.100369

Bányai, F., Zsila, Á., Király, O., Maraz, A., Elekes, Z., Griffiths, M. D., Andreassen, C. S., & Demetrovics, Z. (2017). Problematic social media use: Results from a large-scale nationally representative adolescent sample. *PLoS One*, *12*(1), e0169839. DOI: 10.1371/journal.pone.0169839 PMID: 28068404

Bappy, T. A., & Avi, Md. A. R. (2021). Technological Innovation Application in the Tourism and Hospitality Industry of Bangladesh. In A. Hassan (Ed.), *Technology Application in the Tourism and Hospitality Industry of Bangladesh* (pp. 63–77). Springer Singapore. DOI: 10.1007/978-981-16-2434-6_4

Barber, N., & Scarcelli, J. M. (2009). Clean restrooms: How important are they to restaurant consumers? *Journal of Foodservice*, *20*(6), 309–320. DOI: 10.1111/j.1748-0159.2009.00155.x

Barber, N., & Scarcelli, J. M. (2010). Enhancing the assessment of tangible service quality through the creation of a cleanliness measurement scale. *Managing Service Quality*, *20*(4), 373–392. DOI: 10.1108/09604521011011630

Bargh, J. A., McKenna, K. Y. A., & Fitzsimons, G. M. (2002). Can you see the real me? Activation and expression of the "true self" on the Internet. *The Journal of Social Issues*, *58*(1), 33–48. DOI: 10.1111/1540-4560.00247

Barry, C. T., Reiter, S. R., Anderson, A. C., & Schoessler, B. N. (2019). "Let me take a selfie": Associations between self-photography, narcissism, and self-esteem. *Psychology of Popular Media Culture*, *8*(1), 25–33. DOI: 10.1037/ppm0000162

Baumeister, R. F., Campbell, J. D., Krueger, J. I., & Vohs, K. D. (2003). Does High Self-Esteem Cause Better Performance, Interpersonal Success, Happiness, or Healthier Lifestyles? *Psychological Science in the Public Interest*, *4*(1), 1–44. DOI: 10.1111/1529-1006.01431 PMID: 26151640

Bawden, D., & Robinson, L. (2020). Information overload: An overview. Błachnio, A., Przepiórka, A., & Benvenuti, M. (2022). Social media use and mental health: The role of personality traits, cyberbullying, and emotional intelligence. *Psychiatry Research, 307*, 114340. DOI: 10.1016/j.psychres.2021.114340

Baym, N. K., & boyd, . (2012). Socially mediated publicness: An introduction. *Journal of Broadcasting & Electronic Media, 56*(3), 320–329. DOI: 10.1080/08838151.2012.705200

Becker, C., Murrmann, S. K., Murrmann, K. F., & Cheung, G. W. (1999). A pancultural study of restaurant service expectations in the United States and Hong Kong. *Journal of Hospitality & Tourism Research (Washington, D.C.), 23*(3), 235–255. DOI: 10.1177/109634809902300301

Bełch, P., Hajduk-Stelmachowicz, M., Chudy-Laskowska, K., Vozňáková, I., & Gavurová, B. (2024). Factors Determining the Choice of Pro-Ecological Products among Generation Z. *Sustainability (Basel), 16*(4), 1560. DOI: 10.3390/su16041560

Belk, R. W. (2017). Qualitative research in advertising. *Journal of Advertising, 46*(1), 36–47. DOI: 10.1080/00913367.2016.1201025

Bell, B. T., Taylor, C., Paddock, D., & Bates, A. (2021). Digital Bodies: A controlled evaluation of a brief classroom-based intervention for reducing negative body image among adolescents in the digital age. *The British Journal of Educational Psychology, 91*(1), 280–298. DOI: 10.1111/bjep.12449 PMID: 34350594

Beltramo, R., Duglio, S., & Mascadri, G. (2024). Mountain Tourism: Environmental Management for Fostering Tourism Destinations: From Context Analysis to Tourism Products. In Lagioia, G., Paiano, A., Amicarelli, V., Gallucci, T., & Ingrao, C. (Eds.), *Innovation, Quality and Sustainability for a Resilient Circular Economy* (pp. 509–515). Springer International Publishing., DOI: 10.1007/978-3-031-28292-8_62

Berbegal-Mirabent, J., Mas-Machuca, M., & Marimon, F. (2016). Antecedents of online purchasing behaviour in the tourism sector. *Industrial Management & Data Systems, 116*(1), 87–102. DOI: 10.1108/IMDS-05-2015-0213

Beritelli, P., & Schegg, R. (2016). Maximizing online bookings through a multi-channel-strategy—Effects of interdependencies and networks. *International Journal of Contemporary Hospitality Management, 28*(1), 68–88. DOI: 10.1108/IJCHM-07-2014-0326

Berners-Lee, T. (1999). *Weaving the Web: The original design and ultimate destiny of the World Wide Web by its inventor*. Harper San Francisco.

Bertollo, M., Saltarelli, B., & Robazza, C. (2009). Mental preparation strategies of elite modern pentathletes. *Psychology of Sport and Exercise, 10*(2), 244–254. DOI: 10.1016/j.psychsport.2008.09.003

Best, P., Manktelow, R., & Taylor, B. (2014). Online communication, social media and adolescent wellbeing: A systematic narrative review. *Children and Youth Services Review, 41*, 27–36. DOI: 10.1016/j.childyouth.2014.03.001

Bethune, S. (2019, 01 19). Gen Z more likely to report mental health concerns. *50*(1), p. 20. Retrieved from https://www.apa.org/monitor/2019/01/gen-z

Beyens, I., Pouwels, J., van Driel, I. I., Keijsers, L., & Valkenburg, P. M. (2021). Social Media Use and Adolescents' Well-Being: Developing a Typology of Person-Specific Effect Patterns. *Communication Research, 51*(6), 691–716. DOI: 10.1177/00936502211038196

Bhalla, A., Singh, P., & Singh, A. (2023). Technological Advancement and Mechanization of the Hotel Industry. In Tailor, R. (Ed.), *Application and Adoption of Robotic Process Automation for Smart Cities* (pp. 57–76). IGI Global., DOI: 10.4018/978-1-6684-7193-7.ch004

Bhorkar, R. (2024, November 14). *The influence of social media influencers on youth culture and identity*. Retrieved May 18, 2025, from https://www.linkedin.com/pulse/influence-social-media-influencers-youth-culture-identity-bhorkar-xybzc/

Bhuiyan, M. R. U., & Bhuiyan, M. B. (2023). Crises and Conflicts on the Way to Sustainable Tourism Development: A Study of Cox's Bazar, Bangladesh. *Journal of Environmental Management and Tourism, 14*(2), 320. DOI: 10.14505/jemt.v14.2(66).03

Bienstock, C. C., DeMoranville, C. W., & Smith, R. K. (2003). Organizational citizenship behavior and service quality. *Journal of Services Marketing, 17*(4), 357–378. DOI: 10.1108/08876040310482775

Billah, M. (2022, December 7). The rise of the "influencer" market in Bangladesh. *The Business Standard*. https://www.tbsnews.net/long-read/rise-influencer-market-bangladesh-546854

Bırni, G., & Eryılmaz, A. (2024). Conceptual and Theoretical Review of Self-Worth. *Psikiyatride Güncel Yaklasimlar, 16*(2), 327–346. DOI: 10.18863/pgy.1336880

Birrer, D., & Morgan, G. (2010). Psychological skills training as a way to enhance an athlete's performance in high-intensity sports. *Scandinavian Journal of Medicine & Science in Sports, 20*(s2), 78–87. DOI: 10.1111/j.1600-0838.2010.01188.x PMID: 20840565

Boerman, S. C., & Van Reijmersdal, E. A. (2020). Disclosing influencer marketing on YouTube to children: The moderating role of para-social relationship. *Frontiers in Psychology, 10*, 3042. DOI: 10.3389/fpsyg.2019.03042

Bonfanti, R. C., Melchiori, F., Teti, A., Albano, G., Raffard, S., Rodgers, R., & Lo Coco, G. (2025). The association between social comparison in social media, body image concerns and eating disorder symptoms: A systematic review and meta-analysis. *Body Image, 52*, 101841. DOI: 10.1016/j.bodyim.2024.101841 PMID: 39721448

Bonfils, M. (2022). The Effects of Social Media on Gen Zs' Mental Health (Doctoral dissertation, Doctoral dissertation, School Of Business, Siam University, Bangkok, Thailand).

Bournemouth University. (2023, June 30). *Passive social media use is linked to higher levels of loneliness and psychological distress*. Retrieved July 12, 2025, from Bournemouth University.

boyd, d. (2010). Social network sites as networked publics: Affordances, dynamics, and implications. In Z. Papacharissi (Ed.), A networked self (pp. 39–58). Routledge.

Boyd, D. (2014). *It's complicated: The social lives of networked teens*. Yale University Press.

Boyle, R. (2009). *Power play: Sport, the media and popular culture*. Edinburgh University Press. https://books.google.com/books?hl=en&lr=&id=fQerBgAAQBAJ&oi=fnd&pg=PR2&dq=1.%09Boyle,+R.,+%26+Haynes,+R.+(2009).+Power+play:+Sport,+the+media+and+popular+culture.+Edinburgh+University+Press.&ots=RBFWJLoxhU&sig=8drhFLqOeOy6FMHQQFxyzEldyvo

BRAC Mental Health Strategy 2020-2030. (2021). In https://www.brac.net/program/mental-health/. BRAC Mental Health Strategy Working Group. Retrieved June 7, 2025, from https://www.brac.net/program/wp-content/uploads/2021/09/BRAC-mental_-health_strategy-2020-2030.pdf

Braun, V., & Clarke, V. (2006). Using thematic analysis in psychology. *Qualitative Research in Psychology, 3*(2), 77–101. DOI: 10.1191/1478088706qp063oa

Bronfenbrenner, U. (1979). *The Ecology of Human Development: Experiments by Nature and Design*. Harvard University Press. DOI: 10.4159/9780674028845

Brown, J., & Marshall, M. (2006). The Three Faces of Self-Esteem. In Kernis, M. (Ed.), *Self-esteem: Issues and answers* (pp. 4–9). Psychology Press.

Brown, Z., & Tiggemann, M. (2016). Attractive celebrity and peer images on Instagram: Effect on women's mood and body image. *Body Image*, *19*, 37–43. DOI: 10.1016/j.bodyim.2016.08.007 PMID: 27598763

Bucher, T. (2017). The algorithmic imaginary: Exploring the ordinary affects of Facebook algorithms. *Information Communication and Society*, *20*(1), 30–44. DOI: 10.1080/1369118X.2016.1154086

Buhalis, D., Leung, X. Y., Fan, D., Darcy, S., Chen, G., Xu, F., Wei-Han Tan, G., Nunkoo, R., & Farmaki, A. (2023). Editorial: Tourism 2030 and the contribution to the sustainable development goals: the tourism review viewpoint. *Tourism Review*, *78*(2), 293–313. DOI: 10.1108/TR-04-2023-620

Burr, C., Taddeo, M., & Floridi, L. (2020, August). The ethics of digital well-being: A thematic review. *Science and Engineering Ethics*, *26*(4), 2313–2343. DOI: 10.1007/s11948-020-00175-8 PMID: 31933119

Caine, D., Walch, T., & Sabato, T. (2016). The elite young athlete: Strategies to ensure physical and emotional health. *Open Access Journal of Sports Medicine*, *7*, 99–113. DOI: 10.2147/OAJSM.S96821 PMID: 27621677

Cain, N., & Gradisar, M. (2010). Electronic media use and sleep in school-aged children and adolescents: A review. *Sleep Medicine*, *11*(8), 735–742. DOI: 10.1016/j.sleep.2010.02.006 PMID: 20673649

Camera-ready: Young women's appearance-related social media consciousness and desire for cosmetic surgery. *Body Image, 32*, 212–220. DOI: 10.1016/j.bodyim.2020.01.006

Carvalho de Rezende, D., & Alberto Rodrigues Silva, M. (2013). Eating-out and experiential consumption: A typology of experience providers. *British Food Journal*, *116*(1), 91–103. DOI: 10.1108/BFJ-02-2012-0027

Casaló, L. V., Flavián, C., & Ibáñez-Sánchez, S. (2018, July). The relevance of creativity and emotions in engaging users on Instagram. In *Global Marketing Conference* (pp. 4-5).

Casaló, L. V., Flavián, C., & Ibáñez-Sánchez, S. (2018). Influencers on Instagram: Antecedents and consequences of opinion leadership. *Journal of Business Research*, *117*, 510–519. DOI: 10.1016/j.jbusres.2018.07.005

Cash, T. F. (2005). The influence of sociocultural factors on body image: Searching for constructs. *Clinical Psychology : a Publication of the Division of Clinical Psychology of the American Psychological Association*, *12*(4), 438–442. DOI: 10.1093/clipsy.bpi055

Castells, M. (2000). Globalisation, identity and the state. *Social Dynamics*, *26*(1), 5–17. DOI: 10.1080/02533950008458682

Chae, J. (2018). Explaining females' envy toward social media influencers. *Media Psychology*, *21*(2), 246–262. DOI: 10.1080/15213269.2017.1328312

Chang, A.-M., Aeschbach, D., Duffy, J. F., & Czeisler, C. A. (2015). Evening use of light-emitting eReaders negatively affects sleep, circadian timing, and next-morning alertness. *Proceedings of the National Academy of Sciences of the United States of America*, *112*(4), 1232–1237. DOI: 10.1073/pnas.1418490112 PMID: 25535358

Chang, C.-Y., Jhang, S.-J., Yang, Y.-T., Chang, H.-C., & Chang, Y.-J. (2024). Utilizing Skip-Gram for Restaurant Vector Creation and Its Application in the Selection of Ideal Restaurant Locations. In Deng, D.-J., & Chen, J.-C. (Eds.), *Smart Grid and Internet of Things* (Vol. 557, pp. 141–147). Springer Nature Switzerland., DOI: 10.1007/978-3-031-55976-1_14

Chan, K. T. (2022). Emergence of the 'Digitalized Self' in the Age of Digitalization. *Computers in Human Behavior Reports*, *6*(1), 100191. DOI: 10.1016/j.chbr.2022.100191

Charmaraman, L., Hojman, H., Auqui, J. Q., & Bilyalova, Z. (2025). Understanding Adolescent Self-esteem and Self-image Through Social Media Behaviors. *Pediatric Clinics of North America*, *72*(2), 189–201. DOI: 10.1016/j.pcl.2024.07.034 PMID: 40010860

Chaudhury, S. K., Sarkar, S., Pattnaik, C. S., & Rahman, S. (2023). Assessment of Kerala Tourism Industry-An Economic Perspective. *Dera Natung Government College Research Journal*, *8*(1), 97–110. DOI: 10.56405/dngcrj.2023.08.01.07

Chen, H. T., & Li, X. (2017). The contribution of mobile social media to social capital and psychological well-being: Examining the role of communicative use, friending and self-disclosure. *Computers in Human Behavior*, *75*, 958–965. DOI: 10.1016/j.chb.2017.06.011

Chen, Y. (2025). Navigating the digital mirror: The role of information-seeking orientation and uncertainty tolerance in social media-driven body image anxiety. *Computers in Human Behavior Reports*, *18*, 100665. Advance online publication. DOI: 10.1016/j.chbr.2025.100665

Chettiparamb, A., & Kokkranikal, J. (2012). Responsible tourism and sustainability: The case of Kumarakom in Kerala, India. *Journal of Policy Research in Tourism, Leisure & Events*, *4*(3), 302–326. DOI: 10.1080/19407963.2012.711088

Chhabra, J., Pilkington, V., Benakovic, R., Wilson, M. J., La Sala, L., & Seidler, Z. (2025). Social Media and Youth Mental Health: Scoping Review of Platform and Policy Recommendations. *Journal of Medical Internet Research*, *27*, e72061.

Chiang, Y. T., & Lin, S. S. (2010). Early adolescent players' playfulness and psychological needs in online games. *Social Behavior and Personality*, *38*(5), 627–636. DOI: 10.2224/sbp.2010.38.5.627

Chib, S., Mehta, A. K., Selvakumar, P., Saravanan, A., Mishra, B. R., & Manjunath, T. C. (2025). Mental health challenges and solutions in high-pressure work environments. In Harriott, S. (Ed.), *Innovative Approaches to Managing Conflict and Change in Diverse Work Environments* (pp. 247–272). IGI Global Scientific Publishing., DOI: 10.4018/979-8-3693-9556-1.ch011

Choi, E., King, G. K., & Duerden, E. G. (2023). Screen time in children and youth during the pandemic: A systematic review and meta-analysis. *Global Pediatrics*, *6*, 100080. Advance online publication. DOI: 10.1016/j.gpeds.2023.100080

Chon, K. S. (2012). *The Tourism and Leisure Industry: Shaping the Future* (0 ed.). Routledge. DOI: 10.4324/9780203049853

Choudhary, B., & Qadir, A. (2021). Impact of COVID-19 on wellness and spa industry. *International Journal of Spa and Wellness*, *4*(2–3), 193–203. DOI: 10.1080/24721735.2021.1986970

Chou, H. T., & Edge, N. (2012). They are happier and having better lives than I am: The impact of using Facebook on perceptions of others' lives. *Cyberpsychology, Behavior, and Social Networking*, *15*(2), 117–121. DOI: 10.1089/cyber.2011.0324 PMID: 22165917

Choukas-Bradley, S., Maheux, A. J., Aubrey, J. S., Charmaraman, L., Maas, M. K., Nesi, J., & Yang, C.-c. (2025). Social Media Use, Body Image Concerns, and Disordered Eating Among Adolescents. In Christakis, D. A., & Hale, L. (Eds.), *Handbook of Children and Screens* (pp. 149–156). Springer Nature., DOI: 10.1007/978-3-031-69362-5_21

Choukas-Bradley, S., Nesi, J., Widman, L., & Higgins, M. K. (2020).

Chrisler, J. C., & Ghiz, L. (1993). Body image issues of older women. *Women & Therapy*, *14*(1-2), 67–75. DOI: 10.1300/J015v14n01_07

Chua, B.-L., Al-Ansi, A., Lee, M. J., & Han, H. (2021). Impact of health risk perception on avoidance of international travel in the wake of a pandemic. *Current Issues in Tourism*, *24*(7), 985–1002. DOI: 10.1080/13683500.2020.1829570

Chuc, N. D., & Anh, D. T. (2023). Digital transformation in Vietnam. *Journal of Southeast Asian Economies*, *40*(1), 127–144. DOI: 10.1355/ae40-1f

Common Sense Media. (2022). The impact of social media on youth mental health. Common Sense Media. https://www.commonsensemedia.org

Corbin, J., & Strauss, A. (2008). *Basics of Qualitative Research* (3rd ed.). Techniques and Procedures for Developing Grounded Theory., DOI: 10.4135/9781452230153

Craig, S. L., Eaton, A. D., & McInroy, L. (2020). Navigating negativity online: Exploring the effects of cyberbullying and social networking on LGBTQ youth. *Youth & Society*, *52*(5), 551–573. DOI: 10.1177/0044118X19856139

Craig, V. (2018). The impacts of high-volume massage on spa therapists' physical and mental wellness. *International Journal of Spa and Wellness*, *1*(3), 218–227. DOI: 10.1080/24721735.2019.1596659

Creswell, J. W., & Poth, C. N. (2018). *Qualitative inquiry and research design: Choosing among five approaches* (4th ed.). Sage.

Cristancho Triana, G. J., Cancino Gomez, Y. A., & Ninco Hernandez, F. A. (2024). Factores que influyen en el comportamiento de consumo sostenible en la generación Z. *Retos*, *14*(27), 51–67. DOI: 10.17163/ret.n27.2024.04

Crocker, J., & Wolfe, C. (2001). Contingencies of self-worth. *Psychological Review*, *108*(3), 593–623. DOI: 10.1037/0033-295X.108.3.593 PMID: 11488379

Cronbach, L. J. (1951). Coefficient Alpha and the Internal Structure of Tests. *Psychometrika*, *16*(3), 297–334. DOI: 10.1007/BF02310555

Cropink. (2025). *50+ alarming social media and mental health statistics*. Cropink. https://cropink.com/social-media-mental-health-statistics

Csirmaz, É., & Pető, K. (2015). International Trends in Recreational and Wellness Tourism. *Procedia Economics and Finance*, *32*, 755–762. DOI: 10.1016/S2212-5671(15)01458-6

Cyranski, C. (2017a). *Purifying Purges and Rejuvenating Massages: Ayurvedic Health Tourism in South India*. DOI: 10.11588/HEIDOK.00022342

Dahiya, R., & Selvakumar, P. Vidyadhara, & Manjunath, T. C. (2025). Design and Aerodynamics: Principles and Advances. In M. Mellal (Ed.), Innovations and Developments in Unmanned Aerial Vehicles (pp. 145-170). IGI Global Scientific Publishing. DOI: 10.4018/979-8-3693-8462-6.ch007

Dann, C., & Capdevila, R. (2023). Social Media and Gendered Power: Young Women, Authenticity, and the Curation of Self. In Zurbriggen, E., & Capdevila, R. (Eds.), *The Palgrave Handbook of Power, Gender, and Psychology* (pp. 537–553). Palgrave Macmillan., DOI: 10.1007/978-3-031-41531-9_29

Das, I. R., Talukder, M. B., & Kumar, S. (2024). Implication of Artificial Intelligence in Hospitality Marketing. In Kumar, S., Talukder, M. B., & Pego, A. (Eds.), *Advances in Hospitality, Tourism, and the Services Industry* (pp. 291–310). IGI Global., DOI: 10.4018/979-8-3693-1978-9.ch014

De Barros Neto, J. P., & De Oliveira, L. P. (2023). Study on the perception of Generation Z about robotized selection processes. *International Robotics & Automation Journal*, *9*(3), 99–107. DOI: 10.15406/iratj.2023.09.00271

de Jans, S., Van de Sompel, D., Hudders, L., & Cauberghe, V. (2023). How young children process influencer marketing: The moderating role of media literacy. *Journal of Advertising*, *52*(1), 88–103. DOI: 10.1080/00913367.2023.2172165

De Segovia Vicente, D., Van Gaeveren, K., Murphy, S. L., & Vanden Abeele, M. M. P. (2024). Does mindless scrolling hamper well-being? Combining ESM and log-data to examine the link between mindless scrolling, goal conflict, guilt, and daily well-being. *Journal of Computer-Mediated Communication*, *29*(1), zmad056. Advance online publication. DOI: 10.1093/jcmc/zmad056

De Veirman, M., Cauberghe, V., & Hudders, L. (2017). Marketing through Instagram influencers: The impact of number of followers and product divergence on brand attitude. *International Journal of Advertising*, *36*(5), 798–828. DOI: 10.1080/02650487.2017.1348035

De Veirman, M., Hudders, L., & Nelson, M. R. (2019). What is influencer marketing and how does it target children? A review and direction for future research. *Frontiers in Psychology*, *10*, 2685. Advance online publication. DOI: 10.3389/fpsyg.2019.02685 PMID: 31849783

Debatin, B., Lovejoy, J. P., Horn, A.-K., & Hughes, B. N. (2009). Facebook and online privacy: Attitudes, behaviors, and unintended consequences. *Journal of Computer-Mediated Communication*, *15*(1), 83–108. DOI: 10.1111/j.1083-6101.2009.01494.x

Debord, G. (1967). *Society of the spectacle*. Bureau of Public Secrets.

Deci, E. L., Olafsen, A. H., & Ryan, R. M. (2017). Self-determination theory in work organizations: The state of a science. *Annual Review of Organizational Psychology and Organizational Behavior*, *4*(1), 19–43. DOI: 10.1146/annurev-orgpsych-032516-113108

De, D., El Jamal, M., Aydemir, E., & Khera, A. (2025). Social media algorithms and teen addiction: Neurophysiological impact and ethical considerations. *Cureus, 17*(1). Advance online publication. DOI: 10.7759/cureus.77145 PMID: 39925596

Deepika, M. (2025, March 15). *The impact of social media influencers on youth behavior and culture in India.* The One Liner. Retrieved May 19, 2025, from https://theoneliner.in/the-impact-of-social-media-influencers-on-youth/

Del Chiappa, G., Alarcón-Del-Amo, M.-D.-C., & Lorenzo-Romero, C. (2016). Internet and user-generated content versus high street travel agencies: A latent gold segmentation in the context of Italy. *Journal of Hospitality Marketing & Management, 25*(2), 197–217. DOI: 10.1080/19368623.2014.1001933

Department of Economic and Social Affairs. United Nations. (2015). *THE 17 GOALS.* Retrieved from United Nations: https://sdgs.un.org/goals

Deshmukh, A., T. K. S., Rahul, S., & Medhekar, A. A. (2024). *User generated content and its influence on relationship marketing among Generation Z. Journal of Informatics Education and Research, 4*(1). DOI: 10.52783/jier.v4i1.633

Designed and Developed by Will Earp, South West Grid for Learning Trust Ltd. (n.d.). *Impact of Influencer Culture – How to help young people create a more positive online space.* Retrieved May 19, 2025, from https://swgfl.org.uk/topics/digital-wellbeing/impact-of-influencer-culture-how-to-help-young-people-create-a-more-positive-online-space/

Dewangan, S., & Kumar, S. (2024). AI and Big Data Analytics Revolutionizing Industry 5.0: Unlocking the Power of Smart Manufacturing and Beyond. In Darwish, D. (Ed.), (pp. 398–410). Advances in Business Information Systems and Analytics. IGI Global., DOI: 10.4018/979-8-3693-0413-6.ch016

Dhir, A., Pallesen, S., Torsheim, T., & Andreassen, C. S. (2016). Do age and gender differences exist in selfie-related behaviours? *Computers in Human Behavior, 63,* 549–555. DOI: 10.1016/j.chb.2016.05.053

Dhir, A., Yossatorn, Y., Kaur, P., & Chen, S. (2018). Online social media fatigue and psychological well-being—A study of compulsive use, fear of missing out, and fatigue. *International Journal of Information Management, 40,* 141–152. DOI: 10.1016/j.ijinfomgt.2018.01.012

Dhir, A., Yossatorn, Y., Kaur, P., & Chen, S. (2021). Online social media fatigue and psychological well-being—A study of compulsive use, fear of missing out, and gender differences. *International Journal of Information Management, 61,* 102255. DOI: 10.1016/j.ijinfomgt.2021.102255

Ding, L., & Jiang, C. (2023). The effect of perceived collective efficacy and self-efficacy on Generation Z restaurant customers' food waste reduction intentions. *Journal of Global Responsibility*, *14*(3), 337–359. DOI: 10.1108/JGR-08-2022-0079

Dionne, M. M., & Davis, C. (2012). Body Image and Personality. In Cash, T. F. (Ed.), *Encyclopedia of Body Image and Human Appearance* (pp. 135–140). Academeic Press., DOI: 10.1016/B978-0-12-384925-0.00020-1

Djafarova, E., & Rushworth, C. (2017). Exploring the credibility of online celebrities' Instagram profiles. *Computers in Human Behavior*, *68*, 1–7. DOI: 10.1016/j.chb.2016.11.009

Dodanwala, K. L., & Weerasekera, S. (2023). The impact of westernisation on the purchase intention of cruelty-free products: A study based on the Sri Lankan cosmetic market. *South Asian Journal of Marketing*, *5*(2), 131–148. DOI: 10.1108/SAJM-01-2023-0006

Dogan, S., Mistry, T. G., & Nanu, L. (2024). Revolutionizing getaways: Automation and artificial intelligence's transformative journey in tourism and hospitality. *Worldwide Hospitality and Tourism Themes*, *16*(2), 248–251. Advance online publication. DOI: 10.1108/WHATT-03-2024-0075

Domoff, S. E., Foley, R. P., & Ferkel, R. (2020). Addictive phone use and academic performance in adolescents. *Human Behavior and Emerging Technologies*, *2*(1), 33–38. DOI: 10.1002/hbe2.171

Dorčić, T. M., Smojver-Ažić, S., Božić, I., & Malkoč, I. (2023). Effects of Social Media Social Comparisons and Identity Processes on Body Image Satisfaction in Late Adolescence. *Europe's Journal of Psychology*, *19*(2), 220–231. DOI: 10.5964/ejop.9885 PMID: 37731891

Dores, A. R., Peixoto, M., Fernandes, C., & Marques, A. (2025). The Effects of Social Feedback Through the "Like" Feature on Brain Activity: A Systematic Review. *In Healthcare, 13*(1), 89.

Döring, N., Reif, A., & Poeschl, S. (2016). How gender-stereotypical are selfies? A content analysis and comparison with magazine adverts. *Computers in Human Behavior, 55(Part B)*, 955-962. DOI: 10.1016/j.chb.2015.10.001

Dredge, R., & Che, S. (2020). Chinese online gamers versus nongamers: A difference in social media use and associated well-being and relational outcomes? *Psychology in the Schools*, *57*(9), 1457–1474. DOI: 10.1002/pits.22418

Duffy, B. E., & Hund, E. (2015). "Having it all" on social media: Entrepreneurial femininity and self-branding among fashion bloggers. *Social Media + Society*, *1*(2), 1–11. DOI: 10.1177/2056305115604337

Duffy, B. E., & Schwartz, B. (2018). Digital "women's work?": Job recruitment ads and the feminization of social media employment. *New Media & Society*, *20*(8), 2972–2989. DOI: 10.1177/1461444817738237

Ebrahimpour Sadagheyani, M., & Tatari, F. (2021). Social media's double-edged sword: Mental health perspectives. *Journal of Cyberpsychology*, *7*(2), 24–39.

Ehimuan, B., Akindote, O. J., Olorunsogo, T., Anyanwu, A., Olorunsogo, T. O., & Reis, O. (2024). Mental health and social media in the U.S.: A review: Investigating the potential links between online platforms and mental well-being among different age groups. *International Journal of Science and Research Archive*, *11*(1), 464–477. DOI: 10.30574/ijsra.2024.11.1.0059

Electro, I. Q. (2025). Social Media Mental Health Statistics and Facts. ElectroIQ. https://electroiq.com/stats/social-media-mental-health-statistics/

El-Gohary, H. (2012). Factors affecting e-marketing adoption and implementation in tourism firms: An empirical investigation of Egyptian small tourism organisations. *Tourism Management*, *33*(5), 1256–1269. DOI: 10.1016/j.tourman.2011.10.013

Elhai, J. D., Levine, J. C., Dvorak, R. D., & Hall, B. J. (2016). Fear of missing out, need for touch, anxiety, and depression are related to problematic smartphone use. *Computers in Human Behavior*, *63*, 509–516. DOI: 10.1016/j.chb.2016.05.079

Elkind, D. (1967). Egocentrism in adolescence. *Child Development*, *38*(4), 1025–1034. DOI: 10.2307/1127100 PMID: 5583052

Ellison, N. B., & Boyd, D. M. (2007). Social Network Sites: Definition, History, and Scholarship. *Journal of Computer-Mediated Communication*, *13*(1), 210–230. DOI: 10.1111/j.1083-6101.2007.00393.x

Emory University Rollins School of Public Health. (2024). *Overview of social media's impact on youth mental health, noting rising anxiety, depression, and the role of algorithms.* Retrieved from Rollins School of Public Health.: https://sph.emory.edu

Engel, E., Gell, S., Heiss, R., & Karsay, K. (2023). Social media influencers and adolescents' health: A scoping review of the research field. *Social Science & Medicine*, *340*, 116387. DOI: 10.1016/j.socscimed.2023.116387 PMID: 38039770

Erangi, D. H. N., & Stecenko, I. (2024). Digital transformation in Sri Lanka: Evaluating progress and addressing challenges. Green. *Blue and Digital Economy Journal*, *5*(2), 1–11.

Erikson, E. H. (1968). *Identity: Youth and crisis*. W. W. Norton.

Escobar-Rodríguez, T., & Carvajal-Trujillo, E. (2014). Online purchasing tickets for low cost carriers: An application of the unified theory of acceptance and use of technology (UTAUT) model. *Tourism Management*, *43*, 70–88. DOI: 10.1016/j.tourman.2014.01.017

Etikan, I. (2016). Comparison of convenience sampling and purposive sampling. *American Journal of Theoretical and Applied Statistics*, *5*(1), 1. DOI: 10.11648/j.ajtas.20160501.11

Evangeline, S., Rajkumar, M. R., & Parambath, S. G. (Eds.). (2019). *Recent Advances in Materials, Mechanics and Management* (1st ed.). CRC Press., DOI: 10.1201/9781351227544

Exploring the influence of online platforms on well-being: The intersection of social media and mental health. *Center for Advanced Policy & Development Research*. http://capdr.org/wp-content/uploads/2023/11/60.-Dr.-ABDAL-AHMED-et-al.pdf

Fabris, M. A., & Longobardi, C. (2024). Body image. In Troop-Gordon, W., & Neblett, E. W. (Eds.), *Encyclopedia of Adolescence* (2nd ed., pp. 32–42). Academic Press. DOI: 10.1016/B978-0-323-96023-6.00012-9

Falk, T., Hammerschmidt, M., & Schepers, J. J. (2010). The service quality–satisfaction link revisited: Exploring asymmetries and dynamics. *Journal of the Academy of Marketing Science*, *38*(3), 288–302. DOI: 10.1007/s11747-009-0152-2

Fardouly, J., Diedrichs, P. C., Vartanian, L. R., & Halliwell, E. (2015). Social comparisons on social media: The impact of Facebook on young women's body image concerns and mood. *Body image*, *13*, 38-45.

Fardouly, J., Diedrichs, P. C., Vartanian, L. R., & Halliwell, E. (2015). Social comparisons on social media: The impact of Facebook on young women's body image concerns and mood. *Body Image*, *13*, 38–45. DOI: 10.1016/j.bodyim.2014.12.002 PMID: 25615425

Fardouly, J., & Vartanian, L. R. (2016). Social Media and Body Image Concerns: Current Research and Future Directions. *Current Opinion in Psychology*, *9*(9), 1–5. DOI: 10.1016/j.copsyc.2015.09.005

Farivar, S., & Wang, F. (2022). Effective influencer marketing: A social identity perspective. *Journal of Retailing and Consumer Services*, *67*, 103026. DOI: 10.1016/j.jretconser.2022.103026

Fassi, L., Ferguson, A. M., Przybylski, A. K., Ford, T. J., & Orben, A. (2025). Social media use in adolescents with and without mental health conditions. *Nature Human Behaviour*, *9*(6), 1–17. DOI: 10.1038/s41562-025-02134-4 PMID: 40325198

Feinstein, B. A., Hershenberg, R., Bhatia, V., Latack, J. A., Meuwly, N., & Davila, J. (2013). Negative social comparison on Facebook and depressive symptoms: Rumination as a mechanism. *Psychology of Popular Media Culture*, *2*(3), 161–170. DOI: 10.1037/a0033111

Fekete, M., & Nagy, Á. (2022). Qlimates and Quarantines – Testing the Hypothesis of How Gen Z Transformed into a Generation. In Schutter, S., Harring, D., & Bass, L. E. (Eds.), *Sociological Studies of Children and Youth* (pp. 1–27). Emerald Publishing Limited., DOI: 10.1108/S1537-466120220000030001

Fernandes, T. (2024). Brands as drivers of social media fatigue and its impact on user engagement. *Young Consumers*, *25*(5), 625–642. DOI: 10.1108/YC-11-2023-1763

Festinger, L. (1954). A theory of social comparison processes. *Human Relations*, *7*(2), 117–140. DOI: 10.1177/001872675400700202

Festinger, L. (1957). *A Theory of Cognitive Dissonance*. Stanford University Press. DOI: 10.1515/9781503620766

Firoj, K., & Mohammad, B. T. (2024). Measuring sustainability in the broadcasting media industry in Bangladesh. *I-Manager's. Journal of Management*, *18*(3), 51. DOI: 10.26634/jmgt.18.3.20234

Firth, J., Firth, J. A., Stubbs, B., & Torous, J. (2019). The "online brain": How the Internet may be changing our cognition. *World Psychiatry; Official Journal of the World Psychiatric Association (WPA)*, *18*(2), 119–129. DOI: 10.1002/wps.20617 PMID: 31059635

Fogaca, J. L. (2021). Combining Mental Health and Performance Interventions: Coping and Social Support for Student-Athletes. *Journal of Applied Sport Psychology*, *33*(1), 4–19. DOI: 10.1080/10413200.2019.1648326

Foroudi, P., Gupta, S., Sivarajah, U., & Broderick, A. (2018). Investigating the effects of smart technology on customer dynamics and customer experience. *Computers in Human Behavior*, *80*, 271–282. DOI: 10.1016/j.chb.2017.11.014

Foucault, M., Martin, L. H., Gutman, H., & Hutton, P. H. (1988). *Technologies of the self*. Tavistock.

Fox, J., & Vendemia, M. A. (2016). elective Self-Presentation and Social Comparison Through Photographs on Social Networking Sites. *Cyberpsychology, Behavior, and Social Networking*, *19*(10), 593–600. DOI: 10.1089/cyber.2016.0248 PMID: 27732079

Francis, R. S., Anantharajah, S., Sengupta, S., & Singh, A. (2024). Leveraging ChatGPT and digital marketing for enhanced customer engagement in the hotel industry. In Bansal, R., Ngah, A., Chakir, A., & Pruthi, N. (Eds.), *Leveraging ChatGPT and artificial intelligence for effective customer engagement* (pp. 55–68). IGI Global., DOI: 10.4018/979-8-3693-0815-8.ch004

Fredrickson, B. L., & Roberts, T.-A. (1997). Objectification Theory: Toward Understanding Women's Lived Experiences and Mental Health Risks. *Psychology of Women Quarterly*, *21*(2), 173–206. DOI: 10.1111/j.1471-6402.1997.tb00108.x

Frison, E., & Eggermont, S. (2016). Exploring the Relationships Between Different Types of Facebook Use, Perceived Online Social Support, and Adolescents' Depressed Mood. *Social Science Computer Review*, *34*(2), 153–171. DOI: 10.1177/0894439314567449

Fromm, J., & Read, A. (2018). *Marketing to Gen Z: The rules for reaching this vast–and very different–generation of influencers*. Amacom. https://books.google.com/books?hl=en&lr=&id=kVBLDwAAQBAJ&oi=fnd&pg=PP1&dq=%E2%80%A2%09Fromm,+J.,+%26+Read,+A.+(2018).+Marketing+to+Gen+Z:+The+rules+for+reaching+this+vast--and+very+different--generation+of+influencers.+AMACOM.&ots=fcUFyJ1mMn&sig=SwxIwCKlg-6J-R39h63bPtCVbpE

Fry, R., & Parker, K. (2018). *Early Benchmarks Show Gen Z Is More Diverse, On Track to Be Better Educated Than Previous Generations*. Pew Research Center.

Future Partners. (2025). What's new with Gen Z travelers? Future Partners Blog. Retrieved from https://futurepartners.com/blog/whats-new-with-gen-z/

Gaiswinkler, L., & Unterrainer, H.-F. (2016). The relationship between yoga involvement, https://www.sciencedirect.com/science/article/pii/S096522991630036X. DOI: 10.1016/j.ctim.2016.03.011 PMID: 27261992

Gann, M. C. (2025). Social Media and Mental Health According to Generation Z: A Health Belief Model-Based Cross-Sectional Evaluation of Generation Z Adults' Attitudes and Perceptions of Problematic Social Media Use and Its Relationship with Depression and Anxiety

Gao, M. (2023). Social media's influence on eating disorders. *Modern Economics & Management Forum*, *4*(4), 107. DOI: 10.32629/memf.v4i4.1489

García-Crespo, Á., Colomo-Palacios, R., Gómez-Berbís, J. M., & Ruiz-Mezcua, B. (2010). SEMO: A framework for customer social networks analysis based on semantics. *Journal of Information Technology*, *25*(2), 178–188. DOI: 10.1057/jit.2010.1

Garrido-Moreno, A., Lockett, N., & García-Morales, V. (2014). Social media use and value creation in hotels. *International Journal of Contemporary Hospitality Management*, *26*(1), 104–123.

Gautham, M., Gururaj, G., Varghese, M., Benegal, V., Rao, G., Kokane, A., Chavan, B., Dalal, P. K., Ram, D., Pathak, K., Lenin Singh, R. K., Singh, L. K., Sharma, P., Saha, P. K., Ramasubramanian, C., Mehta, R. Y., Shibukumar, T. M., Deuri, S. P., Krishnatreya, M., & Majhi, G. (2020). The National Mental Health Survey of India (2016): Prevalence, socio-demographic correlates and treatment gap of mental morbidity. *The International Journal of Social Psychiatry*, *66*(4), 361–372. DOI: 10.1177/0020764020907941 PMID: 32126902

Gen Z mental health. The impact of tech and social media. *McKinsey & Company*. https://www.mckinsey.com/mhi/our-insights/gen-z-mental-health-the-impact-of-tech-and-social-media

Geng, X., Zhang, J., Liu, Y., Xu, L., Han, Y., Potenza, M. N., & Zhang, J. (2023). Problematic use of the internet among adolescents: A four-wave longitudinal study of trajectories, predictors and outcomes. *Journal of Behavioral Addictions*, *12*(2), 435–447. DOI: 10.1556/2006.2023.00021 PMID: 37294627

Gentry, J. H., & Campbell, M. (2002). *Developing Adolescents: A Reference for Professionals*. American Psychological Association.

George, A. T., DeLacy, T., & Jiang, M. (2020). 6 Responsible Rural Tourism Initiatives and Local Community Development in Kerala, India. In Nair, V., Hamzah, A., & Musa, G. (Eds.), *Responsible Rural Tourism in Asia* (pp. 87–101). Multilingual Matters., DOI: 10.21832/9781845417529-008

George, L. (2025). Reclaiming agency in an age of digital distraction: Strategies for mindful media engagement. *Journal of Digital Culture & Society*, *12*(1), 45–61. https://www.researchgate.net/publication/388194527_Reclaiming_Agency_in_an_Age_of_Digital_Distraction

Gerbner, G., & Gross, L. (1976). Living with television: The cultivation perspective. *Journal of Communication*, *26*(2), 172–192. DOI: 10.1111/j.1460-2466.1976.tb01397.x PMID: 932235

Geurin-Eagleman, A. N., & Burch, L. M. (2016). Communicating via photographs: A gendered analysis of Olympic athletes' visual self-presentation on Instagram. *Sport Management Review*, *19*(2), 133–145. DOI: 10.1016/j.smr.2015.03.002

Gibbons, F. X., & Buunk, B. P. (1999). Individual differences in social comparison: Development of a scale of social comparison orientation. *Journal of Personality and Social Psychology*, *76*(1), 129–142. DOI: 10.1037/0022-3514.76.1.129 PMID: 9972558

Girard, R. (1972). *La Violence et le sacre*. Bloomsbury Academic.

Girard, R. (1977). *Violence and the Sacred* (Gregory, P., Trans.). Johns Hopkins University Press. DOI: 10.56021/9780801819636

Goffman, E. (1959). *The Presentation of Self in Everyday Life*.

Goffman, E. (1959). *The presentation of self in everyday life*. Anchor Books.

Govindasamy, K., Kaur, D., Elayaraja, M., Sethi, D., Kalidas, S., Karmakar, D., Orhan, B. E., Astuti, Y., & Parpa, K. (2024). Immediate Effect of Uddiyana Bandha on Heart Rate Variability in Patients with Hypertension: A Randomised Controlled Study. *Annals of Neurosciences*, *09727531241299258*, 09727531241299258. Advance online publication. DOI: 10.1177/09727531241299258 PMID: 39678718

Granic, I., Morita, H., & Scholten, H. (2020). Beyond screen time: Identity development in the digital age. *Developmental Psychology*, *56*(5), 1239–1247. DOI: 10.1037/dev0000935

Greenspan, M. J., & Feltz, D. L. (1989). Psychological interventions with athletes in competitive situations: A review. *The Sport Psychologist*, *3*(3), 219–236. https://journals.humankinetics.com/view/journals/tsp/3/3/article-p219.xml. DOI: 10.1123/tsp.3.3.219

Gudka, M., Gardiner, K. L., & Loma, T. (2023). Towards a framework for flourishing through social media: A systematic review of 118 research studies. *The Journal of Positive Psychology*, *18*(1), 86–105. DOI: 10.1080/17439760.2021.1991447

Gulliver, A., Griffiths, K. M., & Christensen, H. (2012). Barriers and facilitators to mental health help-seeking for young elite athletes: A qualitative study. *BMC Psychiatry*, *12*(1), 157. DOI: 10.1186/1471-244X-12-157 PMID: 23009161

Guo, C., Chen, F., & Wang, Y. (2025). The Psychological Impact of Competitive Sports Participation on Adolescent Athletes: An Analysis of Coping Mechanisms and Performance Outcomes. *Journal of Rational-Emotive & Cognitive-Behavior Therapy*, *43*(2), 24. Advance online publication. DOI: 10.1007/s10942-025-00587-0

Gupta, K. P., & Pande, S. (2023). Understanding Generation Z consumers' revisit intentions to robotic service restaurants. *Young Consumers*, *24*(3), 331–351. DOI: 10.1108/YC-09-2022-1598

Gupta, M., & Sharma, A. (2021, July 6). Fear of missing out: A brief overview of origin, theoretical underpinnings and relationship with mental health. *World Journal of Clinical Cases*, *9*(19), 4881–4889. DOI: 10.12998/wjcc.v9.i19.4881 PMID: 34307542

Gustafsson, H., Lundqvist, C., & Tod, D. (2017). Cognitive behavioral intervention in sport psychology: A case illustration of the exposure method with an elite athlete. *Journal of Sport Psychology in Action*, *8*(3), 152–162. DOI: 10.1080/21520704.2016.1235649

Haferkamp, N., & Krämer, N. C. (2011). Social comparison 2.0: Examining the effects of online profiles on social-networking sites. *Cyberpsychology, Behavior, and Social Networking*, *14*(5), 309–314. DOI: 10.1089/cyber.2010.0120 PMID: 21117976

Ha, L., & Yang, Y. (2023). Research about persuasive effects of social media influencers as online opinion leaders 1990–2020: A review. *International Journal of Internet Marketing and Advertising*, *18*(2–3), 220–241. DOI: 10.1504/IJIMA.2023.132562

Hällgren, C., & Björk, Å. (2022). Young people's identities in digital worlds. *The International Journal of Information and Learning Technology*, *40*(1), 49–61. DOI: 10.1108/IJILT-06-2022-0135

Hammad, A. (2024). Factors Influencing the Digital Tourism Marketing of Generation Z Tourists "Applied to the Egyptian Tourist Destination." *International Journal of Tourism. Archaeology and Hospitality*, *4*(1), 15–37. DOI: 10.21608/ijtah.2024.251138.1107

Han, H., & Hyun, S. S. (2015). Customer retention in the medical tourism industry: Impact of quality, satisfaction, trust, and price reasonableness. *Tourism Management*, *46*, 20–29. DOI: 10.1016/j.tourman.2014.06.003

Han, H., Kiatkawsin, K., Jung, H., & Kim, W. (2018). The role of wellness spa tourism performance in building destination loyalty: The case of Thailand. *Journal of Travel & Tourism Marketing*, *35*(5), 595–610. DOI: 10.1080/10548408.2017.1376031

Han, H., & Kim, Y. (2010). An investigation of green hotel customers' decision formation: Developing an extended model of the theory of planned behavior. *International Journal of Hospitality Management*, *29*(4), 659–668. DOI: 10.1016/j.ijhm.2010.01.001

Hanlon, A.-M., & Jones, K. M. (2023). Ethical concerns about social media privacy policies: Do users have the ability to comprehend their consent actions? *Journal of Strategic Marketing*, 1–18. DOI: 10.1080/0965254X.2023.2232817

Harmony Healthcare IT. (2025, June 5). *State of Gen Z Mental Health*. Retrieved from Harmony Healthcare IT: https://www.harmonyhit.com/

Harmony, H. I. T. (2025). State of Gen Z. https://www.harmonyhit.com/state-of-gen-z-mental-health/

Harter, S. (2012). The construction of the self: Developmental and sociocultural foundations (2nd ed.). Guilford Press. Journal of Adolescent Health. (2022). Evaluating digital wellness curricula in schools: Impacts on anxiety and validation-seeking. Journal of Adolescent Health, 71(4), 511–520. DOI: 10.1016/j.jadohealth.2022.06.005

Hartmann, P., Apaolaza, V., Paredes, M. R., & D'Souza, C. (2025). How Greenfluencers boost climate action: Why inspirational green leadership matters. *International Journal of Consumer Studies*, *49*(3), e70050. Advance online publication. DOI: 10.1111/ijcs.70050

Hassan, V. I., Singh, A., Jaboob, A. S., & Sorayyaei Azar, A. (Eds.). (2025). *Revolutionizing healthcare experience with digital medical tourism*. IGI Global., DOI: 10.4018/979-8-3693-7888-5

Hayes, H. (2024, February 8). *The impact of influencers on young adults and teens*. Heather Hayes & Associates. Retrieved May 19, 2025, from https://heatherhayes.com/the-impact-of-influencers-on-young-adults-and-teens/

Hayes, A. F. (2018). *Introduction to mediation, moderation, and conditional process analysis: A regression-based approach* (2nd ed.). Guilford Press.

Hays, K., Thomas, O., Maynard, I., & Butt, J. (2010). The role of confidence profiling in cognitive-behavioral interventions in sport. *The Sport Psychologist*, *24*(3), 393–414. DOI: 10.1123/tsp.24.3.393

Healey, E. (2025, June). *Raw, messy aesthetic and the illusion of authenticity*. Retrieved from The Guardian: https://www.theguardian.com

Helberger, N., Pierson, J., & Poell, T. (2018). Governing online platforms: From contested to cooperative responsibility. *The information society*, *34*(1), 1-14.

Hewamanne, S. (2019). Crafting social change: Former global factory workers negotiating new identities in Sri Lanka's villages. *Identities (Yverdon)*, *26*(2), 165–183. DOI: 10.1080/1070289X.2017.1380942

Hjetland, G. J., Finserås, T. R., Sivertsen, B., Colman, I., Hella, R. T., & Skogen, J. C. (2022). Focus on self-presentation on social media across sociodemographic variables, lifestyles, and personalities: A cross-sectional study. *International Journal of Environmental Research and Public Health*, *19*(17), 11133. DOI: 10.3390/ijerph191711133 PMID: 36078843

Hoang, D. P., Nguyen Hai, D., Nguyen, V. T. N., Nong, H. T., Pham, P. T., & Tran, T. M. (2024). Factors affecting restaurant choices for traditional foods among Gen Y and Gen Z: A multigenerational study on Vietnamese "Pho." *Journal of Hospitality and Tourism Insights*. DOI: 10.1108/JHTI-10-2023-0766

Hogan, B. (2010). The presentation of self in the age of social media: Distinguishing performances and exhibitions online. *Bulletin of Science, Technology & Society*, *30*(6), 377–386. DOI: 10.1177/0270467610385893

Hollander, D., Meyers, M. C., & LeUnes, A. (1995). Psychological factors associated with overtraining: Implications for youth sport coaches. *Journal of Sport Behavior*, *18*, 3–3. https://www.academia.edu/download/109139060/Psychological_Factors_Associated_with_Overtraining.pdf

Holland, G., & Tiggemann, M. (2016). A systematic review of the impact of the use of social networking sites on body image and disordered eating outcomes. *Body Image*, *17*, 100–110. DOI: 10.1016/j.bodyim.2016.02.008 PMID: 26995158

Holman, E. A., Garfin, D. R., & Silver, R. C. (2013). Media's role in broadcasting acute stress following the Boston Marathon bombings. *Proceedings of the National Academy of Sciences of the United States of America*, *111*(1), 93–98. DOI: 10.1073/pnas.1316265110 PMID: 24324161

Holm, J. E., Beckwith, B. E., Ehde, D. M., & Tinius, T. P. (1996). Cognitive-behavioral interventions for improving performance in competitive athletes: A controlled treatment outcome study. *International Journal of Sport Psychology*, *27*, 463–475. https://www.researchgate.net/profile/Timothy-Tinius/publication/232485180_Cognitive-behavioral_interventions_for_improving_performance_in_competitive_athletes_A_controlled_treatment_outcome_study/links/54e8c62e0cf25ba91c7e71aa/Cognitive-behavioral-interventions-for-improving-performance-in-competitive-athletes-A-controlled-treatment-outcome-study.pdf

Houston, S., & Swords, C. (2021). Critical realism, mimetic theory and social work. *Journal of Social Work : JSW*, *22*(2), 345–363. DOI: 10.1177/14680173211008806

Huan, C. (2021). Correlations of online social network size with well-being and distress: A meta-analysis. *Cyberpsychology (Brno)*, *15*(2).

Huang, B., Huang, Y., Zhai, M., Zhou, Q., Ji, S., Liu, H., Zhuang, X., Zhang, Y., & Zhang, J. (2024). Association of Sex With Cardiovascular Outcomes in Heart Failure Patients With Obstructive or Central Sleep Apnea. *Journal of the American Heart Association*, *13*(5), e031186. DOI: 10.1161/JAHA.123.031186 PMID: 38410942

Huang, C. (2017). Time spent on social network sites and psychological well-being: A meta-analysis. *Cyberpsychology, Behavior, and Social Networking*, *20*(6), 346–354. DOI: 10.1089/cyber.2016.0758 PMID: 28622031

Hudson, S., Thal, K., Cárdenas, D., & Meng, F. (2017). Wellness tourism: Stress alleviation or indulging healthful habits? *International Journal of Culture, Tourism and Hospitality Research*, *11*(1), 35–52. DOI: 10.1108/IJCTHR-09-2015-0111

Hunt, M. G., Marx, R., Lipson, C., & Young, J. (2018). No More FOMO: Limiting Social Media Decreases Loneliness and Depression. *Journal of Social and Clinical Psychology*, *37*(10), 751–768. DOI: 10.1521/jscp.2018.37.10.751

Hu, Q., & Cheong, P. H. (2021). Understanding digital generations: Social media habitus, memetic engagements, and digital social inequalities in China. *International Journal of Communication*, *15*, 22.

Hutchins, B., & Rowe, D. (2014). Sport beyond television: The internet, digital media, and the rise of networked media sport. *International Journal of Sport Communication*, *7*(2), 279–281. DOI: 10.1123/IJSC.2014-0029

Hu, W. (2022). Research on the Integration and Development of Folk Art and Cultural Tourism Industry under the Modern Cultural Background. *BCP Education & Psychology*, *7*, 145–150. DOI: 10.54691/bcpep.v7i.2627

Influencer Marketing Hub. (2025, October 1). *What is an Influencer? – Social Media Influencers Defined [Updated 2024]*. Retrieved October 3, 2025, from https://influencermarketinghub.com/what-is-an-influencer/

Influencity. (2024, August 9). Marketing with Kid Influencers: Benefits and Best Practices. *Influencity*. Retrieved May 19, 2025, from https://influencity.com/blog/en/marketing-with-kid-influencers-benefits-and-best-practices

Internet World Stats. (2023). *Internet growth statistics: Today's road to e-commerce and global trade*. Retrieved July 08, 2025, from https://www.internetworldstats.com/emarketing.htm

Ionescu, C. G., & Licu, M. (2023). Are TikTok algorithms influencing users' self-perceived identities and personal values? A mini review. *Social Sciences (Basel, Switzerland)*, *12*(8), 465. DOI: 10.3390/socsci12080465

Islam, M. T. (2023). Disaster Management in Bangladesh: Historical Perspective. In M. T. Islam, *Disaster, Governance and Development* (pp. 33–59). Springer Nature Singapore. DOI: 10.1007/978-981-99-1631-3_3

Islam, A. (2015). Mental Health and the health system in Bangladesh: Situation analysis of a neglected domain. *American Journal of Psychiatry and Neuroscience*, *3*(4), 57. DOI: 10.11648/j.ajpn.20150304.11

Islam, N., & Singh, A. (2025). Role of digitalization into hospitality businesses: Innovations and trends. In Rana, V., Bathla, G., Raina, A., & Chhabra, D. (Eds.), *Transforming the service sector with new technology* (pp. 447–458). IGI Global., DOI: 10.4018/979-8-3693-7447-4.ch027

Isorna-Folgar, M., Leirós-Rodríguez, R., López-Roel, S., & García-Soidán, J. L. (2022). Effects of a cognitive-behavioral therapy intervention on the rowers of the junior spain national team. *Health Care*, *10*(12), 2357. https://www.mdpi.com/2227-9032/10/12/2357 PMID: 36553881

Issa, A. (2025). Digital Anthropology: Navigating Human Experience in the Age of Artificial Intelligence and Social Media. *Digital Humanities, Social Sciences and Cultural Preservation*. https://doi.org/DOI: 10.2139/ssrn.5258483

Izea. (2024, December 13). *Impact and Influence: The Effects of Influencer Culture on Society - IZEA Worldwide, Inc*. IZEA Worldwide, Inc. Retrieved May 19, 2025, from https://izea.com/resources/impact-and-influence-of-influencer-culture-on-society/

Jain, S. (2024, November 8). *Social Media's Impact on Indian Students Well-Being*. Retrieved from India Today: https://bestcolleges.indiatoday.in/news-detail/social-medias-impact-on-indian-students-well-being

Jain, A., & Dutta, D. (2019). Millennials and Gamification: Guerilla Tactics for Making Learning Fun. *SA Journal of Human Resource Management*, *6*(1), 29–44. DOI: 10.1177/2322093718796303

Jalilvand, M. R., & Samiei, N. (2012). The effect of electronic word of mouth on brand image and purchase intention: An empirical study in the automobile industry in Iran. *Marketing Intelligence & Planning*, *30*(4), 460–476. DOI: 10.1108/02634501211231946

James, W. (1890). *The principles of psychology* (Vol. 1). Henry Holt and Co., DOI: 10.1037/10538-000

Janicke-Bowles, S. H., Buckley, T. M., Rey, R., Wozniak, T., Meier, A., & Lomanowsk, A. (2023). Digital flourishing: Conceptualizing and assessing positive perceptions of mediated social interactions. *Journal of Happiness Studies*, *24*(3), 1013–1035. DOI: 10.1007/s10902-023-00619-5

Jennings, R. (2020, July 10). *Doom-scrolling, explained.* Vox. https://www.vox.com/the-goods/21547961/doom-scrolling-meaning-definition-what-is-meme

Jeong, E., & Jang, S. (2011). Restaurant experiences trigger positive electronic word-of-mouth (eWOM) motivations. *International Journal of Hospitality Management*, *30*(2), 356–366. DOI: 10.1016/j.ijhm.2010.08.005

Jeong, M., & Lambert, C. U. (2001). Adaptation of an information quality framework to measure customers' behavioral intentions to use lodging web sites. *International Journal of Hospitality Management*, *20*(2), 129–146. DOI: 10.1016/S0278-4319(00)00041-4

Jia, N., Zhao, X., Gou, L., García, J. A., Liao, Z., Feng, Y., Li, Y., Wang, Y., Li, H., & Wu, J. (2022). Detailed analysis on the reflection component for the black hole candidate MAXI J1348–630. *Journal of Computer-Mediated Communication*, *27*(4). Advance online publication. DOI: 10.1093/jcmc/zmac009

Jiang, S., & Ngien, A. (2020). The Effects of Instagram Use, Social Comparison, and Self-Esteem on Social Anxiety: A Survey Study in Singapore. *Social Media + Society*, *6*(2), 2056305120912488. Advance online publication. DOI: 10.1177/2056305120912488

Jia, Y., & Mvondo, G. (2025). Exploring The Adverse Effects Of The Metaverse On Users' Psychological Well-being and Self-esteem: A Mixed-methods Study. *Journal of Retailing and Consumer Services*, *86*(C), 104321. DOI: 10.1016/j.jretconser.2025.104321

Jiotsa, B., Naccache, B., Duval, M., Rocher, B., & Grall-Bronnec, M. (2021). Social Media Use and Body Image Disorders: Association between Frequency of Comparing One's Own Physical Appearance to That of People Being Followed on Social Media and Body Dissatisfaction and Drive for Thinness. *International Journal of Environmental Research and Public Health*, *18*(6), 2880. DOI: 10.3390/ijerph18062880 PMID: 33799804

Jones, L., Johnson, E., & Kotler, P. (2025). Digital Detox and Self-Comforting Attitudes in Gen Z. Retrieved from https://www.researchgate.net/publication/392967217_Digital_Detox_and_Self-Comforting_Attitudes_in_Gen_Z

Jones, D. C. (2001). Social comparison and body image: Attractiveness comparisons to models and peers among adolescent girls and boys. *Sex Roles*, *45*(9), 645–664. DOI: 10.1023/A:1014815725852

Jones, G. (1993). The role of performance profiling in cognitive behavioral interventions in sport. *The Sport Psychologist*, *7*(2), 160–172. DOI: 10.1123/tsp.7.2.160

Josep, J. (2025). The algorithmic self: How AI reshapes human identity, introspection, and agency. *Frontiers in Psychology*, *16*, 1645795. DOI: 10.3389/fpsyg.2025.1645795 PMID: 40718563

Josiam, B. M., & Monteiro, P. A. (2004). Tandoori tastes: Perceptions of Indian restaurants in America. *International Journal of Contemporary Hospitality Management*, *16*(1), 18–26. DOI: 10.1108/09596110410516525

Joson, G. H. G., Pyke, J., Delacy, T., & Davidson, C. (2024). Wellness in the Spa Industry: An Investigation of Hot Spring Tourism in Australia. In Chhabra, D., Atal, N., & Maheshwari, A. (Eds.), *Sustainable Development and Resilience of Tourism* (pp. 63–79). Springer International Publishing., DOI: 10.1007/978-3-031-63145-0_4

Journal of Medical Internet Research. (2024). Effectiveness of AI-driven digital mental health tools for adolescents. JMIR, 26(7), e54672. DOI: 10.2196/54672

Journal of Youth and Adolescence. (2022). Community service participation and self-esteem among adolescents. Journal of Youth and Adolescence, 51(3), 403–416. https://doi.org/DOI: 10.1007/s10964-021-01523-6

Jung, J., Barron, D., Lee, Y., & Swami, V. (2022). Social media usage and body image: Examining the mediating roles of internalization of appearance ideals and social comparisons in young women. *Computers in Human Behavior*, *135*, 107357. DOI: 10.1016/j.chb.2022.107357

Kabir, K., & Rahman, M. S.-U. -. (2020). General Tourism and Hospitality Education and Research in Bangladesh. In M. S.-U.- Rahman & A. Hassan (Eds.), *Tourism Policy and Planning in Bangladesh* (pp. 179–192). Springer Singapore. DOI: 10.1007/978-981-15-7014-8_11

Kalenjuk Pivarski, B., Grubor, B., Banjac, M., Đerčan, B., Tešanović, D., Šmugović, S., Radivojević, G., Ivanović, V., Vujasinović, V., & Stošić, T. (2023). The Sustainability of Gastronomic Heritage and Its Significance for Regional Tourism Development. *Heritage*, *6*(4), 3402–3417. DOI: 10.3390/heritage6040180

Kalra, S., & Sharma, R. (2025). *Mental toughness and athletic coping skills among young adult athletes*. https://www.researchgate.net/profile/Sakshi-Kalra-4/publication/392126542_Mental_Toughness_and_Athletic_Coping_Skills_among_Young_Adult_Athletes/links/6835d0266b5a287c30465e50/Mental-Toughness-and-Athletic-Coping-Skills-among-Young-Adult-Athletes.pdf

Kanaujia, S., Saraswati, P., Anshu, , Singh, N., Singh, S., Kataria, N., & Yadav, P. (2023). Effect of yoga and mindfulness on psychological correlates in young athletes: A meta-analysis. *Journal of Ayurveda and Integrative Medicine*, *14*(3), 100725. DOI: 10.1016/j.jaim.2023.100725 PMID: 37321018

Kannan, L., & Kumar, T. P. (2022). Social media—the emotional and mental roller-coaster of Gen Z: an empirical study. In *Managing disruptions in business: causes, conflicts, and control* (pp. 81–102). Springer International Publishing. DOI: 10.1007/978-3-030-79709-6_4

Kaplan, A. M., & Haenlein, M. (2010). Users of the world, unite! The challenges and opportunities of social media. *Business Horizons*, *53*(1), 59–68. DOI: 10.1016/j.bushor.2009.09.003

Kapoor, K., Tamilmani, K., Rana, N. P., Patil, P., Dwivedi, Y. K., & Nerur, S. (2022). Advances in social media research: Past, present and future. *Information Systems Frontiers*, *24*, 1–28. DOI: 10.1007/s10796-021-10136-y

Kappes, K. (2021). *#LimitingMyself: The Relationship Between Gender Norms, Self Presentation, and Selfies (Honors Thesis)*. Muhlenberg College.

Katz, R., Ogilvie, S., Shaw, J., & Woodhead, L. (2021). Gen Z, explained: The art of living in a digital age. In *Gen Z, explained*. University of Chicago Press. DOI: 10.7208/chicago/9780226814988.001.0001

Kaur, M., Selvakumar, P., & Dinesh, N. Mohit, Chandel, P. S., & Mnjunath, T. C. (2025). Reconstruction and Preservation Strategies for Cultural Heritage. In S. Oflazoğlu & M. Dora (Eds.), Preserving Cultural Heritage in Post-Disaster Urban Renewal (pp. 385-412). IGI Global Scientific Publishing. DOI: 10.4018/979-8-3693-9097-9.ch016

Kausar, D. R., Damanik, J., & Tanudirjo, D. (2024). Borobudur as priority tourism destination: How political economy affects world cultural heritage site management and heritage preservation. *IOP Conference Series. Earth and Environmental Science*, *1366*(1), 012057. DOI: 10.1088/1755-1315/1366/1/012057

Kearney-Cooke, A., & Tieger, D. (2015). Body Image Disturbance and the Development of Eating Disorders. In Smolak, L., & Levine, M. P. (Eds.), *The Wiley Handbook of Eating Disorders, Assessment, Prevention, Treatment, Policy, and Future Directions* (pp. 283–296). John Wiley & Sons, Ltd., DOI: 10.1002/9781118574089.ch22

Keles, B., McCrae, N., & Grealish, A. (2020). A systematic review: the influence of social media on depression, anxiety and psychological distress in adolescents. *International journal of adolescence and youth, 25*(1), 79-93.

Keles, B., McCrae, N., & Grealish, A. (2020). A systematic review: The influence of social media on depression, anxiety and psychological distress in adolescents. *International Journal of Adolescence and Youth, 25*(1), 79–93. DOI: 10.1080/02673843.2019.1590851

Kelly, Y., Zilanawala, A., Booker, C., & Sacker, A. (2018). Social Media Use and Adolescent Mental Health: Findings From the UK Millennium Cohort Study. *EClinicalMedicine, 6*, 59–68. DOI: 10.1016/j.eclinm.2018.12.005 PMID: 31193561

Kemp, S. (2025, February 25). *Digital 2025: India*. Retrieved from DataReportal: https://datareportal.com/reports/digital-2025-india

Kerr, G. A., & Stirling, A. E. (2012). Parents' Reflections on their Child's Experiences of Emotionally Abusive Coaching Practices. *Journal of Applied Sport Psychology, 24*(2), 191–206. DOI: 10.1080/10413200.2011.608413

Khajuria, A., Gandotra, A., Khajuria, A., Arora, K., Gupta, R. K., Gupta, U., & Babber, S. (2025). Role of Social Media in the Rising Body Dissatisfaction and Dysmorphia Among Adolescents. *Cureus, 17*(1), e78314. DOI: 10.7759/cureus.78314 PMID: 40034880

Khalid, N. L., Jayasainan, S. Y., & Hassim, N. (2018). Social media influencers-shaping consumption culture among Malaysian youth. In *SHS Web of Conferences* (Vol. 53, p. 02008). EDP Sciences. DOI: 10.1051/shsconf/20185302008

Khan, M. M. (2023, July 25). *The Power Of Social Media Influencers On Today's Youth*. Mentoria. Retrieved May 19, 2025, from https://mentoriablog.azurewebsites.net/the-power-of-social-media-influencers-on-todays-youth/

Khan, S. R. (2024, January 1). Traversing the power of digital and influencer marketing in apparel industry. *Textile News, Apparel News, RMG News, Fashion Trends*. https://www.textiletoday.com.bd/traversing-the-power-of-digital-and-influencer-marketing-in-apparel-industry

Khan, I. A., & Shibami, A. H. A. (2019). Generation Z's learning preferences: Impact on organizational learning and development - a study conducted in a vocational institute in UAE. *International Journal of Learning and Change*, *11*(4), 379. DOI: 10.1504/IJLC.2019.105646

Kholmogorova, A., Tarhanova, P., & Shalygina, O. (2018). Standards of physical beauty and mental health in children and young people in the era of the information revolution. *International Journal of Culture and Mental Health*, *11*(1), 87–98. DOI: 10.1080/17542863.2017.1394007

Kiarie, E. (2024). Cultural Heritage Preservation in the Face of Globalization. *International Journal of Humanities and Social Science*, *3*(3), 1–14. DOI: 10.47941/ijhss.2081

Kietzmann, J. H., Hermkens, K., McCarthy, I. P., & Silvestre, B. S. (2011). Social media? Get serious! Understanding the functional building blocks of social media. *Business Horizons*, *54*(3), 241–251. DOI: 10.1016/j.bushor.2011.01.005

Kim, J. S. (2024). BeReal or BeCurated? Examining authenticity cues and self-presentation on ephemeral social media. *Proceedings of the International AAAI Conference on*, 18, pp. 122–134. Web and Social Media. Retrieved July 24, 2025, from https://arxiv.org/abs/2408.02883

Kim, D. H., Seely, N. K., & Jung, J.-H. (2017). Do You Prefer, Pinterest or Instagram? The Role of Image-Sharing SNSs and Self-Monitoring in Enhancing Ad Effectiveness. *Computers in Human Behavior*, *70*, 535–543. DOI: 10.1016/j.chb.2017.01.022

Kim, J., & Kim, M. (2022). Rise of Social Media Influencers as a New Marketing Channel: Focusing on the Roles of Psychological Well-Being and Perceived Social Responsibility among Consumers. *International Journal of Environmental Research and Public Health*, *19*(4), 2362. DOI: 10.3390/ijerph19042362 PMID: 35206553

Kim, S., Chung, J.-E., & Suh, Y. (2016). Multiple reference effects on restaurant evaluations: A cross-cultural study. *International Journal of Contemporary Hospitality Management*, *28*(7), 1441–1466. DOI: 10.1108/IJCHM-05-2014-0220

Kishore Kumar, M., & Priyadarshini, R. G. (2018). Important factors of self-efficacy and its relationship with life satisfaction and self-esteem – with reference to gen y and gen z individuals. *IOP Conference Series. Materials Science and Engineering*, *390*, 012007. DOI: 10.1088/1757-899X/390/1/012007

Kivela, J., Inbakaran, R., & Reece, J. (1999). Consumer research in the restaurant environment, Part 1: A conceptual model of dining satisfaction and return patronage. *International Journal of Contemporary Hospitality Management, 11*(5), 205–222. DOI: 10.1108/09596119910272739

Kleiser, M., & Mayeux, L. (2021). Popularity and gender prototypicality: An experimental approach. *Journal of Youth and Adolescence, 50*(1), 144–158. DOI: 10.1007/s10964-020-01344-5 PMID: 33156453

Kokkinopoulou, E., Papasolomou, I., Porcu, L., & Vrontis, D. (2025). Exploring the impact of online co-creation on eudemonic well-being and sustainable fashion choices among Generation Z. *EuroMed Journal of Business*. Advance online publication. DOI: 10.1108/EMJB-12-2024-0356

Kommineni, M., Chundru, S., Maroju, P. K., & Selvakumar, P. (2025). Ethical Implications of AI in Sustainable Development Pedagogy. In Chinedu, C., Mafarja, N., Hussein, M., & Saleem, A. (Eds.), *Rethinking the Pedagogy of Sustainable Development in the AI Era* (pp. 17–36). IGI Global Scientific Publishing., DOI: 10.4018/979-8-3693-9062-7.ch002

Kularathne, S., Perera, A., Rathnayake, N., Rathnayake, U., & Hoshino, Y. (2024). Analyzing the impact of socioeconomic indicators on gender inequality in Sri Lanka: A machine learning-based approach. *PLoS One, 19*(12), e0312395. DOI: 10.1371/journal.pone.0312395 PMID: 39724101

Kumar, H., Aswathy, V. K., & Kumar, S. (2025). Converging Realms of Social Health, Domestic Workers, and Telemedicine Landscape: Challenges and Prospects. In Özbek, M. F., & Christiansen, B. (Eds.), *Organizational Sociology in the Digital Age* (pp. 165–180). IGI Global., DOI: 10.4018/979-8-3693-7398-9.ch010

Kumar, S., Talukder, M. B., Kabir, F., & Kaiser, F. (2023). Challenges and Sustainability of Green Finance in the Tourism Industry: Evidence From Bangladesh. In Taneja, S., Kumar, P., Grima, S., Ozen, E., & Sood, K. (Eds.), (pp. 97–111). Advances in Finance, Accounting, and Economics. IGI Global., DOI: 10.4018/979-8-3693-1388-6.ch006

Kumar, S., Talukder, M. B., & Pego, A. (Eds.). (2024). *Utilizing Smart Technology and AI in Hybrid Tourism and Hospitality*. IGI Global., DOI: 10.4018/979-8-3693-1978-9

Kunkel, T., Doyle, J., & Funk, D. (2013). Exploring Sport Brand Development Strategies to Strengthen Consumer Involvement with the Product–The Case of the Australian A-League. *Doyle, J., Kunkel, T., Funk, D.(2013). Sport Spectator Segmentation: Examining the Differing Psychological Connections amongst Spectators of Leagues and Teams. International Journal of Sports Marketing & Sponsorship, 14*(2), 95–111.

Kuşcu, F. N., Yorulmaz, M., & Göde, A. (2024). THE EFFECT OF PATIENT EXPECTATIONS AND SATISFACTION ON REGIONAL TRUST IN HEALTH TOURISM: A PRIVATE HOSPITAL EXAMPLE. *Journal of International Health Sciences and Management, 10*(19), 1–12. DOI: 10.48121/jihsam.1323199

Ladhari, R. (2009). Service quality, emotional satisfaction, and behavioral intentions: A study in the hotel industry. *Managing Service Quality, 19*(3), 308–331. DOI: 10.1108/09604520910955320

Ladhari, R., & Michaud, M. (2015). eWOM effects on hotel booking intentions, attitudes, trust, and website perceptions. *International Journal of Hospitality Management, 46*, 36–45. DOI: 10.1016/j.ijhm.2015.01.010

Lajnef, K. (2023). The effect of social media influencers' on teenagers Behavior: An empirical study using cognitive map technique. *Current Psychology (New Brunswick, N.J.), 42*(22), 19364–19377. DOI: 10.1007/s12144-023-04273-1 PMID: 36742063

Lancet Child & Adolescent Health. (2020). Social media use and adolescent mental health: Findings from a UK cohort. The Lancet Child & Adolescent Health, 4(12), 901–909. https://doi.org/DOI: 10.1016/S2352-4642(20)30205-9

Langley, P., & Leyshon, A. (2017). Platform capitalism: The intermediation and capitalisation of digital economic circulation. *Finance and Stochastics, 3*(1), 11–31. DOI: 10.2218/finsoc.v3i1.1936

Lastella, M., Roach, G. D., Halson, S. L., & Sargent, C. (2015). Sleep/wake behaviours of elite athletes from individual and team sports. *European Journal of Sport Science, 15*(2), 94–100. DOI: 10.1080/17461391.2014.932016 PMID: 24993935

Laverty, S. M. (2003). Hermeneutic Phenomenology and Phenomenology: A comparison of historical and methodological considerations. *International Journal of Qualitative Methods, 2*(3), 21–35. DOI: 10.1177/160940690300200303

Lawfluencers. (2024, September 9). Social media influencers impact on youth - positive and negative. *Lawfluencers | Lawyers for Digital & Collaborative Economy*. Retrieved May 19, 2025, from https://lawfluencers.com/social-media-influencers-impact-on-youth/

Leary, M. R. (1996). *Self-presentation: Impression Management And Interpersonal Behavior*. Routledge., DOI: 10.4324/9780429497384

Leary, M. R., & Baumeister, R. F. (2000). In Zanna, M. (Ed.), *The nature and function of self-esteem: Sociometer theory* (Vol. 32, pp. 1–62). Advances in Experimental Social Psychology, DOI: 10.1016/S0065-2601(00)80003-9

Lee, A., & Chung, T. D. (2025). With great power comes great responsibility: The antecedents and outcomes of social media influencers' perceived social responsibility authenticity. *Journal of Business Research, 192*, 115300. DOI: 10.1016/j.jbusres.2025.115300

Lee, J., Wood, E., Vogel, N., Santhosh, E., & Chauhan, P. K. (2023). Burn or balm? Exploring university students' experiences with social media during the COVID-19 pandemic. *Frontiers in Psychology, 14*, 1018334. DOI: 10.3389/fpsyg.2023.1018334

Lee, Y., Jeon, Y., Kang, S., Shin, J. I., Jung, Y.-C., & Jung, S. (2022). Social media use and mental health during the COVID-19 pandemic in young adults: A meta-analysis of 14 cross-sectional studies. *BMC Public Health, 22*(1), 995. Advance online publication. DOI: 10.1186/s12889-022-13409-0 PMID: 35581597

Lee, Y., Lin, H., & Huang, H. (2022). Examining the effects of digital fatigue on mental health and academic performance. *Journal of Educational Technology & Society, 25*(2), 104–116. https://www.jstor.org/stable/48635645

Leng, H. K., & Zhang, J. J. (2023). . In H. K. Leng & J. J. Zhang, *Sports Sponsorship and Branding* (1st ed., pp. 1–18). Routledge. DOI: 10.4324/9781003458890-1

Lhendup, K. (2024). *PhD Thesis Final Draftword-2 3*. DOI: 10.13140/RG.2.2.20121.63849

Liang, M. (2022). The end of social media? How data attraction model in the algorithmic media reshapes the attention economy. *Media Culture & Society, 44*(6), 1110–1131. DOI: 10.1177/01634437221077168

Lim, L. T. S., Regencia, Z. J. G., Dela Cruz, J. R. C., Ho, F. D. V., Rodolfo, M. S., Ly-Uson, J., & Baja, E. S. (2022). Assessing the effect of the COVID-19 pandemic, shift to online learning, and social media use on the mental health of college students in the Philippines: A mixed-method study protocol. *PLoS One, 17*(5), e0267555. DOI: 10.1371/journal.pone.0267555 PMID: 35503779

Lim, Y. S., Ng, T. H., Lam, M. S., & Tan, S. Y. (2023). Communication in the 21st Century: The Effect of Internet Celebrity as the Communication Source in Influencing Generation Z Purchase Intention. *Jurnal Komunikasi: Malaysian Journal of Communication, 39*(4), 507–522. DOI: 10.17576/JKMJC-2023-3904-27

Linardon, J., McClure, Z., Tylka, L. T., & Tyszkiewicz, M. F. (2022). Body appreciation and its psychological correlates: A systematic review and meta-analysis. *Body Image*, *42*, 287–296. DOI: 10.1016/j.bodyim.2022.07.003 PMID: 35878528

Linardon, J., Messer, M., & Tylka, T. L. (2023). Functionality appreciation and its correlates: Systematic review and meta-analysis. *Body Image*, *45*, 65–72. DOI: 10.1016/j.bodyim.2023.02.002 PMID: 36796304

Lin, L., Chang, F., Huang, T., Yu, T., Chen, T., Chiu, C., Chen, P., Miao, N., Chuang, H., Chen, C., & Chen, H. (2025). Body dissatisfaction and unhealthy weight-control behaviors of adolescents: The roles of exposure to influencer marketing and use of dating apps. *Medicine*, *104*(27), e43152. DOI: 10.1097/MD.0000000000043152 PMID: 40629583

Lin, W., Cen, Z., & Chen, Y. (2025). The impact of social media addiction on the negative emotions of adolescent athletes: The mediating role of physical appearance comparisons and sleep. *Frontiers in Public Health*, *12*, 1452769. DOI: 10.3389/fpubh.2024.1452769 PMID: 39926290

Lin, X., Shen, Z., Teng, X., & Mao, Q. (2024). Cultural Routes as Cultural Tourism Products for Heritage Conservation and Regional Development: A Systematic Review. *Heritage*, *7*(5), 2399–2425. DOI: 10.3390/heritage7050114

Li an, D. E. (2025). Online captive: The impact of social media addiction on.... *Behavioral Sciences (Basel, Switzerland)*, *15*(4), 481. DOI: 10.3390/bs15040481 PMID: 40282102

Liu, R., Gupta, S., & Patel, P. (2023, December). The application of the principles of responsible AI on social media marketing for digital health. *Information Systems Frontiers*, *25*(6), 2275–2299. Advance online publication. DOI: 10.1007/s10796-021-10191-z

Liu, Y., & Jang, S. S. (2009). Perceptions of Chinese restaurants in the U.S.: What affects customer satisfaction and behavioral intentions? *International Journal of Hospitality Management*, *28*(3), 338–348. DOI: 10.1016/j.ijhm.2008.10.008

Livingstone, S., & Helsper, E. (2007). Gradations in digital inclusion: Children, young people and the digital divide. *New Media & Society*, *9*(4), 671–696. DOI: 10.1177/1461444807080335

Lora, A., Purba, J. T., Hossain, M. S., Oriana, F., & Seum, C. (2024). The psychological consequences of infinite scrolling: Examining digital fatigue and emotional well-being. *Computers in Human Behavior*, *152*, 108123. DOI: 10.1016/j.chb.2023.108123

Lou, C., & Yuan, S. (2018). Influencer Marketing: How message value and credibility affect consumer trust of branded content on social media. *Journal of Interactive Advertising, 19*(1), 58–73. DOI: 10.1080/15252019.2018.1533501

Lupton, D. (2016). *The quantified self.* Polity Press.

MacIsaac, S., Kelly, J., & Gra, S. (2018). She has like 4000 followers!': The celebrification of self within school social networks. *Journal of Youth Studies, 21*(6), 816–835. DOI: 10.1080/13676261.2017.1420764

Mack, R. W., Snyder, J., Rodgers, W. C., & Love, R. H. (2008). Ethical judgments of marketing professionals: Influences of personal values and organizational factors. *Journal of Business Ethics, 80*(4), 813–826.

Magee, L. (2025). Computational scapegoats: From mimetic to alienated desire in the production of large language models. *Subjectivity, 32*(2), 67–85. Advance online publication. DOI: 10.1057/s41286-025-00212-6

Malik, A., Dhir, A., Kaur, P., & Johri, A. (2021). Correlates of social media fatigue and academic performance decrement: A large cross-sectional study. *Information Technology & People, 34*(2), 557–580. DOI: 10.1108/ITP-06-2019-0289

Mamun, M. A., Hossain, M. S., & Griffiths, M. D. (2019). Mental health problems and associated predictors among Bangladeshi students. *International Journal of Mental Health and Addiction, 20*(2), 657–671. DOI: 10.1007/s11469-019-00144-8

Manhas, P. S., Charak, N. S., & Sharma, P. (2019). Wellness and spa tourism: Finding space for Indian Himalayan spa resorts. *International Journal of Spa and Wellness, 2*(3), 135–153. DOI: 10.1080/24721735.2020.1819705

Marcia, J. E. (1966). Development and validation of ego-identity status. *Journal of Personality and Social Psychology, 3*(5), 551–558. DOI: 10.1037/h0023281 PMID: 5939604

Marciano, L., Ostroumova, M., Schulz, P. J., & Camerini, A.-L. (2022). Digital Media Use and Adolescents' Mental Health During the Covid-19 Pandemic: A Systematic Review and Meta-Analysis. *Frontiers in Public Health, 9*, 793868. DOI: 10.3389/fpubh.2021.793868 PMID: 35186872

Marengo, D., Sindermann, C., Elhai, J. D., & Montag, C. (2022). The association between the Big Five personality traits and smartphone use disorder: A meta-analysis. *Journal of Behavioral Addictions, 11*(1), 77–93. DOI: 10.1556/2006.2021.00086

Marino, C., Gini, G., Vieno, A., & Spada, M. M. (2018). The associations between problematic Facebook use, psychological distress and well-being among adolescents and young adults: A systematic review and meta-analysis. *Journal of Affective Disorders*, *226*, 274–281. DOI: 10.1016/j.jad.2017.10.007 PMID: 29024900

Marques, J., Gomes, S., Ferreira, M., Rebuá, M., & Marques, H. (2025). Generation Z and travel motivations: The impact of age, gender, and residence. *Tourism and Hospitality*, *6*(2), 82. Advance online publication. DOI: 10.3390/tourhosp6020082

Marwick, A. E. (2015). Instafame: Luxury selfies in the attention economy. Public Culture, 27(1 75), 137–160. DOI: 10.1215/08992363-2798379

Marwick, A. E., & boyd, . (2011). To see and be seen: Celebrity practice on Twitter. *Convergence (London)*, *17*(2), 139–158. DOI: 10.1177/1354856510394539

Maslach, C., & Leiter, M. P. (2016). Understanding the burnout experience: Recent research and its implications for psychiatry. *World Psychiatry; Official Journal of the World Psychiatric Association (WPA)*, *15*(2), 103–111. DOI: 10.1002/wps.20311

Massawe, A. (2013). Customer segmentation in full service restaurant business [Bachelor's thesis, Saimaa University of Applied Sciences]. http://www2.uwstout.edu/content/lib/thesis/2003/2003threevitayas.pdf (Note: This appears to be a thesis; the link provided in search results leads to a related document, but the original may be available via institutional repositories.)

Mastroianni, C. (2024). Social Support in the Time of Social Media: Predicting Gen Zers' Preferences for In-Person and Virtual Support (Doctoral dissertation, Seton Hall University).

Mathur, A., & Chhibber, N. (2015). A social media campaign case study: Critical success factors in action. *Chanakya International Journal of Business Research*, *1*(1), 47–56.

Matilda, A. M., Wulandari, B. P., & Darmanto, D. (2025). UNDERSTANDING GEN Z'S MENTAL HEALTH CHALLENGES. PHENOMENON: Multidisciplinary. *Journal Of Sciences and Research*, *3*(1), 38–52.

McComb, C. A., Vanman, E. J., & Tobin, S. J. (2023). A meta-analysis of the effects of social media exposure to upward comparison targets on self-evaluations and emotions. *Media Psychology*, *26*(5), 612–635. DOI: 10.1080/15213269.2023.2180647

McGuire, M. (2023, June 8). *The silent epidemic: Why Gen Z is more anxious than ever—and what we're doing about it. Medium.* Retrieved from https://medium.com/@miamcguire6/the-silent-epidemic-why-gen-z-is-more-anxious-than-ever-and-what-were-doing-about-it-e7fd56149eca

McLean, S. A., Paxton, S. J., Wertheim, E. H., & Masters, J. (2015). Photoshopping the selfie: Self photo editing and photo investment are associated with body dissatisfaction in adolescent girls. *International Journal of Eating Disorders*, *48*(8), 1132–1140. DOI: 10.1002/eat.22449 PMID: 26311205

McRobbie, A. (2009). The aftermath of feminism: Gender, culture and social change. *Sage (Atlanta, Ga.)*.

MDPI. (2024). Generation Z's preferences for virtual tourism and sustainable experiences. *Sustainability*, *16*(24), 10858. Advance online publication. DOI: 10.3390/su162410858

MDPI. (2025). Digital natives on the move: Cross-cultural insights into Generation Z global tourism. *Sustainability*, *17*(14), 6601. Advance online publication. DOI: 10.3390/su17146601

Medanta (2025). The Impact of Social Media on Mental Health. Medanta Hospital. https://www.medanta.org/patient-education-blog/the-impact-of-social-media-on-mental-health

Mede, N. G., & Schroeder, R. (2024). The "Greta Effect" on Social Media: A systematic review of research on Thunberg's impact on digital climate change communication. *Environmental Communication*, *18*(6), 801–818. DOI: 10.1080/17524032.2024.2314028

Media influence on pre-teens and teenagers: social media, movies, YouTube and apps. (2024, December 20). Raising Children Network. Retrieved May 19, 2025, from https://raisingchildren.net.au/pre-teens/entertainment-technology/media/media-influence-on-teens

Mehrabian, A., & Russell, J. A. (1974). *An approach to environmental psychology*. MIT Press.

Meier, A., & Johnson, K. (2022). Social comparison and envy on social media: A critical review. *Current Opinion in Psychology*, *45*, 101302. DOI: 10.1016/j.copsyc.2022.101302 PMID: 35184028

Meinhardt, C., Rajapaksha, D., Oliveira, D. R., & Gultepe, A. (2025). *Scrolling in the deep: Analysing contextual influences on intervention effectiveness during infinite scrolling on social media*. arXiv. https://arxiv.org/abs/2501.11814

Mills, C. (2018). From 'Invisible Problem' to Global Priority: The Inclusion of Mental Health in the Sustainable Development Goals. *Development and Change*, *49*(3), 843–866. DOI: 10.1111/dech.12397

Mills, J. S., Musto, S., Williams, L., & Tiggemann, M. (2018). “Selfie” harm: Effects on mood and body image in young women. *Body Image*, *27*, 86–92. DOI: 10.1016/j.bodyim.2018.08.007 PMID: 30149282

Milmo, D. (2024, November 26). Online influencers need ‘urgent’ fact-checking training, warns Unesco. *The Guardian*. https://www.theguardian.com/media/2024/nov/26/online-influencers-need-urgent-fact-checking-training-warns-unesco?utm_source=chatgpt.com

Ministry of Health and Family Welfare, Government of India. (2014, October). *New Pathways New Hope: National Mental Health Policy of India*. Retrieved from National Health Mission: https://nhm.gov.in/images/pdf/National_Health_Mental_Policy.pdf

Mladenovic, A., Maricic, M., & Ciric, M. (2022). Scroll fatigue and digital well-being: Exploring compulsive browsing behaviors. *Computers in Human Behavior*, *135*, 107373. DOI: 10.1016/j.chb.2022.107373

Mohammad, B. T., & Fahmida, K. (2023). Economic impact of river tourism: Evidence of Bangladesh. *I-Manager's. Journal of Management*, *18*(2), 47. DOI: 10.26634/jmgt.18.2.20235

Mohanty, S., Kashyap, R. S., Katuri, B., Kalal, N., Kodicherla, M., & Choudary, D. (2024). Impact Of Social Media On Adolescents' Self-Esteem And Procrastination. *Educational Administration: Theory and Practice*, *30*(1), 5765–5773. DOI: 10.53555/kuey.v30i1.9244

Molina, L. F. M., & Roja, C. A. R. (2024, May). Exploratory study: Social media impact on mental health perception in Colombian Gen Z. In *Proceedings of a conference hosted by European Conference on Social Media (ECSM 2024)*

Montag, C., Wegmann, E., Sariyska, R., & Brand, M. (2021). How to overcome taxonomical problems in the study of internet use disorders and what to do with ‘smartphone addiction’? *Journal of Behavioral Addictions*, *10*(1), 1–7. DOI: 10.1556/2006.8.2019.59

Morgan, D. L. (1997). *Focus groups as qualitative research* (2nd ed.). Sage. DOI: 10.4135/9781412984287

Muñoz, P., Barton, M., Braun, S., Chowdhury, F., Jayne-Little, N., Rowland, J., Sykes, K., Smith, J., Talbot-Jones, C., Taggart, A., & Komes, J. (2023). The deterioration of self-worth in entrepreneurship. *Journal of Business Venturing Insights*, *20*, e00430. DOI: 10.1016/j.jbvi.2023.e00430

Murtaza, G. (2023, May 24). *Understanding the role of social media influencers on youth*. Retrieved May 18, 2025, from https://www.linkedin.com/pulse/understanding-role-social-media-influencers-youth-ghulam-murtaza

Nadkarni, A., & Hofmann, S. G. (2012). Why do people use Facebook? *Personality and Individual Differences*, *52*(3), 243–249. DOI: 10.1016/j.paid.2011.11.007 PMID: 22544987

Nair, B. B., Sinha, S., & Dileep, M. R. (2022). Exploring the impact of COVID-19 on the travel intermediaries in India: Mapping trends and strategies. *International Journal of Tourism Policy*, *12*(4), 427. DOI: 10.1504/IJTP.2022.128137

Nanayakkara, S. (2021). A descriptive analysis on digital behaviour of young adults in Sri Lanka. *International Journal of Business and Management Invention*, *9*(6). https://www.academia.edu/download/68897491/4._A_Descriptive_Analysis_on_Digital_Behaviour_of_Young_Adults_in_Sri_Lanka.pdf

Nasiche, N. (2024). The Role of Wellness Tourism in the Growth of the Hospitality Industry. *Journal of Modern Hospitality*, *3*(1), 53–64. DOI: 10.47941/jmh.1954

Neff, K. (2011). *Self-compassion: The proven power of being kind to yourself.* Hachette UK. https://books.google.com/books?hl=en&lr=&id=PDAEzLL9mscC&oi=fnd&pg=PT7&dq=3.%09Neff,+K.+D.+(2011).+Self-compassion:+The+proven+power+of+being+kind+to+yourself.+William+Morrow.&ots=Aft5k6lpb-&sig=vQfrlhMdQGl4KAjkJmX57yzU8zo

Neff, K. D., & Vonk, R. (2009). Self-compassion versus global self-esteem: Two different ways of relating to oneself. *Journal of Personality*, *77*(1), 23–50. DOI: 10.1111/j.1467-6494.2008.00537.x PMID: 19076996

Nesi, J., & Prinstein, M. J. (2015, November). Using social media for social comparison and feedback-seeking: Gender and popularity moderate associations with depressive symptoms. *Journal of Abnormal Child Psychology*, *43*(8), 1427–1438. DOI: 10.1007/s10802-015-0020-0

NetGirls. (n.d.). The Internet, Facebook, and body image concern in adolescent girls. *International Journal of Eating Disorders*, *47*(6), 630–643. DOI: 10.1002/eat.22254 PMID: 23712456

Neuts, B., Romão, J., Nijkamp, P., & van Leeuwen, E. (2013). Describing the relationships between tourist satisfaction and destination loyalty in a segmented and seasonal tourism market. *Tourism Economics*, *19*(4), 743–765.

Ni, Y., Ding, Y., Hu, H., & Chu, J. (2023). Research on the influencing factors of public opinion information forwarding behaviour of Generation Z group (Next): Mechanism of action. *Highlights in Science. Engineering and Technology*, *42*, 309–321. DOI: 10.54097/hset.v42i.7110

Noaime, E. (2023). *Historic Syrian Cities in the Post-War Period: Balancing Cultural Preservation and Tourism Investment*. DOI: 10.20944/preprints202303.0457.v1

Nuong Deri, M., Singh, A., Zaazie, P., & Anandene, D. (2024). Leveraging Artificial Intelligence in Higher Educational Institutions: A Comprehensive Overview. *Education and Law Review*, (30). Advance online publication. DOI: 10.1344/REYD2024.30.45777

Nussenbaum, T. (2023, December 14). *Social media causes attention spans to drop*. Retrieved from The Standard: https://standard.asl.org/27705/uncategorized/social-media-causes-attention-spans-to-drop/

Obe, S. M., Von Weiler, J., & Gardner, W. (2024, December 12). *What are the impacts of influencer culture on young people?* Internet Matters. Retrieved May 19, 2025, from https://www.internetmatters.org/hub/question/how-influencer-culture-affects-young-people-online/

Oberst, U., Wegmann, E., Stodt, B., Brand, M., & Chamarro, A. (2020). Negative consequences from heavy social networking in adolescents: The mediating role of fear of missing out. *Journal of Adolescence*, *55*, 51–60. DOI: 10.1016/j.adolescence.2017.11.003

Olorunsogo, T. O., Balogun, O. D., Ayo-Farai, O., Ogundairo, O., Maduka, C. P., Okongwu, C. C., & Onwumere, C. (2024). *Mental health and social media in the U.S.: A review: Investigating the potential links between online platforms and mental well-being among different age groups*. World Journal Of Advanced Research and Reviews. DOI: 10.30574/wjarr.2024.21.1.0015

Ong, E. (Ed.). (2024). *The Emergence of the Digital World: Friend Or Foe to Young Adults in the Post-pandemic Era?* Springer Nature. DOI: 10.1007/978-981-97-3098-8

Orben, A., & Przybylski, A. K. (2019). The association between adolescent well-being and digital technology use. *Nature Human Behaviour*, *3*(2), 173–182. DOI: 10.1038/s41562-018-0506-1 PMID: 30944443

Orel, F. D., & Kara, A. (2014). Supermarket self-checkout service quality, customer satisfaction, and loyalty: Empirical evidence from an emerging market. *Journal of Retailing and Consumer Services*, *21*(2), 118–129. DOI: 10.1016/j.jretconser.2013.07.002

Orgilés, M., Morales, A., Delvecchio, E., Mazzeschi, C., & Espada, J. P. (2020). Immediate Psychological Effects of the COVID-19 Quarantine in Youth From Italy and Spain. *Frontiers in Psychology*, *11*, 579038. DOI: 10.3389/fpsyg.2020.579038 PMID: 33240167

Østergaard, S. D. (2017, November). Taking Facebook at face value: Why the use of social media may cause mental disorder. *Acta Psychiatrica Scandinavica*, *136*(5), 439–440. DOI: 10.1111/acps.12819 PMID: 28940179

Ozdemir-Guzel, S., & Bas, T. (2021). Social media and the transformation of travel experiences: A study on Generation Z. *Tourism Management Perspectives*, *40*, 100888. DOI: 10.1016/j.tmp.2021.100888

Pacewicz, C. E., & Mellano, K. (2024). The Toll of the Scroll: A Path Toward Burnout. *Psychology of Sport and Exercise*, *74*, 102681. DOI: 10.1016/j.psychsport.2024.102681 PMID: 38815779

Palacios-Florencio, B., García del Junco, J., Castilla-Polo, F. J., & Santos-Roldán, L. (2018). Sustainable tourism tags to reward destination loyalty. *Sustainability*, *10*(5), 1544.

Pande, L., & Sengupta, S. (2024). Wellness Tourism in India: Evolution, Perspectives, and Trends. SSRN *Electronic Journal*. DOI: 10.2139/ssrn.4674035

Parida, Y., Bhardwaj, P., & Roy Chowdhury, J. (2018). Effects of economic development and crime on tourism in India. *Anatolia*, *29*(1), 63–73. DOI: 10.1080/13032917.2017.1384742

Park, I., & Jeon, J. (2023). Psychological skills training for athletes in sports: Web of science bibliometric analysis. *Health Care*, *11*(2), 259. https://www.mdpi.com/2227-9032/11/2/259 PMID: 36673627

Park, S. Y., & Baek, Y. M. (2018). Two faces of social comparison on Facebook: The interplay between social comparison orientation, emotions, and psychological well-being. *Computers in Human Behavior*, *79*, 83–93. DOI: 10.1016/j.chb.2017.10.028

Park, S. Y., Do, B., Yourell, J., Hermer, J., & Huberty, J. (2024). Digital Methods for the Spiritual and Mental Health of Generation Z: Scoping Review. *Interactive Journal of Medical Research*, *13*, e48929. DOI: 10.2196/48929 PMID: 38261532

Pataranutaporn, P., ... (2024). Future You: AI-mediated self-connection and reduced anxiety. ArXiv preprint. https://arxiv.org/abs/2405.12514

Pathil, J. M., Kabeer, F., & Anas, A. P. (2024). The Mindful Matrix: Exploring Social Media's Influence on Mental Wellbeing. *Deleted Journal*, *2*(12), 3597–3599. DOI: 10.47392/IRJAEM.2024.0530

Patil, A., Prathibha Raj, M. S., Gowri Shankar, R., & Lakshmi, R. B. (2025). Cultivating Wellness: Synergy of Emerging Technologies in Spiritual and Wellness Tourism. In Tyagi, P. K., Nadda, V., & Singh, A. K. (Eds.), *Meaningful Tourism* (pp. 145–162). Emerald Publishing Limited., DOI: 10.1108/978-1-83797-837-320251022

Peash, M. N. H. (2025, May 26). Influencer culture among our youth on the rise -. *The Daily Observer*. https://www.observerbd.com/news/527197#:~:text=Influencer%20culture%20has%20contributed%20to,fleeting%20fads%20and%20viral%20content%20

Pegoraro, A. (2010). Look who's talking—Athletes on Twitter: A case study. *International Journal of Sport Communication*, *3*(4), 501–514. DOI: 10.1123/ijsc.3.4.501

Pelham, B. W., & Swann, W. B. (1989). From self-conceptions to self-worth: On the sources and structure of global self-esteem. *Journal of Personality and Social Psychology*, *57*(4), 672–680. DOI: 10.1037/0022-3514.57.4.672 PMID: 2795437

Perloff, R. (2023). *The Dynamics of Persuasion: Communication and Attitudes in the 21st Century*. Routledge., DOI: 10.4324/9781003290056

Perloff, R. M. (2014). Social Media Effects on Young Women's Body Image Concerns: Theoretical Perspectives and an Agenda for Research. *Sex Roles*, *71*(11–12), 363–377. DOI: 10.1007/s11199-014-0384-6

Petersen, B., Schinke, R. J., Coholic, D., Larivière, M., & Giffin, C. E. (2024). The social effects of mental ill-health stigma in sport. *Sport, Exercise, and Performance Psychology*, *13*(3), 223–239. DOI: 10.1037/spy0000351

Peters, K., & Hervé Remaud, P. (2020). Factors influencing consumer menu-item selection in a restaurant context. *Food Quality and Preference*, *82*, 103887. DOI: 10.1016/j.foodqual.2020.103887

Pettijohn, L. S., Pettijohn, C. E., & Luke, R. H. (1997). An evaluation of fast food restaurant satisfaction: Determinants, competitive comparisons and impact on future patronage. *Journal of Restaurant & Foodservice Marketing*, *2*(3), 3–20. DOI: 10.1300/J061v02n03_02

Petty, R. E., & Cacioppo, J. T. (1986). Communication and persuasion. In *Springer eBooks*. https://doi.org/ DOI: 10.1007/978-1-4612-4964-1

Pew Research Center. (2019). Gen Z is more diverse and progressive than previous generations. Retrieved from https://www.pewresearch.org/social-trends/2019/01/17/generation-z-looks-a-lot-like-millennials-on-key-social-and-political-issues/

Pew Research Center. (2021). Teens, social media, and technology. Pew Research Center. https://www.pewresearch.org

Pew Research Center. (2024, 12 12). *Teens, Social Media and Technology 2024.* Retrieved from Pew Research: https://www.pewresearch.org/2024/12/12/teens-social-media-tech-acknowledgments/

Pichler, S., Kohli, C., & Granitz, N. (2021). DITTO for Gen Z: A framework for leveraging the uniqueness of the new generation. *Business horizons, 64, no. 5 (*(5), 599-610.

Podlog, L. W., Heil, J., Burns, R. D., Bergeson, S., Iriye, T., Fawver, B., & Williams, A. M. (2020). A cognitive behavioral intervention for college athletes with injuries. *The Sport Psychologist, 34*(2), 111–121. DOI: 10.1123/tsp.2019-0112

Potts, C., & Stebleton, M. J. (2023). Behind the Digital Mask: Examining Social Media and Masculinity. *About Campus: Enriching the Student Learning Experience, 28*(4), 4–13. DOI: 10.1177/10864822231195574

Pounders, K., Kowalczyk, C. M., & Stowers, K. (2016). Insight into the motivation of selfie postings: Impression management and self-esteem. *European Journal of Marketing, 50*(9-10), 1879–1892. DOI: 10.1108/EJM-07-2015-0502

Pouwels, J. L., Valkenburg, P. M., Beyens, I., van Driel, I. I., & Keijsers, L. (2021). Social Media Use and Friendship Closeness in Adolescents' Daily Lives: An Experience Sampling Study. *Developmental Psychology, 57*(2), 309–323. DOI: 10.1037/dev0001148 PMID: 33539132

Prasad, A., Das, D., & Ajith Kumar, N. (2025). A Tourism Potential of Alleppey District: A Study on Vembanad Backwaters. In Fong, S., Dey, N., & Joshi, A. (Eds.), *ICT Analysis and Applications* (Vol. 1162, pp. 21–30). Springer Nature Singapore., DOI: 10.1007/978-981-97-8605-3_3

Prasad, S., Ait Souabni, S., Anugwom, G., Aneni, K., Anand, A., Urhi, A., Obi-Azuike, C., Gibson, T., Khan, A., & Oladunjoye, F. (2023). Anxiety and depression amongst youth as adverse effects of using social media: A review. *Annals of Medicine and Surgery (London), 85*(8), 3974–3981. DOI: 10.1097/MS9.0000000000001066 PMID: 37554895

Preji, M. P., & Lenka, S. K. (2020). Wellness tourism in Kerala: A study on the tourist perception in terms of therapeutic and industry performance indicators. *Siddhant- A Journal of Decision Making, 20*(1and2), 57. DOI: 10.5958/2231-0657.2020.00007.5

Primack, B. A., Shensa, A., Sidani, J. E., Whaite, E. O., Lin, L., Rosen, D., Colditz, J. B., Radovic, A., & Miller, E. (2017). Social media use and perceived social isolation among young adults in the US. *American Journal of Preventive Medicine, 53*(1), 1–8. DOI: 10.1016/j.amepre.2017.01.010 PMID: 28279545

Prince, M., Patel, V., Saxena, S., Maj, M., Maselko, J., Phillips, M. R., & Rahman, A. (2007). No Health Without Mental Health. *Lancet, 370*(9590), 859–877. DOI: 10.1016/S0140-6736(07)61238-0 PMID: 17804063

Pryde, S., & Prichard, I. (2022). TikTok on the clock but the #fitspo don't stop: The impact of TikTok fitspiration videos on women's body image concerns. *Body Image, 43*, 244–252. DOI: 10.1016/j.bodyim.2022.09.004 PMID: 36194987

Przybylski, A. K., Murayama, K., DeHaan, C. R., & Gladwell, V. (2013). Motivational, emotional, and behavioral correlates of fear of missing out. *Computers in Human Behavior, 29*(4), 1841–1848. DOI: 10.1016/j.chb.2013.02.014

Przybylski, A. K., & Weinstein, N. (2017). A large-scale test of the Goldilocks hypothesis: Quantifying the relations between digital-screen use and the mental well-being of adolescents. *Psychological Science, 28*(2), 204–215. DOI: 10.1177/0956797616678438 PMID: 28085574

Putrevu, D. J., & Mertzanis, C. (2025). The Rise of the Wellness Business Sector: A Systematic Literature Review. SSRN *Electronic Journal*. DOI: 10.2139/ssrn.5190935

Qazi, H., Alam, S., & Phulpoto, A. (2023). Motivating Factors Influencing Green Buying Behavior of Generation Z: An Application of Theory of Planned Behavior (TPB). *Pakistan Journal of Humanities and Social Sciences, 11*(3). Advance online publication. DOI: 10.52131/pjhss.2023.1103.0646

Qu, H. (1997). Determinant factors and choice intention for Chinese restaurant dining: A multivariate approach. *Journal of Restaurant & Foodservice Marketing, 2*(2), 35–49. DOI: 10.1300/J061v02n02_03

Qu, H., Kim, L. H., & Im, H. H. (2011). A model of destination branding: Integrating the concepts of the branding and destination image. *Tourism Management, 32*(3), 465–476. DOI: 10.1016/j.tourman.2010.03.014

Radcliffe, J. N., Comfort, P., & Fawcett, T. (2015). Psychological strategies included by strength and conditioning coaches in applied strength and conditioning. *Journal of Strength and Conditioning Research, 29*(9), 2641–2654. DOI: 10.1519/JSC.0000000000000919 PMID: 25719912

Raghavan, S., & Sandanapitchai, P. (2024). The relationship between cultural variables and resilience to psychological trauma: A systematic review of the literature. *Traumatology, 30*(1), 37–51. DOI: 10.1037/trm0000239

Raguseo, E., & Vitari, C. (2017). The effect of brand on the impact of eWOM on hotels' financial performance. *International Journal of Electronic Commerce, 21*(2), 249–269. DOI: 10.1080/10864415.2016.1234287

Rahman, M. (2025, May 23). Social media influencers & the new youth economy. *The Financial Express*. https://thefinancialexpress.com.bd/views/views/social-media-influencers-the-new-youth-economy

Rai, V., & Singh, A. (2026). The digital renaissance of hospitality. In Talukder, M., & Chowdhury, H. (Eds.), *Smart operations in hospitality* (pp. 125–144). IGI Global., DOI: 10.4018/979-8-3373-2145-5.ch005

Rajkumar, E., Julia, G. J., & Sri Lakshmi, K. (2022). Prevalence of mental health problems among rural adolescents in India: A systematic review and meta-analysis. *Scientific Reports, 12*(1), 16573. Advance online publication. DOI: 10.1038/s41598-022-19731-2 PMID: 36195719

Rao, A. L., & Hong, E. (2020). Overcoming the Stigma of Mental Health in Sport. In E. Hong & A. L. Rao (Eds.), *Mental Health in the Athlete* (pp. 1–10). Springer International Publishing. DOI: 10.1007/978-3-030-44754-0_1

Rather, R. A., Hollebeek, L. D., & Rasoolimanesh, S. M. (2021). First-time versus repeat tourism customer engagement, experience, and value co-creation: A comparison of prominent relationship constructs.

Reich, S. M., Subrahmanyam, K., & Espinoza, G. (2012). Friending, IMing, and hanging out face-to-face: Overlap in adolescents' online and offline social networks. *Developmental Psychology, 48*(2), 356–368. DOI: 10.1037/a0026980 PMID: 22369341

Rhee, L., Bayer, J. B., Lee, D. S., & Kuru, O. (2021). Social by definition: How users define social platforms and why it matters. *Telematics and Informatics, 59*, 101538. DOI: 10.1016/j.tele.2020.101538

Roberts, S. R., Maheux, A. J., Ladd, B. A., & Choukas-Bradley, S. (2022). The Role of Digital Media in Adolescents' Body Image and Disordered Eating. In Handbook of Adolescent Digital Media Use and Mental Health. Cambridge University Press. Retrieved 07 4, 2025, from DOI: 10.1080/08164640802680635

Rodgers, R. F., Slater, A., Gordon, C. S., McLean, S. A., Jarman, H. K., & Paxton, S. J. (2020). A Biopsychosocial Model of Social Media Use and Body Image Concerns, Disordered Eating, and Muscle-Building Behaviors among Adolescent Girls and Boys. *Journal of Youth and Adolescence*, *49*(2), 399–409. DOI: 10.1007/s10964-019-01190-0 PMID: 31907699

Rogowska, A. M., & Tataruch, R. (2024). The relationship between mindfulness and athletes' mental skills may be explained by emotion regulation and self-regulation. *BMC Sports Science, Medicine and Rehabilitation*, *16*(1), 68. DOI: 10.1186/s13102-024-00863-z PMID: 38504372

Rosenberg, M. (1965). Society and the adolescent Self-Image. In *Princeton University Press eBooks*. https://doi.org/ DOI: 10.1515/9781400876136

Rosenberg, M. (1979). *Conceiving the self*. Basic Books.

Rosenberg, M., Schooler, C., Schoenbach, C., & Rosenberg, F. (1995). Global Self-Esteem and Specific Self-Esteem:Different Concepts, Different Outcomes. *American Sociological Review*, *60*(1), 141–156. DOI: 10.2307/2096350

Rosen, L. D., Lim, A. F., Carrier, L. M., & Cheever, N. A. (2011). An empirical examination of the educational impact of text message-induced task switching in the classroom: Educational implications and strategies to enhance learning. *Psicología Educativa. Revista de Los Psicólogos de La Educación*, *17*(2), 163–177.

Rosič, J., Janicke-Bowles, S. H., Carbone, L., Lobe, B., & Vandenbosch, L. (2022). Positive digital communication among youth: The development and validation of the digital flourishing scale for adolescents. *Frontiers in Digital Health*, *4*, 975557. DOI: 10.3389/fdgth.2022.975557 PMID: 36120715

Rössler, M. (2023). Balancing Tourism and Heritage Conservation: A World Heritage Context. In Cameron, C. (Ed.), *Evolving Heritage Conservation Practice in the 21st Century* (Vol. 5, pp. 207–218). Springer Nature Singapore., DOI: 10.1007/978-981-99-2123-2_13

Roychowdhury, D. (2021). *Understanding mindfulness in sport, exercise, and performance psychology. Routledge Encyclopedia of Psychology in the Real World* (1st ed.). Routledge., https://api.taylorfrancis.com/content/entry-versions/download?identifierName=doi&identifierValue=10.4324/9780367198459-REPRW220-1&type=webpdf

Roy, M. (2021). Tourism Industry in Bangladesh: An Assessment of Advanced SWOT Model and TOWS Matrix. In Hassan, A. (Ed.), *Tourism in Bangladesh: Investment and Development Perspectives* (pp. 279–310). Springer Nature Singapore., DOI: 10.1007/978-981-16-1858-1_18

Rudman, L. A., & Fairchild, K. (2004). Reactions to Counterstereotypic Behavior: The Role of Backlash in Cultural Stereotype Maintenance. *Journal of Personality and Social Psychology*, *87*(2), 157–176. DOI: 10.1037/0022-3514.87.2.157 PMID: 15301625

Ruiz, N., Molina Leon, G., & Heuer, H. (2024). Design Frictions on Social Media: Balancing reduced mindless scrolling and user satisfaction. *Maedche, M. Beigl, K. Gerling, & S. Mayer (Eds.), Proceedings of Mensch und Computer 2024* (pp. 442–447). Association for Computing Machinery. Retrieved from DOI: 10.1145/3670653.3677495

Rusida, E. (2024, November 24). *Swipe, scroll, get bored: The real reason Gen Z annot focus. Kind to Mind Indonesia.* Retrieved from Medium: https://medium.com/@Kindtomind_id/swipe-scroll-get-bored-the-real-reason-gen-z-cant-focus-3391094d6162

Ryan, R. M., Deci, E. L., Vansteenkiste, M., & Soenens, B. (2021). Building a science of motivated persons: Self-determination theory's empirical approach to human experience and the regulation of behavior. *Motivation Science*, *7*(2), 97–110. DOI: 10.1037/mot0000194

Ryan, R. M., & Deci, L. (2000). Self-determination theory and the facilitation of intrinsic motivation, social development, and well-being. *The American Psychologist*, *55*(1), 68–78. DOI: 10.1037/0003-066X.55.1.68 PMID: 11392867

Ryan, R. M., & Deci, L. (2019). Brick by brick: The origins, development, and future of self-determination theory. *Advances in Motivation Science*, *6*, 111–156. DOI: 10.1016/bs.adms.2019.01.001

Ryan, R. M., & Moller, A. C. (2017). Competence as central, but not sufficient, for high-quality motivation. In Elliot, A. J., Dweck, C. S., & Yeager, D. S. (Eds.), *Handbook of competence and motivation: Theory and application.* The Guilford Press.

Sagioglou,C., & Greitemeyer, T. (2014). Facebook's emotional consequences: Why Facebook causes a decrease in mood and why people still use it. *Computers in Human Behavior, 35*, 359-363.

Sakdiyakorn, M., Golubovskaya, M., & Solnet, D. (2021). Understanding Generation Z through collective consciousness: Impacts for hospitality work and employment. *International Journal of Hospitality Management, 94*, 102822. DOI: 10.1016/j.ijhm.2020.102822

Saldana, J. (2021). *The Coding Manual for Qualitative Researchers.* Sage Publications Limited.

Salmerón-Ruiz, M. A., de Ribera, C. G., Barberán, V. S., Ives, L. E., & Álvarez-Pitti, J. (2025). Impact of digital media on development and physical health. *Anales de Pediatría (English Ed.), 102*(6), 503876. DOI: 10.1016/j.anpede.2025.503876 PMID: 40461313

Samal, A., & Misra, L. I. Mohit, Pougajendy, S., Chandel, P. S., Manjunath, T. C., & Selvakumar, P. (2025). Musealization and Tourism Practices. In S. Oflazoğlu & M. Dora (Eds.), Preserving Cultural Heritage in Post-Disaster Urban Renewal (pp. 115-142). IGI Global Scientific Publishing. DOI: 10.4018/979-8-3693-9097-9.ch006

Sardar, S., Hossain, D. M. E., Kamruzzaman, D. M., & Ray, R. (2021). ICT APPLICATIONS IN TOURISM AND HOSPITALITY INDUSTRY OF BANGLADESH: A RESEARCH REVIEW. *IJRDO -. Journal of Business and Management, 7*(6), 64–74. DOI: 10.53555/bm.v7i6.4404

Sardar, S., Ray, R., Hasan, M., Chitra, S. S., Parvez, A. T. M. S., & Avi, M. A. R. (2022). Assessing the Effects of COVID-19 on Restaurant Business From Restaurant Owners' Perspective. *Frontiers in Psychology, 13*, 849249. DOI: 10.3389/fpsyg.2022.849249 PMID: 35496209

Sarkar, S. (2003). *Gender as a cultural factor influencing mental health among adolescent students in India and Sri Lanka: A cross-cultural study*. State University of New York at Albany.

Sathurusinghe, R. I. T. (2024). An analysis on the impact of digital media devices on child socialization in Sri Lankan society. Proceedings of the International Research Conference of the Open University of Sri Lanka (IRC-OUSL 2024) http://repository.ou.ac.lk/bitstream/handle/94ousl/2676/IRC-OUSL2024_19_Sathurusinghe.pdf?sequence=1

Saura, J. R., Gelashvili, V., & Martínez-Navalón, J. G. (2025). The impact of social media on Gen Z's mental health and privacy. *Cyberpsychology Journal*, 12(3), 145-160. https://www.cjournal.cz/files/573.pdf

Saura, R., Jose, V. G., & Martínez-Navalón, J. G. (2025). The Impact of Social Media on Gen Z's Mental Health and Privacy. *Journal of Competitiveness*, *17*, 1. https://www.cjournal.cz/files/573.pdf

Sawyer, S. M., Azzopardi, P. S., Wickremarathne, D., & Patton, G. C. (2018). The age of adolescence. *The Lancet. Child & Adolescent Health*, *2*(3), 223–228. DOI: 10.1016/S2352-4642(18)30022-1 PMID: 30169257

Saxena, S., Funk, M., & Chisholm, D. (2014). WHO's Mental Health Action Plan 2013-2020: What can psychiatrists do to facilitate its implementation? *World Psychiatry; Official Journal of the World Psychiatric Association (WPA)*, *13*(2), 107–109. DOI: 10.1002/wps.20141 PMID: 24890053

Schachter, S. (1959). *The psychology of affiliation: Experimental studies of the sources of gregariousness*. Stanford University Press.

Schlenker, B. R., & Pontari, B. A. (2000). The strategic control of information: Impression management and self-presentation in daily life. In Tesser, A., Felson, R. B., & Suls, J. M. (Eds.), *Psychological Perspectives on Self and Identity* (pp. 199–232). American Psychological Association., DOI: 10.1037/10357-008

Schlosser, A. E. (2020). Self-disclosure versus self-presentation on social media. *Current Opinion in Psychology*, *31*, 1–6. DOI: 10.1016/j.copsyc.2019.06.025 PMID: 31357096

Scott, H., & Woods, H. C. (2019). Understanding links between social media use, sleep, and mental health. *Sleep Medicine Reviews*, *44*, 1–12. DOI: 10.1016/j.smrv.2018.01.008

Seabrook, E. M., Kern, M. L., & Rickard, N. S. (2016). Social networking sites, depression, and anxiety: A systematic review. *JMIR Mental Health*, *3*(4), e50. DOI: 10.2196/mental.5842 PMID: 27881357

Seemiller, C., & Grace, M. (2016). *Generation Z goes to college*. John Wiley & Sons. https://books.google.com/books?hl=en&lr=&id=xjDvCQAAQBAJ&oi=fnd&pg=PR9&dq=4.+5.%09Seemiller,+C.,+%26+Grace,+M.+(2016).+Generation+Z+goes+to+college.+Jossey-Bass.+6.%09Smith,+A.+(2019).+Digital+fandom:+New+media+studies+of+sport+and+entertainment.+Peter+Lang.&ots=7CLsMBeE9j&sig=3VwETz7GW1fvZYnzZzjQCaDcuFE

Sezgi, N. E., & Uyanik, B. (2022). Priorities of consumers for restaurant preferences: A conjoint analysis study on generation Z. *Journal of Tourism Leisure and Hospitality*, *4*(2), 6–6. DOI: 10.48119/toleho.1187392

Sgroi, F. (2021). Food products, gastronomy and religious tourism: The resilience of food landscapes. *International Journal of Gastronomy and Food Science*, *26*, 100435. DOI: 10.1016/j.ijgfs.2021.100435

Shah, D., Webster, E., & Kour, G. (2022). Consuming for content? Understanding social media-centric consumption. *Journal of Business Research*, *155*, 113408. DOI: 10.1016/j.jbusres.2022.113408

Shah, P., Bhusal, N., & Chettri, K. K. (2023). Influence of Social Media Usage on Generation Z's Choice in Selecting Restaurants in Kathmandu. *Journal of Business and Social Sciences Research*, *8*(1), 95–110. DOI: 10.3126/jbssr.v8i1.56592

Shah, S. R., Bhave, S. Y., Shringarpure, K., & Bhave, Y. (2023). Effect of COVID-19 Lockdown on Lifestyle, Internet Addiction and Media Usage among Adolescents and Young Adults in India - A Cross-sectional Survey. *Indian Journal of Youth and Adolescent Health*, *10*(3), 4–12. DOI: 10.24321/2349.2880.202309

Shan, B., Oh, I., & Rowley, C. (2023). Innovation and entrepreneurship in East Asia during the digital era: Post-pandemic prospects. *Asia Pacific Business Review*, *29*(4), 843–851. DOI: 10.1080/13602381.2023.2256106

Sharifian, N., Zaheed, A. B., & Zahodne, L. B. (2022). The role of envy in linking active and passive social media use to memory functioning. *Psychology of Popular Media*, *11*(1), 80–89. DOI: 10.1037/ppm0000318 PMID: 35402066

Sharma, M., Deepak, K., & Sudhanshu, J. (2023). 5). Adverse effect of social media on generation Z user's behavior: Government information support as a moderating variable. *Journal of Retailing and Consumer Services*, *72*, 103256. DOI: 10.1016/j.jretconser.2023.103256

Sharma, M., Mohapatra, G., & Giri, A. K. (2025). Assessing the role of ICT, governance, and infrastructure on inbound tourism demand in India. *Journal of Economic and Administrative Sciences*, *41*(1), 320–335. DOI: 10.1108/JEAS-03-2022-0064

Sharma, M., & Singh, A. (2024a). Embracing Technological Innovation: A Review of Hi-Tech Services in Hospitality Industry. *Evergreen*, *11*(4), 2818–2830. DOI: 10.5109/7326926

Sharma, R., & Singh, A. (2024b). Blockchain Technologies and Call for an Open Financial System: Decentralised Finance. In Vardari, L., & Qabrati, I. (Eds.), *Decentralized Finance and Tokenization in FinTech* (pp. 21–32). IGI Global., DOI: 10.4018/979-8-3693-3346-4.ch002

Sharma, V., & Tiwari, R. (2016). A Review on "IOT" & It's Smart Applications. *International Journal of Science* [IJSETR]. *Engineering and Technology Research*, *5*(2), 472–476. DOI: 10.17762/ijritcc.v6i9.5295

Shensa, A.. (2017). Social media use and depressive symptoms among U.S. young adults. *Depression and Anxiety*, *34*(4), 323–331. PMID: 28446367

Sherlock, M., & Wagstaff, D. L. (2018). Exploring the relationship between frequency of Instagram use, exposure to idealized images, and psychological well-being in women. *Psychology of Popular Media Culture*, *8*(4), 482–490. DOI: 10.1037/ppm0000182

Sherman, L. E., Hernandez, L. M., Greenfield, P. M., & Dapretto, M. (2018). Peer influence via Instagram: Effects on brain and behavior in adolescence and young adulthood. *Child Development*, *89*(1), 37–47. DOI: 10.1111/cdev.12838 PMID: 28612930

Sherman, L. E., Payton, A. A., Hernandez, L. M., Greenfield, P. M., & Dapretto, M. (2016). The Power of the Like in Adolescence: Effects of Peer Influence on Neural and Behavioral Responses to Social Media. *Psychological Science*, *27*(7), 1027–1035. DOI: 10.1177/0956797616645673 PMID: 27247125

Shi, Y., Kong, F., & Zhu, M. (2024). How Does Social Media Usage Intensity Influence Adolescents' Social Anxiety: The Chain Mediating Role of Imaginary Audience and Appearance Self-Esteem. *International Journal of Mental Health Promotion*, *26*(12), 977–985. DOI: 10.32604/ijmhp.2024.057596

Siddique, M. B., Ovi, M. R., Ahammed, T., Chowdhury, M. B., & Uddin, M. J. (2022). Mental health knowledge and awareness among university students in Bangladesh. *Heliyon*, *8*(10), e11084. DOI: 10.1016/j.heliyon.2022.e11084 PMID: 36303905

Silva, R. C., & Steins, G. (2023). Social media and body dissatisfaction in young adults: An experimental investigation of the effects of different image content and influencing constructs. *Frontiers in Psychology*, *13*, 1037932. DOI: 10.3389/fpsyg.2023.1037932 PMID: 36968719

Simon @ DMI. (2025a, February 5). 9 of the Biggest Social Media Influencers on Instagram. *Digital Marketing Institute*. https://digitalmarketinginstitute.com/blog/9-of-the-biggest-social-media-influencers-on-instagram

Simon @ DMI. (2025b, May 8). 20 surprising influencer marketing Statistics. *Digital Marketing Institute*. https://digitalmarketinginstitute.com/blog/20-influencer-marketing-statistics-that-will-surprise-you

Singh, A., & Bathla, G. (2023). Fostering Creativity and Innovation: Tourism and Hospitality Perspective. In P. Tyagi, V. Nadda, V. Bharti, & E. Kemer (Eds.), Embracing Business Sustainability Through Innovation and Creativity in the Service Sector (pp. 70-83). IGI Global Scientific Publishing. DOI: 10.4018/978-1-6684-6732-9.ch005

Singh, A., & Hassan, S. C. (2024). Identifying the skill gap in the workplace. In A. M. Thake et al. (Eds.), Contemporary challenges in social science management (Vol. 112B, pp. 101–114). Emerald. https://doi.org/DOI: 10.1108/S1569-37592024000112B006

Singh, A., & Singh, V. K. (2022). The impact of ergonomic practices on housekeeping employee retention and efficiency in hotels during COVID-19 in India. Turyzm/Tourism, 32(2), 29–50. DOI: 10.18778/0867-5856.32.2.02

Singh, S. (2025, May). *Gen Z and the pressure to be perfect: Chasing an illusion. Deccan Chronicle*. Retrieved from https://deccanchronicle.com/deccanchronicle.com

Singh, A. (2022). Conceptual framework on Smart Learning Environment- An Indian perspective. *Journal of Education and Law*, (25). Advance online publication. DOI: 10.1344/REYD2022.25.36706

Singh, A. (2024a). Quality of Work-Life Practices in the Indian Hospitality Sector: Future Challenges and Prospects. In Valeri, M., & Sousa, B. (Eds.), *Human Relations Management in Tourism* (pp. 208–224). IGI Global., DOI: 10.4018/979-8-3693-1322-0.ch010

Singh, A. (2024b). Virtual Research Collaboration and Technology Application: Drivers, Motivations, and Constraints. In Chakraborty, S. (Ed.), *Challenges of Globalization and Inclusivity in Academic Research* (pp. 250–258). IGI Global., DOI: 10.4018/979-8-3693-1371-8.ch016

Singh, A. (2024c). Impact of E-learning on Student Motivation in Higher Education Institutions: An Indian Perspective. *Journal of Education and Law*, (29). Advance online publication. DOI: 10.1344/REYD2024.29.43214

Singh, A. (2025). Analysis of perceptions on employment of differently-abled people in the Indian hotel industry. *Pasos (El Sauzal)*, *23*(1), 167–183. DOI: 10.25145/j.pasos.2025.23.011

Singh, A., & Ansari, A. I. (2024). Role of training and development in employee motivation. In Mazurowski, T. (Ed.), *Enhancing employee motivation* (pp. 248–261). IGI Global., DOI: 10.4018/979-8-3693-1674-0.ch011

Singh, A., & Hassan, S. C. (2024). Service Innovation Through Blockchain Technology in the Tourism and Hospitality Industry: Applications, Trends, and Benefits. In Singh, S. (Ed.), *Service Innovations in Tourism: Metaverse, Immersive Technologies, and Digital Twin* (pp. 205–214). IGI Global., DOI: 10.4018/979-8-3693-1103-5.ch010

Singh, A., & Kumar, S. (2021). Identifying Innovations in Human Resources: Academia and Industry Perspectives. In Pathak, A., & Rana, S. (Eds.), *Transforming Human Resource Functions With Automation* (pp. 104–120). IGI Global. DOI: 10.4018/978-1-7998-4180-7.ch006

Singh, A., & Kumar, S. (2024). Effective talent management practices. In Christiansen, B. (Eds.), *Global practices on talent acquisition* (pp. 126–144). IGI Global., DOI: 10.4018/979-8-3693-1938-3.ch008

Singh, A., & Kumar, V. (2025). Organizational innovation and adaptation in hospitality. In Ramos, C. (Eds.), *Open innovation and technology in tourism* (pp. 355–372). IGI Global., DOI: 10.4018/979-8-3693-8633-0.ch018

Singh, A., & Sihmar, P. (2025). Higher education institution sustainability. In Adu-Gyamfi, M. (Eds.), *Green HRM awareness* (pp. 1–14). IGI Global., DOI: 10.4018/979-8-3693-2956-6.ch001

Singh, A., & Supina, S. (2024). Talent Acquisition and Retention in Hospitality Industry: Current Skill Gaps and Challenges. In Christiansen, B., Aziz, M., & O'Keeffe, E. (Eds.), *Global Practices on Effective Talent Acquisition and Retention* (pp. 363–379). IGI Global., DOI: 10.4018/979-8-3693-1938-3.ch020

Singh, A., Tyagi, P. K., & Garg, A. (Eds.). (2024). *Sustainable Disposal Methods of Food Wastes in Hospitality Operations*. IGI Global., DOI: 10.4018/979-8-3693-2181-2

Singh, V., & Singh, A. (2024a). Digital Health Revolution: Enhancing Well-Being Through Technology. In Nadda, V., Tyagi, P., Moniz Vieira, R., & Tyagi, P. (Eds.), *Implementing Sustainable Development Goals in the Service Sector* (pp. 213–219). IGI Global., DOI: 10.4018/979-8-3693-2065-5.ch016

Singh, V., & Singh, A. (2024b). Revolutionizing the Hospitality Industry: How chatGPT Empowers Future Hoteliers. In Bansal, R., Ngah, A., Chakir, A., & Pruthi, N. (Eds.), *Leveraging ChatGPT and Artificial Intelligence for Effective Customer Engagement* (pp. 192–203). IGI Global., DOI: 10.4018/979-8-3693-0815-8.ch011

Small, G. W., Lee, J., Kaufman, A., Jalil, J., Siddarth, P., Gaddipati, H., Moody, T. D., & Bookheimer, Y. S. (2020). Brain health consequences of digital technology use. *Dialogues in Clinical Neuroscience*, *22*(2), 179–187. DOI: 10.31887/DCNS.2020.22.2/gsmall PMID: 32699518

Smith, L. R., & Sanderson, J. (2015). I'm Going to Instagram It! An Analysis of Athlete Self-Presentation on Instagram. *Journal of Broadcasting & Electronic Media*, *59*(2), 342–358. DOI: 10.1080/08838151.2015.1029125

Smith, R. E., & Smoll, F. L. (1991). Behavioral research and intervention in youth sports. *Behavior Therapy*, *22*(3), 329–344. DOI: 10.1016/S0005-7894(05)80370-3

Social media influencers' impact on youth today. (2025, May 29). RTC Networks. https://www.myrtcnetworks.com/news-releases/social-media-influencers-impact-on-youth-today/?utm_source=chatgpt.com

Somerville, L. H. (2013). The Teenage Brain: Sensitivity to Social Evaluation. *Current Directions in Psychological Science*, *22*(2), 121–127. DOI: 10.1177/0963721413476512 PMID: 24761055

Sonnentag, S. (2018). The recovery process: Sleep and recovery. In R. J. Burke & K. M. Page (Eds.), Research handbook on work and well-being (pp. 144–157). Edward Elgar.

Soriano, D. R. (2002). Customers' expectations factors in restaurants: The situation in Spain. *International Journal of Quality & Reliability Management*, *19*(8/9), 1055–1067. DOI: 10.1108/02656710210438122

Sorokowski, P., Sorokowska, A., Oleszkiewicz, A., Frackowiak, T., Huk, A., & Pisanski, K. (2015). Selfie posting behaviors are associated with narcissism among men. *Personality and Individual Differences*, *85*, 123–127. DOI: 10.1016/j.paid.2015.05.004

Spates, C. R., Samaraweera, N., Plaisier, B., Souza, T., & Otsui, K. (2007). Psychological Impact of Trauma on Developing Children and Youth. *Primary Care*, *34*(2), 387–405. DOI: 10.1016/j.pop.2007.04.007 PMID: 17666234

Srivastava, A., Singh, B. M., Singh, A., & Singh, A. (2025). Customer immersiveness and customer retention. In Al Aqad, M. (Eds.), *Navigating AI and the metaverse* (pp. 475–500). IGI Global., DOI: 10.4018/979-8-3373-0340-6.ch023

Stapleton, P., Luiz, G., & Chatwin, H. (2017). Generation Validation: The Role of Social Comparison in Use of Instagram Among Emerging Adults. *Cyberpsychology, Behavior, and Social Networking*, *20*(3), 142–149. DOI: 10.1089/cyber.2016.0444 PMID: 28263682

Statista. (2022). Most used social media platforms by Gen Z worldwide. Statista. https://www.statista.com

Statista. (2023). Average daily screen time among Generation Z worldwide. Statista. https://www.statista.com

Statista. (2023). Number of social media users worldwide from 2010 to 2023. Statista. https://www.statista.com

Steinberg, L. (2010, April). A dual systems model of adolescent risk-taking. *Developmental Psychobiology*, *52*(3), 216–224. DOI: 10.1002/dev.20445 PMID: 20213754

Stern, R. PhD. (2025, March 9). How social media is shaping teen identity. *Psychology Today*. https://www.psychologytoday.com/us/blog/power-in-relationships/202503/likes-and-lies-the-effects-of-influencers-on-teens

Streiner, D. L. (2003). Starting at the Beginning: An Introduction to Coefficient Alpha and Internal Consistency. *Journal of Personality Assessment*, *80*(1), 99–103. DOI: 10.1207/S15327752JPA8001_18 PMID: 12584072

Suban, S. A. (2024a). Spa tourism: Understanding the relationship of tourist's emotional experience, destination image, satisfaction, and intention to recommend using an integrated model. *International Journal of Spa and Wellness*, *7*(1), 1–22. DOI: 10.1080/24721735.2024.2314943

Suciu, S. A., Georgescu, M. I., & Stănciulescu, M. (2024). Exploring the Generation Z travel trends and behavior. *SBE: Economics and Business*, *19*(Special Issue), 189. Advance online publication. DOI: 10.2478/sbe-2024-0010

Suganya, R., & Bawa, S. A. (2024). Exploring the influence of social media influencers' credibility on consumer behavior: An empirical study. *ComFin Research*, *12*(1), 82–92. DOI: 10.34293/commerce.v12i1.6815

Suheryadi, H., Dian Sua Pratama, B., Rahmah Farahdiba, S., & Elya Rohimi, U. (2023). Generation Z's Perception of Dining Experience at Korea Restaurants, South Jakarta. *Journal of Wood Science*, *2*(10), 1696–1702. DOI: 10.58344/jws.v2i10.422

Sultana, N. (2025, January 14). Understanding the rise of influencers. *Dhaka Tribune*. https://www.dhakatribune.com/opinion/op-ed/370760/under-the-rise-of-influencers

Supina, S., & Singh, A. (2024). Exploring the presence and adoption of quality of work-life dimensions. *African Journal of Hospitality, Tourism and Leisure*, *13*(2), 421–429. DOI: 10.46222/ajhtl.19770720.524

Supina, S., & Singh, A. (2025). Accentuating responsible travel in an ecotourism destination. In Tyagi, P. K. (Eds.), *Meaningful tourism* (pp. 269–279). Emerald., DOI: 10.1108/978-1-83797-837-320251035

Supriyadi, Sulistiasih, Rahmi, Pramono, & Fahrudin. (2025). The impact of digital fatigue on employee productivity and well-being: A scoping literature review. DOI: 10.59429/esp.v10i2.3420

Suresh, R. V., Selvakumar, P., Naresh Babu, K., Nithya, G., Manjunath, T. C., & Kartigeyan, J. (2025). Best Practices and Practical Applications. In Çela, E., Paliktzoglou, V., Sengar, S., Eappen, P., & Vajjhala, N. (Eds.), *Enhancing School Counseling With Technology and Case Studies* (pp. 341–362). IGI Global Scientific Publishing., DOI: 10.4018/979-8-3693-8392-6.ch013

Swann, W. B.Jr, Pelham, B. W., & Krull, D. S. (1989). Agreeable fancy or disagreeable truth? Reconciling self-enhancement and self-verification. *Journal of Personality and Social Psychology*, *57*(5), 782–791. DOI: 10.1037/0022-3514.57.5.782 PMID: 2810025

Taber, K. S. (2018). The use of Cronbach's alpha when developing and reporting research instruments in science education. *Research in Science Education*, *48*(6), 1273–1296. DOI: 10.1007/s11165-016-9602-2

Tajfel, H., & Turner, J. C. (1979). An integrative theory of intergroup conflict. In W. Austin & S. Worchel (Eds.), The social psychology of intergroup relations (pp. 33–47). Brooks/Cole.

Tajfel, H., & Turner, J. C. (1979). An integrative theory of intergroup conflict. In Austin, W. G., & Worchel, S. (Eds.), *The social psychology of intergroup relations* (pp. 33–37). Brooks/Cole.

Talukder, M. B., Kabir, F., & Mia, Md. N., & Khan, M. R. (2024). Application of Smart Technologies in the Development and Promotion of Religious Tourism Destination: In R. A. Castanho & M. Franco (Eds.), *Advances in Hospitality, Tourism, and the Services Industry* (pp. 71–88). IGI Global. DOI: 10.4018/979-8-3693-3158-3.ch003

Talukder, M. B., Kumar, S., Kaiser, F., & Mia, Md. N. (2024). Pilgrimage Creative Tourism: A Gateway to Sustainable Development Goals in Bangladesh. In M. Hamdan, M. Anshari, N. Ahmad, & E. Ali (Eds.), *Advances in Public Policy and Administration* (pp. 285–300). IGI Global. DOI: 10.4018/979-8-3693-1742-6.ch016

Talukder, M.B., & Kumar, S. (2024). Revisiting intention in food service outlet of five-star hotels:A quantitative approach based on food service quality. Sport i Turystyka. Środkowoeuropejskie Czasopismo Naukowe, 7(1), 137–156. https://doi .org/_DOI: 10.16926/sit.2024.01.08

Talukder, M. B. (2020). The Future of Culinary Tourism: An Emerging Dimension for the Tourism Industry of Bangladesh. I-Manager's. *Journal of Management*, *15*(1), 27. DOI: 10.26634/jmgt.15.1.17181

Talukder, M. B. (2021). An assessment of the roles of the social network in the development of the Tourism Industry in Bangladesh. *International Journal of Business, Law, and Education*, *2*(3), 85–93. DOI: 10.56442/ijble.v2i3.21

Talukder, M. B. (2025). Climate change adaptation strategies for a tourism destination: A study of Kuakata beach. *Acta Scientiarum Polonorum. Administratio Locorum*, *24*(1), 165–179. DOI: 10.31648/aspal.10073

Talukder, M. B., & Das, I. R. (2024). The Technology Impacts and AI Solutions in Hospitality. i-manager's Journal on Artificial Intelligence &. *Machine Learning*, *2*(1), 56–72. DOI: 10.26634/jaim.2.1.20291

Talukder, M. B., Hossain, S. E., Al Ferdous, F., & Khan, M. R. (2024). Exploring the Rise of Wellness Tourism: Trends, Benefits, and Market Potential. In Jermsittiparsert, K., & Marzo, R. R. (Eds.), (pp. 351–378). Advances in Computational Intelligence and Robotics. IGI Global., DOI: 10.4018/979-8-3693-9158-7.ch013

Talukder, M. B., Kumar, S., & Das, I. R. (2024a). Implications of blockchain technology-based cryptocurrency in the cloud for the hospitality industry. In *Emerging trends in cloud computing analytics, scalability, and service models* (pp. 340–358). IGI Global Scientific Publishing. DOI: 10.4018/979-8-3693-0900-1.ch018

Talukder, M. B., Kumar, S., & Das, I. R. (2024b). Perspectives of digital marketing for the restaurant industry. In *Advancements in socialized and digital media communications* (pp. 118–134). IGI Global Scientific Publishing. DOI: 10.4018/979-8-3693-0855-4.ch009

Talukder, M. B., Kumar, S., & Das, I. R. (2024c). *Food Wastage on the Economic Outcome: Evidence From the Hotel Industry. Sustainable Disposal Methods of Food Wastes in Hospitality Operations*. IGI Global., DOI: 10.4018/979-8-3693-2181-2.ch005

Talukder, M. B., Kumar, S., & Khan, M. R. (2024). The Integration of Sustainable Practices in Cultural and Gastronomic Tourism. In Munuhwa, S. (Ed.), (pp. 467–484). Advances in Civil and Industrial Engineering. IGI Global., DOI: 10.4018/979-8-3693-3755-4.ch017

Talukder, M. B., Kumar, S., Sood, K., & Grima, S. (2023). Information Technology, Food Service Quality and Restaurant Revisit Intention. *International Journal of Sustainable Development and Planning*, *18*(1), 295–303. DOI: 10.18280/ijsdp.180131

Talukder, M. B., Swarna, D. A., Kumar, S., & Kabir, F. (2025). Leveraging Technology for Employee Wellness in Hospitality: Smart Solutions for a Vibrant Service Culture. In Baez, M. D. (Ed.), (pp. 221–246). Advances in Logistics, Operations, and Management Science. IGI Global., DOI: 10.4018/979-8-3373-1687-1.ch008

Tapera, J., Hamunakwadi, P., Mashapure, R., & Mukurazita, E. (2024). African Tourism and Hospitality Experience. In B. Nyagadza, F. Chigora, & A. Hassan, *Agritourism in Africa* (1st ed., pp. 119–144). Routledge. DOI: 10.4324/9781032696188-7

Tavakoli, R., & Wijesinghe, S. N. R. (2019). The evolution of destination branding: A review of literature on destination branding. *Journal of Hospitality and Tourism Insights*, *2*(3), 269–280.

Tavitiyaman, P., Qu, H., & Zhang, H. Q. (2011). The impact of industry force factors on resource competitive strategies and hotel performance. *International Journal of Hospitality Management*, *30*(3), 648–657. DOI: 10.1016/j.ijhm.2010.11.010

Taylor, J., & Armes, G. (2024). Social comparison on Instagram, and its relationship with self-esteem and body-esteem. *Discover Psychology*, *4*(1), 126. DOI: 10.1007/s44202-024-00241-3

Thaloor, S. (2024). Metaverse and Wellness Tourism: An Investigation on Mixed Reality (MR) Health Care Approaches in the Tourism Industry. In Krishnan, C., Behl, A., Dash, S., & Yadav, P. D. (Eds.), *The Metaverse Dilemma: Challenges and Opportunities for Business and Society* (pp. 183–203). Emerald Publishing Limited., DOI: 10.1108/978-1-83797-524-220241011

Thangavel, P., Pathak, P., & Chandra, B. (2021). Millennials and Generation Z: A generational cohort analysis of Indian consumers. *Benchmarking*, *28*(7), 2157–2177. DOI: 10.1108/BIJ-01-2020-0050

The importance of crisis management in tourism. (2022). USF M3 Publishing, LLC. DOI: 10.5038/9781955833080

The influencer impact - children and screens. (2024, August 16). Children and Screens. Retrieved May 19, 2025, from https://www.childrenandscreens.org/learn-explore/research/the-influencer-impact-a-parents-guide-to-influencers/

Thompson, J. K., Heinberg, L. J., Altabe, M. N., & Tantleff-Dunn, S. (1999). *Exacting beauty: Theory, assessment, and treatment of body image disturbance.* American Psychological Association., DOI: 10.1037/10312-000

Thornton, D. A., & Arrowood, A. J. (1966). Self-evaluation, self-enhancement, and the locus of social comparison. *Journal of Experimental Social Psychology, 1*(1), 40–48. DOI: 10.1016/0022-1031(66)90064-3

Threevitaya, S. (2003). Factors that influence the decisions of customers to dine at selected restaurants in Bangkok, Thailand [Master's thesis, University of Wisconsin-Stout]. http://www2.uwstout.edu/content/lib/thesis/2003/2003threevitayas.pdf

Tiggemann, M., & Slater, A. (2013). NetGirls: The Internet, Facebook, and body image concern in adolescent girls. *International Journal of Eating Disorders, 46*(6), 630–633. DOI: 10.1002/eat.22141 PMID: 23712456

Tiggemann, M., & Slater, A. (2014). NetTweens: The Internet and Body Image Concerns in Preteenage Girls. *The Journal of Early Adolescence, 34*(5), 606–620. Advance online publication. DOI: 10.1177/0272431613501083

Tirocchi, S. (2024). Generation Z, values, and media: From influencers to BeReal, between visibility and authenticity. *Frontiers in Sociology, 8*, 1304093. Advance online publication. DOI: 10.3389/fsoc.2023.1304093 PMID: 38274837

Tremblay, M. S., LeBlanc, A. G., Kho, M. E., Saunders, T. J., Larouche, R., Colley, R. C., Goldfield, G., & Gorber, S. (2011). Systematic review of sedentary behaviour and health indicators in school-aged children and youth. *The International Journal of Behavioral Nutrition and Physical Activity, 8*(1), 98. DOI: 10.1186/1479-5868-8-98 PMID: 21936895

Turk, Y. (2021). *Active and Passive Instagram Use: Female Undergraduate's Social Comparison Behaviors, Self-Esteem, and Contingent Self-Worth (Honors Thesis).* Muhlenberg College.

Turner, A. (2015). Generation Z: Technology and Social Interest. *Journal of Individual Psychology, 71*(2), 103–113. DOI: 10.1353/jip.2015.0021

Twenge, J. M. (2017). *iGen: Why today's super-connected kids are growing up less rebellious, more tolerant, less happy–and completely unprepared for adulthood–and what that means for the rest of us*. Simon and Schuster. https://books.google.com/books?hl=en&lr=&id=HiKaDQAAQBAJ&oi=fnd&pg=PT2&dq=%E2%80%A2%09Twenge,+J.+M.+(2017).+iGen:+Why+today%E2%80%99s+super-connected+kids+are+growing+up+less+rebellious,+more+tolerant,+less+happy%E2%80%94and+completely+unprepared+for+adulthood.+Atria+Books.&ots=aRXXiVfNR-&sig=8_irlFitzXZvaqNTEc-cKJXkQpI

Twenge, J. M., & Campbell, W. K. (2018). Associations between screen time and lower psychological well-being among children and adolescents: Evidence from a population-based study. *Preventive Medicine Reports*, *12*, 271–283. DOI: 10.1016/j.pmedr.2018.10.003 PMID: 30406005

Twenge, J. M., Haidt, J., Joiner, T. E., & Campbell, W. K. (2018). Increases in depressive symptoms, suicide-related outcomes, and suicide rates among U.S. adolescents after 2010. *Clinical Psychological Science*, *6*(1), 3–17. DOI: 10.1177/2167702617723376

Twenge, J. M., Martin, G. N., & Spitzberg, B. H. (2019). Trends in U.S. adolescents' media use and associations with mental health. *Journal of Adolescence*, *79*, 1–13. DOI: 10.1016/j.adolescence.2019.12.018

Tylka, T. L., & Wood-Barcalow, N. L. (2015). The Body Appreciation Scale-2: Item refinement and psychometric evaluation. *Body Image*, *12*, 53–67. DOI: 10.1016/j.bodyim.2014.09.006 PMID: 25462882

Uhlmann, L., Donovan, C., & Zimmer-Gembeck, M. (2020). Beyond the Thin Ideal: Development and Validation of the Fit Ideal Internalization Test (FIIT) for Women. *Psychological Assessment*, *32*(2), 140–153. DOI: 10.1037/pas0000773 PMID: 31535875

UNICEF. (1995). *Convention on the Rights of the Child.* United Nations. Retrieved from https://www.unicef.org/media/52626/file

United Nations Children's Fund. (2021, October). *The State of the World's Children 2021: On My Mind – Promoting, protecting and caring for children's mental health.* Retrieved from UNICEF: https://www.unicef.org/reports/state-worlds-children-2021

United Nations. (n.d.). *Global issues- Children*. Retrieved from United Nations: https://www.un.org/en/global-issues/children

Vainre, M., Dalgleish, T., Bendriss-Otiko, T., Butler, M., Kirkpatrick, A., Kosugiyama, N., Martinez-Sosa, C., Mariscotti, F., Sideri, A., & Soenksen, S. (2022). *Mindfulness training for work performance: A systematic review and meta-analysis of randomised controlled trials*. https://osf.io/preprints/psyarxiv/2vkru/

Vaishnav, M., Javed, A., Gupta, S., Kumar, V., Vaishnav, P., Kumar, A., & Ashurov, Z. (2023). Stigma towards mental illness in Asian nations and low-and-middle-income countries, and comparison with high-income countries: A literature review and practice implications. *Indian Journal of Psychiatry*, *65*(10), 995–1011. DOI: 10.4103/indianjpsychiatry.indianjpsychiatry_667_23 PMID: 38108051

Valkenburg, P. M. (2022). Theoretical Foundations of Social Media Uses and Effects. In Nesi, J., Telzer, E. H., & Prinstein, M. J. (Eds.), *Handbook of Adolescent Digital Media Use and Mental Health* (pp. 39–60). Cambridge University Press. DOI: 10.1017/9781108976237.004

Valkenburg, P. M., Beyens, I., Pouwels, J. L., van Driel, I. I., & Keijsers, L. (2021). Social media use and adolescents' self-esteem: Heading for a person-specific media effects paradigm. *Journal of Communication*, *71*(1), 56–78. DOI: 10.1093/joc/jqaa039

Valkenburg, P. M., Meier, A., & Beyens, I. (2022). Social media use and its impact on adolescent mental health: An umbrella review of the evidence. *Current Opinion in Psychology*, *44*, 58–68. DOI: 10.1016/j.copsyc.2021.08.017 PMID: 34563980

Valkenburg, P. M., & Peter, J. (2009). The effects of instant messaging on the quality of adolescents' existing friendships: A longitudinal study. *Journal of Communication*, *59*(1), 79–97. DOI: 10.1111/j.1460-2466.2008.01405.x

Valkenburg, P. M., & Peter, J. (2013). The differential susceptibility to media effects model. *Journal of Communication*, *63*(2), 221–243. DOI: 10.1111/jcom.12024

Valkenburg, P. M., Peter, J., & Schouten, A. P. (2006). Friend networking sites and their relationship to adolescents' well-being. *Cyberpsychology & Behavior*, *9*(5), 584–590. DOI: 10.1089/cpb.2006.9.584 PMID: 17034326

Van Den Bergh, J., De Pelsmacker, P., & Worsley, B. (2024). Beyond labels: Segmenting the Gen Z market for more effective marketing. *Young Consumers*, *25*(2), 188–210. DOI: 10.1108/YC-03-2023-1707

Van Dijck, J., Poell, T., & De Waal, M. (2018). *The Platform Society: Public Values in a Connective World*. Oxford University Press. DOI: 10.1093/oso/9780190889760.001.0001 van Dorssen-Boog, P., van Vuuren, T., de Jong, J., & Veld, M. (2021). Facilitating health care workers' self-determination: The impact of a self-leadership intervention on work engagement, health, and performance. *Journal of Occupational and Organizational Psychology*, *94*(2), 259–281. DOI: 10.1111/joop.12352 PMID: 34149206

Van Manen, M. (2016). *Researching lived experience: Human Science for an Action Sensitive Pedagogy*. Routledge.

Vandello, J. A., Bosson, J. K., Cohen, D., Burnaford, R. M., & Weaver, J. R. (2008). Precarious manhood. *Journal of Personality and Social Psychology*, *95*(6), 1325–1339. DOI: 10.1037/a0012453 PMID: 19025286

Vannucci, A., & McCauley Ohannessian, C. (2019). Social media use subgroups differentially predict psychosocial well-being during early adolescence. *Journal of Youth and Adolescence*, *48*(8), 1469–1493. DOI: 10.1007/s10964-019-01060-9 PMID: 31256313

Vealey, R. S. (1988). Future directions in psychological skills training. *The Sport Psychologist*, *2*(4), 318–336. DOI: 10.1123/tsp.2.4.318

Verduyn, P., Gugushvili, N., Massar, K., Täht, K., & Kross, E. (2020). Social comparison on social networking sites. *Current Opinion in Psychology*, *36*, 32–37. DOI: 10.1016/j.copsyc.2020.04.002 PMID: 32387840

Verhoef, P. C., Reinartz, W. J., & Krafft, M. (2010). Customer engagement as a new perspective in customer management. *Journal of Service Research*, *13*(3), 247–252. DOI: 10.1177/1094670510375461

Vidal, C., Lhaksampa, T., Miller, L., & Platt, R. (2020). Social media use and depression in adolescents: A scoping review. *International Review of Psychiatry (Abingdon, England)*, *32*(3), 235–253. DOI: 10.1080/09540261.2020.1720623 PMID: 32065542

Vidani, J., & Jaiswal, P. (2024). A comparative study on social media's positive and negative effects on Gen Z. *SSRN*. DOI: 10.2139/ssrn.4848123

Vikram, A., & Sutar, D. (2024). Self-Esteem, Body Image and Social Media Usage Among the Adolescents. *International Journal of Indian Psychology*, *12*(2), 137–150. DOI: 10.25215/1202.015

Vissenberg, J., d'Haenens, L., & Livingstone, S. (2022). Digital literacy and online resilience as facilitators of young people's well-being? *European Psychologist*, *27*(2), 76–85. https://econtent.hogrefe.com/doi/abs/10.1027/1016-9040/a000478?journalCode=epp. DOI: 10.1027/1016-9040/a000478

Viţelar, A. (2019, 6). Like Me: Generation Z and the Use of Social Media for Personal Branding. *Management Dynamics in the Knowledge Economy, 7*(2), pp. 257–268. Retrieved 7 4, 2025, from DOI: 10.25019/mdke/7.2.07

Vogel, E. A., Rose, J. P., Okdie, B. M., Eckles, K., & Franz, B. (2015). Who compares and despairs? The effect of social comparison orientation on social media use and its outcomes. *Personality and Individual Differences, 86*, 249–256. DOI: 10.1016/j.paid.2015.06.026

Vogel, E. A., Rose, J. P., Roberts, L. R., & Eckles, K. (2014). Social comparison, social media, and self-esteem. *Psychology of Popular Media Culture, 3*(4), 206–222. DOI: 10.1037/ppm0000047

Walker, J. R. (2011). *The restaurant: From concept to operation* (6th ed.). John Wiley & Sons.

Wall Street Journal. (2021). Facebook knows Instagram is toxic for teen girls, company documents show. The Wall Street Journal. https://www.wsj.com

Walsh, S. (2025, January 31). *The top 30 social media influencers worldwide*. Search Engine Journal. Retrieved May 27, 2025, from https://www.searchenginejournal.com/top-social-media-influencers/475776/

Wan Sulaiman, A. W., Malek, M. D. H., Yunus, A. R., Ishak, N. H., Mohamad Safir, D., & Fahrudin, A. (2024). The Impact of Social Media on Mental Health: A Comprehensive Review. *South Eastern European Journal of Public Health*, 1468–1482. DOI: 10.70135/seejph.vi.2564

Wang, D., Park, S., & Fesenmaier, D. R. (2012). The role of smartphones in mediating the touristic experience. *Journal of Travel Research, 51*(4), 371–387. DOI: 10.1177/0047287511426341

Wang, W., Wang, M., Hu, Q., Wang, P., Lei, L., & Jiang, S. (2020). Upward social comparison on mobile social media and depression: The mediating role of envy and the moderating role of marital quality. *Journal of Affective Disorders, 270*, 143–149. DOI: 10.1016/j.jad.2020.03.173 PMID: 32339106

Wang, X. (2023). The Effect of Service Marketing Mix (7Ps) on Purchase Intention in the Script Killing Industry. *Academic Journal of Management and Social Sciences, 4*(2), 57–62. DOI: 10.54097/ajmss.v4i2.12087

Wang, Y., Zhu, X., & Li, J. (2023). Passive social media use and mental health: A systematic review and meta-analysis. *Cyberpsychology, Behavior, and Social Networking, 26*(2), 79–87. DOI: 10.1089/cyber.2022.0061

Warfield, K. (2014). Making selfies/making self. *Studies in Social Justice*, *8*(2), 206–223. DOI: 10.26522/ssj.v8i2.1144

Webb, J. B., Wood-Barcalow, N. L., & Tylka, T. L. (2015). Assessing positive body image: Contemporary approaches and future directions. *Body Image*, *14*, 130–145. DOI: 10.1016/j.bodyim.2015.03.010 PMID: 25910972

Weigle, P. E., & Shafi, R. M. A. (2024, January). Social media and youth mental health. *Current Psychiatry Reports*, *26*(1), 1–8. DOI: 10.1007/s11920-023-01478-w PMID: 38103128

Wei, S., Teo, T., Malpique, A., & Lause, A. (2022). Parental autonomy support, parental psychological control, and Chinese university students' behavior regulation: The mediating role of basic psychological needs. *Frontiers in Psychology*, *12*, 735570. DOI: 10.3389/fpsyg.2021.735570 PMID: 35250687

West, M., Rice, S., & Vella-Brodrick, D. (2024). Adolescent Social Media Use through a Self-Determination Theory Lens: A Systematic Scoping Review. *International Journal of Environmental Research and Public Health*, *21*(7), 862. DOI: 10.3390/ijerph21070862 PMID: 39063439

Whittemore, R., & Knafl, K. (2005). The integrative review. *Journal of Advanced Nursing*, *52*(5), 546–553. DOI: 10.1111/j.1365-2648.2005.03621.x PMID: 16268861

Wickramanayake, L. (2022). Social media use by adolescent students of Sri Lanka: Impact on learning and behavior. *Global Knowledge, Memory and Communication*, *71*(1/2), 70–85. DOI: 10.1108/GKMC-08-2020-0123

Wickramasurendra, J. M., Jagoda, D. J., & Rathnayake, R. M. L. (2021). Factors influencing social media addiction among GCE advanced level students in Sri Lanka: A case study in Colombo district, Sri Lanka. *Sri Lanka Journal of Social Sciences and Humanities*, *1*(2), 1–11. DOI: 10.4038/sljssh.v1i2.33

Wiekens, C. J. (2009). *Self awareness (Doctoral thesis).* Tilburg University.

Wiekens, C. J., & Stapel, D. A. (2008). The Mirror and I: When private opinions are in conflict with public norms. *Journal of Experimental Social Psychology*, *44*(4), 1160–1166. DOI: 10.1016/j.jesp.2008.02.005

Wies, B., Landers, C., & Ienca, M. (2021). Digital mental health for young people: A scoping review of ethical promises and challenges. *Frontiers in Digital Health*, *3*, 697072. DOI: 10.3389/fdgth.2021.697072 PMID: 34713173

Williams, J., & Chinn, S. J. (2010). Meeting relationship-marketing goals through social media: A conceptual model for sport marketers. *International Journal of Sport Communication, 3*(4), 422–437. DOI: 10.1123/ijsc.3.4.422

Wood, A. (2024). Essay on the Impact of Media Influencers on Youth. *EssayGenius AI Essay Writer.* https://essaygenius.ai/essay/essay-on-the-impact-of-media-influencers-on-youth

Woods, H. C., & Scott, H. (2016). #Sleepyteens: Social media use in adolescence is associated with poor sleep quality, anxiety, depression and low self-esteem. *Journal of Adolescence, 51*(1), 41–49. DOI: 10.1016/j.adolescence.2016.05.008 PMID: 27294324

Worb, J. (2025, March 13). *15 types of social media influencers you need to know in 2025.* Retrieved May 26, 2025, from https://later.com/blog/types-of-social-media-influencers/

World Health Organization. (2013, January 6). *Mental health action plan 2013-2020.* Retrieved from World Health Organization: https://www.who.int/publications/i/item/9789241506021

World Health Organization. (2020). Adolescent mental health. WHO. https://www.who.int

World Health Organization. (n.d.). *Adolescent health.* Retrieved from World Health Organization: https://www.who.int/southeastasia/health-topics/adolescent-health

Wunsch, K., Nigg, C., Niessner, C., Schmidt, S. C. E., Oriwol, D., Hanssen-Doose, A., Burchartz, A., Eichsteller, A., Kolb, S., Worth, A., & Woll, A. (2021). The Impact of COVID-19 on the Interrelation of Physical Activity, Screen Time and Health-Related Quality of Life in Children and Adolescents in Germany: Results of the Motorik-Modul Study. *Children (Basel, Switzerland), 8*(2), 98. DOI: 10.3390/children8020098 PMID: 33540824

Wu, Y., Wei, Y., Li, Y., Pang, J., & Su, Y. (2022). Burnout, negative emotions, and wellbeing among social workers in China after community lockdowns during the COVID-19 pandemic: Mediating roles of trait mindfulness. Frontiers in Public Health, 10, 952269.

Yamamiya, Y., Cash, T. F., Melnyk, S. E., Posavac, H. D., & Posavac, S. S. (2005). Women's exposure to thin-and-beautiful media images. *Body Image, 2*(1), 74–80. DOI: 10.1016/j.bodyim.2004.11.001 PMID: 18089176

Yang, C. C. (2016). Instagram use, loneliness, and social comparison orientation: Interactions between individual and social factors. *Cyberpsychology, Behavior, and Social Networking*, *19*(9), 522–526. DOI: 10.1089/cyber.2016.0201

Yang, C. C., Pham, T., Ariati, J., Smith, C., & Foster, M. D. (2021). Digital social multitasking (DSMT), friendship quality, and basic psychological needs satisfaction among adolescents: Perceptions as mediators. *Journal of Youth and Adolescence*, *50*(12), 2456–2471. DOI: 10.1007/s10964-021-01442-y PMID: 33991272

Yang, Y., Chen, J., & Zhuang, X. (2025). Self-determination theory and the influence of social support, self-regulated learning, and flow experience on student learning engagement in self-directed e-learning. *Frontiers in Psychology*, *16*, 1545980. DOI: 10.3389/fpsyg.2025.1545980 PMID: 40207130

Yau, J. C., & Reich, S. M. (2019). "It's just a lot of work": Adolescents' self-presentation norms and practices on Facebook and Instagram. *Journal of Research on Adolescence*, *29*(1), 196–209. DOI: 10.1111/jora.12376 PMID: 29430759

Yılmaz, H. A. (2022). Self-Awareness and Self-Consciousness: A Review from a Social Psychology Perspective. *Psikiyatride Güncel Yaklaşımlar -. Psikiyatride Güncel Yaklasimlar*, *14*(4), 437–445. DOI: 10.18863/pgy.1029405

Yilmaz, K. (2013). Comparison of Quantitative and Qualitative Research Traditions: Epistemological, theoretical, and methodological differences. *European Journal of Education*, *48*(2), 311–325. DOI: 10.1111/ejed.12014

Yoo, K. H., & Gretzel, U. (2008). What motivates consumers to write online travel reviews? *Information Technology & Tourism*, *10*(4), 283–295. DOI: 10.3727/109830508788403114

Young, S., Adamo, N., Ásgeirsdóttir, B. B., Branney, P., Beckett, M., Colley, W., Cubbin, S., Deeley, Q., Farrag, E., Gudjonsson, G., Hill, P., Hollingdale, J., Kilic, O., Lloyd, T., Mason, P., Paliokosta, E., Perecherla, S., Sedgwick, J., Skirrow, C., & Woodhouse, E. (2020). Females with ADHD: An expert consensus statement taking a lifespan approach providing guidance for the identification and treatment of attention-deficit/ hyperactivity disorder in girls and women. *BMC Psychiatry*, *20*(1), 404. Advance online publication. DOI: 10.1186/s12888-020-02707-9 PMID: 32787804

Youper. (2024). Digital therapy outcomes report. Youper Research Lab. https://www.youper.ai

Yuan, Y.-H., & Wu, C. (2008). Relationships among experiential marketing, experiential value, and customer satisfaction. *Journal of Hospitality & Tourism Research (Washington, D.C.)*, *32*(3), 387–410. DOI: 10.1177/1096348008317392

yusralodi3@gmail.com & yusralodi3@gmail.com. (2024, February 29). *Influencer culture and its impact*. Youth Ki Awaaz. https://www.youthkiawaaz.com/2024/02/influencer-culture-and-its-impact/

Zeithaml, V. A., Parasuraman, A., & Berry, L. L. (1990). *Delivering quality service: Balancing customer perceptions and expectations*. Simon and Schuster.

Zeng, B., & Gerritsen, R. (2014). What do we know about social media in tourism? A review. *Tourism Management Perspectives*, *10*, 27–36. DOI: 10.1016/j.tmp.2014.01.001

Zhang, L. (2011). *An assessment of contemporary dining out behaviour: The moderating factors of culture and food selection within Chinese full-service restaurants in Shanghai, China* (Doctoral dissertation, University of Waikato).

Zhang, G., Chong, L., Kotovsky, K., & Cagan, J. (2022). Trust in an AI versus a Human teammate: The effects of teammate identity and performance on Human-AI cooperation. *Computers in Human Behavior*, *139*, 107536. DOI: 10.1016/j.chb.2022.107536

Zhao, S., Grasmuck, S., & Martin, J. (2008). Identity construction on Facebook. *Computers in Human Behavior*, *24*(5), 1816–1836. DOI: 10.1016/j.chb.2008.02.012

Zheng, Y. (2024). To Access or Not to Access: Influencing Factors for Government Microblogging Information Seeking and Avoidance among Chinese Generation Z. *Human Behavior and Emerging Technologies*, *2024*, 1–14. DOI: 10.1155/2024/8288503

Zhou, L.. (2021). Youth digital identity and mental health. *The Journal of Adolescent Health*, *69*(1), 15–22.

Zhou, Y., & Wang, Z. (2022). Digital fatigue: Psychological antecedents and behavioral consequences. *Journal of Consumer Psychology*, *32*(1), 50–67. DOI: 10.1002/jcpy.1245

Zhou, Z., & Dong, Y. (2024). The Mediating Roles of Beauty Ideals and Upward Comparison in Social Media's Influence on Body Image Anxiety Among Chinese High School Students. *Psychology and Behavioral Sciences (New York, N.Y.)*, *13*(4), 106–110. DOI: 10.11648/j.pbs.20241304.13

Zhuang, X. (2023). The Impact of Social Media on Self-Image Control in Adolescents and Relevant Factors. *Journal of Education. Humanities and Social Sciences*, *22*, 41–46. DOI: 10.54097/ehss.v22i.12283

Zimmer-Gembeck, M., Hawes, T., & Pariz, J. (2021). A closer look at appearance and social media: Measuring activity, self-presentation, and social comparison and their associations with emotional adjustment. *Psychology of Popular Media*, *10*(1), 74–86. DOI: 10.1037/ppm0000277

About the Contributors

Viana Hassan is actively involved in academic and research work in Tourism & Cultural Management in Lebanon and Malta. She is the Founder and CEO of European Tourism and Events training Academy, She got her Ph.D. in Tourism Management and Cultural from Saint Joseph University, Beirut. Her Thesis was entitled "Medical Tourism in Lebanon". She has more than 19 years of tourism experience in many related Travel and Tourism Fields, varying from airline sales experience (MEA), to Co-management several Lebanese Travel agencies. She is an Experienced Lecturer with more than 16 years' experience at several universities in Lebanon (Lebanese University, A.U. L, Lebanese International University, Islamic University), the Institute of Tourism Studies, STC higher education partner of Wolverhmapton University UK and University of Malta (Malta), GBS Malta, Scholars School system (UK) with a demonstrated history of working in the Higher education industry, Skilled in Tourism Management, Customer service, Branding, Event Management, Airline Business Management, Niche Tourism, Business operations management, Customer acquisition and Medical Tourism. Dr. Viana has participated in international conferences (Expo Dubai 2020, 7th Medical Tourism World Summit) including Athens, Paris, Vienna, Dubai, Valencia, India, Turkey etc....

Amrik Singh is a Professor and Head at Lovely Professional University. He has over 20 years of experience in teaching, researching, and innovating in the hospitality domain, with a focus on accommodation and tourism management. He holds a Ph.D. and a Master's in Hospitality Management from Kurukshetra University. As a leader and educator, Dr. Singh oversees the curriculum, faculty, and student development, and strives to enhance the quality and relevance of hospitality education. He is also a prolific researcher and innovator, with a passion for advancing the hospitality industry through research, innovation, and education. He has authored 130+ Scopus indexed publications, 12 books, 21 copyrights and 12 patents in various areas of hospitality management. He is also a certified HACCP, room care, and floor care professional, and an award-winning teacher and educator.

A. R. Kanagaraj is a seasoned academic and Professor in the Department of Corporate Secretaryship at Dr. N.G.P. Arts and Science College, Coimbatore, Tamil Nadu. With an impressive teaching career spanning over 26 years at the institution, he has made significant contributions to both academia and research. Dr. Kanagaraj has published more than 45 articles in various national and international journals, reflecting his deep expertise and ongoing commitment to the advancement of knowledge in his field. His longstanding dedication and scholarly output have earned him a respected place in the academic community.

Kingsley Obioma Anyanwu is a business strategist, academic researcher, and higher education professional with over a decade of experience spanning banking, education, and International Trade. He holds a B.Sc. in Accountancy from Imo State University, an MBA from Charisma University, and an M.Sc. in Marketing and Brand Management from Bath Spa University, UK, delivered through GBS Malta. Kingsley currently serves as an Assessment Officer at GBS Malta, where he specializes in academic administration, quality assurance, and student support. His research interests include business strategy, innovation, marketing, and the sociocultural impact of digital technologies on Generation Z. He has contributed scholarly work to peer-reviewed publications and is passionate about leveraging strategic thinking and research to improve organizational performance and societal well-being.

Namchan Norbu Bhutia is currently pursuing his Ph.D. in Physical Education at Jadavpur University, Kolkata, with a specialization in Sports Training and Research Methodology. He completed his Master's degree in Physical Education from the same university in 2020 and has qualified the UGC NET in Physical Education. His research interests lie in sports performance analysis, emotional intelligence in sports, and the psychological aspects of athletic performance. He has actively contributed to the academic community through participation in national and international conferences, publication of research papers, and chapter contributions to edited volumes. He is a recipient of the prestigious National Fellowship for Higher Education of Scheduled Tribe Students (NFST), which has supported his research journey. In addition to his academic pursuits, he has completed several workshops and training programs related to research methodology, statistics, and data analysis. Passionate about advancing the field of sports science, Namchan is committed to impactful research and continuous academic growth.

Anindita Das is an esteemed Associate Professor at the Lakshmibai National Institute of Physical Education (LNIPE), Gwalior, with a distinguished career in teaching, research, and sports. Since joining LNIPE in 2007, she has been actively engaged in teaching core subjects such as Health Education, Physiology, and Football (practical). Dr. Das has made significant academic contributions through her authorship of numerous research papers in Scopus, patents, books and chapters in the field of physical education and sports sciences. She has published over twenty research articles in reputed national and international journals and has presented her work at a wide array of conferences. Notably, she presented papers at the Pre-Olympic Congress in Liverpool, UK (2012) and the World Congress on Kinanthropometry in Santiago, Chile (2018). A recipient of international training, Dr. Das completed a 3-month International Coaching Course (ICC) in General Conditioning at Semmelweis University, Budapest, Hungary, in 2009, further enriching her academic and practical expertise. Beyond academics, Dr. Das is a former athlete who has passionately contributed to women's football. She was a four-time member of her university's intervarsity women's football team and won a bronze medal in the All India Intervarsity Women Football Tournament in 2002. She also represented Madhya Pradesh in the National Women's Football Championship and played a key role when her team participated in the 1st Khelo India University Games (KIUG) held in Bhubaneswar, Odisha, in February 2020.

Karuppasamy Govindasamy is a dedicated researcher in Physical Education and Sports Sciences at the Department of Sports, Recreation and Wellness, Symbiosis International (Deemed University), Hyderabad Campus, Telangana. He has authored over 99 publications in Scopus and 48 in Web of Science journals, along with patents, book chapters, and books. His research focuses on innovative training methodologies and the integration of theory and practice in sports science. Dr. Govindasamy is UGC- NET and JRF qualified, has received multiple Best Paper Presentation awards, and was honoured with a national- level Young Researcher Award. He also serves as a reviewer for 15 top- ranking international journals.

Firoj Kabir is a researcher, Lecturer of the Department of "Tourism and Hospitality Management" at the Daffodil International University, Dhaka, Bangladesh, with a solid academic background in BBA and MBA majoring in Tourism and Hospitality Management from the University of Dhaka. His passion lies in exploring the intersection of travel and culture. His diverse areas of interest include archaeological tourism, sustainable tourism, and the unique characteristics of Generation Z travelers. Through extensive research and insightful writing, he sheds light on the intricate connections between historical sites, responsible tourism, and the evolving preferences of the next generation of travelers. His work not only enriches the field of tourism but also inspires readers to engage with the world around them in meaningful and responsible ways.

Debajit Karmakar is a dedicated Ph.D. scholar in Physical Education Pedagogy at Lakshmibai National Institute of Physical Education (LNIPE), Gwalior. An accomplished researcher, Mr. Karmakar has authored numerous research papers, patents, and books, contributing significantly to sports education and physical fitness. His work focuses on advancing training methodologies and innovative approaches in physical education, aligning both theory and practice. He brings his passion for sports into his academic pursuits, making impactful contributions to sports science and education. Mr. Karmakar's achievements mark him as a promising figure in physical education and sports science.

Akanksha Kathuria is an accomplished academician with over 15 years of teaching and research experience in Marketing and Management. She is currently serving as an Assistant Professor at the School of Management and Commerce, K.R. Mangalam University, Gurugram. Currently pursuing her Ph.D. in Management from JC Bose University of Science & Technology, YMCA Faridabad, Ms. Kathuria also holds an MBA, an MA in English Literature, and an MA in Yoga. She is certified in Digital Marketing, POSH, and Yoga Trainer. Ms. Kathuria has published extensively in Scopus- and ABDC-indexed journals and has authored a book titled An Introductory Approach to Research Methodology. Her research spans green marketing, consumer behavior, AI applications, and sustainable mobility. In addition to academics, she has conducted Management Development Programs (MDPs) and corporate training in Digital Marketing and Workplace Wellness for reputed organizations. She also holds three patents, reflecting her innovative approach to applied research.She serves on the editorial board of the Journal of Research in Business Management and is actively engaged in community service and wellness initiatives.

Varun Kesavan is a research scholar in the VIT Business School, VIT (Vellore Institute of Technology) University, Vellore, Tamil Nadu, India. He is a prolific and voracious researcher in the areas of financial technologies, digital payment systems, banking, corporate finance, financial management, green finance, artificial intelligence, sustainability, tourism, and quantum computing domains. He was a gold medallist at graduation and postgraduation. He authored 41 books, 12 Scopus articles, published 36 articles, case studies, and book reviews in leading international and national journals, published more than 300 articles on leading websites, published more than 1000 newspaper articles in an English daily from Hyderabad, India, and published a couple of articles in a reputed English daily based in Odisha, Bhubaneshwar, India, on various managerial domains.

Zarjina T. Khalil is a Senior Lecturer at the Department of Marketing and International Business at North South University, where she combines rigorous scholarship with a commitment to real-world impact. With 17+ years of experience, she specializes in Services Marketing, Brand Management, and Emerging Economies, while actively shaping the future of business education through her role on the Assessment and Curriculum Planning Committee. Over the years, along with her academic journey, she has been instrumental in ensuring multiple successful events at NSU. Key Contributions - Academic Leadership: Designed and launched cutting-edge courses like Digital Marketing, ensuring curriculum aligns with global industry trends. Served as Chair in Charge of her department, fostering industry collaborations and student-centered learning. - Women's Empowerment: As Executive Director of the World Bank-funded Business Management Training Program for Women Entrepreneurs, she helped equip Bangladeshi women with strategic business skills, expanding access to cohorts nationwide. - Sustainability: Certified Social Business Fellow from HEC Paris, integrating sustainable and inclusive practices into research, teaching, and community projects. - Research & Thought Leadership: Published widely on technology-driven branding, post-pandemic tourism, and healthcare innovation with renowned publishers like Emerald, SAGE and journals IGI Global. Has also been a guest lecturer at international institutions (e.g., BML Munjal University, India; Padang State University, Indonesia). Education & Honors - Master of Marketing (Griffith University, Australia) – Griffith Award for Academic Excellence - BBA (North South University) – Magna Cum Laude (Marketing & Information Systems).

Awesh Khati is a dedicated Ph.D. scholar specializing in Physical Education Pedagogy at the Lakshmibai National Institute of Physical Education (LNIPE), Gwalior. He has qualified for the UGC-NET JRF in Physical Education, contributed to a few research papers, written multiple books, and participated in numerous seminars, conferences, and workshops related to physical education and sports. An accomplished athlete, he has competed in inter-university football tournaments and holds coaching licenses from the All India Football Federation and Athletics Federation of India. With a diverse academic background in International Relations and Physical Education, he brings a unique perspective to sports education. Passionate about advancing physical education in India, he blends theoretical knowledge with practical expertise to promote holistic athletic and academic development.

Sanjeev Kumar is a Professor in Lovely Professional University Punjab India. He received Undergraduate in Hotel Management from Osmania University, Postgraduate in Tourism Management from Madurai Kamaraj University. He completed Doctor of Philosophy in Hospitality Management in 2019 from Amity

University Jaipur India. His research areas lies in food Service Industry, his research focuses on Alcoholic beverages, Event management and Sustainable Management Practices, Metaverse, AI Machine Learning and Artificial Intelligence. He published more than 60 research papers, articles and chapters in Scopus Indexed, UGC Approved and peer reviewed Journals and books. Dr. Sanjeev Kumar participated and acted as resource person in various National and International conferences, seminars, session chair, research workshops and industry talks and his work has been widely cited. Dr. Sanjeev also edited more than 12 books with various International Publishers such as IGI Global, Cambridge Scholars, Emerald, CABI, Bentham Science, Taylor & Francis. Dr Sanjeev is an active researcher and has published numerous research articles in prestigious national and international journals and books.

Sarala Hemanth Kumar is an esteemed Assistant Professor at Padmashree Institute of Management and Sciences, bringing over 14 years of distinguished teaching experience. She specializes in Human Resource Management and holds an MBA from Visvesvaraya Technological University (VTU). In addition to her academic qualifications, she has garnered valuable industry exposure and is currently pursuing a Ph.D. in Management from a reputed university, reflecting her commitment to continuous professional development. Prof. Kumar's academic journey exemplifies a dedication to scholarly excellence and pedagogical innovation. She has extensive experience in teaching and mentoring MBA students in HRM and related disciplines, with a focus on people management and organizational behavior. Her teaching philosophy emphasizes experiential learning, practical insights, and the development of future managers equipped to excel in dynamic organizational environments. Dedicated to fostering academic excellence, student growth, and research-driven teaching methodologies, Prof. Kumar remains committed to contributing meaningfully to the field of management education.

T.C. Manjunath was born on 6th February 1967. He did his B.E. from RV College of Engg. in 1989 (B'lore Univ), M.E. in Robotics & Automation from Govt.'s LD College of Engg., (Gujarat Univ., Ahmedabad) in 1992 with FCD-First Rank & PhD in Systems & Control Engg. from IIT Bombay in the year 2007, got best research scholar award for the entire IITB. He is currently working as the Dean Research (R & D) and as Professor in Dept. of Computer Science & Engg. with specialization in IoT, Cyber Security, Blockchain Technology in Rajarajeswari College of Engineering, Bengaluru, Karnataka. He has got a teaching (academic), research & administrative experience of more than 35+ years (10 years as Principal & 8 years as HoD, 1 year as Dean Research & rest as faculty) and has published more than 1500+ research papers in various national & international journals &

conferences, with 175+ patents, 100+ book-chapters, 25 awards, 100s of Keynote talks and also published 25 text books in various field of science, engineering & technology, completed projects worth Rs. 9 Crores till date & guided 10 PhD scholars in VTU. He is a member of 30 Professional Society Chapters and is a fellow of IE, IETE, AMIEE, Sr. Member of IEEE and a chartered engineer.

Anumeha Mathur is a dynamic and accomplished academic professional with over 18 years of extensive experience in teaching, research, and curriculum development in the field of marketing. Currently serving as Assistant Professor (Marketing) and Program Coordinator – BBA at the School of Management and Commerce, KR Mangalam University, she brings deep expertise in Consumer Behaviour, Brand Management, and Integrated Marketing Communication. Her academic journey includes teaching role at esteemed institutions like St. Kabir Institute of Professional Studies, Nirma University, and Skylark School of Business Technology, among others. She has consistently contributed to student success through the development of innovative and practical teaching methodologies and corporate readiness programs. Dr. Mathur is also an active researcher, with multiple publications, conference presentations, and patents to her credit. She holds important institutional roles, including SRC Member, University IPR Cell Member, and Editorial Board Member of the SOMC Newsletter. Throughout her career, she has designed and delivered a wide range of courses such as Marketing Management, Global Marketing, Product and Brand Management, Sales and Distribution Management, Services Marketing, and Integrated Marketing Communication. Her commitment to academic excellence and student mentoring continues to make a significant impact in shaping future marketing professionals.

Richa Nangia is an academician, researcher and author. An alumnus of University of Rajasthan, she holds a Masters (MBA) and Doctorate (Ph. D.) in Management. She is also a gold medallist in her master's programme. Presently, Dr. Richa Nangia is an Associate Professor at School of Business, Sushant University, Gurugram with more than 15 years of experience in teaching and research. She is an author of the book titled ——Research Methodology|| written for postgraduation courses. She is also the Reviewer of Business Ethics and Corporate Governance book published by McGraw Hill. Fourteen students have been awarded their doctoral degree under her guidance and many more are in queue. She has published numerous papers in UGC Care listed Journal, ABDC indexed, and Scopus indexed journals. She has also published one book on -Research Methodology and reviewed one book titled ——Business Ethics and Corporate Governance|| of Tata McGraw Publishing House. She has also presented various research papers in numerous International and National Conferences including IIM Indore, MDI Gurugram and others. She is the member of editorial board of various Scopus indexed journals and reviewer of various UGC Care listed journal. She has also won best paper award in at various International Conference and National Conference and one of them was organized by Padamshree Dr. D Y Patil Institute of Management Studies, Pune. She has convened various International and National Conferences and FDPs on Research Methods and Qualitative Research Analysis. She has chaired various International and National conferences as session chair. Her areas of interest include Organization Behaviour, Training and Development, Human Resource Development and Values and Ethics.

P. Selvakumar is currently an Associate Professor in the Department of Science and Humanities at Nehru Institute of Technology, Coimbatore, Tamil Nadu, India. Prior to joining Nehru Institute of Technology, he held positions as an Assistant Professor in the Department of Science and Humanities various engineering colleges in Coimbatore, Tamil Nadu, India, spanning from 2011 to 2023. Dr.P. Selvakumar's academic and research interests lie primarily in the field of phytochemistry. He has made significant contributions to his field, with an impressive record that includes 30 journal publications, 12 patents, and 20 conference papers. Additionally, he has organized 5 seminars and conferences, further demonstrating his commitment to academic and scientific exchange. Throughout his career, Dr. P.Selvakumar has been recognized for his dedication and excellence in teaching, having been honored with several awards, including the Best Teacher Awards. He holds a prominent position in the academic community, contributing actively to research.

Madura Thivanka Pathirana is research fellow for Grifith Institute for Tourism at Griffith University and a Senior Lecturer in Strategic Management at Edith Cowan University Sri Lanka, specializing in sustainable business management, with a particular focus on tourism. He holds a Doctor of Business Administration (DBA) from the University of Wales Trinity Saint David, UK, and his research centers on integrating sustainability into business practices, especially within small island developing states (SIDS). Dr. Pathirana has contributed significantly to the field of sustainable tourism through his research and practical initiatives, including his funded projects such as "Learning for Survival" and the "Sri Lankan Delights Initiative." He has supervised numerous postgraduate theses and developed courses on sustainable tourism and strategic management. Dr. Pathirana is actively engaged in the academic community as an editorial board member for the Journal of Management & Organization and a co-chair for international symposia. He also contributes to community engagement through projects like the Sorabora Tourism Village and training programs for local youth in sustainable business practices, supported by DFAT Australia.

Aruna Polisetty is an Associate Professor at VIT University. Her research interests include Sustainability, Technology Adoption, Tourism, and Psychology. She has research contributions and publications in reputed journals and books. She is a prolific Case study developer and has build numerous case studies on a wide range of topics.

Samira Rahman is an accomplished academic and researcher with over 14 years of experience in teaching and curriculum development at North South University. Specializing in International Business (INB), she has taught courses such as Global Business Strategy, International Trade and Finance, and International Business Negotiation, equipping students with practical insights into global markets. Her research focuses on the transformative role of social media influencers, particularly their impact on consumer purchasing behavior and the mental health of followers—a critical area in today's digital economy. As a committed academic leader, Samira has served as BBA Coordinator and played pivotal roles in the ACPC Committee, contributing to accreditation efforts (ACBSP), curriculum design, and standardized case development for INB capstone courses. Her administrative excellence includes coordinating departmental assessments, class visits, and academic catalogs. Beyond teaching, she has co-authored publications on post-pandemic tourism and healthcare innovation in emerging economies (Emerald, Crown Publishing), reflecting her interdisciplinary approach. With an MSc in International Management (University of Sheffield, UK) and an MBA in HRM (CGPA: 3.95/4), Samira blends theoretical rigor with real-world relevance. Her accolades include Summa Cum Laude honors and merit scholarships, underscoring her dedication to excellence. Long-term, she aims to expand research on digital consumer behavior while fostering industry-aligned education. https://orcid.org/0009-0005-3386-6358.

S. Jyothirmaye Reddy is a distinguished academician in the Faculty of Management Studies at Marwadi University, Rajkot, Gujarat. With over 24 years of experience in the Human Resources domain, Dr. Reddy has made significant contributions to the field through both research and teaching. She has published 26 research articles in reputed journals, including Scopus, WoS, ABDC (C & B category), and other peer-reviewed publications. In addition to her research, Dr. Reddy has actively participated in various International and National conferences, where she has presented her papers, further contributing to the global academic community. Currently, she is supervising four PhD scholars, guiding the next generation of researchers in the HR field. Her vast experience and commitment to academia have made her a respected figure in her field.

Jai Balaji is an Assistant Professor with 4 years of teaching experience and 12 years of industry exposure. He specializes in Marketing subject for MBA students at VTU University. Committed to delivering practical and industry-relevant knowledge, he focuses on equipping students with the skills needed for successful careers in these fields. With a blend of academic expertise and real-world insights, Mr. Jai Balaji aims to foster a dynamic learning environment that encourages critical thinking and practical application.

Sohom Saha is a dedicated academic and sports psychology scholar currently pursuing his Ph.D. in Physical Education at LNIPE, Gwalior. He holds an M.P.Ed. from LNIPE and a B.P.Ed. and B.A. in Physical Education from Visva-Bharati University, Shantiniketan. Specializing in Sports Psychology, Volleyball, and Yoga, he blends scientific insight with hands-on experience. Mr. Saha has competed in national-level sports, including All-India Inter-University events and NCC championships. He has published extensively in Scopus, Web of Science, and peer-reviewed journals, with research interests in emotional resilience, psychological well-being, and performance enhancement. He has also authored books on sports psychology and technology and serves as a reviewer for international journals. A member of the Sports Psychology Association of India, his work advocates mental toughness, inclusivity, and athlete development, aiming to inspire future educators and researchers in the sporting field.

Rintu Saibya is a dedicated Physical Educationist and football coach, currently pursuing his Ph.D. in Physical Education at the University of Kalyani. He holds an M.Phil in Physical Education and an M.P.Ed from Jadavpur University, along with a B.P.Ed and a B.A. from the University of North Bengal. He also completed a Post Graduate Diploma in Yoga Education from Ramakrishna Mission Shikshanamandira. Rintu has served as a football coach at The BGES School (ICSE), Kolkata, and as Assistant Football Coach for East Zone Inter-University Football. His qualifications include the State Eligibility Test (SET) for Assistant Professor in West Bengal and a Six-Week Certificate Course in Football Coaching from NSNIS. Actively involved in sports, he has participated and won several state and inter-college football championships. Passionate about promoting academic excellence and athletic development, he continues to contribute significantly to the field of physical education.

Anshul Saluja has a PhD in Educational Policy from the National Institute of Educational Planning and Administration (NIEPA), New Delhi and has also attained M.Phil. from NIEPA, New Delhi. She holds UGC-NET (JRF) in Education. She has been a recipient of the University Grants Commission-Junior Research Fellowship,

University Grants Commission-Senior Research Fellowship and MHRD-NIEPA Senior Research Fellowship during her M.Phil. and PhD. Her area of specialization is School Participation of Children at the Elementary Level of Education. She did her Master's in Psychology with a specialisation in Counselling Psychology. Her other academic possessions are Master in Education (M.Ed.), Bachelor of Education (B.Ed.) and Bachelor of Science (H) Botany. Besides, she has also cleared CTET (Central Teacher Eligibility Test) and HTET (Haryana Teacher Eligibility Test). She is working as an Assistant Professor in the School of Education, K. R. Mangalam University. She teaches the subjects like Child Development, Childhood and Growing Up, Cognition and Learning, Basic Concepts and Thoughts in Education, Contemporary India and Education, Biology etc. She has been guiding students in writing research papers and some of my students have presented their papers at national seminars and conferences. She has been the speaker and moderator of various webinars organized by K. R. Mangalam University. She has organized FDPs and seminars at the school level as co-ordinator. Besides, being an assistant professor at the School of Education, she has been assigned an additional charge of Assistant Dean, Student Welfare, K.R. Mangalam University. Being on this post, she has been the convener of the Induction-cum-Orientation Programme for Freshmen (2021-22), Induction Programme for Freshmen and various annual fests and inter-university events. She is also heading NAAC Criteria 5 at the university level and is a member of various important committees (like the university discipline committee, and grievance redressal cell). She has published papers in UGC care-listed journals and Scopus journals. She has attended several seminars/conferences and has presented many papers on issues related to education in various national and international seminars/conferences and has also attended several workshops. She is the Editorial Board Member of the International Journal of Education, Culture, and Society (http://www.ijecs.org/editorialboard).

Amrik Singh is working as Professor in the School of Hotel Management and Tourism at Lovely Professional University, Punjab, India. He obtained his Ph.D. degree in Hotel Management from Kurukshetra University, Kurukshetra. He started his academic career at Lovely Professional University, Punjab, India in the year 2007. He has published more than 40 research papers in UGC and peer-reviewed and Scopus/Web of Science) journals. He has published 12 patents and 01 patent has been granted in the inter-disciplinary domain. Dr. Amrik Singh participated and acted as a resource person in various national and international conferences, seminars, research workshops, and industry talks. His area of research interest is accommodation management, ergonomics, green practices, human resource management in hospitality, waste management, AR VR in hospitality, etc. He is currently guiding 8Ph.D. scholars and 2 Ph.D. scholars have been awarded Ph.D.

Mohammad Badruddoza Talukder is an Associate Professor, College of Tourism and Hospitality Management, IUBAT - International University of Business Agriculture and Technology, Dhaka, Bangladesh. He holds PhD in Hotel Management from Lovely Professional University, India. He has been teaching various courses in the Department of Tourism and Hospitality at various universities in Bangladesh since 2008. His research areas include tourism management, hotel management, hospitality management, food & beverage management, and accommodation management, where he has published research papers in well-known journals in Bangladesh and abroad. Mr. Talukder is one of the executive members of the Tourism Educators Association of Bangladesh. He has led training and consulting for a wide range of hospitality organizations in Bangladesh. He just became an honorary facilitator at the Bangladesh Tourism Board's Bangabandhu international tourism and hospitality training institution.

Mansi Yadav is an Assistant Professor at K.R. Mangalam University, Gurugram, Haryana, India. She holds a Ph.D. with a specialization in Digital Financial Literacy and personal financial behavior, with her research published in reputed journals indexed by Scopus, ABDC, and Web of Science. She teaches both undergraduate and postgraduate students, offering expertise in Predictive Modeling, Econometrics, and Data Visualization. Her academic interests extend to interdisciplinary research that bridges economics, finance, and technology, reflecting her commitment to exploring the evolving dynamics of the digital era. Passionate about digital empowerment and inclusion, her current work focuses on promoting informed digital decision-making applicable across diverse technology-driven contexts. She has presented her work at national and international platforms and continues to contribute actively to academia through research, teaching, and scholarly publications.

Index

E

F

G

I

L

M

O

P

R

S

T

V

W

Y

Z